NURSING CARE OF
Survivors of Family Violence

ALIVE

A shattered heart, and shattered dreams.
Silent prayers, unheard screams.
Fires of ice is what I feel,
others laughing, can my heart even heal?

Crying as a child, nowhere to go,
breaking in half, don't let it show . . .

Fall to the ground and desperately cry,
knowing only pain, wanting to die.
A dark hole, feel no light, hanging on with all my might.

Letting go, slipping away, never to awake at the break of day. . .
Something continues to make me survive, face the truth,
I am alive . . .

Anonymous

NURSING CARE OF
Survivors of Family Violence

Jacquelyn Campbell, RN, PhD

Associate Professor
College of Nursing
Wayne State University
Detroit, Michigan

Janice Humphreys, RN, C, PhD

Associate Professor
Department of Nursing Education
Eastern Michigan University
Ypsilanti, Michigan

*with **4** illustrations*

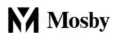

St. Louis Baltimore Boston Chicago London Philadelphia Sydney Toronto

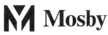
Mosby

Dedicated to Publishing Excellence

Executive Editor: Linda L. Duncan
Developmental Editor: Teri Merchant
Project Manager: Gayle May Morris
Production Editor: Lisa Nomura
Designer: Susan Lane
Cover illustration: Glenn Myers

SECOND EDITION

Printed in the United States of America

Mosby-Year Book, Inc.
11830 Westline Industrial Drive
St. Louis, Missouri 63146

Library of Congress Cataloging in Publication Data

Nursing care of survivors of family violence / [edited by] Jacquelyn Campbell, Janice Humphreys. —2nd ed.
    p.   cm.
    Rev. ed. of: Nursing care of victims of family violence / [edited by] Jacquelyn Campbell, Janice Humphreys.
    Includes bibliographical references and index.
    ISBN 0-8016-6378-4
    1. Victims of family violence. 2. Nursing. I. Campbell, Jacquelyn. II. Humphreys, Janice. III. Nursing care of victims of family violence.
    [DNLM: 1. Child Abuse—nurses' instruction. 2. Elder Abuse--nurses' instruction. 3. Family—nurses' instruction. 4. Nursing Care 5. Spouse Abuse—nurses' instruction. 6. Violence—nurses' instruction. WY 150 N97145]
RC569.5.F3N872 1992
362.82'928—dc20
DNLM/DLC   92-48726
for Library of Congress   CIP

93   94   95   96   97   CA/DC   9 8 7 6 5 4 3 2 1

Contributors

James Bannon, PhD
Detroit Police Department
Detroit, Michigan

Sara Barrett, RN, MA
ABC Home Health Services
Medicaid Waivered Services Division
Detroit, Michigan

David G. Blocker
Child Abuse Unit
Detroit Police Department
Detroit, Michigan

Diane K. Bohn, BNSc, CNM, RN
Hennepin County Medical Center
Minneapolis, Minnesota

Doris Campbell, PhD, RN
University of Florida
Gainesville, Florida

Jacquelyn C. Campbell, PhD, RN,
FAAN
School of Nursing
Wayne State University
Detroit, Michigan

Janet Elizabeth Findlater, JD
Wayne State University Law School
State of Michigan Violence and
   Treatment Board
Detroit, Michigan

Nancy Fishwick, MSN, RN, C
Planned Parenthood of Greater
   Cleveland
School of Nursing
Case Western Reserve University
Cleveland, Ohio

Terry T. Fulmer, PhD, RN, C, FAAN
Columbia University
New York, New York

Patricia Hanrahan, MS, MA, RA
Department of Sociology
School of Nursing
University of Massachusetts
Amherst, Massachusetts

Janice Humphreys, PhD, RN, C
Department of Nursing Education
Eastern Michigan University
Ypsilanti, Michigan

William O. Humphreys, JD
Horton, Barbaro, and Reilly
Santa Ana, California

Karen Landenburger, PhD, RN
Nursing Program
University of Washington
Tacoma, Washington

Judith McFarlane, DrPH, RN, FAAN
College of Nursing
Texas Women's University
Houston, Texas

Laura Smith McKenna, DDNSc,
RNC
Department of Nursing
Samuel Merritt College
Oakland, California

Isaiah McKinnon, PhD
Renaissance Center Venture
Security Fire and Safety Department
Detroit, Michigan

Joyce Underwood Munroe, JD
Department of English
College of Liberal Arts
Wayne State University
Detroit, Michigan

Barbara Parker, PhD, RN, FAAN
School of Nursing
University of Maryland
Catonsville, Maryland

Ann Marie Ramsey, MSN, RN
CS Mott Children's Hospital
Department of Otolaryngology
University of Michigan
Ann Arbor, Michigan

Mary Cay Sengstock, PhD, CCS
Department of Sociology
Wayne State University
Detroit, Michigan

Daniel Sheridan, MS, RN
Oregon Health Sciences
University Trauma Program
Portland, Oregon

Yvonne Campbell Ulrich, PhD,
ARNP
College of Health Professions
Department of Nursing
The Wichita State University
Wichita, Kansas

Joan C. Urbancic, PhD, RN, CS
MacAuley School of Nursing
University of Detroit Mercy
Detroit, Michigan

To *Christy* and *Brad*
with love
*and in memory of **Connie Morrow**,*
a woman who exemplified caring.

J.C.

To *Rick, Bill,* and *Jack*
with love.

J.H.

Preface

heartless
is the cold empty carcass
of a world
once full of love
we must go back
to the time of the female
eons
and
eons
ago
back to caress
of the great mother
nurture and care we need
she's calling

Susan Venters*

A woman enters the emergency room with facial bruises and severe abdominal pain. She is asked perfunctorily how her injuries occurred, and she mumbles that she fell down a flight of stairs. Her male companion glowers in the doorway of the cubicle. The nurse firmly asks him to wait outside and gently proceeds with obtaining a detailed history from the woman, including assessment for family violence. In another part of the hospital, a newly postpartum battered mother in the obstetrical unit fears going home and does not know where to go. Her primary care nurse helps arrange her discharge directly to a wife abuse shelter. A 14-year-old daughter of a woman who has five other children is being seen in the outpatient clinic with her mother.

*Reprinted from *Every Twelve Seconds*, compiled by Susan Venters (Hillsboro, Oregon: Shelter, 1981) by permission of the author.

The mother voices the concern, "I don't want to have to 'do time' for what I might do to her." Mother and daughter are counseled by the nurse.

These are three illustrations of the multitude of possible interfaces of nursing and family violence. Family violence is a significant health problem, widespread in American society. "A person is more likely to be hit or killed in his or her home by another family member than anywhere else or by anyone else" (Gelles & Straus, 1979, p. 15). Nursing has an important role to play in the prevention, detection, treatment, and scholarly investigation of this health concern.

A violent act is one of physical force that results in injury or abuse to the recipient. Within the family, violence can be directed toward any member by another and can include sexual acts as well as other forms of physical aggression. Regardless of whether the violent action is perpetrated by the father against the mother, the mother against the child, or the adolescent against the grandfather, violence in the family is a profound event that affects the whole family. To look at wife abuse, child abuse, or abuse of elderly family members in isolation views only a portion of the effects of violence in American families. The problem must be addressed in its totality to see the full picture with all its ramifications.

Campbell (1988) has presented a plea for recognition of nursing and for its potential and actual contribution to the needs of survivors of family violence. She clearly describes the unique role that nurses can play in assisting battered children, women, and elders as they respond to the trauma of physical and psychological assaults. Beginning with the scientific basis for nursing first described by Nightingale, Campbell argues that nursing as a predominantly female profession, and as a discipline based on holistic and client-based theories and models, is ideally suited to understand the needs of family violence survivors. Although many reports in the literature fail to separate nursing from medicine, which Campbell notes may in itself have sexist implications, this text specifically addresses the role of nursing in response to family violence.

Since the first edition of this text was published, hundreds of nurses have become involved in a variety of ways in the care of survivors of family violence. Nurses provide direct care to survivors in shelters, homes, hospitals, and community settings. Nurses are frequently members of boards of directors at shelters and other agencies assisting survivors. Nursing research on family violence has evolved rapidly and is reported in the literature with ever greater frequency. One of the most visible outcomes of nursing's greater awareness and contribution to the area is the development of the Nursing Network on Violence Against Women. This group was a direct outgrowth of the 1985 Surgeon General's Workshop on Violence and Public Health. Immediately following that meeting and every 2 years since, the Nursing Network on Violence Against Women (NNVAW) has held a conference where the formal exchange of research, theory, and ideas is only one of the many highlights. At the last conference those in attendance were so energized

that new Co-Chairs and the next two conference locations (Tampa in 1993, Seattle in 1995) were decided. A quarterly column from the NNVAW also can be found in the journal, *Response*. The American Nurses' Association has also adopted a resolution against violence against women and the American Academy of Nursing has formed a policy task force on violence. Exciting developments—yet much more can be done. (See Chapter 15, Future Directions for Nursing, for further discussion of nursing education, research, and social policy issues.)

All the clients in the introductory examples are "victims" of family violence in that they are "subjected to oppression, deprivation or suffering" within violent families, whether or not they are the actual recipients of the aggressive acts. At the same time, the philosophy of this text is that these people and their family units have significant strengths on which appropriate nursing care will build. This is why the term *survivor* has replaced *victim* in the title of this book. We wish to move from a nursing care perspective of feeling sorry for victims to nursing care that forms partnerships with survivors and potential survivors. The other basic assumptions of the book are that nursing care of survivors of family violence considers the whole family, is based on a firm theoretical foundation, and can be a significant force at all levels of prevention. The main objective of this book is to integrate nursing practice in family violence with existing theory and research. The need for increased nursing theoretical development and nursing research in this area is also a consistent theme.

Culture and Family Violence

Because of the increased availability of information on racial, ethnic, and cultural aspects of family violence, we have made a concerted effort to discuss these variables in each chapter. While there are obvious similarities to the plights of all survivors of family violence, there are, nevertheless, aspects that are unique to certain racial and cultural groups. For example, while Gondolf, Fisher, and McFerron (1988) found great similarities in abuse and help-seeking variables in Anglo, black, and Hispanic women in shelters, they also reported that Hispanic women were in need of additional economic and educational supports. These beginning research efforts shed light on the unique needs of diverse groups of women with the common problem of family violence.

Goodwin (1985) identified the necessary components of a comprehensive program to treat family violence:

A coordinated reporting system
Coordinated training among health care and law enforcement personnel and others likely to encounter family violence
Crisis facilities
    24-hour hotlines
    Emergency shelters
    Surrogate families
Adequate treatment systems
    Long-term relationships with helpers
    Treatment and self-help groups
    Time-intensive treatment involving coordinated use of many agencies, day and institutional care, and trained volunteers
Outreach to potential survivors
Outreach to potential abusers
Use of mass media to inform the general public
Promotion of legislative and community programs to provide services and decrease stress on families, to facilitate access to treatment, to provide education and training, and to encourage research.*

Relevance to Nursing

The definition of nursing given by the American Nurses Association in its Social Policy Statement is, "the diagnosis and treatment of human responses to actual or potential health problems." Nursing care of survivors of family violence fits well within the scope of this definition and thereby includes the prevention of family violence, as well as detection and treatment.

Nursing from the time of Nightingale has been concerned with the individual, the family, and the community. Professional nurses develop a plan of care only after thorough consideration of the client's community. In turn, nursing as a profession must adapt to the ever-changing needs of the community and society. For example, if violence in the family is common and possibly increasing, then the professional nurse must alter the process by which she develops, initiates, and evaluates her care to include the likelihood of violence in families. The actual and potential alterations in individual and family health that are associated with violence are immense, complex, and in need of nursing consideration if maximum levels of wellness are to be achieved. Stress on the family is a major contributing factor to the occurrence of violence in families. The professional nurse, aware of this influence and practicing in an area of increasing unemployment, would be remiss if she failed to consider and adapt to the increased potential for family violence when conducting her assessment.

The mere awareness of the problem of family violence is not enough. Nurses must act as client advocates. In the case of family violence, the nurse may begin by educating other professionals of the dynamics of the problem. For instance, she may help others who become involved in a case of child abuse to understand that physical harm inflicted on a dependent child by a parent is really just an isolated act in the interactions of a complex family unit.

Nursing is furthermore in an excellent position to prevent, identify, or intervene against family violence. In hospitals nurses may administer nursing care to patients with a wide range of needs related to potential or actual family violence (such as the teenage boy with a gunshot wound, the infant who has been abandoned, and the chronically ill elderly woman who is preparing to move in with her daughter's family.) Mental health and obstetrical inpatient units are also areas where patient needs arising out of violence can be found if nurses know how to look for them. Client advocacy, in the clinic, community, and the hospital, involves active searching for victims and attention to prevention, as well as education and direct intervention.

The professional nurse has always focused primarily on the client rather than "the problem."

---

*From Goodwin, J.: Family violence: Principles of intervention and prevention. *Hospital and Community Psychiatry,* 36, 1074-1079.

Such a focus allows the nurse to be perceived as more helping and better prepared than many other professionals to assist clients who experience family violence. Nursing's ability "to conceptualize the familial and social context of problems of violence" has recently been identified by other health professionals as well (Newberger & Bourne, 1978).

Because of their sheer numbers, variety of practice locations, and client needs, and in particular the nature of their practice, nurses are in an ideal position to take action to decrease the likelihood of family violence and to mitigate its effects. Nurses provide care to families in more settings than probably any other health care provider. Nurses see family members in the hospital, clinic, school, community, and in private practice. They have traditionally provided care to whole families, even though the initial request for care may have come from an individual. The nurse routinely includes information about the individual's family, culture, and health attitudes and practices when doing an assessment. She is frequently seen as help by families when they can trust no other health professional (Hiberman & Munson, 1978).

The Nurse as Coordinator of Care

The problem of family violence is multidimensional. The professional nurse cannot be expected to meet the needs of every member of a violent family in every respect without help. Rather, violent families require a broad range of interventions and teamwork. Many other professionals are likely to have contact with the members of the violent family. Social workers, physicians, lawyers, police officers, and dentists all may be involved in their own form of intervention with the violent family. According to Newberger, a physician, the necessary involvement of professionals from different backgrounds can result in difficulties. "Each professional does what he or she can, within the ethical definition of his domain. Yet the family and its individual members can be harmed—not helped—by these well-intended, independent acts" (1976, p. 15). It is thus necessary that one professional coordinates these varied interventions. The professional nurse is in a prime position in many instances to initiate, coordinate, and

evaluate the multidisciplinary approach to the care of violent families. She is in a much less threatening position to elicit information from a battered woman or abusing parent and to ensure that the individual client and/or family has the paramount role in decision making beyond what the law requires. When the setting, agency, family, or situation indicates that another professional would be better suited as coordinator, the nurse, when well informed and aware, is still an integral member of the team. This book is designed to give the nurse the necessary background to understand, identify, assess, coordinate care of, and provide interventions for potential and actual victims of family violence.

Unit of Focus: Family

The purpose of this book is to address the nursing care of survivors of family violence, including victims of child abuse, wife abuse, and abuse of the elderly. Violence therefore will be examined as an indicator of family needs and issues. Often abuse of a family member is viewed as an isolated interaction involving at the most the survivor and the perpetrator. As will be shown, every violent act within a family affects each of its members. The family and its functioning are the major unit of focus.

If the violent family is to be the major focus of the present work, it is necessary to examine the consequences of violence on each family member. Literature on child abuse is far more extensive than that on abuse of any other family member. The present text includes violence against children, and the facets less commonly discussed, abuse of women and the elderly, and the effects of violence in the home on all the children. The kind of abuse perpetrated against all family members is not limited to physical violence. Sexual abuse, emotional abuse, incest, and neglect are discussed where appropriate.

Family Violence from a Nursing Perspective: Prevention

This book approaches care of violent families in a manner heretofore not found, a nursing perspective. The nursing care of violent families is presented from a holistic, preventive standpoint. First, holism requires that the nurse be concerned with any factor that affects the client's health. Second, prevention has long been "the heart of community health nursing" (Shamansky & Clausen, 1980, p. 104). It therefore seems appropriate to present the nursing care of a problem that involves families and the community in such a manner.

Some confusion exists as to what is meant by "levels of prevention." In this text levels of prevention are used as defined by Shamansky and Clausen (1980). Briefly, "primary prevention is prevention in the true sense of the word, it precedes disease or dysfunction and is applied to a generally healthy population. It does not require identification of a problem and may be a generalized enhancement of overall health approach or be specifically aimed at a particular health problem" (Shamansky & Clausen, 1980, p. 106). "The purpose is to decrease the vulnerability of the individual to illness or dysfunction. Health promotion encourages optimum health and personality development to strengthen the individual's capacity to withstand physical and emotional stressors" (Shamansky & Clausen, 1980, p. 106). Primary prevention takes place before dysfunction exists; however, it may involve interventions with individuals or families who are considered "at risk."

Secondary prevention occurs when some kind of disease or dysfunction has been identified or is suspected. "Secondary prevention emphasizes early diagnosis and prompt intervention to halt the pathological process, thereby shortening its duration and severity and enabling the individual to regain normal functioning at the earliest possible point" (Shamansky & Clausen, 1980, p. 106). Secondary prevention includes screening programs, problem identification, and treatment that attempts to decrease the severity of impact of a problem.

Finally, "tertiary prevention comes into play when a defect or disability is fixed, stabilized, or irreversible. Rehabilitation, the goal of tertiary prevention, is more than halting the disease process itself; it is restoring the individual to an optimum level of functioning within the constraints of the disability" (Shamansky & Clausen, 1980, p. 106).

The application of each level of prevention in the nursing care of abused women, abused children, and the abused elderly can be found in the appropriate subsequent chapters.

Review of Book Contents

This text attempts to provide the professional nurse with information needed to confidently and successfully provide nursing care to violent families. By virtue of the contribution of chapters by several different authors of diverse backgrounds, certain variations exist in the format of individual sections. Each chapter is relevant to the overall text theme, theory, research, and practice in nursing care of survivors of family violence. The differing perspectives on violence in the family offer the reader valuable assistance in viewing the central issues from multiple stylistic as well as cognitive perspectives. The overall goal is a unique presentation that is comprehensive, informative, and thought provoking.

The reality of the nature of nursing practice results in nurses who are most often specialists in one or more areas. Family violence, in contrast, can occur with any family member, of any age, in any stage of development or wellness state. To provide both a generalist nursing approach and a text from which a nurse can select certain relevant sections, each chapter thoroughly addresses its topic and may briefly restate discussions from other chapters.

The book is divided into five main sections, the first presenting essentially the theory components of family violence (Chapters 1, 2, and 3). The second section addresses both the theory and clinical application of specific areas of family violence (Chapters 4 through 7). The third section focuses on the nursing care of abused children, abused women, and families experiencing violence (Chapters 8, 9, and 10). The fourth section has four chapters written by law enforcement and legal professionals (Chapters 11 through 14). Nursing is well versed in the need for collaboration with other disciplines in its approach to most health problems. However, the interface of nursing with law enforcement and the legal profession regarding family violence is an unexplored area that these chapters address. The final chapter provides a look to the future and examines nursing education, practice, and research implications in the area.

Summary

Violence in the American family is a common health problem of possibly tremendous magnitude. Violence occurs against all family members and is an indicator of complex family needs and issues. Nursing is in an excellent position to be actively involved with other professionals by initiating, coordinating, and evaluating the multidisciplinary approach to violent families, but has a limited knowledge base about family violence. This text conveys knowledge to nurses in a format that covers nursing interventions based on existing theories and research about families and violence, extends nursing care to all members of violent families and all forms of family violence, and emphasizes the strengths and health potential of victims and families so that nursing can contribute to the prevention of this major health concern.

Acknowledgments

This book evolved out of our professional interest in and commitment to survivors of family violence. For the existence of this text we owe a great many thanks.

To our many friends and colleagues who provided support and indulgence.

To our expert contributing authors who share our concern for survivors of family violence.

To Barbara Scheffer for her expert consultation on the sample nursing processes.

To our invaluable funding sources.

The research conducted by Jacquelyn Campbell was supported by two grants from the National Center for Nursing Research, National Institutes of Health. The research conducted by Janice Humphreys was supported by Department of Health and Human Services, National Research Service Award 1F31 NU-05708-01 from the Division of Nursing.

To Linda Duncan, Executive Editor, Nursing Division, Mosby–Year Book for her advice, counsel, and commitment to the needs of families.

To our students who have challenged us to grow.

To the battered women and children who freely shared their problems and concerns.

To the profession of nursing for providing an opportunity to care about the needs of other human beings.

To each other for continuing friendship, and sharing of ideas.

Jacquelyn Campbell
Janice Humphreys

REFERENCES

Campbell, J. C. (1988). Nursing and battered women. *Response, 11*(2), 21–23.

Gelles, R. J., & Straus, M. A. (1979). Violence in the American family. *Journal of Social Issues, 35*, 13–17.

Gondolf, E. W., Fisher, E., & McFerron, J. R. (1988). Racial differences among shelter residents: A comparison of Anglo, black, and Hispanic battered women. *Journal of Family Violence, 3*, 39–51.

Goodwin, J. (1985). Family violence: Principles of intervention and prevention. *Hospital and Community Psychiatry, 36*, 1074–1079.

Hiberman, E., & Munson, K. (1978). Sixty battered women. *Victimology: An International Journal, 2*, 469.

Newberger, E. H. (1976). A physician's perspective on the interdisciplinary management of child abuse. *Psychiatric Opinion, 13*, 14–17.

Newberger, E. H., & Bourne, R. (1978). The medicalization and legalization of child abuse. *American Journal of Orthopsychiatry, 48*, 604.

Shamansky, S. L., & Clausen, C. L. (1980). Levels of prevention: Examination of the concept. *Nursing Outlook, 28*, 104–108.

Contents

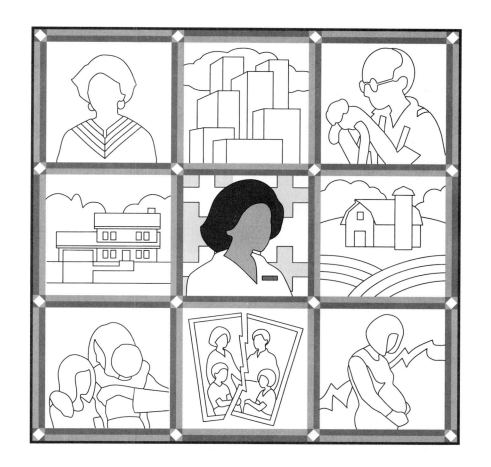

PART

I

Theory

CHAPTER

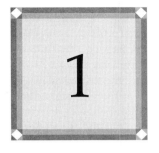

1

Theories of Violence

Patricia Hanrahan, Jacquelyn Campbell, *and* Yvonne Ulrich

Joanne Dewey

as a young girl i played
with my cousins
in sun lit country fields
amazons in the jungles
fearless women
brave and strong
no harm could ever come to us
in these journeys that we made
through forests fields and over mountains
across the horizon as far as we could see
sometimes we were birds
flying floating gliding free as the wind
until
we came upon a country grave yard
a picture on a grave stone
stared out from the lonely

oh the solemn eyes
of the dark haired spirit staring
i remembered a story
that the news papers carried
of a young girls body
found by hunters in a stream
joanne dewey murdered
raped is what they said
etched beneath the picture
in the cold marble stone
here lies joanne dewey
born 1937 died 1953
and we as young girls ran
ran for our lives
birds with broken wings
freedom left behind

Susan Venters*

Violence in the family cannot be fully understood without analysis of the broader picture of violence in general. This chapter provides a background of the major theoretical frameworks found in the current literature and used to explain violence in our society. Concept analysis, historical background, and a summary of the perspectives on violence from biology, psychology, sociology, and anthropology are presented as a basis for nursing conceptualization of violence as a health problem.

One way to estimate the magnitude of the health concern that violence represents is to examine homicide statistics. Among advanced capitalist countries, the United States has the highest murder rate at 7.9 per 100,000 of the population for a total of 18,980 homicides (Federal Bureau of Investigation, 1985). Only Mexico and Paraguay have a higher incidence of murder than the United States. In addition, one's lifetime risk of being murdered has been estimated at a probability of 1 in 133 (FBI, 1985). For

*Reprinted from *Every Twelve Seconds*, compiled by Susan Venters (Hillsboro, Oregon: Shelter, 1981) by permission of the author.

3

black men, this risk has been estimated at an alarming 1 in 21; homicide as the leading cause of death for black males between the ages of 15 to 35 (U.S. Dept. of Health & Human Services, 1986). The leading cause of death for young black women in the same age group is also homicide. Furthermore, the rate of murder victims who are related to their assailants is 1.2 per 100,000 of the population (FBI, 1985). Finally, in family homicides that are committed between husbands and wives, women are the victims 62% of the time (FBI, 1985).

If nursing identifies prevention of health problems as a major area of concern, an examination of causes of violence is mandated. To approach the research literature on the causes of violence, an examination of the concepts involved is necessary.

CONCEPT ANALYSIS

Chinn and Jacobs (1978) emphasize the importance of concept analysis as "the beginning examination of phenomena important to the area of inquiry." What seem to be relatively simple ideas, used frequently in common language, need to be carefully scrutinized as the basis for further study. When literature reports of violence are studied, there is striking disagreement among authors about definitions of even the most frequently used terms and more importantly, the values and connotations attached to them. Is aggression bad or good? Can violence be useful in achieving moral human aspirations or is it always negative? An abbreviated concept analysis is presented of the two most important ideas in understanding this field—aggression and violence.

Aggression

Aggression is defined in Webster's Third New International Dictionary as "an offensive action or procedure." The root is Latin from the word *aggressus,* which means attack (Webster's Third New International Dictionary, 1988). From these beginnings there is a variety of definitions used in the literature and in common usage. The viewpoint that aggression is an instinct or drive common to all human beings softens the negative connotations of the definition. The

synonyms listed for the adjective form, aggressive, reflect two different perspectives. Synonyms include hostile, belligerent, assailant, pugnacious, vicious, contentious; the second group includes self-assertive, forceful, bold, enterprising, energetic, zealous. The disparate definitions reflect the ambivalence about aggression in American society.

However, connotations of aggression as negative or positive are well grounded in the sex-role stereotypes held about male and female behavior. Psychoanalytical perspectives allow for healthy expressions of aggression as drives for accomplishment and mastery. However, typically this meaning of aggression has applied only to men. Aggressive men are often described as bold, forceful, enterprising, energetic, zealous, and/or self-assertive. For women, aggression has not been viewed as positively. Schur (1983) writes that aggression in women violates gender norms. These norms dictate and determine what is considered to be appropriate male and female behavior within a society. When a woman acts in an aggressive manner, her behavior is often judged as hostile, belligerent, or contentious because it does not reflect stereotypical assumptions about women's nature as kind or nurturing. These opposing interpretations of the term *aggression* suggest that perceptions of this concept are well grounded in the social context of the behavior. Views of aggressive behavior are derived from how males and females are expected to act in society.

However, there has been a shift from regarding aggression as innate or as a personality characteristic. Currently the majority of researchers (see for example, Ball-Rokeach, 1980; Berkowitz, 1983; or both) studying aggression view it as behavior that is a deliberate attempt to harm others, regardless of gender. A representative definition of this school of thought is Moyer's description of aggression as "overt behavior involving intent to inflict noxious stimulation or to behave destructively toward another organism (1987, p. 18). These scholars include psychological injury as one of the possible results of aggression. Nursing has also addressed aggression in the work attempting to distinguish assertiveness from aggression. Herman (1978) describes aggression as getting what is wanted at the expense of others. Aggressive behavior is seen as dominating, deprecating, humiliating, and embarrassing to others, whereas "assertion is the direct, honest, and appropriate expression of one's thoughts, feelings, opinions and beliefs . . . and without infringing on the right of others." (1978). This distinction seems useful and is accepted as a basic premise of this book. Aggression therefore is seen as destructive in intent either physically or psychologically and as infringing on the rights of others.

Violence

Aggression can be seen on a continuum with violence at the extreme end, encompassing destructive results, as well as aggressive intent. Webster defines violence as the "exertion of any physical force so as to injure or abuse (Webster's Third New International Dictionary). The word originates from the Latin *violare*, to violate, rape, or injure. Consistent with the official definition and its Latin root, common associations with violence are much more negative. Haber and Seidenberg (1978) conducted a small survey in which they found the following associations included in a list elicited by the word violence: "murder, crime, gangs, men, torture, hate, uneducated, unsocialized, disgusting animals." Yet much violence is socially tolerated; for instance, police violence, war, self-defense, and in some cases, riots. As Haber and Seidenberg point out, whether violence is deemed appropriate depends on the agent, the circumstances, the status of the victim, and the degree of harm inflicted. Some authors have even insisted that violence is necessary as a reflection of conflicting groups and interests in any society. Yet there are cultures that are totally nonviolent and wherein violence in any form is absolutely disallowed (Levinson, 1989).

American culture officially condemns violence, but it is covertly sanctioned in many ways. Violent characters are glorified on television and in books; threats to hurt and kill each other are made in jest as a constant part of common language. Wolfgang states, "When war is glorified in a nation's history and included as part of the child's educational materials, a moral judgement about the legitimacy of violence is firmly made" (1978). American society is undecided whether hitting a child is legitimate punishment or a form of violence. Societal ambivalence about attitudes and values toward violence are undoubtedly reflected in the high rate of violent crime and in problems with violence in the family.

HISTORICAL BACKGROUND

Anthropologists are uncertain about the prevalence of violence in early civilizations. Some scholars have used the historical record to argue in favor of the inevitability of violence. For instance, Kolb (1971) observes that "at best, only ten generations in the era of recorded history have avoided war." Freeman (1964) argues that peoples of peace are relatively rare in the ethnographic record, and states they were usually backward and submissive to a powerful and overtly aggressive neighbor. In refutation, Malinowski (1973) shows that wars cannot be traced back to the earliest beginnings of human culture, only to the start of written history. Andreski (1964) adds that only a small percentage of the population took part in the early wars and that people have to be indoctrinated for war. As for the contention that peaceful peoples were always in the minority, there is evidence that the majority of the peoples living in the "cradle of civilization" (Asia Minor) from approximately 9000 to 5000 b.c. were hunter-gatherers and apparently lived in a predominantly peaceful manner. For the 800 years explored to date in the excavations of the Catal Hüyük neolithic peoples, none of the hundreds, of skeletons unearthed shows evidence of violent death. Far from being backward, this culture was one of the most advanced of its time (Eisler, 1988).

It has often been noted that the United States has a long history of violence used as a means to achieve socially acceptable ends. The favorite period of many Americans is the era of the "Old West," which is characterized as violent as much as anything else. In a survey for the National Commission on Violence, Harris found that 51% of Americans agreed or strongly agreed with the statement: "Justice may have been a little rough and ready in the Old West, but things worked better than they do today with all the legal red tape'' (Mulvehill & Tumin, 1969). Americans also tend to romanticize their early wars and to admire the violent heroes of the past. Some scholars have correlated the fascination with the violent past with the fact that there are only four countries that have a higher homicide rate (per 100,000 population) than the United States (Archer & Gartner, 1984).

Thus historical examination of violence shows a predilection for violence among human beings from at least very early in civilization, but a propensity that is by no means equally distributed among cultures nor among all periods of time. Historical background gives an overview to the problem of violence, but does not illuminate causation. (See the box below for summaries of explanations of violence).

Summaries of Explanations of Violence

- Biological

  Aggression is an innate characteristic that is either an instinctual drive (the instinctivist school of thought) or neurologically based (neurophysiological theories). The latter examines how brain functioning and/or hormones influence degrees of aggressive tendencies and/or violent behaviors. Research evidence links increased testosterone levels to increases in aggression, but the studies do not indicate a causal relationship and factors such as mood, sampling difficulties, and environment must be considered as intervening characteristics.

- Role of alcohol

  Research indicates that alcohol seems to facilitate aggression because of the negative affect it has on conscious cognitive processing, yet violence occurs as frequently *without* the presence of alcohol. Alcohol is often used as an excuse or a justification for violence.

- Psychoanalytical viewpoint

  This position, espoused by Freud and followers, states that violence results from ego weaknesses and the internal need to discharge hostility. Frustration is the stimulus that leads to the expression of aggression. Catharsis or the expression of the aggression results in a decrease of subsequent aggressive behaviors.

- Social-learning theory

  Aggression and violence are learned responses and may be considered adaptive or destructive depending on the situation. The family, television, and environmental conditions serve as models for children to learn how to be aggressive and/or violent.

- Cultural attitudes fostering violence

  Tacit acceptance of violence as a means to resolve conflict. War and weapons are justified as protection. In everyday language, we jokingly threaten to ''kill'' people or ''beat them up.'' We accept physical punishment as a way to discipline children under ''certain circumstances.'' Pornographic depictions of women are legal and deemed as erotica.

- Power and violence

  Violence or its threat is often used as a method of persuasion, as in rape or incest. Fear of being a victim of violence keeps people, primarily women, in positions of submission.

- Poverty

  Being poor is a condition of oppression, and aggression and violence are methods of expressing such oppression. Poverty needs to be considered as a circumstance in which violence occurs rather than as factor causing such behaviors.

- Subculture of violence

  There is a theme of violence that permeates the life-style values of the individuals who are party of this ''cultural group.'' Violence is a fairly typical method of resolving conflict.

THEORETICAL FRAMEWORKS EXPLAINING VIOLENCE

The theoretical frameworks that attempt to illuminate the causative factors of violence can be divided in a variety of ways. The broad categories chosen to organize this material for this text are biological, psychological, sociological, and anthropological. This review of theoretical frameworks cannot be considered exhaustive, but indicates the problems with determining causality of problems of violence and points out some of the inconsistencies, gaps, and difficulties in the traditional theoretical field. It also serves to underpin the theoretical information concerned with specific aspects of violence in the family.

The Biological Perspective

The biological theories of violence can be explored in two main sections: instinctivist and neurophysiological. The two frameworks, although derived from at least two very different disciplines, share the idea that violence is biologically determined, and both draw heavily from studies of animals (ethology).

Instinctivist

Lorenz's (1966) theory on aggression is the best known in the field. He views aggression as a fighting instinct that is common to men and animals and serves important species preservation functions by favoring genes for strength and preventing too much population density. Ardrey (1966), who also sees aggression as innate and within species, uses observations of animals to postulate that dominance and subordination are inevitable, and aggression and competition ensure the genetic transmission of useful traits. He believes that humans and animals are fundamentally motivated by aggression and the acquisition and defense of territory. Much time and space has been used to refute the simplistic theories of Ardrey and Lorenz from all perspectives. They have been criticized severely for poor scholarship, for anthropomorphizing, for equating hunting with aggression, for ignoring evidence of cultures where

violence is unknown, for failing to recognize that the fighting of animals of the same species (highly ritualized, defensive, stereotyped, and seldom fatal) cannot be compared to the cruel, destructive, and attacking violence of humans, and for disregarding the evidence that the early hunting and gathering populations were predominantly peaceful (Montagu, 1976). It has also been found that in nonhuman primates, male aggression, territoriality, and dominance battles are only a small fraction of the total interactions, and the group cohesively strives to keep these disruptive incidents to a minimum (Tracy & Crawford, 1992). Wallace (1973) points out that there are many animals that are almost entirely passive and yet are thriving as species. Aggression leading to violence has been shown by other anthropologists to be maladaptive in early human civilizations and thereby hardly genetically favored (Leavitt, 1975).

However, there is some evidence that evolutionary psychology can help explain some of the patterns of homicide (Wilson & Daly, 1988). These researchers interpret much of the homicide between young men and between spouses in terms of men's need to control women and their reproduction to ensure their genetic continuation. However, Wilson and Daly also emphasize that their analysis is not designed to provide an answer to homicide questions in terms of motive, nor do they claim that biological theory should replace social or circumstantial explanations for violence.

Neurophysiological

In contrast to the instinctivist theories, the neurophysiological approach is characterized by controlled laboratory research and generally by a recognition that many factors, both environmental and physical, contribute to violence. Neurophysiologists also draw extensively from studies of animals, but these have been conducted in the laboratory, mainly because of the ethical considerations involved in research with human subjects, not because they fail to grasp the problems in generalizing findings to human beings. Neurologists also point out that the neuroanatomically specific pathways in the human brain involved in the integration of aggressive behavior do not differ substantially in "distribution and general topography" from those of experimental animals (Valzelli, 1981). This perspective is important in addressing violence from a holistic viewpoint because it explains the physical basis of the aggression and violent behavior that is seen. The literature in this area is frequently technical in nature and relies heavily on graphs, charts, and schematic drawings of the brain. Readers may refer to anatomy and physiology texts for a more detailed clarification of neurophysiology. One of the most comprehensive overviews of the subject is provided by Moyer (1987). He maintains that aggression is "determined by an interwoven complex of internal, external and experiential factors" that are constantly interacting. Aggression equates with hostility for most of the neurophysiologists like Moyer and includes violence, as opposed to achievement or assertiveness. Moyer and other brain researchers are in general agreement that:

> . . . impulses generated in the sensory systems, the cerebral cortex and still undetermined neural structures may activate triggering mechanisms that in turn excite visceral and semantic systems whose activities in concert provide physiologic expression of aggressive behavior (Goldstein, 1974).

Moyer is careful to note that the sensorimotor feedback is also important because changes in the stimulus disrupt aggressive behavior. This shows that aggression is "stimulus bound" in contrast to the conceptualization of the instinctivists, who view it as spontaneous (Moyer, 1987). Studies of animals seem to indicate that there are several different neural systems for different kinds of aggression. Electrical stimulation of parts of the limbic system in humans has also produced evidence of different, although somewhat overlapping, neurological representations in the brain for different kinds of hostility (Goldstein, 1974; Moyer, 1987). Generalizing from these studies, brain researchers have concluded that many different neuroanatomical centers also exist for specific types of human aggression (Valzelli, 1981).

However, as neurologist Valzelli (1981) cautions, "electrical stimulation of the brain produces no strange or distorted behavior but acts only as a trigger or modulator of cerebral functions by influencing the processing of sensory inputs and the release of previously acquired behavior patterns." When perceived, appropriate stimulus (that is, pain, danger) activates the sensory system involved and alerts the animal (or person), leading to a generalized state of arousal that includes increased sensitivity of the sensory systems (greater responsiveness to the environment) and increased muscle tone. When one of the specific neural systems is active, all neural activity in one area is facilitated. Such substances as amphetamines enhance the activity in the area, but do not by themselves initiate activity in the aggressive systems. If any of the systems for aggression is active, the organism is more likely to respond aggressively to appropriate stimulus (Moyer, 1987). Studies in animals indicate that there are both facilitatory and inhibitory neural mechanisms for different kinds of aggression. Both surgical interruption of the neural systems for aggression and electrical stimulation of inhibitory systems in humans have decreased the tendencies toward hostility, resulting in neurologists reaching the same conclusions about humans. The activation of one system may involve the inhibition of another, as in animals when stimulation of the escape system inhibits aggression. Other neural systems (that is, higher brain centers in humans) are constantly interacting with the aggressive system, and the ultimate behavior is a function of those interactions not under control of the limbic system alone (Moyer, 1987).

Hormonal influences. Blood chemistry is also responsible for both inhibiting and facilitating the aggressive neural systems. Again, at least in animals, levels of certain endocrines (that is, norepinephrine, acetylcholine, dopamine, and serotonin) seem to selectively affect different kinds of aggression. Goldstein (1971) has concluded that the "specific neural systems in the central nervous system that synthesize, store and release these agents are differentially engaged" for different kinds of aggression. The action of these agents may explain the relationship of stress to aggression since both norepinephrine and acetylcholine have been identified as part of the stress reaction (Seyle, 1956). Deprivation states (that is, food and sleep deprivation and morphine withdrawal in addicted rats) have been associated with increased aggression and also cause a stress reaction. Although there has been no experimental verification, Moyer (1987) also hypothesizes that the hormone balance characterizing the stress system may sensitize the aggressive systems in the brain.

Other hormones affect both the facilitating and inhibitory mechanisms. It has been shown that testosterone sensitizes the brain system involved with intermale aggression in animals so that it is more easily activated by adequate stimuli. Testosterone has also been studied extensively in relationship to human assertiveness, dominance, and aggression.

In 1985 Mazur hypothesized that a feedback loop existed between testosterone levels and assertiveness in humans. This "biosocial theory of status" contends that as an individual's testosterone level rises, he or she is assumed to become activated and increasingly willing to compete in contests for higher status. Such status gains are postulated to either produce testosterone increases or maintain elevated levels, thus sustaining the person's readiness for continued pursuit of higher status. Alternatively, status losses produce decreases in testosterone levels. Mazur (1985) and others (Booth, Shelly, Mazur, Tharp, & Kittock, 1989) believe that this feedback loop accounts for winning and losing "streaks" because each win reinforces the high testosterone, which subsequently encourages further competitiveness. Conversely, losses diminish testosterone, perhaps acting to inhibit persons from continuing to engage in situations when they might potentially lose. Empirical testing of this model has been completed primarily with athletes (Booth et al., 1989; Mazur, 1985; Mazur, Mazur, & Keating, 1984), and the evidence indicates that links do exist between testosterone levels and assertiveness.

However, a person's mood also plays an important role. That is, testosterone levels were higher in those athletes who were happy about their wins compared with those who were indifferent or upset about their victories. Thus it can be concluded from this evidence that there is a relationship between assertiveness and testosterone levels, yet mood is

an important intervening variable that also merits consideration.

This point is not surprising if the relationship between aggression and pain is considered. Berkowitz (1984) argues that people who are in pain or feeling "bad" (emotionally or physically) are more likely to be aggressive than those who are in good moods or pain free, although aggression is not usually an initial response. Based on extensive evidence from both animal and human research, Berkowitz concludes that avoidance seems to be the first reaction to painful stimuli. However, humans or animals respond with aggression if the painful stimuli continue or if avoidance is not possible, particularly if the person believes that by attacking the pain will cease. In addition, Berkowitz cites evidence suggesting that strength of the aggressive response may be heightened by continual exposure to pain. The victim of wife abuse in the film *The Burning Bed* exemplifies how one battered woman, determined not to endure continual physical abuse and pain any longer, killed her husband by setting him on fire. The strength of her aggressive response is heavily influenced by the intense and long-suffering pain this woman endured at the hand of her husband.

The evidence cited by Berkowitz does not identify testosterone levels as being elevated or depleted in association with the painful stimuli and aggression. However, there is compelling empirical evidence that links elevated testosterone levels with aggression. In one study, Olweus (1984) measured testosterone levels of adolescent boys and found that those with higher levels of the androgen tended to respond more to provocation. In addition, these boys were more impatient and irritable than a comparative group of adolescent boys who had substantially lower levels of the hormone. Other studies examining testosterone, aggression, and violence have also identified that a positive relationship exists between the hormone level and aggressive/violent behavior.

Testosterone levels are equal in preadolescent girls and boys, but boys are still more aggressive (Rosoff & Tobach, 1991). The relationship between high violent crime rates and adolescent boys has often been noted even though the testosterone levels have started to fall during the period of highest violence (age 18 to 25) (Persky, Smith, & Basu, 1971). The correlations among testosterone levels, hostility, aggression, and dominance found in young men and in criminal populations, as well as the high serum testosterone levels found in especially aggressive hockey players, have led some researchers to postulate that although gonadal hormones do not regulate aggressive behavior, they may play a role in sustaining these actions (Valzelli, 1981).

Archer's (1991) comprehensive literature review on this subject details a number of studies comparing the testosterone levels of violent and nonviolent offenders. These studies are quite dissimilar, either because of research design or statistical techniques employed; however, results of all clearly identify that those prisoners convicted of violent crimes had higher testosterone levels than those who committed nonviolent wrongdoing. Although most of the studies reviewed by Archer used samples of male offenders, research completed with female convicts had similar findings, but these studies were significantly fewer in number. In contrast, a study of 23 girls who were accidentally given androgens postnatally showed no difference in aggressive behavior from normal females, although an increase in "tomboyishness" was noted (Persky, Smith, & Basu, 1971).

Progesterone, as an androgen inhibitor, and estrogen have also been studied in relation to aggression. Feelings of irritability and hostility and reports of increased violence in women have been linked to the fall of progesterone premenstrually in women (Moyer, 1987). However, Moos et al. (1969) found that premenstrual symptoms are not the same for all women, that the mood changes were consistent with the general personality. Only generally more aggressive or irritable women showed consistent increases in these affective states premenstrually.

Thus the majority of recent empirical evidence points to a relationship between elevated testosterone levels and aggression or violence. Yet several caveats are in order. First, as indicated, mood seems to play a role with elevated testosterone levels and assertiveness. It is less clear how mood influences testosterone and aggression, yet this connection may be an important one. It is known that the physical body, mood, and emotions are inextricably linked, thus how a person feels may also mediate effects of testosterone and violence. Empirical evidence on aggression and elevated testosterone levels has not consistently measured mood, and this omission is a critical one. Second, the studies reviewed here represent only a small proportion of the testosterone research and generally have been conducted on select samples, primarily prisoners and offenders. Most have been correlational. Thus increased testosterone may be the result rather than the cause of aggressive behavior. Indeed, there is experimental evidence that competitive sports and combat do raise testosterone levels (Rosoff & Tobach, 1991).

The few studies of voluntary castration of violent men showed that although the procedure decreased the problematic behavior of sexually deviant men, it neither inhibited the aggression of severely violent men nor helped their resocialization (Goldstein, 1974). Additional aggression/testosterone research has been completed in significant amounts, but samples consist primarily of rodents and other animals (Flannelly, Flannelly, & Blanchard, 1984). Therefore it is impossible to generalize any of these findings to the general population.

Whether aggression and violence are socially or biochemically determined has been the subject of long and often acrimonious debate (see Berkowitz (1984) and/or Flannelly, Flannelly, & Blanchard (1984) for further discussion on this matter). As the empirical evidence suggests, there is some credence to the position that hormones do influence aggressive behavior. However, the researchers add that direct causal links cannot be established and assert that social and environmental factors are more clearly linked to violence. Thus how both biological and social factors interact with each other in the expression of aggression must be considered.

The role of alcohol and drugs. Other substances in the blood can affect the inhibitory or facilitating neural mechanisms for aggression. The role of alcohol in this regard is not completely clear. Violent crime and alcohol are associated in both research and our personal experience, but neither are most criminals alcoholics nor the majority of alcoholics violent criminals (Moyer, 1987). Gerson and Preston (1979) analyzed the correlations among violent crime, age, sex, income, population density, and sales of alcohol in urban areas. The alcohol sales accounted for only 16% of the rate variations in violent crime. Laboratory experiments have shown increased aggression with alcohol ingestion, but there is variability in the studies and not all subjects react the same. In her careful review of the literature, Graham (1980) concluded that research has not substantiated a "direct cause paradigm," the theory that alcohol directly causes aggression by disinhibition. However, alcohol does produce psychological and physiological changes that seem to increase the probability of aggression under certain conditions. Because alcohol is frequently implicated in family violence, some examination of these changes is warranted.

The cognitive effects of alcohol ingestion have been examined in several studies. Not all research shows intoxication resulting in decreased intellectual functioning, but a decrease in verbal fluency is well established, an increase in expectation of attack from others has been noted in several studies, and higher doses of the substance do result in a variety of impairments (Schmutte, Leonard, & Taylor, 1979). Increased risk taking, time distortions, and a decreased awareness of the drinker's own actions and environment have also been documented (Graham, 1980; Kutash et al., 1978). The facilitation of aggressive behavior by alcohol is most likely related to these negative influences of alcohol in conscious, higher-level cognitive processing (Hillbrand et al., 1991). However, it is difficult to establish a direct relationship between those changes and aggressive behavior.

Physiological results of long-term ingestion, such as brain damage, disruption of rapid eye movement (REM) sleep, and poor nutrition leading to hypoglycemia, have all been related to aggression in themselves, but not directly in relation to alcohol ingestion (Graham, 1980). The immediate effects of alcohol are both sedative and arousing, depending on both internal and external circumstances. It has been hypothesized that increased testosterone levels interact with alcohol to produce increased facilitation of aggression, but this has not been corrob-

orated in research (Graham, 1980). Alcohol has been shown to cause temporal lobe dysrhythmia, which has been associated with aggressivity under laboratory conditions, but the subjects had all committed acts of violence previously (Abel, 1977). The substance has also produced abnormal electroencephalograms (EEGs) in some men with ordinarily negative readings (Gross, 1971). Bach-Y-Rita et al. (1971) found 25 of 30 violent criminals hospitalized for psychiatric illness to have problems with "pathological intoxication," characterized as loss of control early in the course of intoxication and leading to an outburst of explosive violence for which the man was amnesic afterward, suggesting neurologic predisposition. From these findings, it has been hypothesized that the aggression apparently stemming from physiological causes is related to a prior susceptibility to alcohol's effects or an already neurologically or environmentally established tendency to aggression (Abel, 1977). Such pathological intoxication seems rare, and stressful environmental conditions appear necessary for such states to result in violence (Kutash, 1978). The emotional lability sometimes cited as stemming from alcohol consumption and leading to aggression is not well documented in research. People seem to drink for a variety of reasons, including a desire to reduce anxiety and tension that does not fit with an aggressive behavior model. However, some men have been documented to drink to feel stronger or increase their sense of personal power, which may be expressed in sexual and aggressive conquests. A subset of the population may be predisposed to aggression and use drinking occasions as an acceptable time to express this behavior. There is ambivalence in our culture about whether people are less guilty for violent acts when drunk (Graham, 1980). Gelles (1972) has observed that there are other cultures where drunkenness is not followed by so-called disinhibited behavior, concluding that "drunken deportment is situationally variable and essentially a learned affair."

Alcohol abuse often is implicated in family violence. Okun (1986) cites a number of studies in which 48% to 85% of abuse has been documented as occurring in the presence of alcohol. However, on closer examination of these figures, it is evident that violence occurs *as frequently* when alcohol is not a factor, suggesting that cause and effect are not directly established.

Although alcohol ingestion and aggression and violence are linked in American society, cause and effect are not directly established. Such factors as preexisting physical and personality factors, dosage, expectations, settings, and other circumstances surrounding the drinking are as important as the neurophysiological effects of the substance.

Association between violence and other drug use is varied and inconclusive. At the turn of the century, postulates about the connections between violence and cocaine use were common, yet these claims were never demonstrated empirically (Helmer, 1983). More recently, in their literature review Gelles and Straus (1988) concluded that although drugs such as crack and marijuana have been associated with violence, this is not true with opiates. As with alcohol, effects of drugs on violent behavior appear to be associated with social, individual, and situational factors rather than neurophysiological causes. A possible exception to this are amphetamines. In studies completed with nonhuman primates, stump-tail macaques (monkeys) were given protocol *d*-amphetamines. After receiving the drug, it was noted that the monkeys' aggressive behaviors increased significantly. According to Gelles and Straus (1988), there are some investigators pursuing the link between human amphetamine use and violence, but presently there is no conclusive evidence suggesting a causal link between this drug and violence.

However, nicotine apparently has a suppressing effect on aggressive behavior. Cherek (1984) found that increased nicotine levels from smoking cigarettes were associated with lower levels of aggressive behaviors when compared with nonsmokers. These results are consistent with earlier studies examining this relationship.

Effects of heredity. The effects of heredity on the neural bases of aggression are equally debatable. Animal breeding for aggression has been done successfully in bulls and fighting cocks in natural settings and in mice in the laboratory (Moyer, 1987).

Valzelli (1981) uses these findings plus his research on brain levels of serotonin, which is a genetically determined characteristic related to emotional stability, to conclude that there are multiple genetic determinants to aggression. There may be genetic variability in the sensitivity of specific neural systems and in the determination of hormonal levels in humans, but research has not definitely established the connections (Valzelli, 1981).

Brain disorders. The interaction between epilepsy and aggression has been carefully studied. Usually aggressive acts are not part of temporal lobe seizures. When they do occur, they are described as "bad moods" rather than destructive or assaultive behavior (occurring in only about 5% of epileptics); when such behavior does occur, it is frightening to the family, but rarely results in criminal acts and does not occur without provocation (Blumer, 1976).

The periodic or episodic dyscontrol syndrome has been associated with violence. Russell R. Monroe et al. (1976) defines the disorder as

> . . . precipitously appearing maladaptive behavior that interrupts the life style and life flow of the individual; the behavior is out of character for the individual and out of context for the situation.

This behavior is contrasted with psychopathic behavior that is a way of life for an individual. Monroe et al. characterized the syndrome as the result of both "faulty learning and faulty equipment." The neurological basis is theorized to be excessive neuronal discharges in the limbic system that often do not appear on routine (scalp) EEGs, but may be manifested using deeply implanted electrodes.

"Soft" neurological signs, such as impaired psychomotor and perceptual ability, history of altered status of consciousness, history of febrile convulsions, and headaches, have been associated with episodic dyscontrol (Maletzky, 1973; Morrison & Minkoff, 1975; Spellacy, 1977). In addition, hyperactivity has been associated with aggressiveness in children. Violent male criminals frequently describe a history of this indication of minimal brain damage (Morrison & Minkoff, 1975; Bach-Y-Rita et al., 1971). However, Allen, Safer, and Covi (1975) note that aggressiveness may be only secondary to the effects of overactivity and may only reflect the way these boys have been treated and/or their need for constant stimulation and ways to expend their energy. The favorable response of some patients to anticonvulsant medications has been used as evidence for the neurological epileptic-like basis for the episodic dyscontrol syndrome (Bach-Y-Rita et al., 1971). However, most of the studies were not blind, and in one blind study, there were few dramatic changes with anticonvulsant medication, and the most therapeutic response was from the placebos (Maletzky, 1973; Monroe et al., 1976). It has been definitely established that some serious brain damage may cause otherwise unexplainable violent and aggressive behavior (that is, brain tumors in the limbic system and temporal lobes, brain trauma, and encephalitis), showing that human beings' "neural systems for aggression can be activated by internal physiologic processes" (Moyer, 1987). It is therefore theorized that minimal brain damage can have the same effect, but the exact neural mechanisms have been variously explained as lack of integration of the nervous system, extra activity in the neural cells responsible for aggression, increased sensitivity to aggressive cues because of general arousal, destruction of inhibitory systems, or destruction of learning systems (Kolb, 1971; Moyer, 1987; Spellacy, 1977). The results could also be explained by a combination of two or more of the variables. Moyer (1987) describes four variables that may interact in some not yet completely understood manner to explain chronic behavioral tendencies toward aggression: (1) a lowered threshold for activation of the neural systems of aggression (caused by heredity); (2) normal threshold, but increased sensitization of neurons (by hormones, activation from other systems, blood chemistry changes from stress and frustration, structural damage) facilitating their activation; (3) normal aggression system activation with decreased inhibition system activation (from decrease in some hormones and other blood substrates and alcohol); and (4) learning. Most of the researchers of episodic dyscontrol have noted other psychological and sociological correlates with the syndrome (Maletzky, 1973; Monroe et al., 1976). Researchers of aggressive neurophysiology usually stress the im-

portance of the interaction of social, environmental, and hereditary influences. They are all convinced of the aggressive potential in all human brains, but as Moyer (1987) states:

> Man, of course, learns better and faster than any other animal. It is therefore reasonable to expect that the internal impulses to aggressive behavior would be more subject to modification by experience in man than in any other animal. In addition, because of man's additional ability to manipulate symbols and to substitute one symbol for another, one would expect to find a considerable diversity in the stimuli that elicit or inhibit activity in the aggression system. One would expect that the modes of expression would be more varied, diverse and less stereotyped in man than in other animals (p. 18).

Only a few brain researchers imply that most violence could be prevented by surgery, pharmacological agents, or electrical pacemakers, or that violence is completely determined by biological mechanisms. The few that do, for instance Mark and Ervin (1970), are severely criticized by the rest, as well as by social scientists. It must be remembered that the biological mechanisms detailed underlie aggression, not necessarily violence. When applied to violence, these mechanisms may only explain potential for problems, not the violent behavior itself. Aggressive people are rarely always aggressive, and their hostile behavior may or may not be superimposed on a background of hostility. There are also no automatically elicited behavior patterns of aggression from environmental or electrical stimulus for humans as there are for animals (Moyer, 1987). Kolb (1971) points out that the neocortex in humans has "both a facilitatory and inhibitory influence on aggressive behaviors characterized by rage" and that it also influences the direction and timing.

Limitations of the neurophysiological approach. It should be noted that most of the brain research has been conducted with men, that men are inexplicably more likely to display episodic dyscontrol, and that the researchers use "man" in all of their descriptions of human beings. It is difficult to tell if they are referring only to the male sex in describing conclusions. Except for the evidence on the influence of hormones that we have seen is fragmentary and not totally conclusive, the neurophysiologists have not adequately explained the differences between male and female behavior. Females of all species are generally more difficult to stimulate to aggression, and once stimulated, express hostility somewhat differently (Rosoff & Tobach, 1991). It has been found that previous social experience and acquired learning of hierarchical rules are more important than sexual hormones in aggressiveness and dominance pattern formation in monkeys (Laborit, 1978).

The most important determining factor in aggressive behavior in humans is gender, and although gender is obviously a physical factor, the explanation of that difference is primarily found in the fields of sociology and psychology. Sociologists and psychologists generally acknowledge the neuronal and blood chemistry basis for aggression, but differ in their perspectives on the major determinants of violence. Sociologists point to the peaceful cultures that exist, and wonder why persons with minimal brain damage in those societies do not behave aggressively if socialization is not more important than brain disorders. Delgado (1971) asserts that patients with implanted electrodes display hostility when stimulated, "but it is always expressed according to the subject's previous experience and evaluation of his present environment." Brain researchers have also been criticized for diverting attention from our social dilemmas that "contributes to unwillingness to undertake the political solutions to violence which promise to achieve much more" (Coleman, 1974). However, neurophysiological bases for aggression are important for holistic understanding and can be viewed as background for psychological, sociological, and cultural influences that may lead to violent expression of the aggression.

Psychological Theories of Violence

Psychological explanations of violence vary greatly. Many psychologists echo Freud's theories that aggression is a basic instinct or drive (Freud, 1932). Others deemphasize or refute that view and identify other psychological traits that characterize the violent person. The basic premise of most psycho-

analytical frameworks is that some basic need or needs have been thwarted in the violent individual, usually by some form of faulty child-raising (Warren & Hindelang, 1979). The other major branch of psychological theories is derived from behavioral psychology. This includes Bandura's social-learning theory (1973) and Eysenck's biologically rooted conditioning framework (1977).

Psychoanalytical viewpoints

The psychoanalytical instinctivists derive their theories from basic Freudian concepts. Freud is not a modern theorist and his views have been analyzed extensively elsewhere (Fromm, 1973; Kutash et al., 1978). By the end of his career, Freud had reluctantly concluded that aggression was a basic instinct, as part of the death instinct and opposed to eros (Freud, 1932). His influence in this regard has pervaded psychoanalytic thought.

MacDonald, a relatively modern psychoanalyst, also writes from the same perspective of an "internal need to discharge hostility." He theorizes that murderers are likely to have ego weaknesses resulting in erratic control over aggressive impulses (MacDonald, 1961). Abrahamsen (1960) postulates that human behavior has four roots: (1) society at large, (2) community and its subcultures, (3) family, and (4) individual (psychological and physical). Thus he acknowledges the multiplicity of causative factors for criminal behavior, but still insists that all people have "criminal tendencies," "murderous impulses," and "hidden violence," which are activated when influenced by internal and external events. A corollary of the psychological instinctivists is that frustration is the instigation or stimulus that leads to the expression of aggression. This part of the theory was first advanced in 1939 and was linked to early behavioral psychology language. Dollard et al. (1970) hypothesized that the occurrence of aggression always presupposes frustration. Since then it has been determined by research that frustration does not *always* lead to aggression and that aggression does not always stem from frustration, nor is it the most potent instigator (Fromm, 1973). There is also ambiguity about the meaning of Dollard's terms. However, this concept has been adopted widely because of its simplicity, and there are references to it in sociological literature. One of the basic premises of the drive theory is that since aggression is a basic instinct, its appearance in behavior reduces accumulated hostility and decreases the amount of aggression shown in response to further frustration (Dollard et al., 1970). This is the catharsis premise first formulated by Freud and conceptualized by Hokanson (1970) as "the idea that the expression of aggression reduces the aggressor's internal state of anger and his general level of physiological tension." The catharsis theory is one aspect of psychoanalytical theory that lends itself to empirical testing, and the literature abounds with such research. Discriminatory studies have shown "clearly that overt aggression does not inevitably lead to either physiological tension reduction or a reduction in subsequent aggression" (Hokanson, 1970). Evidence against the catharsis hypothesis comes from other perspectives. In both experimental and natural settings, verbal aggression has not been shown to decrease subsequent physical attack; in fact, the opposite tends to occur (Moyer, 1987; Straus, 1974). The watching of violent films, seen by catharsis proponents as a substitution for aggressive behavior, has been shown to increase rather than decrease later aggression (Donnerstein, 1983; Donnerstein & Berkowitz, 1981; Malamuth, 1983). It has also been observed that watching violent sports tends to instigate aggression rather than lessen it (Moyer, 1987). One of the weakest points of the psychoanalytic view of aggression as a drive that must be expressed is therefore the catharsis assumption. One of the outgrowths of the catharsis concept is Megargee's (1966) concept of "overcontrolled personality types" who display extreme violence. Megargee theorizes that these persons are instilled with such excessive inhibitions against aggression in childhood that their hostile impulses build up. Although the instigation for aggression must be much stronger finally to elicit aggressive behavior, when it does appear it is likely to be excessively violent (Megargee, 1966). Much work has been done to identify these overcontrolled personalities. Behavioral and psychological tests in prison populations of murderers and violent criminals

have been developed, and a subscale of the Minnesota Multiphasic Personality Inventory (MMPI) was developed (OH—"overcontrolled hostility"—scale) for identification (Megargee, 1966; Hanley, 1979). The OH scale has not proved to be valid and the whole catharsis concept is controversial, so this explanation of violence must be highly questioned (Megargee, 1966; Hokanson, 1970).

Limitations of the psychoanalytical perspective. It is difficult not to be alienated by the blaming of mothers for violent sons rampant in psychoanalytical literature. Whether it is because of a "loveless" home, "emotional deprivation," "maternal symbiosis," "mother domination," "maternal deprivation," or "paternal neglect," the implication is that the mother has the primary responsibility for childrearing and she has failed in her task (Abrahamsen, 1970; Sendi & Blongren, 1975; Seyle, 1956; Storr, 1972). These theorists also note that the violent men have also frequently been exposed to abusive and alcoholic fathers (Maletzky, 1973; Satten et al., 1960; Sendi & Blongren, 1975). The mechanisms the psychoanalysts believe to be operating vary. The general theme is that the violent individual is acting out some form of emotional problems. Terms such as "psychotic," "neurotic," "psychopathic," "personality disorder," "passive aggressive," "self-destructive," "paranoid," etc., are used to describe almost every violent individual evaluated in psychoanalytical literature (Bach-Y-Rita & Veno, 1974; Sendi & Blongren, 1975; Storr, 1972). The triad of youthful enuresis, fire setting, and cruelty to animals has been identified as common in the childhood of habitually violent men (Bach-Y-Rita & Veno, 1974). The "individual psychology of the murderer" or violent person is considered the most important factor, and as Abrahamsen states, "emotional disturbances are always at the root of antisocial or criminal behavior" (Abrahamsen, 1960; Lunde, 1976; Saul, 1976).

There are problems with this conceptualization. The theories are usually derived from small case studies of violent men (rarely any women), and research involving larger groups often uses psychiatric hospital patients as controls (if there are any controls when identifying psychological traits "causing" violence (Bach-Y-Rita & Veno, 1974; Satten et al., 1960; Sendi & Blongren, 1975). The prisoners given psychiatric diagnoses by psychoanalysts have seldom been identified as mentally ill by the courts or other psychiatrists; the literature often indicates attempts to make the men "fit" into categories even when symptoms and testing show minimal aberrations (Hanley, 1979; McGurk, 1978). It has been found that the rates of violence for those patients labeled criminally insane (by the courts) are "not remarkably different" from the normal population, and the actual psychiatric pathology in criminal populations is estimated at only 18% (Mesnikoff & Lauterbach, 1975). If violence and psychiatric illness are so interwoven, it is difficult to explain why former mental patients commit fewer crimes, including violent crimes, than the normal population (Kolb, 1971). Psychiatrists and psychologists have not been able to consistently and accurately predict dangerousness or violence using psychological tests, psychiatric examination, or identification of the childhood "triad" (Buck & Graham, 1978; Mesnikoff & Lauterbach, 1975). The theories do not account for the preponderance of males committing violent offenses, and they share the assumption of the instinctivists (although not as forcefully) that aggression is an innate drive.

Derivations of psychoanalytical theory. A derivative branch of psychoanalytical theory is represented mainly by Fromm (1973), May (1972), and Kaplan (1975). They each conceptualize aggression as a result of the thwarting of some basic human need, differing somewhat in the need identified. These three theorists have shifted from the instinctivist position.

Fromm (1973) considered benign forms of aggression that are biologically adaptive and life serving (that is, self-assertive aggression, defensive aggression), to be innate, whereas malignant aggression (sadism and necrophilia) is not. The basic need that Fromm considers as thwarted when malignant aggression appears is the need "to transcend the triviality of life" to find greater meaning. He thinks that although pathological child-rearing and genetics can play a part, the primary determinant of malignant aggression is the "dry, banal, pedantic, dishonest, unalive atmosphere" characterizing many families

and social situations. Fromm's analysis is more philosophical in nature than research oriented. The ideas are interesting and useful for approaching the meaning of violence, but difficult to apply to specific situations.

May (1972) also discusses the basic need for a sense of significance, but in terms of self-affirmation and self-assertion. His theory can be summarized in the following quote:

> Deeds of violence in our society are performed by those trying to establish their self-esteem, to defend their self-image and to demonstrate that they, too, are significant.

May characterizes aggression as "moving into position of power or prestige" and feels that violence is the expression of powerlessness. He views power on a continuum from energy to force to violence, depending on the amount of blockage the person encounters.

Kaplan's (1975) theory is similar to May's in that he ascribes a basic need for self-esteem to human beings and thinks that when a person has a history of low self-esteem and self-devaluing experiences, he is more likely to develop hostile and retreating defenses. People with "negative stable self-attitudes" are "predisposed or motivated to seek out and adopt deviant patterns." The deviant patterns alleviate the subjective distress associated with what the person perceives as the critical attitude associated with the normative environment. Such people also satisfy the need for self-esteem by the "avoidance of, attacks upon or substitution for the normative environment." The person reacting to a history of self-devaluing experiences with hostile defenses is suspicious of and lacks identification with others and is thereby more likely to use violence.

Kaplan cites Toch's study (1969) of 69 male inmates and parolees as support for his theory. Toch found that almost one half of the offenders had used violence to buttress feelings of inadequacy. Even though their self-esteem was considered normal, another large group of convicts showed evidence of dehumanizing their victims, which is associated with Kaplan's hostile defenses (Toch, 1969). Kaplan (1975) maintains that many criminals do not show low self-esteem, because their deviant behavior has resulted in a reduction of negative self-feelings. Thus it is difficult to prove or disprove his theory by studying criminal populations. Yelsma and Yelsma (1977) gave the Coopersmith self-esteem inventory to 62 inmates (60 male, 2 female) of a county jail and a forensic center. They found that those who were destructive only to themselves (convicted of alcohol-related charges) had the lowest scores; those directly violent to others (murder, rape, or robbery) also had lower than normal scores, whereas those who were only indirectly destructive (forgery, drug sales) had higher than normal scores. From this evidence it can be postulated that there is some support for Kaplan's association of deviance and retreating defenses with low self-esteem, but the reason that the behavior had resulted in more positive self-concept for some and not for others is unclear. A small study of 10 homicidal adolescents (nine male, one female) found "vacillations" in self-esteem and a "lack of cohesion of self" (McCarthy, 1978). Other psychologists postulate that negative self-concept accounts for violence in some violent individuals but not in others, or that threatened self-esteem always results in aggression, but the aggression is not necessarily destructive (Grant, 1978).

Other psychoanalytical formulations about aggression should be considered. Adler viewed the drive for power as a source of aggression, postulating that those who needed to attack to get power usually acted out of inadequacy. Jung perceived violence as the "unleashing of primordial archetypical behavior inherent in the collective unconscious." Horney conceptualized destructive aggression as part of the behavior of those who "move against" rather than those who "move toward" or "move away." Sullivan was more apt to view violence and aggression as arising from disturbances in interpersonal relationships (Kutash, 1978).

Many ego psychologists do not conceptualize aggression as an independent drive and clearly differentiate benign aggression, a trait similar to what has been defined here as assertion, from malignant aggression or violence. They maintain that the healthy individual has strong ego boundaries that allow for the use of "reality testing, accurate appraisal of

threat, learning, conflict resolution and the use of defense mechanisms" by the ego to ensure that aggression is dealt with without harming others (Kutash, 1978). These conceptualizations are all useful in understanding the emotional context of violent behavior but have generally not been operationalized for empirical testing. As has been noted, the psychoanalytical theories and those derived from this framework are characterized by less support from empirical research than those of the biologists and a general reliance on some of the highly disputed assumptions of Freud. They generally fail to account for the preponderance of males committing violence, suffer from a primarily male orientation, and do not explain predominantly peaceful cultures.

The emotional conditions supporting violence are important in a holistic framework, but the psychoanalytical viewpoint has failed to prove that psychological mechanisms are mainly responsible for causing violence. However, there are violent individuals who must be considered mentally ill. Although "the incidence of psychosis among murderers is no greater than the incidence of psychosis in the total population," occasionally psychotic individuals, especially paranoid schizophrenics, are directed by auditory hallucinations or other delusionary systems to act violently. Even in these cases, psychological and sociological mechanisms affecting the "normal" murderer also influence the one who is labeled insane (Lunde, 1976).

Social-learning theory

Bandura (1973) is the originator and best known proponent of social-learning theory as an explanation for aggression. He calls the theory *psychological* because it grows out of the school of behavioral psychology, yet it obviously also combines aspects of sociological frameworks. In a review of the literature by Newcombe in 1978, it was found that the "majority of social scientists" agreed that aggression and violence are learned rather than instinctive. Okun (1986) notes that the majority of the general violence literature and more specifically, the research on abuse of women, use learning theory either explicitly or implicitly to explain why violence occurs. It is also not uncommon to find theorists combining aspects of the social learning theory with neurophysiological research (Laborit, 1978). Bandura defines aggression as "behavior that results in personal injury and in destruction of property," including that the injury "may be psychological." He also notes that the behavior must be labeled as aggressive by society, this labeling determined by the action's intensity, the intentions attributed to the performer by others, and the characteristics of the labelers (Laborit, 1978). Bandura (1979) thinks that aggressive behavior may be considered adaptive or destructive depending on the situation in which it is used. He acknowledges the role of biological subcortical structures in producing destructive behavior, but believes that the social situation is most important in determining the frequency, form, circumstances, and target of the action. He states:

> In the social learning view, people are endowed with neurophysiological mechanisms that enable them to behave aggressively, but the activation of these mechanisms depends on appropriate stimulation and is subject to cognitive control.

Bandura postulates that rather than arising from instinct or frustration, aversive experiences result in emotional arousal, which is perceived in the individual as fear, anger, sorrow, or even euphoria, depending on prior learning, cognitive interpretation, and other people's reaction to the same experience. Moreover, "frustration or anger arousal is a facilitative but not a necessary condition for aggression" (Bandura, 1973). Bandura concludes that the majority of events that stimulate aggression (that is, insults, status threats, unjust treatment) "gain activating capacity through learning experiences." To illustrate this, he notes the many people who have experienced divorce, parental rejection, poverty, mental illness, brain damage, etc. who have never become violent. He perceives the motivation for aggression as reinforcement based, not biologically determined. "The social learning theory of aggression distinguishes between acquisition of behaviors that have destructive and injurious potential and factors that determine whether a person will perform what he has learned . . . because not all that people learn is exhibited in their actions.

The acquisition of aggressive behavior can be learned through modeling or observational learning or by direct experience or practice. Performance is determined by both internal (biological and cognitive) and external instigators (Bandura, 1973; 1979). This has been confirmed in laboratory experiences with children (Bandura, 1973). Models for aggressive behavior can be found in the family, the subculture, and the media. Using analysis of a nationwide self-report sample of violent behavior and attitudes toward violence, Owens and Straus (1975) concluded that the more a child sees or is the victim of violence in his or her home or social structure, the more violence the child will perform as an adult, since he or she has seen the behavior modeled. Observation of others' behavior also provides clues as to whether the action will be rewarded or punished when it occurs. If a child sees a parent or peer gain status, dominance, resources, or power by using violence, he or she will be more likely to use it (Bandura, 1973). It has often been noticed that violent men are more likely to have been abused as children, and these ideas also help to explain why some peer groups (that is, gangs) and subcultures are known for violence (Bandura, 1973). Bandura found that parents of aggressive boys from middle-class homes, although they neither abused their children nor displayed antisocial violence, "repeatedly modeled and reinforced combative attitudes and behavior" (Bandura, 1973). The long-term effects of modeling were shown in an experiment where nursery school boys could imitate aggressive behavior shown 6 months previously. The girls, however, showed much less imitative behavior in this study (Hicks, 1965). Parental use of physical punishment is also considered a strong model for the use of force in other contexts. A recent study by Jerry Neopolitan (1981) suggests that the more juvenile males identify with their fathers, the greater the correlation between aggressive behavior and frequent use of physical punishment by male parents.

The effects of childhood family aggression on marital violence in the next generation were examined by Kalmuss (1984). This investigator studied

2143 adults attempting to discern whether the present level of violence with a spouse was more related to the observation of hitting between parents or to the actual experience of being hit as a child. Kalmuss found that those adults who witnessed hitting were more likely to abuse as adults than those who had been hit. In addition, observing one's father hit one's mother increased the likelihood that both men and women would be victims as well as perpetrators of violence. From these data, Kalmuss concluded that the transmission of family violence across generations was related to the modeling effects of the parental roles. That is, childhood exposure to violence teaches children that violence is an acceptable way to mediate conflict within the family.

The role of the media and especially television in modeling aggressive behavior has often been noted in theories of violence. Empirical evidence is beginning to show considerable substantiation. McCarthy et al. (1975) conducted a 5-year follow-up on a random sample cross-section of 732 children in Manhattan and Houston. They found that heavy viewing of violent programs was associated with two (of three) measures of aggression, fighting, and delinquency, as well as with regressive anxiety, mentation problems, and depression. However, Milgram and Shotland (1973) found no more imitative results from a television program showing a man stealing watched by male adult subjects who were then given an easy opportunity to do the same, in comparison to a matched control group who watched a neutral film. Several other studies have shown no effects or unreliable effects of television on violence or aggression (Kaplan & Singer, 1976; Milgram & Shotland, 1973). The effects of violent television viewing seem to be more apparent in children, suggesting that there is a critical period when aggressive patterns are learned and when television has the most impact. Singer and Singer (1980) found impressive correlations between extensive violent television watching and aggressive behavior in preschoolers. Eron's (1980) longitudinal study of more than 400 children showed that the single best predictor of the boys' aggressive behavior at age 19 was how much violent television they were watching at 8 years old. In an extensive review

of literature (1956-1976) of 153 studies, Andison (1977) found a weak positive overall correlation between viewing violence and subsequent aggressive behavior and noted that the more recent studies show increasingly positive results. This may be related to a cumulative effect of increasingly violent television watching, more emphasis on the effects on children, and/or better methods used in the later studies.

Much television programming, especially children's programs, depicts violence, and shows violent males as heroes who gain power by its use (Gerbner et al., 1979). Researchers postulate that in addition to the modeling effect, heavy violence viewing disinhibits aggressive behavior by showing good triumphing over evil with the use of violence, and by desensitizing and habituating people to violence (Bandura, 1979; McCarthy et al., 1975). Goldstein's study of people exposed to more violence in real life showed that they also were more likely to prefer violent portrayals in media (Goldstein, 1974). A study by Fenigstein (1979) suggested that previous aggressive thoughts and actions increase preferences for viewing violence, which further increases aggressive behavior. Leyens et al. (1975) found that only previously aggressive boys in their study were increasingly aggressive after watching filmed violence; the less aggressive boys were not. However, the more violent boys showed a modeling effect, because their physical aggression closely paralleled the types shown in the movies.

The other postulated effect of televised violence is the production of a concept of the world as a dangerous place. Viewers who watch television heavily have been shown to have more feelings of mistrust and suspicion, which may increase their tendencies to use violence in marginally appropriate situations (Bandura, 1979; Gerbner et al., 1979). Gerbner et al., with extensive research on the results of television watching, concludes that only 1 to 2 per 1,000 "heavy" watchers actually imitate the violence on television and threaten society, but that the majority become more fearful, insecure, and dependent on authority.

Bandura (1979) explains that behavior learned from models is reinforced if the imitative actions are perceived as useful to the person. Laborit (1978) explains that if aggression is successful and dominance achieved by it, "then the aggression will in itself constitute reinforced behavior because of the gratification that followed." This mechanism was illustrated in a study showing that fifth-grade boys who were measured as aggressive were more likely to reward themselves with tokens for aggressive behavior even when the victim expressed pain, than those who showed low aggression on the inventory (Perry & Bussey, 1977). Laborit also notes that "society's rewards tend to go to the least compassionate members," which is a strong reinforcement for aggression. Extending this model to women is problematic; however, the social-learning theorists postulate that aggressive behavior is a product of the cognitive structure that either inhibits or disinhibits the performance of the activity (Bandura, 1979; Megargee, 1971). They believe that the socially learned inhibitors to aggression are much stronger for women and that violence is less useful to women (Owens & Straus, 1975). But, it must be remembered that violence is not socially sanctioned in women as it is in men. Thus it is difficult to separate the links between the individual and the social meaning of violence.

Empirical verification. Much laboratory research has been done to identify and determine the relative strength of the inhibitors, disinhibitors, and facilitators of learned aggressive behavior. Most of the studies involve subjects being given the opportunity to be aggressive by using shock machines. The intensity, duration, and number of shocks given is measured to determine the amount of aggression shown. There is much controversy among researchers regarding which conditions are the most powerful in affecting aggression. Most studies use male college students, and it is questionable whether these laboratory results can be generalized to the rest of the population (Fromm, 1973; Leyens, 1975). For the purposes of this review, these studies can be summarized stating that the effects of: (1) generally arousing films (not necessarily violent), (2) the presence or firing of guns, (3) violence depicted as justified, (4) lowered responsibility for actions, (5) dehumanization of victims, (6) continued aggressive action as self-reinforcement, (7) competition, (8) sexual arousal especially when subjects are angered, (9) pain cues given by the victim, (10) anticipated punishment, (11) empathy, and (12) prior social contact with the victim have all been studied (Hartman, 1969; Goldstein, 1975). The relative strengths of these factors are controversial, but the evidence suggests that the first eight may facilitate or disinhibit aggression and the last three have some inhibiting effect. Pain cues or other signs of victim suffering seem to increase aggression when the subject is angered or reinforced for such behavior (Sanders & Baron, 1975; Sebastian, 1978).

The social-learning theory does incorporate biological, psychological, and sociological factors of causation of violence. Other theorists have modified and/or amplified Bandura's basic propositions, but the thrust of the arguments remains the same (Goldstein, 1974; Straub, 1971). These authors think that aggressive behavior, the instigations for hostile activity, the factors that facilitate or inhibit its expression, the appropriate targets, and the mechanism used to display aggression are all learned, although somewhat influenced by neurophysiological and psychological mechanisms. As previously noted, there is much empirical evidence to support these conclusions, although the details have not yet been conclusively established. These theories account for the effects of different sociological factors in terms of learning.

Sociological Forces Affecting Violence

The sociological theories of violence generally consider some of the biological and psychological aspects of causation, but their basic proposition is that social structure and conditions are more important (West, 1979). They vehemently reject the idea that aggression is an instinct or drive, and postulate that most violent offenders are basically normal and generally do not act destructively (Chatterton, 1976). Except for these areas of agreement, the sociologists vary widely in their approach. There are theorists who emphasize any one of the following aspects: cultural attitudes fostering violence, the structural violence inherent in our society, the role of power, the influence of poverty, a subculture of violence, and machismo.

Cultural attitudes fostering violence

The United States has a long history of violence used as a means to achieve socially approved ends. American culture reflects at least a covert acceptance of violence in the media, in attitudinal surveys, and in choice of heroes. Blumenthal et al. (1972) interviewed 1374 American men with a variety of socioeconomic characteristics and found that one half to two thirds could justify the police shooting in situations not involving self-defense or protection of innocent people from bodily harm, situations only requiring social control (conditions like campus protests or riots or gangs inflicting property damage). Twenty percent to 30% would advise the police to shoot to kill in these instances. These researchers believe such attitudes are a "covert message that it is socially acceptable to use violence for instrumental reasons" (Blumenthal et al., 1972). A variation on this theme in different terminology is Lundsgaarde's (1969) view of homicide as reflecting the sanctions in a culture. "A sanction is a reaction on the part of a society or a considerable number of its members to a mode of behavior which is thereby approved (positive sanctions) or disapproved (negative sanctions)." Lundsgaarde used an analysis of homicide in Houston, Texas, in 1969 to show that official negative sanctions (the police, courts, and laws) against killing can be overcome by covert positive sanctions defining homicide as more permissible in such cases as husband-wife killings, homicides among friends and associates, or those among the poor and black (Lundsgaarde, 1969).

Similarly, in a cross-cultural analysis of wife beating, Counts, Brown, and Campbell (1992) found that sanctions against wife battering at the community level were extremely important in keeping occasional acts of violence against wives from escalating to severe abuse.

There is also some evidence to suggest that both negative and positive sanctions may be mediated either by the gender of the aggressor and the crime. Saunders (1988) contends that a double standard exists with regard to the types of sentences men and women receive for murdering a spouse, particularly when the crime has been motivated by sexual infidelity. Saunders writes that "men are traditionally given light sentences if they kill an unfaithful wife 'in the heat of passion.' Women are not afforded the same leniency" (p. 100). Brienes and Gordon (1983) maintain that this double standard exists for men and women with regard to any type of violent behavior. They argue that there is a cultural expectation for women to be nonviolent, whereas this does not exist with men. When women deviate from the norm and commit violent acts or heinous crimes, their behavior is seen as much more severe than men's and is judged more harshly.

Structural violence of society

A closely related theme is that violence in America reflects the violence inherent in our way of life. Gil (1978) notes that the structure of our society results in "acts and conditions which obstruct the spontaneous unfolding of innate human potential, the inherent drive toward development and self-actualization." He believes that capitalism fosters an "all pervasive, exploitative attitude" that is necessary to "get ahead" in the system, and that families act as agents of the structure in their stress on hierarchical patterns and arbitrary authority, which transmits those violent attitudes to each succeeding generation. Bergen and Rosenberg (1976) echo these sentiments when they describe our culture as "brutalizing" and our society represented by "competitive striving and lust for power and control over one's fellows, and mutual exploitation." Wolfgang (1966) also speaks of the society legitimizing violence by "the labels of virtue" it attaches to methods of social control and the use of military force.

Power and violence

When considering both the cultural and structural elements of society that nourish violent behaviors, the role of power must also be considered. Power is a subject of interest to sociologists because the manifestations of power indicate a great deal about the social conditions in which people interact with each other. For example, someone has a gun and tells the other person to turn over his or her valuables. It is likely that the person will comply in order not to be hurt. The threat of physical force is a powerful tool in controlling the interaction. Similarly, a supervisor tells a worker that a particular task must be finished before leaving work that night. Although the threat of physical force is absent in this situation, the outcome is similar because the boss is shaping what the worker will do. Power also operates beyond the level of the individual. The Supreme Court has the power to determine the continued legality of abortion. This legislative body is in a position of shaping the decisions that American women make about childbearing. Power is an integral aspect of social life and is continually used to influence the outcomes of situations, whether at the individual level or more generally, as a component of the social structure.

There are many scholars who believe that violence and/or its threat are manifestations of power. For example, Straus (1980) contends that the use of violence on a governmental level (strategic arms, war) reinforces the notion that violence is an appropriate exhibition of power. Goode (1971) argues that violence occurs in all types of social systems because it is a set of resources by which people can move others to serve their ends. Some view violence as a manifestation of the unequal power relations between men and women (see for example, Barry, 1979; Daly, 1978; and/or Kurz, 1989). Sheffield (1989) asserts that men use violence to control or dominate women. She states "Violence and its corollary, fear, serve to terrorize females and to maintain the patriarchal definition of women's place" (p. 3). Women who are afraid to go out by themselves or who are worried about being alone in public places are being terrorized, Sheffield argues. It is this sexual terrorism that serves as a mechanism of social control by shaping how women organize their lives. Sheffield believes that sexual terrorism is a common characteristic in all forms of violence against women because it frightens and controls women to act in ways that are socially acceptable. Thus women are dependent on men to be their escorts, as well as being encouraged to be timid in the face of danger and not self-assured. In turn, these behaviors by women re-

inforce men's roles as protectors of women, which further highlights the unequal power balance between men and women. Another aspect of unequal power relations between men and women can be seen clearly in discussions of wife abuse, a topic discussed in Chapter 3.

There are other sociological frameworks that attempt to explain why violence occurs, such as strain theories, role theory, social disorganization, and theories of population density. These explanations are among some of the older ones in sociology and may be described as being primarily *macrosociological* in nature. They do not explain *why* violence occurs between individuals, but why violence exists at a more general societal level. The strain theories postulate that crime and delinquency result when material possessions cannot be achieved through conventional means and illegal activities are chosen as an alternative means of obtaining desired ends. Social disorganization theory explains violence by suggesting that violence occurs when there is a confusion or disorganization of social values or norms. The population density ideas are grounded in the notion that overcrowding causes violent behaviors, thus violence is more likely to occur in larger cities. These theoretical frameworks are accompanied by empirical evidence that affirms their tenets. However, they are less likely to explain the social forces that affect individuals within a small group, namely the family, which is the main focus of this book. Strengths and weaknesses are listed on the box on the next page.

Poverty

In an effort to further explain the greater amounts of urban violence, especially among poor young black men, sociologists have proposed extensive theories (Rose, 1979). In a study of the 17 largest U.S. cities, Curtis (1974) found that reported urban criminal homicide and aggravated assault is most frequently committed by black males in their teens and twenties who victimize other black male friends, acquaintances, or strangers, the same age or older, living in close proximity, in the course of relatively trivial altercations. Instead of postulating that any single factor causes this violence, the social scien-

Strengths and Weaknesses of Theoretical Approaches

Biological

Strength

- Aggression and violence are brain or hormonal imbalances, thus are treatable or manageable with treatment.

Weaknesses

- Social or environmental conditions that may influence or mediate violence or aggression are not considered.
- Human research has been done primarily on men and prisoners.
- Minimal effort has been made to include women into the research.

Psychological

Strength

- Aggression and violence are individual characteristics resulting from basic needs or drives that have been thwarted, usually by some form of childrearing. Thus through psychological treatment, the individual can be "cured."

Weaknesses

- The mother is usually blamed for the faulty child-rearing.
- Social or environmental conditions that may influence or mediate violence or aggression are not considered.
- Much of the research has been completed with the mentally ill or prisoners and has been generalized to unrelated populations.

Social-learning theory

Strength

- Incorporates how environmental influences such as television and exposure to violence affect behavior. By monitoring such societal influences, violence can be mediated.

Weaknesses

- Suggests a causal relationship between amount of violence observed and subsequent behavior, yet direct causal link not established.
- Minimizes the role that power has in violent interactions.
- Implies that once the violence is modeled and observed, then violent actions will automatically follow. Individuals are not allowed to change or grow after examining *how* the violence affects the victims.

Sociological explanations

Strength

- Conditions such as unequal power relations and poverty create situations where violence is an outcome. Structural level changes, such as equal status between men and women and minimizing the financial gap between the rich and the poor, will eradicate the need for violence actions to occur.

Weaknesses

- Solutions are long term and don't address the immediate health concerns resulting from violent behaviors.
- The explanations tend to be focused on the general "macrosociological" level and do not hold individuals accountable for their violent behaviors.

Cultural explanations

Strength

- Violent behaviors in certain cultures tend to be associated with factors such as child-rearing techniques and beliefs, attitudes about women, and warfare and crime. By examining cultural practices, we can gain understanding of how violence fits and what purposes it serves.

Weakness

- Analysis of culture does not offer any solutions about how to change specific behaviors of individuals or groups.

tists tended to note various circumstances associated with the cultural setting of the inner city. Many have noted the anger generated by discrimination and racism (Wolfgang, 1964). Liston (1974) says in this regard, ''violence is simply a message, a desperate one, that a situation of inequality, frustration and rage exists that badly needs correction. Parker and Smith (1979) found that the highest correlation between noninstrumental homicide (murder during heated conflict rather than for a specific purpose) and other factors was poverty, although race and young adult status were also related. However, another study found unemployment not related to the incidence of violent crime (Spector, 1975). Curtis (1974) held socioeconomic class constant and found no significant correlation between race and violence within poverty areas in Boston, Atlanta, and San Francisco, but did find a correlation in Chicago and Philadelphia.

There is much discussion in the literature as to whether the association between poor black men and violence is related to poverty and lack of opportunity, social characteristics specific to race, or lower-class values (Hawkins, 1990; Rose, 1979). From a study of all the homicide cases reported from across the nation in *The New York Times* from 1955 to 1975 that were committed by middle-class and upper-class citizens (119 cases), Greene and Wakefield (1979) report that there were no black offenders. This finding strongly suggests that the dynamics that operate to cause the young black male to kill frequently have less to do with his race than with his condition of oppression. Luchterhand and Weller (1976) found white inner-city boys to be significantly more verbally aggressive, whereas blacks were more physically aggressive, but the black students were more likely to control aggressive behavior of either kind in the research situation. Balkwell et al. (1978) also found white high school students in Georgia from all social classes more verbally expressive of all emotions than black students. In contrast, Coles (1967) found black inner-city children ''active, vigorous and more outgoing than the middle class child but quick to lose patience and feel wronged.'' He attributes these characteristics to the violence and uncertainty of their world and the

amount of freedom the poor child has in the street compared to the strict physical punishment he or she encounters at home.

The idea of social disintegration on the family level is reflected by theorists writing in this area. Moynihan (1969) describes the disorganization of the black family, and Scarpitti (1969) identifies stability of the home as the most important factor in keeping poor black children from becoming delinquent. However, these are white theorists making assumptions about a culture that they usually do not understand. Nobles (1978) notes that the black family is a unique cultural form and what may appear to be disintegration to white observers is actually an elastic structure that includes family beyond one household and not necessarily blood-related, has flexible and interchangeable role definitions and performance, and is child centered. Bartz and Levine (1978) supported these conclusions when they found that black families provided more emotional support than Hispanic and white Anglo families in the same lower-working-class neighborhood. However, they found all three groups advocating early autonomy for children, strict controls of behavior, and purposeful use of time for children, suggesting that class-related values may be more important in terms of child-rearing practices than ethnic group membership.

Generally, the sociological literature reviewed to date in regard to the violence of young urban African-American males is unsatisfactory in terms of causal theory. As Rose (1979) states:

> The situation of this segment of the population has become increasingly dire and/or the ability to cope with both internal and external forces has become so burdensome that violent acting out, leading to death, has emerged as an adaptive mechanism. Our lack of understanding of what has become the fifth ranking killer of all black males and the ranking killer of those 15-24 bodes ill for the scientific community (p. 7).

Subculture of violence

This lack of understanding has been addressed differently by other sociologists who work from a framework of the subculture of violence. Cloward and Ohlin (1960) were the first to develop this theory, which they used with "anomie" to explain the behavior of delinquent male gang members. They defined the delinquent subculture as "one in which certain forms of delinquent activity are essential requirements for the performance of dominant roles supported by the subculture." These theorists postulated that the gang members either: (1) follow norms of criminality by imitating deviant characteristics that usually the most outwardly successful men in their environment display, (2) follow the "retreatist" model of being "cool" like the hustlers or drug addicts, or (3) commit violence to maintain status or a reputation of being tough.

Wolfgang and Ferracuti (1967) further refined the theory by extending it from a subculture of delinquency to a subculture of violence. They define subculture as "value judgments or a social value system which is apart from and a part of a larger or central value system." They further explain that a subculture has major values in common with the dominant culture, but also has values that vary and may conflict with those of the larger culture. These values are transmitted through the learning process of socialization, and they are incorporated into the personality structure through strict, physical childhood discipline, "reinforced in juvenile peer groups and confirmed in the strategies of the street." Wolfgang and Ferracuti identify the subculture of violence as a "potent theme of violence current in the cluster of values that make up the life style, the socialization process, the interpersonal relationships of individuals living in similar conditions." The person's integration into the subculture can be measured by his or her records of arrest rate, especially for crimes of assault. Participants in the subculture do not necessarily express violence in all situations, but certain stimuli are expected to be responded to with violence.

Wolfgang and Ferracuti do not account for the causes of a subculture of violence, but postulate that it is present wherever homicide rates are high, such as in urban ghetto areas in the United States and other countries such as Mexico, Columbia, and parts of Italy. They also note that crime rates are as high as in the black urban areas of America, in slums of Italy, Germany, Poland, and other predom-

inantly caucasian cultures. Therefore they conclude that the subculture of violence is based more on poverty, urban blight, and cultural prescriptions than race.

Figures from Wolfgang's 1958 study of criminal homicide in Philadelphia were used to substantiate the subculture of violence thesis, but these were only descriptive in nature and the theory lacks explanatory power. The problem with blaming the culture of a race or class for violence without identifying the antecedents of that culture is that it becomes a way of subtly blaming the victims (and perpetrators) for creating the culture (Letcher, 1979). It can be argued that any subculture of violence in the lower class and/or black culture is related to the systematic denial of opportunity by the majority of society.

Moran (1971) synthesized the subculture hypothesis with the idea that "the more fully low status groups or individuals seek to occupy or maintain status positions based on achievement, the more likely they are to commit criminal homicide." Using homicide data from Boston (1962-66), Moran found that age had a stronger relationship to homicide than sex or race, suggesting that in low-status populations the age group committing the largest proportion of homicide (20 to 29 years) does so because this is the age group with the most emphasis on achievement. When he studied homicide rates among ethnic groups, Moran found that the association between gender and homicide was stronger than that between race and homicide and believed that this "suggests the presence of a subculture of violence among males." Moran's conclusion was that "a subcultural normative system sanctioning the use of violence during social interaction exists mainly among low status groups of individuals experiencing subjective external restraint."

Moran accounts for gender differences in homicide in terms of males being more frustrated by occupational status blocking than females. He thinks that black women are more achievement oriented than other ethnic groups; which, according to Moran, explains why in America black women commit more homicides than white, Italian, Puerto Rican, or Irish females. In the face of evidence that black women are the lowest paid group in the United States, and considering their supposed achievement orientation, it is difficult to understand why their homicide rate is only one fourth that of black men. Moran also fails to provide a reason why the majority of low-status males do not act out the subculture of violence.

An interesting corollary to the subculture of violence theory is the controversy about the existence of a southern version of these values that has diffused into the urban centers by way of migration patterns. Gastil (1971) first advanced this idea by noting the high statistical rates of homicide in the South and by linking this with the southern values of exaggerated sense of honor and a historical predilection for violence, which is usually only lightly punished. Much controversy was raised about whether southerners actually were more likely to own guns (versus handguns), whether less available and lower-quality medical care in the South accounts for the higher homicide rates, and whether it was southerners who had migrated who were committing northern urban violence (Erlanger, 1974). The conclusions varied widely according to the measures used to indicate southernness and violence approval, the statistical methods, and the populations studied, making meaningful comparisons difficult.

Curtis (1975) used the subculture of violence concept as a base and developed a theory that perhaps best explains sociologically the preponderance of poor black urban males committing homicides. Curtis joins the other subcultural theorists in noting the strong influence of violence as a characteristic of the masculine ethic (Curtis, 1975; Erlanger, 1974; Wolfgang & Ferracuti, 1967). Recently Bernard (1990) has suggested that the subculture of violence premises be combined with cognitive aggression theories that emphasize cognitive interpretations of events and physiological arousal, as well as intention. In other words, in certain subcultural groups, young men learn to interpret certain cues as inflammatory and become angrily physiologically aroused because of cognitively originated mechanisms. This integration has the potential to better explain the violence in

society than the original subcultural premises. (See Chapter 3 for further explanations of the role of machismo in wifebeating.)

INSIGHTS FROM ANTHROPOLOGY
Meaning of Violence Cross-Culturally

The meaning of the term *violence* within a culture varies through time as well as from culture to culture. Historically in the United States, the *Journal of Marriage and the Family* first mentioned family violence after 1970 and not until after 1973 were there references to wife abuse in "*The New York Times*" (O'Brien, 1971; Tierney, 1982). Behaviors generally understood as abuse in one culture may be considered legitimate in another. Torres' (1991) comparison of Mexican-Americans and Anglo-Americans demonstrated differences in behaviors that were considered abusive. Although there was no difference in the severity and frequency of violence between the two groups, Mexican-Americans labeled their experience of being battered as abuse less frequently. Whether the differences were related to ethnicity or to sociocultural factors such as religion, education, and economic factors that are characteristic of each group, it is apparent that abuse occurs within a context that influences interpretation (Lee, 1984; Newberger & DeVos, 1988; Torres, 1991).

The absence of reports of abuse in a culture does not mean it does not exist. An unstated assumption in much of the literature is that if the persons interviewed or observed did not know, acknowledge, or admit there was abuse, it was not classified as abuse (Korbin, 1991). If abuse is a function of the person's perception of being victimized (Newberger & DeVos, 1988; Torres, 1991), the culture's beliefs and norms become important in understanding the influence of culture on recognition of violence as well as the culture's definition of violence. In fact, because of different cultures' perceptions of what constitutes *abuse* and the complexity of different cultural systems, it may not be possible to attain a universal definition of family violence that is culturally specific (Korbin, 1991).

Sensitivity of the observer may also reflect societal differences about the meaning of violence. Female anthropologists may be more sensitive to the occurrence of violence against women or may have had women more readily disclose violence to them (Campbell, 1985). An ethnographer may report only the positive either because she or he has "fallen in love" with the people or because he or she wants to maintain the trust with the society that has been established over time (Erchak, 1984).

However, there are societies that are totally nonviolent both interpersonally and in terms of warfare, according to many different anthropologists and other reporters. The fact that there are such cultures provides powerful evidence that cultural forces and learning are at least as important as biology in explaining the occurrence of violence. The characteristics of such societies are important in identifying possible primary prevention approaches. Nonviolent societies tend to be more egalitarian (either in terms of power or economics) than hierarchical in sex roles and ethnic groups arrangements, treat children with kindness and without corporal punishment, value cooperation over competition, and have definitions not tied to violence and control of women (Campbell, 1985; Eisler, 1988; Fromm, 1973; Levinson, 1989; McConahay & McConahay, 1977; Paddock, 1975; Whiting, 1965).

In this discussion, *culture* refers to nations, political subdivisions within nations, ethnic groups, or small-scale societies (Levinson, 1989). The culture of an individual is one's "social heredity" (Gelles, 1974). The role of culture in violence within the culture must be understood (Campbell, 1985; Gelles & Cornell, 1983; Levinson, 1983; Torres, 1991). The problem of understanding is a complex one because there are probably a multiplicity of mingled antecedents associated with violence (Minturn, Grosse, & Haider, 1969).

Theoretical frameworks purporting to explain the cultural influence on violence are: (1) sexual inequality, (2) social organization, (3) cultural patterning, and (4) the cultural spillover hypothesis. Each theoretical frame is described briefly with support for its claims. Although cultural determinants of violence have not been totally established, there is beginning support for each of these theories.

Sexual inequality

Traditionally the patriarchal society has viewed violence toward wives as the man's right, stemming from the idea that a woman is his property (Dobash & Dobash, 1979). There has been no link established cross-culturally between the status of women and violence against women specifically except by Lester (1980), who does not identify the measures he used to determine status of women. Yet within the United States there is support for the hypothesis that low status of women is related to violence against women.

Violence to women is greater in the states where women's status, measured by economic, educational, political and legal rights, is low or high (Yllo, 1983; 1984). Economic dependency has been implicated in another study to be related to the frequency of wife beating (Kalmuss & Straus, 1982) in the United States. Similarly, in a cross-cultural analysis of less complex societies, control of the wealth and authority in the home were also related to frequency of wife beating (Levinson, 1989), Counts, Brown, and Campbell (1992) also found support for women's economic autonomy being associated with less wife battering in a sample of 14 societies.

The concept of women's status is complex and cannot be described by only one factor (Campbell, 1985; Sanday, 1981; Whyte, 1978; Yllo, 1983, 1984). Status may differ between the public and private spheres of culture (Sanday, 1981), as well as among dimensions of power, prestige, and rewards, which are indicators of status in the United States. Cross-cultural indicators are too numerous to list (Whyte, 1978), but some components related to status that have been implicated as associated with wifebeating are: low female autonomy, no matrilocality, virtue as honor, females perceived as male property, male sexual jealousy, strong association of women and nature, cultural sanctions allowing wife beating, other violence against women, female entrapment in marriage (divorce restrictions) (Campbell, 1985; Levinson, 1989), male control of production, and male domestic decision making.

The effect of gender inequality can also be seen cross-culturally in the maltreatment of female children. Female infants and small children are more likely to be malnourished and receive inadequate medical care than their brothers in societies where there is male gender preference (Korbin, 1991). According to the Global Fund for Women, in India, amniocentesis is used for sex determination, followed by abortion of female fetuses (Boston Women's Health Collective, 1984).

The question of the relationship of sexual equality to violence is broad because sexual equality is made up of varied and elaborate factors. Focusing on the status of women sidesteps the issue of why gender inequality exists (Levinson, 1989). Understanding these complex questions is important to prevention of violence.

Social organization

Social organization is defined in sociology as the pattern of relationships between and among individuals and social groups and how the individuals are related to each other and the whole group (Straus, 1974). Social organization theories of family violence claim causes of violence can be found in the structure of the society and its effect on how the family members relate to each other (Levinson, 1988). Levinson (1989) found more severe physical punishment of children in more complex societies and in societies with more single-parent families. He also noted more wife beating and child beating in societies where men have multiple wives (polygynous households).

Cultural patterning

Cultural patterning means that although persons have an innate drive for aggression, they are patterned culturally to discharge their aggression in particular ways. Cultural patterning assumes social-learning theories that allow violence in a particular way for a culture or in subcultures. According to the subculture of violence theory, subcultures have norms related to the extent and conditions of the occurrence of violence that are consistent with the values of the culture (Wolfgang & Ferracuti, 1967). Cultural patterning and the theories subsumed under cultural patterning are based on the notion that the antecedents of violence are complex and always occur in the context of the culture (Minturn, Grosse, & Haider, 1969; Torres, 1991).

Cultural Consistency Theory of Violence

Elements of a culture tend to be interdependent (Lester, 1980). Knowledge of the interdependent factors within a culture and their relationship to violence can ultimately provide a topology of family subcultural norms. This knowledge not only provides a greater understanding of what leads to abuse, it can also help influence the development of cultures that are free of violence (Levinson, 1989).

The cultural consistency theory explains that even cultural norms that are not directly related to violence can have an effect on violence that occurs within the culture. An example of this idea is that Mexican-American boys may be so afraid of their father's punishment that there is little communication between the two. Because of the poor communication, the boys unwittingly act in such a way that they offend their fathers and are punished severely (Carroll, 1980). Family structure that contains stress and physical abuse models violence, which is then acted out by the next generation (Carroll, 1977).

In the cultural consistency theory the norms of this family behavior reflect the values of the society as a whole. The norms are tied to the structure of the systemic properties of the culture (Whyte, 1974). In this way violence tends to be consistent with the norms and values of the society (Carroll, 1980). This explanation thus helps understanding the causation of violence within a culture.

Paddock's (1976) description of antiviolent communities in Mexico is consistent with the cultural consistency theory. Paddock reported differences in child-raising practices between violent and antiviolent communities, including differences in punishment. Attitudes of men in the less violent community reflected less machismo. The antiviolent community was authoritarian, but in the cultural system the authority was shared. The consensus of the group reflected a shared attitude against interpersonal violence. Peterson, Lee, and Ellis (1982) found a relationship between a high value on child conformity (versus self reliance) and physical punishment in a cross-cultural analysis.

Cultural Spillover Hypothesis

According to the cultural spillover hypothesis (Baron & Straus, 1985), the more a society tends to use physical force toward socially approved ends, the greater the likelihood that this legitimization of force will be generalized to other areas of life. Examples of the use of force in a society are in maintaining order in schools, controlling crime, or dominating international events for one's own interest.

ETHNIC GROUPS IN THE UNITED STATES

There are many different cultures in the United States. All of the theories presented may explain the effect of culture on abuse, yet studies of differences among ethnic groups within the United States indicate the complexity of their content. Variables that are implicated in abuse must have explanatory power both within and between cultures (Minturn & Lambert, 1964). We cannot assume that members of ethnic groups can be characterized similarly for the effect of their culture on abuse (Keefe, 1982). The evidence suggests that it is important to con-

sider the level of acculturation of the family into the United States and the socioeconomic status.

Gelfand and Fandetti (1986) show via literature reports and vignettes that an interactional approach is needed to understand the effect of cultural differences on ethnic groups. Their review supports assessing ethnic groups for: (1) language, generation of the immigrant, cultural homogeneity of the neighborhood, degrees of activity in traditional religions, socioeconomic status, and (2) the interaction of these factors with the institutions of work, school, social services, medical services, and community.

Several authors implicate socioeconomic status accounting for differences in husband to wife abuse between African-American and Anglo-American, Mexican-American and Anglo-American, and black, Hispanic, and white (DeMaris, 1990; Lockhart, 1987). Torres' (1991) findings suggested that there may not be a significant difference between Mexican-Americans and Anglo-Americans in the United States when socioeconomic class is the same. The box summarizes key points concerning theories of violence.

SUMMARY

The meaning of *abuse* cannot be understood out of context. The complexity of factors related to violence

---

Summary of Important Points about Theories of Violence

- Aggression is not an instinctual drive, but must be viewed as destructive with intent to harm physically or emotionally. Our notions of aggression are grounded in our perceptions of men and women. We often see aggressive behavior as different depending on the gender of the person.
- Violence is a complex and multifaceted phenomenon that is tolerated and socially sanctioned throughout American society. We justify war and physical punishment of children.
- Biological, psychological, social, and cultural explanations of violence add to a growing body of knowledge about violence, yet none of the explanations alone answer satisfactorily the question of why violence occurs. Each approach has strengths and weaknesses, all of which should be considered.
- Social and cultural explanations about aggression and violence are the most comprehensive, because they consider factors that are beyond the individual and address issues of how our social world influences behaviors.
- Race and poverty are correlated variables, thus in studies of poverty and violence faulty assumptions must be avoided about violence occurring more frequently in certain racial groups, with an understanding that poverty is a condition that often sustains violence.

is magnified by varied cultural systems. Complicating factors within the United States are that members of the various cultures and ethnic groups differ in their level of acculturation and oppression. Membership in a culture or ethnic group cannot forecast the person's perception or reaction to violence.

There is a probability that there will be important differences between your beliefs and those of persons from other cultures or ethnic groups. It is important to consider your assumptions (Torres, 1987). Caregivers can consider the influence of spiritual, moral, somatic, psychological, and metaphysical as well as the economic, kinship, and territoriality issues (Gibbs, 1984) to discern the person's views of abuse. Only then can the caregivers structure their approaches to ethnic groups for perception and management of the problem (Flaskerud, 1984).

REFERENCES

Abel, E. L. (1977). The relationship between cannabis and violence: A review. *Psychological Bulletin, 84,* 202-208.

Abrahamsen, D. (1960). *The psychology of crime.* New York: Columbia University Press.

Abrahamsen, D. (1970). *Our violent society.* New York: Funk & Wagnalls.

Allen, R., Safer, D., & Covi, L. (1975). Effects of psychostimulants on aggression. *Journal of Nervous and Mental Diseases, 160,* 138-145.

Andison, F. S. (1977). TV violence and view aggression: A cumulation of study results, 1956-1976. *Public Opinion Quarterly, 41,* 318, 319.

Andreski, S. (1964). Origins of war. In J. D. Carthy & F. J. Ebling (eds.). *The natural history of aggression* (pp. 6-13). London: Academic Press.

Archer, D., & Gartner, R. (1984). *Violence and crime in cross-national perspective.* New Haven, CT: Yale University Press.

Archer, J. (1991). The influence of testosterone on human aggression. *British Journal of Psychology 82,* 1-28.

Ardrey, R. (1966). *The territorial imperative.* New York: Antheneum.

Bach-Y-Rita, G. et al. (1971). Episodic dyscontrol: A study of 130 violent patients. *American Journal of Psychiatry, 127:* 1475.

Bach-Y-Rita, G., & Veno, A. (1974). Habitual violence: A profile of sixty-two men. *American Journal of Psychiatry, 131:* 1016.

Balkwell, C. et al. (1978). On black and white family patterns in America: Their impact on the expressive aspect of sex-role socialization. *Journal of Marriage and the Family, 40,* 744-756.

Ball-Rokeach, S. J. (1980). Normative and deviant violence from a conflict perspective. *Social Problems, 28*(1), 45-60.

Bandura, A. (1973). *Aggression: A social learning analysis.* Englewood Cliffs, NJ: Prentice Hall.

Bandura, A. (1979). The social learning perspective. In H. Toch (Ed.), *Psychology of crime and criminal justice* New York: Holt, Rinehart and Winston.

Baron, L., Strauss, M., & Jaffee, D. (1988). A test of the cultural spillover theory. *Annals of the New York Academy of Sciences, 528,* 79-110.

Barry, K. (1979). *Female sexual slavery.* New York: Avon.

Bartz, K. W., & Levine, E. S. (1978). Childrearing by black parents: A description and comparison to anglo and chicano parents. *Journal of Marriage and the Family, 40,* 909-720.

Bergen, B., & Rosenberg, S. (1976). Culture as violence. *Humanitas, 12,* 196, 197.

Berkowitz, L. (1983). The goals of aggression. In R. Gelles, G. Hotaling, M. Straus, & D. Finkelhor (Eds.), *The dark side of families* (pp. 166-181). Beverly Hills: Sage.

Berkowitz, L. (1984). Physical pain and the inclination to aggression. In R. B. Blanchard & D. Blanchard & K. Flannelly, (Eds.), *Biological perspectives on aggression* (pp. 27-48). New York: Alan R. Liss.

Bernard, T. (1990). Angry aggression among the "truly disadvantaged." *Criminology, 28*(1), 73-96.

Blumenthal, M. et al. (1972). *Justifying violence.* Ann Arbor, MI: Broun-Brumfeld.

Blumer, D. (1976). Epilepsy and violence. In D. J. Madden & J. R. Lion (Eds.), *Rage, assault, and other forms of violence* (pp. 209-220). New York: Spectrum.

Booth, A., Shelly, G., Mazur, A., Tharp, G., & Kittock, R. (1989). Testosterone and winning and losing in human competition. *Hormones and Behavior, 23,* 556-571.

Boston Women's Health Collective (1984). *Our bodies ourselves: A book by and for women.* New York: Simon & Schuster.

Brienes, W., & Gordon, L. (1983, Spring). The new scholarship on family violence. *Signs,* 490-530.

Buck J. A., & Graham, J. R. (1978). The 4-3 MMP, profile type: A failure to replicate. *Journal of Consulting and Clinical Psychology, 46,* 344-356.

Campbell, J. (1985). The battering of wives: A cross cultural perspective. *Victimology, 10,* 174-185.

Chatterton, M. R. (1976). The social contexts of violence. In M. Borland (Ed.), *Violence in the family* (pp. 15-36). Atlantic Highlands, NJ: Humanities Press.

Cherek, D. (1984). Effects of cigarette smoking on human aggressive behavior. In K. Flannelly, et al. (Eds.), *Biological perspectives on aggression.* New York: Alan R. Liss.

Chinn, P. L. & Jacobs, M. K. (1978). A model for theory development in nursing. *Advances in Nursing Science, 1,* 1, 41.

Cloward, M. & Ohlin, L. (1960). *Delinquency and opportunity.* Glencoe, IL: Free Press.

Coleman, L. S. (1974). Perspectives on the medical research of violence. *American Journal of Orthopsychiatry, 44,* 685-692.

Coles, R. (1967). Violence in ghetto children. *Children, 14,* 101-104.

Counts, D., Brown, J., & Campbell, J. C. (1992). *Sanctions and sanctuary: Cultural perspectives on the beating of wives.* Boulder, CO: Westview Press.

Curtis, L. A. (1974). *Criminal violence.* Lexington, MA: D.C. Heath.

Curtis, L. A. (1975). *Violence, race, and culture.* Lexington, MA: D.C. Heath.

Daly, M. (1978). *Gyn/ecology the metaethics of radical feminism.* Boston: Beacon.

Delgado, J. (1971). The neurological basis of violence. *International Social Science Journal, 33,* 33-48.

DeMaris, A. (1990). The dynamics of generational transfer in courtship violence: A biracial exploration. *Journal of Marriage and the Family, 52,* 219-231.

Denton, R. K. (1978). Notes on childhood in a nonviolent context: The Semai case. In A. Montagu (Ed.), *Learning non-aggression* (pp. 18-35). New York: Oxford Press.

Dobash, R. E., & Dobash, R. P. (1979). *Violence against wives.* New York: The Free Press.

Dollard, J. et al. (1970). Frustration and aggression. In E. L. Magargee, & J. E. Hokanson (Eds.) *The dynamics of aggression* (pp. 18-36). New York: Harper & Row.

Donnerstein, E. (1983). Aggressive pornography: Can it influence aggression against women? In Albee G. et al. (Eds.). *Promoting sexual responsibility and preventing sexual problems* (pp. 46-68). Hanover, NH: University of New England Press.

Donnerstein, E., & Berkowitz, L. (1981). Victim response in aggressive erotic films as a factor in violence against women. *Journal of Personality and Social Psychology, 36,* 1270-1277.

Eisler, R. (1988). *The chalice and the blade: Our history, our future.* San Francisco: Harper & Row.

Erchak, G. M. (1984). Cultural anthropology and spouse abuse. *Current Anthropology, 25*(3), 331-336.

Erlanger, H. S. (1974). The empirical status of the subculture of violence thesis. *Social Problems, 22,* 280-292.

Eron, L. (1980). Prescription for reduction of aggression. *American Psychologist, 35,* 244-252.

Eysenck, H. J. (1977). *Crime and personality.* (3rd ed.) London: Routledge & Kegan Paul.

Federal Bureau of Investigation. (1985). *Crime in the United States.* Washington, DC: Government Printing Office.

Fenigstein, A. (1979). Does aggression cause a preference for viewing media violence? *Journal of Personality and Social Psychology, 37,* 2307-2317.

Flannelly, K., Flannelly, L., & Blanchard, R. (1984). Adult experience and the expression of aggression: A comparative analysis. In L. F. Blanchard, D. Blanchard, & K. Flannelly (Eds.), *Biological perspectives on aggression* (pp. 207-259). New York: Alan R. Liss.

Flaskerud, J. H. (1984). A comparison of perceptions of problematic behavior by six minority groups and mental health professionals. *Nursing Research, 33*(4), 190-197.

Freeman, D. (1964). Human aggression in anthropological perspective. In J. D. Carthy & F. J. Ebling (Eds.), *The natural history of aggression* (pp. 12-26). London: Academic Press.

Freud, S. (1932). Why War? In R. Maple & D. R. Matheson (Eds.), *Aggression, hostility and violence* (pp. 118-132). New York: Holt, Rinehart and Winston.

Fromm, E. (1973). *Anatomy of human destructiveness.* New York: Fawce Crost Books.

Gastil, R. (1971). Homicide and a regional culture of violence. *American Sociological Review, 36,* 412-414.

Gelfand, D. E., & Fandetti, D. V. (1986, November). The emergent nature of ethnicity: Dilemmas in assessment. *Social Casework: The Journal of Contemporary Social Work,* 542-550.

Gelles, R. (1974). *The violent home.* Beverly Hills: Sage.

Gelles, R. J., & Cornell, C. P. (1983). *International perspectives on family violence.* Lexington, MA: Heath.

Gelles, R., & Straus, M. (1988). *Intimate violence.* New York: Simon & Schuster.

Gerbner, G. et al. (1979). The demonstration of power: Violence profile no. 10. *Journal of Communications, 29,* 180-196.

Gerson, L., & Preston, D. A. (1979). Alcohol consumption and the incidence of violent crime. *Journal of Studies on Alcohol, 40,* 307-312.

Gibbs, J. L. Jr. (1984). Cultural anthropology and spouse abuse. *Current Anthropology, 25*(3), 533.

Gil, D. G. (1978). Societal violence and violence in families. In J. M. Eckelaar, & S. N. Katz (Eds.), *Family violence* (pp. 16-27). Toronto: Butterworth.

Goldstein, M. (1971). Brain research and violent behavior. *Archives of Neurology, 30,* 2-81.

Goode, W. (1971). Force and violence in the family. *Journal of Marriage and the Family, 33,* 624-636.

Graham, K. (1980). Theories of intoxicated aggression. *Canadian Journal of Behavioral Science, 12,* 2, 143-148.

Grant, D. (1978). A model of violence. *Australian and New Zealand Journal of Psychiatry, 12,* 123-132.

Greene, E., & Wakefield, R. (1979). Patterns of middle and upper class homicide. *Journal of Criminal Law and Criminology, 70,* 175-187.

Gross, M. A. (1971). Violence associated with organic brain disease. In J. Fawcett (Ed.), *Dynamics of violence* (pp. 196-210). Chicago: American Medical Association.

Haber, S., & Seidenberg, B. (1978). Society's recognition and control of violence. In Kutash I. L. et al. (Eds.), *Violence: perspectives on murder and aggression* (pp. 7-30). San Francisco: Jossey-Bass.

Hanley, C. (1979). The gauging of delinquency potential. In H. Toch (Ed.), *Psychology of crime and criminal justice* (pp. 176-191). New York: Holt, Rinehart & Winston.

Hartman, D. P. (1969). Influence of symbolically modeled instrumental aggression and pain cues on aggressive behavior. *Journal of Personality and Social Psychology, 11,* 285-296.

Hawkins, D. F. (1990). Explaining the black homicide rate. *Journal of Interpersonal Violence, 5*(2), 151-163.

Helmer, J. (1983). Blacks and cocaine. In B. M. Shapiro, T. Shapiro, & M. Kelleher (Eds.), *Drugs and Society* (pp. 14-29). Dubuque, IA: Kendall/Hunt.

Herman, S. J. (1978). *Becoming assertive: a guide for nurses.* New York: Van Nostrand Reinhold.

Hicks, D. J. (1965). Imitation and retention of film-mediated aggressive peer and adult models. *Journal of Personality and Social Psychology, 2,* 97-100.

Hillbrand, M. et al. (1991). Alcohol abuse, violence and neurological impairment: A forensic study. *Journal of Interpersonal Violence, 6*(4), 411-422.

Hokanson, J. E. (1970). Psychophysiological evaluation of the catharsis hypothesis. In E. L. Megargee, & J. E. Hokanson (Eds), *The dynamics of aggression* (pp. 37-50). New York: Harper & Row.

Kalmuss, D. (1984). The intergenerational transmission of marital aggression. *Journal of Marriage and the Family, 46,* 11-19.

Kalmuss, D. S., & Straus, M. A. (1982). Wife's marital dependency and wife abuse. *Journal of Marriage and the Family, 44,* 277-286.

Kaplan, H. B. (1975). *Self-attitudes of deviant behavior.* Pacific Palisades, CA: Goodyear.

Kaplan, R. M., & Singer, R. D. (1976). Television violence and viewer aggression: A reexamination of the evidence. *Journal of Social Issues, 32,* 62-71.

Keefe, S. E. (1982). Help-seeking behavior among foreign-born and native-born Mexican Americans. *Social Science Medicine, 16,* 1467-1472.

Kolb, L. (1971). Violence and aggression: An overview. In J. Fawcett, (Ed.), *Dynamics of violence* (pp. 40-50). Chicago: American Medical Associations.

Korbin, J. E. (1991). Cross-cultural perspectives and research directions for the 21st century. *Child Abuse and Neglect, 15,* 67-77.

Kurz, D. (1989). Social science perspectives on wife abuse: Current debates and future directions. *Gender & Society, 3*(4), 489-505.

Kutash, I. L. et al. (1978). *Violence: Perspectives on murder and aggression.* San Francisco: Jossey-Bass.

Laborit, H. (1978). Biological and sociological mechanisms of aggression. *International Social Science Journal, 30,* 738-745.

Leavitt, R. (1975). *Peaceable primates and gentle people: Anthropological approaches to women's studies.* New York: Harper & Row.

Lee, G. R. (1984). The utility of cross-cultural data. *Journal of Family Issues, 5*(4), 519-541.

Lester, D. (1980). A cross-culture study of wife abuse. *Aggressive Behavior, 6,* 361-364.

Letcher, M. (1979). Black women and homicide. In H. M. Rose (Ed.), *Lethal aspects of urban violence* (pp. 50-61). Lexington, MA: Lexington Books.

Levinson, D. (1989). *Family violence in cross cultural perspective.* Newbury Park, CA: Sage.

Levinson, D. (1983). Physical punishment of children and wifebeating in cross-cultural perspective. In R. J. Gelles & C. P. Cornell (Eds.), *International perspectives on family violence.* Lexington, MA: Lexington Books.

Leyens, J. P. et al (1975). Effects of movie violence on aggression in a field setting as a function of group dominance and cohesion. *Journal of Personality and Social Psychology, 32,* 353-362.

Liston, R. (1974). *Violence in America.* New York: Julian Messner.

Lockhart, L. L. (1987). A reexamination of the effects of race and social class on the incidence of marital violence: A search for reliable differences. *Journal of Marriage and the Family, 49,* 603-610.

Lorenz, K. (1966). *On aggression.* New York: Bantam Books.

Luchterhand, E., & Weller, L. (1976). Effects of class, race, sex, and educational status on patterns of aggression in lower class youth. *Journal of Youth and Adolescence, 5,* 63, 65.

Lunde, D. T. (1976). *Murder and madness.* San Francisco: San Francisco Press.

Lundsgaarde, H. (1977). *Murder in space city.* New York: Oxford University Press.

MacDonald, J. M. (1961). *The murderer and his victim.* Springfield, IL: Charles C Thomas.

Malamuth, N. (1983). Factors associated with rape as predictors of laboratory aggression against women. *Journal of Personality and Social Psychology, 45,* 432-442.

Maletzky, B. M. (1973). Episodic dyscontrol syndrome. *Diseases of the Nervous System, 34,* 178-185.

Malinowski, B. (1973). An anthropological analysis of war. In E. Maple and D. Matheson (Eds.), *Aggression, hostility and Violence* (pp. 76-100). New York: Holt, Rinehart and Winston.

Mark, V. H., & Ervin, F. A. (1970). *Violence and the brain.* New York: Harper & Row.

May, R. (1972). *Power and innocence.* New York: W. W. Norton.

Mazur, A. (1985). A biosocial model of status in the face-to-face primates. *Social Forces, 67,* 377-402.

Mazur, A., Mazur, J., & Keating, C. (1984). Military rank attainment of a West Point class: Effects of cadets' physical features. *American Journal of Sociology, 90,* 125-150.

McCarthy, J. B. (1978). Narcissism and the self in homicidal adolescents. *American Journal of Psychoanalysis, 38,* 25-36.

McCarthy, E. D. et al. (1975). Violence and behavior disorders. *Journal of Communications, 25,* 72, 77.

McConahay, S. A. & McConahay, J. B. (1977). Sexual permissiveness, sex-role rigidity, and violence across cultures. *Journal of Social Issues, 33,* 139, 140.

McGurk, B. J. (1978). Personality types among "normal" homicides. *British Journal of Criminology, 18,* 158, 159.

Megargee, E. L. (1966). Undercontrolled and overcontrolled personality type in extreme antisocial aggression. *Psychological Monographs, 80,* 3-20.

Megargee, E. L. (1971). The role of inhibitor in the assessment and understanding of violence. In J. Singer (Ed.), *The control of aggression and violence* (pp. 130-146). New York: Academic Press.

Mesnikoff, A. M., & Lauterbach, C. D. (1975). The association of violent dangerous behavior with psychiatric disorders: A review of the research literature. *Journal of Psychiatry and the Law, 3,* 440.

Milgram, S., & Shotland, R. L. (1973). Television and antisocial behavior: Field experiments. New York: Academic Press.

Minturn, L., Grosse, M., & Haider, S. (1969). Cultural patterning of sexual beliefs and behavior. *Ethnology, 8,* 301-318.

Minturn, L., & Lambert, W. (1964). *Mothers of six cultures: Antecedents of child rearing.* New York: John Wiley & Sons.

Monroe, R. et al. (1976). Brain dysfunction in aggressive criminals. Lexington, MA: D.C. Heath.

Montagu, A. (1978). Learning non-aggression. New York: Oxford Press.

Moos, R. H. et al. Fluctuations in symptoms and moods during the menstrual cycle. *Journal of Psychosomatic Research, 13,* 43.

Moran, R. (1971). Criminal homicide: External restraint and subculture of violence. *Criminology, 8,* 358-372.

Morrison, J. R., & Minkoff, K. (1975). Explosive personality as a sequel to the hyperactive child syndrome. *Comprehensive Psychiatry, 16,* 346-358.

Moyer, K. E. (1987). *The psychobiology of aggression.* New York: Harper & Row.

Moyer, K. E. (1987) *Violence and aggression.* New York: Paragon House.

Moynihan, D. P. (1969). *Violent crime.* New York: George Braziller.

Mulvehill, D. J., & Tumin, M. M. (1969). *Crimes of violence* (Vol. 12). A staff report submitted to the National Commission on the Causes and Prevention of Violence. Washington, DC: U.S. Government Printing Office.

Neopolitan, J. (1981). Parental influence on aggressive behavior: A social learning approach. *Adolescence, 16,* 831-840.

Newberger, C. M., & DeVos, E. (1988). Abuse and victimization: A life-span developmental perspective. *American Journal of Orthopsychiatry, 58*(4), 505-511.

Newcombe, A. (1978). Some contributions of the behavioral sciences to the study of violence. *International Social Science Journal, 30,* 750-768.

Nobles, W. W. (1978). Toward an empirical and theoretical framework for defining black families. *Journal of Marriage and the Family, 40,* 680, 687.

O'Brien, J. E. (1971). Violence in divorce prone families. *Journal of Marriage and the Family, 33*(4), 692-698.

Okun, L. E. (1986). *Woman abuse: Facts replacing myths.* Albany, NY: SUNY Press.

Olweus, D. (1984). Development of stable aggressive reaction patterns in males. In R. Blanchard & D. Blanchard (Eds.), *Advances in the study of aggression* (Vol. 1) (pp. 51-72). New York: Academic Press.

Owens, D. J., & Straus, M. A. (1975). The social structure of violence in childhood and approval of violence as an adult. *Aggressive Behavior, 1,* 195, 196, 210.

Paddock, J. (1975). Studies on antiviolent and "normal" communities. *Aggressive Behavior, 1,* 217-33.

Paddock, J. (1976). Values in an antiviolent community. *Humanitas, 12,* 183-92.

Parker, R. N., & Smith, M. D. (1979). Deterrence, poverty, and type of homicide. *American Journal of Sociology, 85,* 622-630.

Perry, D. G., & Bussey, K. (1977). Self-reinforcement in high- and low-aggressive boys following acts of aggression. *Child Development, 48,* 653, 655.

Persky, H., Smith, K. D., & Basu, G. K. (1971). Relationship of psychologic measures of aggression and hostility to testosterone production in men. *Psychosomatic Medicine, 33,* 265-271.

Petersen, L. R., Lee, G. R., & Ellis, G. J. (1982). Social structure, socialization & disciplinary techniques: A cross cultural analysis. *Journal of Marriage and the Family, 44,* 131-142.

Rose, H. M. (1979). *Lethal aspects of urban violence.* Lexington, MA: Lexington Books.

Rosoff, B. & Tobach, E. (1991). *On peace, war and gender: A challenge to genetic explanations.* New York: The Feminist Press.

Sanders, G. S., & Baron, R. S. (1975). Pain cues and uncertainty as determinants of aggression in a situation involving repeated instigation. *Journal of Personality and Social Psychology, 32,* 495-502.

Sanday, P. R. (1981). *Female power and male dominance.* Cambridge: Cambridge University Press.

Satten J. et al. (1960). Murder without apparent motive: A study in personality disorganization. *American Journal of Psychology, 117,* 49-56.

Saul, L. (1976). A psychoanalytic view of hostility: its genesis, treatment, and implications. *Humanitas, 12,* 171-181.

Saunders, D. G. (1988). Wife abuse, husband abuse, or mutual combat? A feminist perspective on the empirical findings. In K. Yllo & M. Bograd (Eds.), *Feminist perspectives on wife abuse* (pp. 90-113). Newbury Park, CA: Sage.

Scarpitti, F. R. (1969). The good boy in a high delinquency area: Four years later. *American Sociological Review, 25,* 556.

Schmutte, G., Leonard, K., & Taylor, S. (1979). Alcohol and expectations of attack. *Psychological Reports, 45,* 1, 164.

Schur, E. (1983). *Labeling women deviant gender stigma and social control.* Philadelphia: Temple University Press.

Sebastian, R. J. (1978). Immediate and delayed effects of victim suffering on the attacker's aggression. *Journal of Research in Personality, 12,* 312-328.

Sendi, I. B., & Blongren, P. G. (1975). A comparative study of predictive criteria in the predisposition of homicidal adolescents. *American Journal of Psychiatry, 132,* 425, 426.

Seyle, H. (1956). *The stress of life.* New York: McGraw-Hill.

Sheffield, C. (1989). Sexual terrorism. In J. Freeman (Ed.), *Women: A feminist perspective* (pp. 3-19). Mountain View, CA: Mayfield.

Singer, J., & Singer, D. (1980). Television viewing, family style and aggressive behavior in preschool children. In M. R. Green (Ed.), *Violence and the family* (pp. 23-36). Boulder, CO: Westview Press.

Spector, P. (1975). Population density and unemployment. *Criminology, 12,* 400-410.

Spellacy, F. (1977). Neuropsychological difference between violent and nonviolent adolescents. *Journal of Clinical Psychology, 33,* 168-173.

Storr, A. (1972). *Human destructiveness.* New York: Basic Books.

Straub, E. (1971). The learning and unlearning of aggression. In J. Singer, (Ed.), *The control of aggression and violence.* New York: Academic Press.

Straus, M. (1974). Leveling, civility, and violence in the family. *Journal of Marriage and the Family, 36,* 18, 25.

Straus, M. (1980). The marriage license as a hitting license. In M. Straus & G. Hotaling (Eds.), *The social causes of husband-wife violence* (pp. 465-479). Minneapolis: University of Minnesota Press.

Tierney, K. J. (1982). The battered women movement and the creation of the wife beating problem. *Social Problems, 29*(3), 207-220.

Toch, H. (1969). *Violent men.* Chicago: Aldine.

Torres, S. (1987). Hispanic-American battered women: Why consider cultural differences? *Response to the Victimization of Women and Children, 12*(1), 20-21.

Torres, S. (1991). A comparison of wife abuse between two cultures: Perceptions, attitudes, nature, and extent. *Issues in Mental Health Nursing, 12*(1), 113-131.

Tracy, K. K., & Crawford, C. B. (1992). Wife abuse: Does it have an evolutionary origin. In D. A. Counts, J. K. Brown, & J. C. Campbell, (Eds.) *Sanctions and Sanctuary: Cultural perspectives on the beating of wives* (pp. 19-42). Boulder, CO: Westview Press.

U.S. Deptment of Health and Human Services. (1986). *Health—United States.* Washington, DC: Government Printing Office.

Valzelli, L. (1981). *Psychobiology of aggression and violence.* New York: Raven Press.

Wallace, C. (1973). Why do animals fight? In T. Maple & D. R. Matheson, (Eds.), *Hostility and violence* (pp. 126-135). New York: Holt, Rinehart & Winston.

Warren, M. Q., & Hindelang, M. J. (1979). Current explanation of offender behaviory. In H. Toch, (Ed.), *Psychology of crime and criminal justice* (pp. 62-80). New York: Holt, Rinehart and Winston.

Webster's Third New International Dictionary. (1988). Springfield, MA: Merriam-Webster.

West, D. J. (1979). The response to violence. *Journal of Medical Ethics, 5,* 128-136.

West, L. J. (1980). Discussion: Violence and the family in perspective. In M. R. Green, (Ed.), *Violence and the family* (pp. 236-242). Boulder: Westview Press.

Whiting, B. B. (1965). Sex identity conflict and physical violence: A comparative study, Part 2. *American Anthropologist, 67,* 128-135.

Whyte, M. K. (1978). Cross-cultural code dealing with the relative status of women. *Ethnology, 17,* 214-225.

Wilson, M., & Daly, M. (1988). *Homicide.* Hawthorne, NY: Aldine de Gruyter.

Wolfgang, M. (1964). *Crime and race.* New York: Institute of Human Relations Press.

Wolfgang, M. (1966). A preface to violence. *Annals of the American Academy of Political and Social Science, 364,* 1-7.

Wolfgang, M. (1978). Violence in the family. In I. L. Kutash, et al. (Eds.), *Violence: perspectives on murder and aggression.* San Francisco: Jossey-Bass.

Wolfgang, M., & Ferracuti, F. (1967). *The subculture of violence.* London: Tavistock.

Yelsma, P., & Yelsma, J. (1977). Self-esteem of prisoners committing directly versus indirectly destructive crimes. *Perceptual and Motor Skills, 44,* 375, 378.

Yllo, K. (1983). Sexual equality and violence against wives in American states. *Journal of Comparative Family Studies, 14*(1), 67-86.

Yllo, K. (1984). The status of women, marital equality, and violence against wives. *Journal of Family Issues, 5* (3), 307-320.

CHAPTER

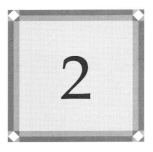

Child Abuse

Janice Humphreys *and* Ann Marie Ramsey

"Thoughtless"
  enjoying the lush warmth
  looking forward to more
  who is this
  ripping thoughtlessly
  tearing at my sensitive branch?
  oh my tree soon to die
  hurry patch it
  grab a wrap
  heal the wound
  so my tree
  may be precious
  thriving and strong
                    Elizabeth Roth*

Child abuse and neglect is a common area of concern for the nurse who cares for families. The problem is that child abuse and neglect is so common. The literature of several different professions (nursing, law, medicine, dentistry, social work, etc.) abounds with research reports, opinions, case studies, literature reviews, incidence reports, and theories of child abuse and neglect of varying degrees of scholarliness. The task for the nurse who wishes to stay abreast of the knowledge and practice in the area of child abuse and neglect is monumental, if not impossible. This chapter provides an overview of the knowledge and controversies to date on child abuse and neglect.

The theoretical foundations of child maltreat-

ment exist in both violence and family literature. The attempt is to update the nurse on the current theoretical understanding of child abuse and neglect, and to provide a basis for development of nursing research and application to practice (see Chapter 9).

DEFINITION OF CHILD ABUSE AND NEGLECT

The spectrum of maltreatment of children is broad and often defined by time, perpetrator, situation, professional conducting the study, and the law (see Chapter 14). To study all acts of violence against children and consider them in some manner equally damaging is an attitude that is not generally accepted or practical. What then is meant by *child abuse?* The state of Michigan defines child abuse as "harm or threatened harm to a child's health or wel-

---

*Reprinted from *Every Twelve Seconds*, compiled by Susan Venters (Hillsboro, Oregon: Shelter, 1981) by permission of the author.

fare by a person responsible for the child's health or welfare which occurs through nonaccidental physical or mental injury, sexual abuse, or maltreatment." In Michigan, and many other states, child abuse means actual physical violence against a child or the threat of such an act. The child need not experience physical injury to be considered abused. In addition, the injury to the child need not be physical, it can be mental or emotional. Here the problem of defining just what is mental or emotional abuse becomes evident.

Equally difficult to define is child neglect. To use the Child Protection Law (1975) in Michigan as an example, "child neglect" means "harm to a child's health or welfare by a person responsible for the child's health or welfare which occurs through negligent treatment, including the failure to provide adequate clothing, shelter, or medical care." The child who is obviously abandoned by its parents is undoubtedly neglected. However, the child who has not received quite enough food to satisfy his or her hunger may not be considered neglected. If, in addition, the reason for the lack of food is the extreme poverty of the family, who is at fault? Must the parent of a child provide adequate shelter, food, and clothing at any cost? The problem is difficult.

C. Henry Kempe coined the phrase "battered child syndrome" to describe the most severe form of child abuse. However, such a phrase imposes limitations, including the fact that many consider only the severely physically assaulted child to have experienced abuse (Kempe, Silver, Steele, Droegemueller, & Silver, 1962). Kempe and Helfer (1972) have altered their definition, asserting that "the battered child is any child who received nonaccidental physical injury (or injuries) as a result of acts (or omissions) on the part of his parents or guardians" (p. XI).

Newberger and Bourne (1978) assert that for professionals to view child abuse as only physical battering is a disservice to the children they sought to assist. By identifying severe physical abuse from the medical perspective, many of the maltreated children do not receive the multifaceted care they need. Theories of causation and interventions are also based on a limited and medical model. The reality is

that the severely battered, tortured child is at the extreme end of the abuse spectrum. Unfortunately, it is often only when the discovery of such profoundly abused children is reported in the media that some people give thought to the general maltreatment of children.

In 1974 the Child Abuse Prevention and Treatment Act was signed into law. The Act's passage included the creation of the National Center on Child Abuse and Neglect (NCCAN) and mandated the secretary of this body to make a full and complete study of the national incidence of child abuse and neglect. The first national study (NIS-1) was conducted in 1979 and 1980. To measure the entire spectrum of child abuse and neglect, this study operationally defined child maltreatment as demonstrable harm incurred to a child that was nonaccidental, avoidable, and committed by a parent(s), parent substitutes, or other adult caretakers (NCCAN, 1988). This definition was rather narrow. Hence, in the second national study (NIS-2) the definition was broadened considerably by defining child maltreatment as both demonstrable harm *and* child endangerment, specifically including children whose health and well-being were endangered, through acts that are nonaccidental, avoidable, committed by parent(s)/parent substitutes, other adult, *and*/or adolescent caretakers. The broadening of these definitions for the NIS-2 study resulted in a greater number of cases of child maltreatment included in the study results. The complete study results are presented in the next section.

In their investigations Gelles and Straus (1979) do not use the phrase "child abuse." Rather, they define violence as "an act carried out with the intention or perceived intention of physically hurting another person" (p. 20). Their reason for using this broad definition was to include in their study those acts, such as slapping or spanking, that many people might consider appropriate as discipline. If such acts were carried out against someone not in the family, they would be considered assaultive. Their concern was also primarily centered on the act of violence and not the outcome. Such a broad definition of maltreatment is useful if the researchers are interested in the tendency of violence to escalate within the family. Although broad in its definition of violence, this definition completely overlooks nonviolent neglect of children. Therefore the usefulness of such a definition on a day-to-day basis for the practitioner is limited.

Child abuse and neglect are on a continuum from the extreme to the mild and every degree in between. Child maltreatment exists and is well documented; unfortunately, professionals spend much of their time trying to decide what it is and is not. As Gil (1976) states, "The inability to reach closure on the issue of defining abuse (particularly moving beyond the restricted phenomenon of physical injury to include 'emotional' abuse and other operationally ambiguous concepts) reveals the lack of coherent prochild ideology among Americans" (p. 30). Further hesitancy about a commitment to one definition of child abuse and neglect may be due to deeper insecurities. "The broader the definition of abuse, the more clear is its relation to 'normal' caregivers and their behavior with children, and the more serious the 'indictment' against society and its institutions" (p. 34).

For the purpose of this and subsequent chapters by these authors, the definitions of child abuse and neglect quoted from the State of Michigan Child Protection Law will apply.

SCOPE

The scope of the problem of child abuse is difficult to ascertain. Few people are willing to admit that they cause physical and/or psychological injury to their children. Hence, professionals must rely on a variety of agencies that provide statistics of current child abuse incidence. Examples of such agencies include state agencies, such as the Department of Protective Services, and private agencies, such as the American Association for Protecting Children, the American Humane Society, and numerous government-funded studies. The National Association of Children's Hospitals and Related Institutions (NACHRI, 1989) based on data from the American Association for Protecting Children and Select Committee on Children, Youth, and Families Survey, reported that child abuse has increased from 1.1 mil-

lion cases in 1980 to 1.9 million in 1985, representing a 55% increase in a 5-year period. Although this statistic is disturbing, further analysis of the actual numbers and the societal milieu during this time is necessary to determine the actual scope of the problem.

The inherent limitation of any statistic that is based on "reported" accounts is that not all cases of child abuse are reported; hence, authors frequently designate statistics as estimated cases or incidence. Although every state has mandated that all health care professionals are responsible for reporting suspected child abuse, and there is considerable medical nomenclature surrounding abuse (Vaughn-Switzer, 1986), the reporting of abuse continues to remain sporadic and subjective (Dukes & Kean, 1989; Gelles, 1980; Hampton & Newberger, 1985; Knudsen, 1988). Factors that contribute to this phenomenon include inconsistencies between state guidelines. For example, Arizona defines child abuse as unexplained injury, whereas South Dakota defines abuse as including "threatened harm" (Vaughn-Switzer). Theoretically, in South Dakota a person could be reported for threatening to "beat your bottom until it shines like an apple," but would not be reported at all in Arizona.

These definitions contribute to another problem inherent in reporting of abuse. The decision to report abuse is determined subjectively by the individual doing the reporting. Hampton and Newberger (1985) recognized that hospitals report the largest numbers of child abuse and became interested in what factors and biases, if any, existed within this population. To assess this, they designed several scenarios of abuse or neglect and asked 805 physicians to describe how they should treat such situations. They found that physical abuse (including sexual) was more likely to be reported than emotional or psychological abuse. This is not surprising because the abuse most likely to be seen in a hospital would be abuse resulting in physical injury. Interestingly, however, they found that hospital personnel were reporting higher numbers of lower-income, black, single parents. Hampton and Newberger attributed this to the apparent aversion of the subjects to the label, "child abuser." The research subjects found child abusers so aversive that they did not want to be associated with such individuals; hence, the medical caregivers showed unconscious bias of reporting only persons socially, culturally, and economically different from themselves. Hampton and Newberger found the following factors influential in reporting of abuse in the hospital setting: type of abuse (physical reported most frequently), race of abusers (blacks and Latinos were more likely to be reported than white families), income (families with incomes of less than $25,000 per year had a greater chance to be reported), age of child (the younger the child, the more likely the incident to be reported), and perpetrator of the abuse (the abuse was more likely to be reported if the mother was not the perpetrator of the crime). Factors such as gender of the child, method of payment (private versus public), or marital status were not significantly related to reporting of abuse.

Dukes and Kean (1989) were also interested in child abuse reporting trends. However, they observed that while hospitals reported the majority of child abuse cases, individuals who report child abuse in hospitals (i.e., physicians, nurses, and social workers) constitute a fraction of the adult population. They became interested in the factors that contribute to individuals', other than those who are mandated by law, decisions to report child abuse. The study method was similar to that of Hampton and Newberger in that the subjects responded to scenarios that depicted different types of child abuse and different surrounding circumstances. One hundred forty-four non-health care professionals were randomly selected from college sociology classes. They represented a variety of ages, cultures, and both sexes. Some were parents and some were not. The results of the study were both surprising and disturbing. Neglect was more likely to be reported than abuse, and of 124 persons who perceived the abuse as severe, only 50 people planned to report it. Furthermore, when abuse was perceived as less severe, only four of 20 people planned to report it. Contrary to the medical personnel in the study by Hampton and Newberger, these subjects were more likely to report psycholog-ical abuse than physical abuse. Within this variable, psychological abuse was seen as more detrimental to older children than younger children. Finally, subjects were asked what action they would take based on their assessments. In contrast to the previous study, Dukes and Dean found that females were more likely to be reported if the subject perceived abuse, and males were more likely to be reported if the subject perceived neglect. The majority of respondents stated they would speak to the parent immediately; some even stated that they would restrain the parent if necessary (Dukes & Kean).

Nationally Based Statistics

Although statistics of child maltreatment have limitations, their importance cannot be negated. As discussed earlier, The Child Abuse Prevention and Treatment Act mandated a national study to determine the incidence of child abuse and neglect. The first study (NIS-1) was conducted in 1979 and 1980 and the second study (NIS-2) was conducted late in 1986. It is important to understand that this study did *not* collect data on *all* the cases of child abuse in the United States that occurred during the study period. Rather, 26 representative counties were included in NIS-1 and 29 representative counties were included in NIS-2. The study sample comprises cases of child maltreatment reported in these counties. By using statistical methods it is possible to estimate how many cases of child maltreatment per 1,000 children occur in the United States.

Much can be learned from comparing the results of NIS-1 with NIS-2. In reporting the results, the investigators were careful to compare cases based on the same definitions. As mentioned earlier, NIS-2 defined child maltreatment more broadly than NIS-1. To compare results based on two different definitions would result in erroneous findings. Hence, NIS-2 results are reported as two figures, one based on the NIS-1 definition and one based on the broader NIS-2 definition.

The overall incidence of maltreatment increased from 9.8 cases per 1,000 children in 1980 to 16.3 cases in 1986. This is a 66% increase in incidence in the 6-year period, which, incidentally, is very similar to the NACHRI findings. The investigators stressed that they thought this increase was partly the result of increasing professional awareness of child maltreatment, thus increasing the likelihood of reporting. When the NIS-2 definition of child maltreatment was used, 25.2 cases per 1,000 were identified.

Study results were further divided into categories of abuse, neglect, and sexual abuse. Child abuse was further subdivided into categories of fatal, serious, moderate, and probable abuse. Overall abuse rose from 5.3 cases per 1,000 in 1980 to 9.2 cases per 1,000 in 1986, representing a 58% increase. Moderate physical abuse was the most frequently reported type of abuse, with 5.5 cases per 1,000 reported by NIS-1 definition and 15.1 cases per 1,000 (representing 72% of all abuse cases) by NIS-2 definitions. This is an especially significant finding for health care professionals because moderate abuse is defined as bruises, depressions, or emotional distress *not* serious enough to require medical treatment. Hence, the most frequent type of abuse is not likely to present in the emergency room; rather, these children must be identified via nonemergency assessment, such as routine health screening at schools and clinics and by community/public health nurses assessing children in their homes.

Like child abuse, the category of child neglect also showed a significant increase from 4.9 cases per 1,000 in 1980 to 7.9 cases per 1,000 in 1986 by NIS-1 definitions. The significance of definitions became evident with 15.9 cases per 1,000 reported on the basis of NIS-2 definitions. The expanded definitions of NIS-2 also affected subcategories of neglect. Using only NIS-1 definitions, the most frequent type of neglect reported is educational neglect, with 4.6 cases per 1,000, followed by physical neglect, with 2.9 cases reported per 1,000 children. However, based on NIS-2 definitions the categories reversed, with 9.1 cases per 1,000 of physical neglect reported versus 4.6 cases per 1,000 of educational neglect.

Statistics from Individual Studies

Straus and Gelles (1986) and Knudsen (1988) studied the apparent increase in the statistics of child abuse in this country and assessed the reality be-

hind the numbers. Straus and Gelles used the data from the National Study of Child Neglect and Abuse Reporting supported by the American Humane Association in 1976 and 1986 to determine a 10-year trend. After correcting for demographics, they found a *decrease* in the overall violence and severe violence. They credit this decrease to an increasing public awareness of the problem of violence within the family. It must be remembered that Straus and Gelles only included families where the parent was at least 18 years of age, married, living with a partner, divorced, separated, or single with a child under the age of 18 as subjects in their survey.

Knudsen's study (1988) over 20 years of child abuse reporting in an Indiana county found a genuine increase in violence, molestation, or neglect of children. The data that Straus and Gelles (1986) used were self-reports solicited from telephone interviews of a randomly selected group of families selected on the basis of marital status (must be married, or living with significant other, have at least one child ages 3 to 17 years old), whereas Knudsen used reports of child abuse in a specific county over a specific period of time. It must also be considered that there is a probability that the families that Straus and Gelles contacted would not admit publicly to child abuse. Perhaps a more realistic interpretation of these data would infer that child abuse is increasing among at-risk populations, whereas child abuse is remaining steady or mildly decreasing among the general public. The study by Straus and Gelles has particular merit—unlike the majority of research in the area of violence against children, because it involves a "healthy" sample. Straus and Gelles interviewed and recorded the self-reports of violence from individuals who were not currently being followed by a child protective service agency. The violence committed by parents against their children is also categorized (from "slapped" to "used knife or gun") and reveals a broad range of violent acts, not all generally accepted as child abuse.

HISTORICAL BACKGROUND ON THE MALTREATMENT OF CHILDREN

Children have been mistreated by adults historically, for a variety of reasons (see the box on p. 41).

Historical Background on the Maltreatment of Children

1. Children have been sacrificed to please the god of their parents.
2. Children who experienced health disturbances have been thought to be possessed.
3. "Beating some sense into him" is often considered necessary to ensure that children learn.
4. In medieval times the lack of value placed on children is reflected in the art of the times.
5. During the seventeenth century, until the time of puberty children were not considered to be worthy of the same considerations given to adults.
6. According to the 1879 census, one in eight children between 10 and 15 years of age was employed in the United States. The majority were employed in agriculture.
7. From the 1880s to the Depression of the 1930s, efforts to curb child labor were intensive.
8. By 1899, 28 states had passed some child labor legislation. However, most laws applied only to manufacturing and set the age limit to 12 years.
9. The National Child Labor Committee was formed in 1904.
10. By 1914, 35 states had a 14-year-age limit and an 8-hour day for workers under 16.
11. In 1916 the Keating-Owen Act was passed, prohibiting child labor in manufacturing for children under the age of 16.

Sacrifice of children to please the god of their parents was a common practice among certain ancient cultures (Radbill, 1980). Children who were born with a birth defect were killed to protect the parents because it was thought that the child surely had been affected by some demon to have acquired such an anomaly. Children who experienced seizures, were mentally retarded, or mentally ill were also often thought to be possessed or in some form controlled by evil. These children were most likely exposed to all kinds of torture under the guise of "ridding their bodies of demons."

A more contemporary notion is that physical abuse of children is important in the education process. The idea of "beating some sense into him" was considered necessary to ensure that the child learned the lesson. Even the Supreme Court (*Ingram v. Wright*) ruled that schools had the right to corporally punish disobedient students (Knitzer, 1977). This implies that although adult criminals have some safeguards against the administration of cruel and unusual punishment, children's rights are distinctly different.

Treatment of Children in the Middle Ages

By reviewing artwork, Aries (1962) observed "medieval art until the twelfth century did not know childhood or did not attempt to portray it. It is hard to believe that this neglect was due to incompetence or incapacity; it seems more probable that there was no place for childhood in the medieval world" (p. 33). According to Aries, children were not particularly valued during this time and therefore their images and activities were not worthy of reproduction in art. Their treatment by adults in daily life reflected the low value placed on childhood. The rearing of children during the seventeenth century is reported to have routinely included the practice of playing with the child's genitals. The stroking of the genitals and exhibiting them to various family members and neighbors was considered acceptable and necessary for the young child. Circumcision of males was treated as a festival and for religious reasons, a joyous occasion. Children during this time were treated, according to Aries, as if they were incapable of being aware of or affected by sex. Such treatment and low opinion of children imply that until the time of puberty, children are not worthy of the same considerations given to adults.

Childhood during the seventeenth century was virtually not acknowledged. Instead, "the idea of childhood was bound up with the idea of dependence" (Aries, 1962, p. 26). Terms like "boy" and "lad" were used to describe even adults who were not independent, and therefore not really "men."

Furthermore, adolescence was not recognized as being any different from the rest of childhood.

Until the individual was able to independently function and literally protect himself or herself, he or she was not accorded equal treatment and certainly not protected by adults. When childhood finally began to be accepted as a time of life different from adulthood, it was to no advantage to children. "The concept of the separate nature of childhood, of its difference from the world of adults, began with the elementary concept of its weakness, which brought it down to the level of the lowest social strata" (Aries, 1962, p. 262). Elements of the continued low value placed on childhood in the past can still be seen.

Child Labor

According to the 1879 census, approximately one in eight children between 10 and 15 years of age was employed in the United States. By 1900, one in six children was employed, 60% in agriculture and 40% in industry. Over one half of the children employed were of immigrant families (Bremner, 1970). The growing number of children who were sent to work resulted from the rapid industrialization after the Civil War. More than one half of the child labor force was between 10 and 13 years of age; many were under age 10. Although the majority of children were employed in agriculture, it was the general understanding of most Americans that child labor was a problem predominantly of urban industry. The work done by children was as difficult, if not more difficult, than that done by adults. Al Priddy describes part of his mill at approximately 13 years:

> The mule-room atmosphere was kept at from eighty-five to ninety degrees of heat. The hardwood floor burned my bare feet. I had to gasp quick, short gasps to get air into my lungs at all. My face seemed swathed in continual fire. The tobacco chewers expectorated on the floor, and left little pools for me to wade through. Oil and hot grease dripped down behind the mules, sometimes falling on my scalp or making yellow splotches on my overalls or feet. . . . To open a window was a great crime, as the cotton fiber was so sensitive to

wind that it would spoil. (Poor cotton fiber!) (Bremner, 1970, p. 616).

The pay was also much less for the work done by children. The younger siblings of the paid, employed child might be found "helping their brothers and sisters," an explanation that provided numerous unpaid assistants (Bremner, 1970, p. 615).

From the 1880s to the Depression of the 1930s, efforts to curb child labor held the attention of the American public. By 1899, 28 states had passed some legislation regulating child labor; however, most legislation applied only to manufacturing and set the age limit to 12 years (Bremner, 1970). The majority of children, those older than 12 years working in agriculture, remained unaffected by legislation.

In the twentieth century, opposition to child labor became an organized crusade. In 1904 the National Child Labor Committee was formed by several prominent people in the reform movement. The committee was successful to the extent that "by 1914 35 states had a fourteen-year age limit and an eight hour day for workers under sixteen; 34 states prohibited night work under age sixteen, and 36 states had appointed factory inspectors to enforce the laws" (Bremner, 1970, p. 603). The attempt to pass a constitutional amendment was unsuccessful. However, in 1916 the Keating-Owen Act was passed and established federal law prohibiting child labor in manufacturing for children under the age of 16 (Bremner).

The difficulties faced by child advocates who attempted to stop child labor are somewhat reminiscent of more recent efforts to improve the plight of children and families:

> One of the major difficulties of child labor reform in the early twentieth century was the cultural and economic gap between middle class reformers, who in their zeal to refute the stereotype of the poor widow dependent on her little boy's earnings, may have underestimated the economic necessity of child labor among large segments of the working class. . . . The attack on child labor was one of the converging lines of reform which, even before the Great Depression, led to realization that solving problems of childhood required *comprehen-*

sive efforts to promote economic security for families (our emphasis) (Bremner, 1970, p. 604).

(For a detailed outlining of childhood in America from 1600 to 1932 the reader is referred to the extensive two-volume work edited by Bremner.)

Culture and Child Maltreatment

Most often culture is associated with one's ethnicity and ethnic heritage. Although this is true, culture also includes one's values, mores, and societal norms (Long, 1986). Certainly culture has a tremendous impact on child-rearing practices and the value placed on children (Korbin, 1977, 1979; Levinson, 1989). Cultural values influence what is thought to be optimal with regard to child-rearing and to what is viewed as child abuse and neglect. This presents a dilemma: Although it is important to provide culturally sensitive care, one cannot justify child maltreatment on the basis of cultural values. To assist the professional delivery of culturally sensitive care, Korbin (1991) has developed three levels for determining culturally appropriate definitions of child maltreatment. On level one, cultural behavior would demonstrate child-rearing practices that are considered appropriate within the given culture, but are viewed as child maltreatment outside the culture. For example, Turkish mothers view kissing and public praising of their infants' genitals as positive mothering; this same behavior would be considered sexual abuse in Western culture. Level two encompasses behavior that is universally considered abusive or neglectful. All cultures have standards that dictate acceptable child treatment and what determines child maltreatment, and such behaviors are universally considered maltreatment. Physical punishment to the point of dysfunction of the child and withholding of food are two such examples. Finally, level three classifies child maltreatment precipitated by societal insufficiencies, such as extreme poverty, unemployment, hopelessness and hunger, that occur separate and distinct from any parental control.

Korbin (1991) also identifies classifications or groupings of children who are more likely to be maltreated based on a summation of cultural variables.

The child with a poor health status is more likely to be maltreated than his or her healthy counterparts. In underprivileged or developing areas, sick children are viewed as a burden and considered a poor caregiving investment; hence, they are often undercared for and left to die. Disfigured and physically disabled children fall into a similar undervalued category. The handicap reduces their value to their family and community and again, they are viewed as a poor caregiving investment. Children born under stigmatized or difficult conditions are at increased risk for maltreatment. Children born out of wedlock in Western cultures are viewed as less worthy than those born into a marital relationship. Children whose developmental stages predispose them to difficult behaviors, such as toddlers or adolescents, are also at increased risk for maltreatment. Finally, gender can be a significant risk factor in many cultures. Male children are viewed as more valuable in many cultures because they carry on family lines. In India, for example, a male child is desired, since female children require dowries to be married. A poor Indian family cannot afford many female children because of this requirement. Hence, female infants may be cast into rivers to avoid the long-term cost to the family.

Societal norms also influence the trends of child maltreatment. The urbanization of many Nigerian cities has resulted in the evolution of a severe child maltreatment problem, one of "throwing away babies." The urbanization of Nigeria has resulted in a large number of males relocating to the cities to seek their fortune. There has not been an equal number of women entering the cities; hence, men frequently turn to prostitutes or mistresses for sexual gratification. The monetary gain from such work in Nigeria is impressive and conditions such as pregnancy and motherhood threaten the woman's economic viability. When abortion either is unavailable or ineffective, these women elect to give birth, then cast their infants into rivers or bushes to be rid of the burden (Nkpa, 1980). Another form of child maltreatment that has arisen from the "throwing away of babies" has been the evolution of a charm-making business in which charms are made of the parts of murdered infants and sold for good luck.

Societal norms and kin relationships also influence the reporting of child maltreatment. Long (1986) reports that among Native Americans the reporting of child maltreatment is rare because of kin relationships. In one example, a neighbor reported a mother for abusing her 7-year-old child with a broken bottle. Subsequently the mother was charged with child abuse. Despite promised confidentiality, the name of the reporter was revealed and he was subsequently harassed, abused, and beaten by members of the abusive mother's clan; the reporter required medical attention and police protection. This type of kin protection is also evident in Anglo-American culture. In another example, Long cites a case of sexual abuse that occurred to a 13-year-old daughter of a prominent surgeon. A local psychiatrist was treating the child for depression in an inpatient setting when the child revealed the abuse to a nurse. When confronted with this revelation, the psychiatrist refused to believe or report it, stating that he played golf with the child's father and he was not capable of such behavior. The psychiatrist was subsequently removed from the case and the child received proper treatment.

Western culture endorses several rituals that may be considered child maltreatment in other cultures. For example, newborn males are often routinely circumcised without anesthesia before discharge from the hospital (Lubchenco, 1980). Recently, the American Academy of Pediatrics issued a position statement that maintains that circumcision has questionable medical value. Other routine, painful procedures administered to children are ear piercing and orthodontic bands on the teeth. The point to be made here is not whether such cosmetic procedures should be discontinued, but rather that they are culturally dictated, and that they continue to be painfully administered to children by adults who supposedly love them.

Child Protection in the United States

The origin in the United States of societies concerned about the pathetic lot of many children begins with the historic case of Mary Ellen Wilson in April 1874. Briefly, organized efforts for the protection of children developed as an outgrowth of humane work for animals. Mary Ellen was born of Frances (Fanny) Conner Wilson and Thomas Wilson, who died in the Civil War before Mary Ellen was born (Lazoritz, 1990). Shortly after her birth she was abandoned. At the age of 8 years, Mary Ellen was taken from her adoptive parents who routinely beat, starved, imprisoned, and kept her in rags. Neighbors were outraged over the child's mistreatment and feared the family would move before action could be taken on Mary Ellen's behalf. None of the several institutions contacted by concerned neighbors would remove Mary Ellen from the abusive home. As a last resort, the Society for the Prevention of Cruelty to Animals (SPCA) was contacted. Henry Bergh, founder and president of the SPCA, acknowledged that "though the case was not within the scope of the special act to prevent cruelty to animals, (it was) recognized as being clearly within the general laws of humanity. . . . " (Bremner, 1970, p. 186). Mary Ellen was removed from her adoptive parents. Subsequently, in December 1874 the New York Society for the Prevention of Cruelty to Children (NYSPCC) was organized.

Recently, an article has updated the story of Mary Ellen (Lazoritz). It seems that Mary Ellen's case was noteworthy not only for the attention it received. After her removal from her adoptive parents, no suitable relative could be found to care for her, so Mary Ellen was placed in a home for adolescent girls, some of whom were disturbed. Thus Mary Ellen was not only the inspiration for the legal protection of children, she was also the first inappropriate placement from such a case (Lazoritz, 1990). However, Mary Ellen also went on to be a survivor of the horrors she experienced at the hands of her adult caretakers. She completed school, married at age 24, had two daughters and two stepsons, and lived the rest of her life in a poor but loving family. Although she did not become active in the child protection movement, she did provide foster care to a child for many years. Mary Ellen's own daughters attended college and become well-respected teachers. Despite her notoriety, Mary Ellen survived her early experiences and provided nurturance to her own and other children, a remarkable example of resilience and hope for other abused children.

From the NYSPCC grew many organizations in other cities. Initially SPCC actions were policelike; the representatives wore "badges and were duly constituted officers of the law" (Bremner, 1970, p. 116). Originally, the SPCC supported institutional care for abused and neglected children. After the turn of the century, however, the goal of concerned organizations was directed more toward case finding and rehabilitation of parents and the return of the child to the home. In 1882, Massachusetts enacted a "neglect law" no longer limiting the community's concern to the severely physically abused child (Bremner).

Studies of unexplainable injuries to children were first widely recognized in the professional literature in 1946 when Dr. John Caffey identified curious x-rays of certain children. The article was entitled "Multiple Fractures in the Long Bones of Infants Suffering from Chronic Subdural Hematoma" and gives no evidence of the possible causes of the multiple injuries. As Lynch (1985) points out in a review of the medical literature, providers had long recognized that adults might harm children. She cites a Persian pediatric treatise (dated AD 900) that refers to intentional striking of children along with other common health concerns. Lynch cites multiple medical references that cite (1) "How to recognize the newborn that is worth rearing," (2) wet nurse characteristics associated with child abuse and neglect, and (3) clear descriptions of children's injuries that are directly the result of intentional injuries. Although some physicians advocated trauma as the cause of children's unexplained bony lesions visible in the newly invented x-ray films, other physicians were unconvinced.

In 1962, Kempe, a physician, is given credit for having introduced the "battered child syndrome" to the American Academy of Pediatrics (Kempe et al.). Many attribute Kempe's "call to arms" with the passage of laws in all 50 states within a 4-year period mandating identification and reporting of suspected victims of abuse (Newberger & Bourne, 1978). The Child Abuse and Treatment Act of 1974 (PL-93237) went even further and called for a full and complete study on the incidence of child abuse and neglect. Some results of that and other national studies and problems associated with their findings have already been reported in the "Scope" section in this chapter.

Public Concern in the 1970s

Social scientists explain the increased concern about violence committed by parents against children in the 1970s differently. According to Straus (1974), the public's concern about violence in general was the result of three cultural and social forces. First, the public and social scientists were exposed daily to the violence of Southeast Asia, assassinations, civil disturbances, and increasing homicide rates. Second, the women's movement increased the public's awareness of violence against women and children. Third, social scientists were moving toward the conflict or social action model to examine phenomenon. The result of the combination of these forces was said to be the identification, examination, and systematic study of violence in families. The consciousness of professionals and the public alike was raised and brought to action.

THEORETICAL FRAMEWORKS

No single theoretical framework has been recognized as the definitive explanation of the cause of child abuse and neglect. However, there now appears to be considerable consensus that child maltreatment is stimulated by a complex interaction of personal, social, and environmental factors. There is also growing evidence that certain factors can mediate the effects of being an abused child. This section provides an overview of theories/models of child abuse and neglect. Various formulations are included because they are commonly held, have received support in the literature, or otherwise have significance to nursing. See the box on p. 46 for summaries of theoretical models of abuse and neglect of children.

Summaries of Theoretical Models of Abuse and Neglect of Children

Mental illness model

Generally outdated theory that parents who abuse their children are mentally ill. Research suggests that only 5% of all abusive parents are psychotic.

Social-psychological model

First proposed by Helfer and Kempe (1968), this model hypothesizes that three factors must be present: (1) a special parent, (2) a special child, and (3) stress. Parent characteristics, child characteristics, and acute or chronic stress combine to result in child abuse or neglect. The model fails to recognize the role of cultural tolerance for violence. It also fails to explain why some families are abusive and others in similar circumstances are not. More recent research has not supported this model.

Multifactorial models

Although no single framework has been accepted, these models recognize the complex interaction among personal, interpersonal, and environmental factors.

Sociological models

Environment and stress. This model hypothesizes that child abuse and neglect occur within an environment that tolerates, even encourages, violent conflict resolution and child-rearing. Acute or chronic stress becomes unmanageable to parents, who respond with violence. This model fails to explain why some families are abusive and others in similar circumstances do not.

Social-learning model. This model hypothesizes that aggression is learned behavior. Learning may occur through observation or direct experience with violent or aggressive behavior. This model addresses only child abuse, not neglect. Research supports the intergenerational transmission of abuse proposed by this model. However, this model fails to explain why some abused children grow up and do not abuse their own offspring, or why some nonabused children become abusive adults.

Human ecological model

Based on the general ecological model of human development, this model incorporates culture, family, parent, child, and stress. Child abuse is viewed as an outcome of pathological adaptations by the caregiver and (to a lesser extent) the child. These relationships are viewed as part of the larger family relationship. Thus the family is viewed as a system in dysfunction. This model includes major factors considered essential to any useful explanation of child abuse and neglect and has received support from research. However, the model is limited by its separation of patterns of abuse into two types: the mentally ill parent and all others.

Nursing framework

This complex model incorporates child factors, parent factors, stress, child-rearing practices (discipline), and cultural tolerances for violence. Child abuse and neglect is viewed on a continuum as the opposite end from normative/nurturant child-rearing. The model incorporates major factors considered essential to any useful explanation of child abuse and neglect. However, it has not been tested empirically.

MENTAL ILLNESS MODEL

The mental illness model or psychiatric approach was probably the first contemporary theory used to deal with parents who abused their children. In reviewing the literature, significantly fewer examples of its use are evident than formerly. The untested acceptance of the relationship between mental illness and child abuse is likely related to the "discovery" of child abuse by the medical community (Gelles, 1987). As Gelles points out, much of the early writing attempted to delineate a profile of abusers to determine "what kind of a person" would abuse a child. The mental illness model is addressed in this section because its basis—that the child abuser is mentally ill—is still commonly held, and remnants of this model can sometimes be found in recommendations for interventions with child abusers.

Essentially the mental illness model theorizes that parents who abuse their children are mentally ill. The adult who inflicts bodily harm on his or her child is a psychologically "sick" person. No other factor is considered to contribute to the occurrence of child abuse and neglect, and the obvious goal of treatment is to "cure." The implication in the mental illness model is that the fault for the abuse inflicted on the child rests in the poor mental health of the individual adult. In turn, the prospect for overcoming this illness in the parent rests within the parent. The professional, most likely a psychiatrist or psychologist, is merely assisting the parent in his or her treatment. To some extent, organizations like Parents Anonymous still label abusive parents as "sick" and responsible for their own cure (Newberger & Bourne, 1978).

With the publication of an increasing number of investigations in the area of child abuse and neglect, the actual incidence of psychosis among abusive parents was found to be quite small—5% (Justice & Justice, 1976). Attempts to develop a profile of abusers failed to explain a significant amount of variance in the abusive behavior of caretakers (Gelles, 1987).

There is little doubt that some mentally ill adults do abuse their children. Estroff et al. (1984) report that when mothers of abused and neglected children were compared with demographically matched mothers seen in a child psychiatric clinic, differences in maternal psychopathology were found. Abusive mothers were found to experience more psychiatric symptoms (as measured by the Brief Symptom Inventory and Global Severity Index) than mothers in the comparison group, and had low IQs (i.e., dull normal). Evidence of current modes of treatment of mentally ill, abusive parents are still found in the literature (Panter, 1977). However, the majority of abusive parents are not psychotic. To attribute all cases of child abuse and neglect to mental illness will greatly lessen the number of interventions and the effectiveness of the nurse.

Social-Psychological Model

The Helfer and Kempe theoretical framework of child abuse and neglect was the first to receive serious study and is still widely recognized (Helfer, 1973; Helfer & Kempe, 1968; Kempe & Helfer, 1972). They have combined both social and psychological variables in explaining why child abuse and neglect occur.

Helfer and Kempe hypothesize that three factors must be present for a parent to abuse a child: (1) a special parent, (2) a special child, and (3) stress (Helfer, 1973). A special parent is an adult with any number of characteristics that predispose him or her to abuse (Helfer, 1973, pp. 77–78). The adult may be immature, inexperienced, lack self-esteem, have unrealistic expectations of the child, etc. Studies of abusive parents have identified that some manifest such characteristics (see Patterns of Behavior section).

The special child may be perceived as special by the parent, or the child may actually be "special" (Helfer, 1973, pp. 77–78). "Special children" may be handicapped (Friedrich & Boriskin, 1976), small at birth (Goldson, Fitch, Wendell, & Knapp, 1978), chronically ill (Berger, 1980), or in some other way require unique parenting skills. For example, some authors have noted that abused children are described as more difficult to care for (Friedrich & Boriskin) and more demanding or aggressive than other children (George & Main, 1979). Others have suggested that an unplanned pregnancy or delayed mother-child contact after birth or after premature delivery may cause problems in the formation of a bond between mother and child, thereby making the child "special" in either parent's mind (Klaus & Kennell, 1976). Children perceived to be special are equally easy for the nurse to identify; the nurse need only listen to the parent, who will frequently make statements like "he's not like the rest of my kids," "she's always been different," etc.

The stress, identified by Helfer and Kempe, may be acute or chronic (Berger, 1980; Helfer, 1973). "Stress" is perceived by the parent. The necessary amount, kind, and timing of the necessary stress varies according to the individual. An intermingling can occur among the three factors. For example, an adolescent parent may abuse her premature 6-month-old child who will not stop crying in the middle of the night so the mother can sleep. In this example it is easy to identify several sources of stress: parenthood, adolescence, prematurity, lack of sleep, crying, etc.

Helfer and Kempe acknowledge the role of more than one variable in the occurrence of child abuse and neglect. Both the parent and the child contribute to child abuse and neglect, however unwittingly. They do not, however, consider the influence of culture on child abuse and neglect. Green (1968) added a fourth factor necessary for child abuse and neglect: cultural tolerance for familial use of corporal punishment. In addition, although initially Helfer and Kempe's model seemed to have face validity, it tends to view child abuse and neglect in a rather simplistic fashion. Furthermore, research has questioned the notion of a "special child." For example, in a detailed review of the literature, Caplan and Dinardo (1986) conclude that there is no evidence that abused children are more likely to have a learning disability than nonabused children. Nursing research has reported that siblings of abused children are likely to be abused as well, refuting the notion of a single "special child" (Corey, Miller, & Widlak, 1975).

Multifactorial Models

Despite differences in emphasis, most studies agree that child abuse and neglect results from a complex interaction of personal, interpersonal, and environmental factors. Although no single framework has been accepted as the definitive explanation of child abuse and neglect, several models have received considerable study and/or offer insights especially for nursing. Overviews of these models are presented.

Sociological models

Sociologists have written extensively about family violence. Often the primary focus of research was conflict resolution (active, passive, aggressive) rather than abusive relationships. Nevertheless, sociological models have been widely applied to all types of violence and have been extensively researched. The examination of the concepts of stress and environment precedes discussion of causal models. In addition, the developing concept of resilience is examined because it appears to mediate the effects of child abuse and neglect.

Environment and stress

The concepts of environment and stress appear throughout the child abuse and neglect literature. Analysis of the role of the environment in explaining child abuse and neglect generally focuses on the high level of violence in the United States. The environment of the abusive parent is generally violent and approves using physical violence against children under certain circumstances (see Chapter 1 for a discussion of aggression in America). A particularly unruly child or a child who has committed an act of great danger to himself may appropriately be physically punished. "Such phrases as 'this will hurt me more than it will hurt you,' 'beat some sense into you,' and 'teach you a lesson you won't forget' are part of the language of discipline and subordination" (Witt, 1987). Straus, Gelles, and Steinmetz (1980) report that 70% of the Americans in their study viewed spanking and slapping a 12-year-old as necessary, normal, and good. In one study, abusive behavior was justified by abusers if they thought the child had been defiant and they themselves had been under considerable stress (Dietrich, Berkowitz, Kadushin, & McGloin, 1990). The environment accepts that parents must at times use physical punishment for the child's own good.

Stress may be chronic or acute. "In addition to reporting that violence is related to general measures of stress, investigators report associations between various forms of family violence and specific stressful situations and conditions" (Gelles, 1980, p. 879). The parent may experience an unlimited number and/or variety of stresses. The child may or may not contribute to these stresses on the parent (Friedrich & Boriskin, 1976). The stress experienced by the abusive parent is theorized to reach a point of unmanageability. The parent is fraught with overwhelming stress and can no longer control himself or herself. Some have theorized that the desperate parent relieves the stress by physically abusing his or her child (Morse, Hyde, Newberger, & Reed, 1977).

There also is evidence to suggest that an interaction exists between stress and environmental violence. Conger, Burgess, and Barrett (1979) found that abusive parents were more likely than controls to experience both rapid life change and a history of punitive child-rearing. The data suggest that it is primarily when parents are subject to rapid life changes that a punitive childhood history correlates with abusive or neglectful behavior in adulthood.

Conceptualizations that include both the environment and stress do not approve of child abuse nor does the culture in which it occurs. Rather, the approved level of violence and aggression in the culture on a day-to-day basis is so great that it is implied that violence is an acceptable means of problem solving. Child abuse or the physical harming of a child for no good reason is not socially acceptable. Instead, according to some postulations, it is inevitable when stress becomes too great. In a study of the recollections of familial violence from 216 subjects (none known abusers), Gully, Dengerink, Pepping, and Bergstrom (1981) identify that even a sibling's vicarious experiencing of violence can result in an individual who considers physical violence against children acceptable under certain circumstances. The proposed relationship between the environment and stress gains additional support when American violence and child abuse statistics are compared with less violent societies. The incidence of child abuse in Japan, for example, is much less than in the United States (Wagatsuma, 1981). If poverty is considered a source of many stressors, then according to the proposed environmental-stress relationship it would be expected that the poor would experience a higher incidence of child abuse. Statistics reported earlier in this chapter support the greater number of cases of reported child abuse at the poverty level.

The significant roles of stress and environmental acceptance for violence are generally recognized. However, these two factors alone do not completely explain the causes of child abuse and neglect. Poverty exposes parents to many, varied stressors over extended periods of time; however, the majority of poor people do not abuse their children. Many parents who were abused or neglected as children maltreat their own offspring. However, many abused parents do *not* use violence against their children. There is no doubt that violence and aggression are daily demonstrated in the media as methods of dealing with stress and/or problem solving. Nevertheless, many American parents never use aggression or violence of any kind in dealing with their children. Belsky (1980) suggests that tolerance for stress and the ability of a family to call on resources allow nonabusive/neglectful families to function without maltreatment of children. Farrington (1986) suggests that family resources, social support, and combined personal resources of individual family members influence families to respond without violence. In a literature review Seagull (1987) concludes that there is little evidence that social support plays a significant role in the cause of child abuse. She further concludes that greater support can be found for a relationship between child neglect and lack of social support. Neither the concepts of stress nor environment consider the role of family functioning or stress tolerance. However, stress and environment are clearly important and included in all multifactorial models of child abuse and neglect.

Social-learning model

The social-learning model attempts to explain child abuse based on the same principles previously used to describe aggression (see Chapter 1). Briefly restated, the social-learning model hypothesizes that aggression is learned behavior. Learning may occur through observation or direct experience with violent or aggressive behavior. Among the best-known works applying the social learning model to child abuse and neglect is that of Straus, Gelles, and Steinmetz (1980). Their investigations are used herein to describe child abuse in terms of the social-learning model.

Straus, Gelles, and Steinmetz do not mention child neglect; rather, their interest is in aggression, both physical and verbal. In 1976 and subsequently in 1986 Straus, Gelles, and Steinmetz studied the extent and dynamics of violence in the American home (Straus, Gelles & Steinmetz, 1980; Straus & Gelles, 1986). In the 1986 study a nationwide sample of 1,428 households with children between the ages of 3 and 17 years living at home was surveyed. The adults were interviewed and given the Conflict Tactics Scale. Although both studies have weaknesses, the results are useful in explaining child abuse in terms of social learning.

If aggressive behavior is learned, as the social-learning model describes, then the use of violence against one's offspring was most likely taught through the generations. Violent parents likely experienced violence from their own parents. The data from both studies support the notion of transmission of violence through the family generations from parent to child. "Each generation learns to be violent by being a participant in a violent family" (Straus et al., 1980). Violence against children can be taught either through direct experience or by observation (Steinmetz, 1977; Ulbrich & Huber, 1981). The more violent the grandparents, the more violent the parents. The more violent the parents, the more violent the siblings to each other.

The investigators identify that a childhood in a violent home is particularly instructive. "Over one out of every four parents who grew up in a violent household were violent enough to risk seriously injuring a child" (Straus et al., 1980, p. 237). Violent and aggressive behavior is learned primarily, but not totally, from one's family. The social-learning model also acknowledges the societal role in teaching and condoning violence. The fact that violence is glorified in the media, observed on the street, and acceptable in the schools is evidence of the cultural tolerance for violence that the social-learning model identifies as contributing to ongoing violence.

Much of the available data on child abuse supports the social learning model. The social-learning model of child abuse has received much attention primarily because of the productivity of several of its proponents (Finkelhor, Gelles, Hotaling, & Straus, 1983; Gelles, 1972; Gelles & Harrop, 1989; Straus & Gelles, 1990; Straus, Gelles, & Steinmetz, 1980). A major weakness of the formulation is its inability to explain why some abused parents do not abuse their children (Hunter & Kilstrom, 1979). Do some parents "unlearn" the use of violence against their children? Does something else intervene or mediate the effects of growing up in an abusive home? Recently, several authors have suggested that mediating factors do indeed exist.

Human ecological model

In 1977 Garbarino presented a human ecological model to explain child abuse and neglect. The model is based on the general ecological model of human development (Bronfenbrenner, 1979), is complex, and incorporates the major components deemed by many to be involved in child abuse and neglect: culture, family, parent, child, and stress (Belsky, 1980). Garbarino uses the human ecological model to explain physical abuse of children "as part of a larger problem of maltreatment which includes neglect, sexual abuse, and a variety of unhealthy patterns of parent-child relations"(p. 721). Belsky further suggests that "since the parent-child system (the crucible of child maltreatment) is nested within the spousal relationship, what happens between husbands and wives—from an ecological point of view—has implications for what happens between parents and their children (1980, p. 326) (see Chapter 4).

Briefly, the human ecological model explains that "abuse is created by a confluence of forces which lead to a pathological adaptation by caregiver and (to a lesser extent) child" (Garbarino, 1977, p. 723). In turn, complementary relationships of other family members contribute to the existence of abuse. There are not just two malfunctioning dyads, parent and abused child, within the family, but rather multiple interacting systems containing more than two persons. The family then can really be viewed as a system, with patterns of abuse described as system dysfunction. Garbarino states that there are two types of patterns of abuse: the kind perpetrated by pathological adults (a small percentage in general but a large percentage of the lethal abuse), and abuse that results from the compilation and intensification over time of minor parent-child problems and use of physical punishment. The "healthy" parent may, according to the human ecological model, experience "situationally defined incompetence in the role of the caregiver" (McClelland, 1973, p. 2). The parent may experience a situationally defined low level of caregiver skill and/or the child's demand may not "match" (Belsky, 1980). In the majority of cases, therefore, the abusive parent is not mentally ill or sick; instead, the parent who maltreats his or her child is experiencing role malfunction.

To assist the adult in the transition to the role of parent, three factors have been identified: rehearsal of the role, clarity of expectations, and minimal normative change (Elder, 1977). Studies that seek to identify the characteristics of abusive parents frequently identify difficulties in these three areas (see Patterns of Behavior section). Garbarino uses the human ecological model to identify areas of child abuse and neglect in need of scientific research.

The ecological model is supported by a growing number of researchers and has been used by others to explain health-related family behavior (Frey, 1985). Previously cited research has supported the importance of culture (environment), stress, and their interaction in the occurrence of child abuse and neglect. Garbarino and Gillian (1980) and others have described the influence of child, parent, and family characteristics in interaction as contributors to child abuse and neglect (see also Patterns of Behavior section) (Ammerman, 1990; Crittenden, 1988; Dumas, 1984; Hamilton, 1989; Vondra & Toth, 1989; Wolfe, 1987). Ammerman, Van Hasselt, and Hersen (1988) have identified "abuse-provoking" characteristics that have particular significance for the handicapped child, frequently overrepresented

in incidence statistics. These are early separation from parents, disruption in attachment, and vulnerability.

The human ecological model is multifactorial in its explanation of abuse and includes the major concepts generally considered to contribute to abuse. Of particular note is Garbarino's inclusion of the abused child and other family members in the explanation of child abuse. The fact that other members of the family may assist in the initiation and/or perpetuation of child maltreatment should not always be construed, although it sometimes is the case that the nonabused members knew about the violent acts. Garbarino emphasizes that child abuse and neglect occur within a dysfunctional family. The human ecological model is the first of the models presented that considers child abuse and neglect in the larger group, the family.

The major weakness of the human ecological model is that the separation of patterns of abuse into two types—the mentally ill parent and all others—seems a "holdover" from the psychiatric approach. If, as Garbarino states, maltreatment of children represents parent role malfunction, why distinguish those few parents who are psychotic? Would not the individual parent's qualities and difficulties be identified at the time of assessment by the professional? Each parent is unique and would require individualized interventions, regardless of psychosis. To place abusive parents on a continuum from situationally incompetent to chronically abusive and then to isolate the mentally ill parents seems artificial and weakens the human ecological model.

Nursing Framework

All previously described frameworks were developed by non-nurses, and although they have been successfully used by nurses as theoretical bases for practice, none were developed with the role of nursing in mind. In 1981, Millor, a nurse researcher, described a nursing framework for research in child abuse and neglect. The framework is complex and incorporates the major concepts widely recognized as necessary to any comprehensive causal model, as well as viewpoints from other disciplines (psychology, sociology). However, it is unique in its development by and for nursing. Unfortunately, empirical testing of Millor's framework has not yet been reported. The framework is presented here to familiarize the reader with a nursing theory on child abuse and neglect.

Millor's framework borrows from the following theories: symbolic interaction, stress, and temperament theory of personality. The interaction of concepts in Millor's framework is depicted in Figure 2–1. Millor presents child abuse and neglect as a multifactorial phenomenon within an environment (cultural tolerance for physical punishment) that results in family tolerance for physical punishment and establishes the framework for family transactions. The family tolerance for physical discipline is the result and is altered by the parent's own child-rearing history and attitudes. Parent experiences as a child direct the parent's own characteristics and in turn parenting role expectations.

Millor states that the child also plays an important part in child abuse and neglect. Clearly certain children do not "deserve to be beaten," but each child brings to the parent-child interaction certain self-characteristics that interrelate with the child's role behavior (acceptable and unacceptable). According to Millor, stress is interrelated to both the parent and the child. Parents have long been identified as subject to the effects of stress. Millor asserts that stress has its impact on the child as well. The behavioral outcome of the complex interaction of culture, family, parent, child, and stress falls on a continuum: normative/nurturance, normative discipline, neglectful, and abusive. Millor's framework seemingly describes the interaction among nonabusive/nonneglectful, neglectful, and abusive families. The "healthy" family that uses occasional physical

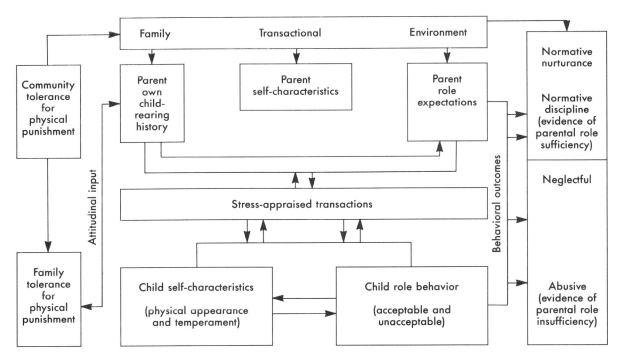

FIGURE 2-1

Self-role definition of the situation model. (Copyright © 1981, American Journal of Nursing Company. Reproduced with permission from: A theoretical framework for nursing research in child abuse and neglect, by G. K. Millor, *Nursing Research 30*, p. 80.)

discipline of its children need not automatically be labeled "high risk." The professional nurse may, by detailed assessment of all contributing factors of the framework, more clearly understand the strengths and resources of the families.

Resilience

Garmezy (1983) examined the role of resilience and other factors in children's responses to stressful life events. He defines these factors as "attributes of persons, environments, situations, and events that appear to temper predictions of psychopathology based upon an individual's at-risk status" (p. 73). His review of the literature consistently identifies a constellation of three factors that mediate the effects of even chronic stress on children. They are (1) dispositional attributes in the child, (2) family milieu, and (3) supportive environment. Although Garmezy does not speak specifically of abused and neglected children, his conclusions may reasonably apply to them.

Dispositional attributes refers to a child's temperament (e.g., flexibility of response, a positive mood, positive sense of self, active), personality (e.g., cooperative, nonaggressive), and cognitive style (e.g., reflectiveness, not impulsive). *Family milieu* refers to family warmth (e.g., protective, praising, close), support (e.g., assistance with problems and school), and organization (e.g., orderliness of roles and home, rules setting). It is important to note that "an intact family was *not* an identifiable consistent correlate" (p. 75). According to Garmezy, there was a striking lack of any consistent evidence in the studies reviewed that father-absence had an adverse effect on children. However, mothers' styles of coping with and compensating for absent fathers had a powerful positive effect. Finally, *supportive environment* refers to external support (e.g., from peers, significant adults, school system) and a sense of identification with the community. "Significant adults provided for the children a representation of their efficacy and ability to exert control in the midst of upheaval" (p. 76). According to Garmezy, in multiple studies using different methods with various groups, these factors have been shown to mediate

the detrimental effects of stressful life even on children. Knowledge of these factors offer suggestions for nursing practice with abused children.

In a critical review of literature on intergenerational transmission, Kaufman and Zigler (1987) conclude that the experience of family violence as a child does not necessarily result in later abuse of one's own children. These findings have significance for nursing practice with abused children. Kaufman and Zigler concluded that although methodological variations in the current research limit the integration of findings, certain factors do appear to influence the effects of family violence on children. To summarize those factors, parents whose families of origin were violent, but who did not subsequently experience abuse with their children, were characterized as follows: (1) they had more extensive social supports (Hunter & Kilstrom, 1979), (2) they had fewer ambivalent feelings about their children (Hunter & Kilstrom), (3) their children were healthier (Hunter & Kilstrom) or they reported fewer life stressors (Egeland, Jacobvitz, & Sroufe, 1988), (4) they were more openly angry about their earlier abuse and better able to give detailed accounts of those experiences (Hunter & Kilstrom; Egeland, et al.) (5) they were more likely to have been abused by only one of their parents (Hunter & Kilstrom), (6) they were more apt to report a supportive relationship with one parent (Hunter & Kilstrom) or foster parent (Egeland et al.), (7) they were more likely to be involved in an emotionally supportive relationship with their partner (Egeland, et al.) and (8) they resolved not to repeat the pattern of abuse with their own children (Egeland, et al.).

Mrazek and Mrazek (1987) identify several generic and three abuse-specific protective factors. Access to good health, education, and social services foster resilience in children regardless of the specific nature of the stressor. Abuse-specific factors include the quick and full acknowledgment of the offender regarding abuse, or timeliness and permanence of legal actions affecting a child's custody. The authors conclude that a history of abuse does not automatically mean that a child will grow into an abusive adult. Rather, there are multiple determinants of future abuse (e.g., history of abuse, poverty, stress,

---

Characteristics of Abusive Parents

1. Immaturity
2. Inexperience with and/or impaired child-rearing
3. Low self-esteem
4. Unrealistic expectations of the child
5. Equally likely to be male or female
6. All ages, with young adolescents at high risk
7. From all socioeconomic groups, with low-income parents at high risk
8. Possibly abused as children themselves

---

lack of support) rather than one determinant. The impact of abuse can be minimized by early recognition and timely response to the child. When there is a history of abuse, the presence of significant positive relationships with one or more persons (support) can mediate the detrimental effects of family violence.

PATTERNS OF BEHAVIOR

Regardless of the theory or model used to explain child abuse and neglect, certain characteristics have been associated with the parent who abuses and/or neglects his or her child. Much of the research in the area of child abuse and neglect is retrospective, involves no controls, or selects "abusive families" based on their identification by social agencies. However, parents who abuse, neglect, or occasionally use violence against their children and who are not known by public agencies generally go unexamined. The box above summarizes characteristics of abusive parents.

Parent Characteristics

When reviewing reports of characteristics associated with adults who abuse and/or neglect their children, it is important to remember that a parent is only one individual within a larger group, the family, who is experiencing difficulty. In their landmark work, *The Battered Child,* Helfer and Kempe (1968)

identified three characteristics that must be present for child abuse to occur: a special parent, a special child, and stress. They listed several of the characteristics of the special parent. These characteristics include immaturity, inexperience with child-rearing, low self-esteem, and unrealistic expectations of the child. von Koss Krowchuk (1989) conducted a study that examined nurses' perceived characteristics of child abusers. The subjects were registered nurses with an average of 14.3 years of clinical experience. The subjects listed emotional and psychological disturbances as the primary characteristics of abusive parents. In addition, the subjects listed drug use, adolescent parents, poor education, male sex, welfare status, and single parents as characteristics of this population. The current research in this area lends varying degrees of support to these claims.

Early reports suggested that women are more frequently reported to have abused or neglected their children than men (Gil, 1970). This was explained by acknowledging that mothers spend more time with their children, and in this society with an ever-increasing number of female-dominated, single-parent homes, mothers also assume more of financial, emotional and child-rearing responsibilities than do fathers. More recently, a national survey indicated no gender differences (Wauchope & Straus, 1990). Interestingly, men, specifically the mother's boyfriend, were more likely to commit fatal child abuse, followed closely by the natural mother and the natural father.

In almost 34% of the reported cases of child abuse and neglect in 1977, the mother or a mother substitute was the only adult in the home. The women in these homes probably had to spend a preponderance of their time with their children because they had total responsibility for those children. In two-parent homes, women are generally still the primary caretakers of children, a task that involves more than just minutes and hours.

Women who work in the United States earn significantly less income on the average than men. The woman who works all day at a job must go home and likely work some more as a parent. For the woman to work at all she must, additionally and with sufficient advanced planning, find an adequate baby-sitter, daycare center, or other source of child care.

For the single female parent, this situation adds the stress of worrying about her ability to afford child care. When she finally returns home, she may or may not receive assistance in child care from a male partner. It is interesting to note that in a review of the literature, Maden and Wrench (1977) found that if the father is unemployed he is as likely as the mother to abuse the children. Gil (1970) reports that when the data are adjusted to allow for homes where no father or father-substitute is present, mothers actually perpetrated child abuse only one-third of the time. Fathers or father-substitutes committed the majority of child abuse. (Showers, Apolo, Thomas, & Beavers, 1985; Jason & Anderec, 1983).

Adolescent mothers are also often reported to be more likely to abuse or neglect their children. In the 1983 study by Jason and Anderec, parenthood before age 20 was associated with a higher degree of fatal child abuse. More recently, the relationship between adolescent mothers and child abuse and neglect has been called into question. It is, however, true that many adolescent mothers are also poor; one study found that families who had experienced an adolescent birth had a mean annual income of $6,608 (Kinard & Klerman, 1980).

Parent development

Many researchers suggest that parents who abuse their children have suffered some kind of developmental trauma as children. Evans (1981) administered an instrument, based on Eriksonian developmental outcomes, to 20 child-abusing and 20 non-child-abusing, low-income mothers. The abusive mothers scored significantly lower on measures of the first six developmental stages. The study used a previously untested instrument and identified abusive mothers through the local protective services unit. It is not known whether having abused their children within the previous 6 months, having been identified by a social service agency as abusive, or having experienced some other developmental trauma resulted in the abusive mothers' lower scores.

Blumberg (1980) suggests that women (note that the study was only of women) who maltreat their children do so because they experience "impairment of proper ego development and later superego evolution, leaving a basically id individual who is, therefore, prone to develop character disorders and emotional aberrations" (p. 353). The source of the developing females' impairment is not identified. Furthermore, the concepts of id, ego, and superego are very abstract and are not verifiable in research. Using nonpsychoanalytical terminology, however, other investigators have reached similar conclusions. Many reports identify that abusive adults were themselves abused as children and therefore never received adequate parenting. Much of this research studies only parents known to be abusive. Similar results with many of the same limitations are used by other researchers to conclude that abusive adults maltreat their children because they lack knowledge of adequate child-rearing practices (Azar, Robinson, Hekimian & Twentyman, 1984). Support for the conclusion that abusive parents are ignorant of normal child development has been provided by additional studies. Systematic analysis of study results is impaired because of the many flaws apparent in the research. However, there does appear to be some evidence suggesting that abusive and neglectful parents frequently come from violent families and demonstrate inadequate parenting skills themselves.

The issue of mental health status has been examined in current research. In a study comparing abusive mothers, depressed mothers, and normal (nondepressed) mothers, Susman, Trinkett, Lannotti, Hollenbeck, and Zahn-Waxler (1985) found abusive mothers to have the greatest degree of variation from the other two groups. Abusive mothers were found to use authoritarian control, anxiety induction, guilt induction, and inconsistency in discipline in their child-rearing. These mothers also reported little enjoyment of the parental role and did not have a rational framework for their child-rearing practices. They reported that they worried more about their children and were less likely to express affection openly to their children. Normal mothers and the depressed mothers had similar scores on child-rearing practices. Hence, it appears from this study that abusive mothers have alterations in parenting skills, and that they are not similar to clinically-depressed mothers. Egeland, et al. (1988), in a study that identified characteristics of previously-abused parents that would act as predicting factors of which individuals would break the cycle of abuse, found that mothers who continued the abuse score high on The Profile of Mood States, indicating a state of depression. Perhaps the fact that all the subjects in the study by Egeland et al. had a previous history of abuse, whereas this factor was not controlled in the study by Susman et al. may be the rationale for this finding.

Personality traits

Numerous personality traits have been associated with abusive and neglectful parents. However, Gil (1970) noted that very little consistency in the identified traits exists among reports. Low self-concept (Mash, Johnston, & Kovitz, 1983; Milner, 1988) and poor impulse control (Elliott, 1988) are characteristics frequently associated in adults who abuse and neglect children.

The issues of psychopathology and personality disorders have been extensively studied in the literature (Oates, Forrest, & Peacock, 1985; Egeland et al., 1989; Martin & Waters, 1982; Susman et al., 1985; Hamilton, 1989; Gaines, Sandgrund, Green, & Power, 1978). A frequent theme among these studies is low self-esteem in many abusive parents. In 1985 Oates et al. compared mothers of abused children with nonabusive mothers. This study is of particular merit because caution was taken to match the subjects on social class. The investigation revealed that abusive mothers were more likely than the control mothers to have received help for an emotional disorder, to have higher expectations of their children, and to perceive their children as having a greater number of personality problems than other children. In addition, Oates et al. found significance in the issue of parental development and attachment. These concepts have been related to the concept of low self-esteem (Evans, 1981, Oates et al., 1985). Egeland et al. concluded that mothers who were able to break the cycle of abuse were able to

form satisfying relationships with partners and others. To do this, they must see themselves as worthy of this type of relationship; in other words, they have a higher sense of self-esteem than those who were unable to break the cycle of abuse. In the study by Hamilton (1989), abusive parents were found to have lower self-esteem than controls (as measured by the Tennessee Self-Concept Scale) in almost every aspect of their lives. In addition, Hamilton found abusive parents to be more impulsive and hostile, as measured by the MMPI, than controls. The Hamilton study is of interest because it included both parents in the data collection.

It is not surprising that current research does not include data collected on nonmaternal child abusers. Martin and Waters (1982) have identified the most likely nonmaternal perpetrator to be the mother's cohabitating boyfriend. This population would be nearly impossible to reach considering: (1) the nonsanctioned relationship to the child and mother, (2) the relative instability of such a relationship making it difficult to find the individual, and (3) the hesitancy of the mother to admit the boyfriend's guilt.

CHARACTERISTICS OF ABUSIVE FAMILIES

Until recently, child abuse has been identified in the literature as a problem that occurred at all socioeconomic levels. Typically, child abuse and neglect have been identified as occurring more often in poor families, but only secondary to reporting source bias and the increased opportunity for "outsider" investigation uniquely associated with poverty. In reporting the higher incidence of child abuse and neglect in poor families, researchers frequently included a disclaimer that poor people were more often involved with public agencies, used the emergency room and public clinics for health care, and were thereby more subject to professional investigation. The box on p. 57 lists characteristics of abusive families.

During assessment by the professional, the poor family was also more likely to be labeled as child abusive than the middle- or upper-class family. Middle- and upper-class families have been thought

Characteristics of Abusive Families

1. From all socioeconomic groups, with low-income parents at high risk
2. Increasing risk of child abuse with increasing numbers of children (Families with one child were least likely to be abusive and families with four or more children were the most likely to be abusive.)
3. More likely to be urban families than rural families

to be less frequently reported as committing child abuse and neglect because of their use of private physicians, who hesitate to label a family peer or acquaintance. Middle- or upper-class families also had the financial resources to seek health care and assistance outside their immediate area, thereby further decreasing their likelihood of identification as child abusers.

The results of NIS-1, NIS-2, and other studies do not support the premise that child abuse is classless. For the purpose of both NIS-1 and NIS-2, families were divided into two groups: those earning less than $15,000 annually and those earning more than $15,000 annually. The differences between groups is astounding with both the original and revised definitions. Using the original definitions, overall maltreatment occurs in approximately 32.3 cases per 1,000 in the less than $15,000 category, whereas it only occurs in 6.1 cases per 1,000 in the more than $15,000 group. This trend continues into the subcategories of abuse, where 16.6 cases per 1,000 occurred in the lower-income range, while only 4.1 cases per 1,000 occurred in the upper-income range. Neglect demonstrates similar significance, with 17.3 cases per 1,000 reported in lower-income levels compared with 2.2 cases per 1,000 in higher-income levels. When the revised definition of maltreatment is used, the difference becomes even more astonishing: 54.0 cases per 1,000 of child maltreatment were reported in lower-income ranges, whereas 7.9 cases per 1,000 were reported in the higher-income ranges. This means the child living in poverty is

seven times more likely to be a victim of maltreatment than his or her upper-income counterpart.

Pelton (1979) presents a persuasive argument why child abuse and neglect is not "classless." In light of Pelton's study and other evidence, child abuse and neglect must be considered a problem with increased incidence in poor families. The main points of Pelton's study are outlined in the following section.

Families receiving general assistance have been consistently reported as experiencing more child abuse and neglect than those who do not (Gil, 1970). In particular, some studies reported that the very poor had an even higher incidence of child abuse and neglect than those still at the poverty level but with more income: as poverty increased, so did child abuse and neglect (Giovannono & Billingsley, 1970).

As child abuse and neglect reporting laws have come into existence and public awareness has grown, the incidence of reported child abuse and neglect has also increased. It would be expected that not just the public agency professional but every concerned citizen would be more likely to report child abuse and neglect, thereby increasing the percentage of nonpoor reported cases. However, the socioeconomic data over time have remained relatively unchanged (National Center on Child Abuse and Neglect, 1988). The poor continue to be over-represented in child abuse and neglect statistics. In the cases of child abuse and neglect that resulted in death, a difficult fact to hide at any socioeconomic level, the poor continue to contribute an unequal number of cases (National Center on Child Abuse and Neglect, 1988).

According to Pelton, the reason for the persistence of the "myth of classlessness" lies with the individuals who are supposedly working for the public good—health professionals who practice in the context of a medical model and politicians. Failure to associate child abuse and neglect with being poor, according to Pelton, increases the likelihood of monies available to "search out the real cause" and avoids the identification of the problem with something unlikely to get many votes, poverty.

Concerned health professionals may have some

difficulty in accepting Pelton's treatise. Many labels already are attached to people at the bottom of the socioeconomic stratum. Acknowledging the high incidence of child abuse and neglect among the poor at first appears to be just another label to keep "the poor in their place." Conversely, if poverty is viewed as a large contributor to the stress experienced by the child-abusing and neglectful family (see Theoretical Frameworks section), the high incidence can be understood and no "blame" attached. In two studies examining child health and social status, the number and degree of severity of specific health problems (other than abuse) was also significantly associated with poverty (Elmer, 1977; Egbuonu & Starfield, 1982). If poverty is a major factor inhibiting the ability of individuals to achieve and maintain life, health, and well-being, failure to acknowledge its role prevents the identification of truly helpful interventions.

Whereas Pelton's theory of poverty-associated abuse focuses on a single precipitating factor, Trinkett, Aber, Carlson, and Cicchetti (1991) proposes an environmental approach framework. This study compared abused and nonabused children from low-income (predominantly single-parent) families with children from two-parent, working-class families. The findings identify that abusive homes have additional developmental problems other than those related to lack of income. Parents in abusive homes reported experiencing little enjoyment in parenting, being worried a majority of the time, using authoritarian controls, and having high expectations for their children. One would expect that as income increases, families would have fewer worries and enjoy parenting more. This did not occur in the abusive families in this study. Even as income increased, parents still reported little enjoyment of parenting and many worries. This evidence suggests that socioeconomic status may not have as great a role in the cause of abuse as Pelton indicated.

Family size has also shown significance in terms of child maltreatment, based on NIS-2 findings using the revised definitions. Families with four or more children demonstrated the greatest degree of maltreatment, followed closely by families with two or three children. Families with only one child showed the lowest incidence of maltreatment. This trend deviates slightly when maltreatment is divided into abuse and neglect categories. Families with four or more children show the greatest frequency of both abuse and neglect; however, in the area of abuse, single-child families abuse with a greater frequency than families with two or three children. In terms of neglect, both single-child families and families with two or three children report similar occurrence rates (12.5 cases per 1,000 versus 12.6 cases per 1,000 respectively).

The type of community the family resided in (rural vs. urban) did not demonstrate any significant difference in either the NIS-1 or NIS-2 study. However, if NIS-1 values are compared with NIS-2 values, a higher number of abuse cases occurred in urban areas in the NIS-2 study. This finding suggests that although the family's community is not a significant risk factor, in the last 6 years, child abuse has increased at a greater rate in urban areas than in rural areas.

TYPES OF CHILD MALTREATMENT

In recent years attention has been given to the similarities and differences in child abuse and child neglect. Initially, child abuse and neglect were conceptualized as different points along the same continuum. Child neglect was more subtle, less obvious, and more common, and child abuse was a more visible form of child maltreatment. Admittedly, the majority of reports on child maltreatment continue to group child abuse and neglect together. Causative theoretical formulations generally still are the same for child abuse and neglect. Treatment approaches in the past varied only in their intensity. More recently, additional research has begun to suggest that various types of child maltreatment may be the result of different factors with different outcomes. Literature reports examining these various issues are examined briefly.

Neglectful parents have been described as socially isolated (Seagull, 1987), younger, experiencing great financial stress, and unlikely to be receiving any income supplement (Bolton & Laner, 1986). Educational achievement has been shown to mediate the effects of teenage motherhood on child neglect. The picture of the neglectful parent is one with too great a burden and little or no way to provide sufficient child care (Steele, 1986).

Ney (1987) has proposed that verbal abuse leaves deeper scars than physical abuse or neglect. Acknowledging that few pure forms of verbal abuse exist, Ney stresses that the problem is nevertheless serious. "There are some parents who use verbal abuse but would not hit their children, neglect them, or involve them in sex" (Ney, 1987, p. 371). Children are particularly susceptible to verbal abuse, according to Ney, because they lack the ability to defend themselves and perhaps use parental verbal attacks as a way of abusing themselves. Ney admonishes for greater study of verbal abuse as parents seek physically nonviolent ways of disciplining children.

Claussen and Crittenden (1991) studied the effects of psychological and physical abuse on children. They define psychological abuse as rejecting, terrorizing, isolating, exploiting, degrading, corrupting, and denying emotional responsiveness. They report that psychological maltreatment was almost always concurrent with physical abuse, that psychological abuse can occur alone, that psychological abuse was highly correlated with negative child outcomes, and that family income was related.

Watters, Parry, Caplan, and Bates (1986) report that in their study of child maltreatment identified by hospitals and social service agencies, children who experienced both abuse and neglect suffered the most severely. These abusive and neglectful families also were most likely to have multidisciplinary involvement, often including nurses, physicians, social services, and law enforcement.

These beginning reports urge the need for additional study. Nevertheless, they suggest that neglectful parents may lack the resources to meet the demands for child-rearing, that subtle forms of abuse (psychological, verbal) can have serious consequences for children, and that children who experience more than one type of abuse are at greatest risk.

Characteristics of Abused Children

1. All ages, with greatest risk of fatality under 2 years of age
2. All ages, with increasing risk until middle adolescence (approximately 14 years)
3. Both boys and girls, with adolescent girls at greatest risk for physical, emotional, and sexual abuse
4. Boys and girls equally likely to be neglected
5. All races

CHARACTERISTICS OF ABUSED CHILDREN

As previously identified, children under the age of 5 years are often reported to be the group most likely to experience child abuse and neglect. See the box above for a list of characteristics of abused children. Showers et al. (1985) studied fatal child abuse, using social service records from a Midwest children's hospital, and found that children ages 0 to 3 years were at greatest risk for fatal child abuse. It must be remembered that the younger the child, the more fragile he or she is likely to be, and the more susceptible to fatal injury. This may explain why this group was reported by earlier sources to have a greater risk of abuse.

Interestingly, however, the data from NIS-1 and NIS-2 found that overall child maltreatment increased with age. When maltreatment is divided into subcategories of abuse and neglect, significant age differences appear. The overall incidence of child abuse increases with age until middle adolescence (approximately 14 years of age), when it plateaus. The incidence of abuse rises slowly from birth to approximately age 6, with a plateau between ages 6 and 11, then demonstrates a sharp rise until middle adolescence.

Age was also found to be significant in terms of the type of injury incurred. Younger children (age 0 to 2 years) were more likely to incur fatal injuries, whereas older children (ages 3 and older) were more likely to incur moderate injuries.

Children over the age of 5 years experienced a greater degree of neglect than children under the age of 5 years, according to the NIS-1 definition findings. This can be attributed to the high incidence of educational neglect found, partly as a result of the restrictive NIS-1 criteria. Children under age 5 are not mandated by law to attend school, and hence, cannot be educationally neglected.

The sex of the child was not found to be significant in the overall incidence of maltreatment; however, when divided into subcategories, there were obvious differences. Girls demonstrated higher levels of abuse (11.1 per 1,000 NIS-1 definition) than boys (7.4 per 1,000). Similarly, females were more likely than males to experience physical, emotional, and sexual abuse, with significantly higher incidence per 1,000 cases than males in all three subcategories. Considering that it was previously reported that abuse rises with age, and that abuse incidence peaks in middle adolescence, then the adolescent female is at greatest risk for physical, emotional, and sexual abuse.

Sex of the child was not significant in the area of neglect. Males experienced an approximately equal incidence of abuse and neglect (NIS-1 definition), whereas females experienced slightly less neglect in comparison with abuse. When comparing NIS-1 with NIS-2 findings using both the original and revised definitions, no significant differences were found.

The child's race was not found to be a significant in either child abuse or neglect. Findings were based on both NIS-1 and NIS-2 definitions and a comparison of the two.

Effects of Abuse on Child Health Status

It would seem obvious that abuse has deleterious effects on the child's health and well-being. This fact is well documented in the literature (Aber & Allen, 1987; Keurouac, Taggart, Lescop, & Fortim, 1987; King & Taitz, 1985; Oates et al., 1982; Sherrod, O'Connor, Vietze, & Altemeier, 1984). These effects range from the potentially life-threatening incidence of physical abuse to the long-term effects of abuse, such as the reported increased incidence of male

victims of child abuse becoming abusers as adults (Straus, 1980).

Current literature reports have shown that children who are abused have a higher incidence and frequency of physical illness than their nonabused counterparts. Sherrod et al. (1984) investigated the temporal relationship between onset of illness and onset of child abuse in a 3-year longitudinal study of 80 children, 11 of whom were identified to be at risk for abuse. The children were followed from birth to age 3 to answer the following question: Does the frequency and degree of illness cause abuse, or is the abuse the cause for the frequency of illness? The resulting frequent illness is not the cause per se of abuse in families that have been identified as low risk; however, in families that have been identified as high risk, the frequency of illness may precipitate an abuse incident. These conclusions were based on the finding that some children were both ill and members of abusive families and themselves not abused, and the finding that siblings of the study subjects had lower frequencies of illness than the subject and were found to be abused. Perhaps an interpretation of such findings could include the parents' feeling very protective of the ill family member and dedicating a great deal of time and energy to that child, therefore the only way the sibling may see to get attention is through negative behavior, hence the negative reinforcement in the form of abuse.

In a 1985 study of children of battered women who themselves had been victims of battering, Keurouac et al. found in a sample of Canadian children (ages 12 years and under) an incidence of hearing and sight problems 8% higher than the Canadian average for this age group. Recall that Sherrod et al. found the majority of illness in abused children to occur in the first year of life and decreasing thereafter, and also observed that children in the at-risk-for-abuse category experienced twice the number of accidents than the not-at-risk control group.

Abused children demonstrate health deviations in the areas of development, readiness to learn, psychological well-being, and attachment (Aber & Allen, 1987; Keurouac et al., 1987; Oates et al.,

1985). The mothers in the study by Keurouac et al. reported that their children had experienced nervousness, sadness, unhappiness, withdrawal, and aggressiveness in the past 3 months. In addition, mothers in this study reported that over half the children had missed a significant amount of school. In this group, 24.6% of the children were found to have learning disabilities and 16.1% were found to have disciplinary problems. In a study comparing abused children with welfare children and middle-class children, Aber and Allen found that abused children scored lower on readiness to learn indicators than either of the two comparison groups. Others (Hoffman-Plotkin & Twentyman, 1984) have found that abused children perform poorly on standardized measures of cognitive ability.

All the news in this area is not bad, however. In a study following 95 children referred to the social work department in England, King and Taitz (1985) found that children can "catch up" on lost growth if placed in the appropriate environment. The most optimal environment identified by the investigators was foster placement. The children placed in foster care demonstrated the greatest levels of advancement in the areas of height and weight. The authors hypothesize that when the child is left in the home, despite the interventions of social services and support systems, the dysfunctional environment continues to exist, and hence, the cause of the failure to thrive remains.

SOCIAL SUPPORT AND CHILD ABUSE

In reviewing the child abuse literature on the characteristics of abusive individuals, the common themes of isolation and stress are often found. There has been support in the literature of the relationship between stress and child abuse (Cobb, 1976; Helfer & Kempe, 1968; Kempe & Kempe, 1978; Parke & Collmer, 1975; Straus, 1980). In addition, abusive parents are often noted to be socially isolated for reasons hypothesized as embarrassment, poverty, and lack of transportation, among others (Kempe & Kempe, 1978; Garbarino, 1977). These observations have raised the subject of social support and its role in child abuse.

In a study comparing 41 abusive and 59 nonabusive mothers their perception of the degree of social support they received, Gaudin and Pollane (1983) found that abusive mothers reported their social support systems to be weaker and less supportive than the nonabusing group. The study also included an empirical measure of the amount of stress each participant was experiencing and found no relationship between abuse and degree of stress—the mothers experiencing high levels of stress did not necessarily abuse their children. However, there is a negative correlation between degree of social support and child abuse—as the mother's social support increased, the incidence of child abuse decreased. The authors attribute this finding to the fact that optimal social support networks provide mothers with alternate child care providers to allow time away from the child, feedback on the effectiveness of parenting, and assistance with problem solving in addition to the provision of material resources.

Among the problems identified with child abuse were developmental and social deviations (Aber & Allen, 1987; Keurouac et al., 1987; Oates et al., 1985; Adamakos, Ryan, Ullman, Pascoe, Diaz, & Chessare, 1986). Adamakos et al. studied this problem in a social support context. They found that the measure of maternal social support was the best indicator of stress in the maternal-child relationship. In addition, they found a negative correlation between the number of people the mother could rely on in a time of need and maternal stress. The investigators also found that as maternal social support increased, so did the amount of stimulation that the child received. It was hypothesized that those children who received the greater degree of stimulation would perform better on cognitive measures. The authors used the Bayley Scales to measure cognitive and motor development and found no statistical differences. It should be noted that only 38 of the 198 initial subjects completed the 3-year study and that the large attrition rate may have influenced this finding.

The impact of social support on family function can best be appreciated through implementation of a child abuse prevention program. Schinde, Schilling, Barth, Gilchrist, and Maxwell (1986) implemented such a program for teenage parents. The pretest-posttest design evaluated the effectiveness of a comprehensive stress management program that included the topics of problem solving, self-instruction, self-reinforcement, interpersonal communication, relaxation, and social support. Subjects were posttested immediately after the program, and again 3 months later. Immediately after the program, the subjects scored higher on the Social Support inventory than pretest. At the 3-month posttest the subjects who returned continued to score high in the areas of social support and self-esteem. The long-term consequences of such an experimental program remain unknown.

Kugler and Hansson (1988) became interested in the observation that when all variables were equal (martial status, socioeconomic status, age, etc.), some parents appeared to have adequate social support and others did not. They chose to examine parental personality characteristics as a potential indicator of the degree of social support received. They defined those characteristics that influence a person's ability to achieve and maintain interpersonal relationships as "interrelational competence." Their sample consisted of 54 men and women in a Parents Anonymous treatment program. The results of the study showed that parents who scored low on relational competence measures also scored low on social support measures. They found that these individuals were shy, had low self-esteem, were less assertive, were less controlled emotionally, and scored significantly higher on depression indicators than those parents who scored high on relational competence measures. This is a significant finding and should be considered in intervention strategies. These findings suggest that primary interventions in the treatment of child abuse should address these intrapersonal issues before attempting to link these individuals with a social support network.

Zuravin (1988a; 1988b; 1989) attempted to view social support in a macrosystem context by identifying characteristics of communities where child abuse and neglect is prevalent. This idea was based on the observation by Garbarino (1977) that child maltreatment is more likely to occur in socially impoverished neighborhoods where individuals and families are not embedded in a social network. Through an analysis of seven community characteristics thought to contribute to child abuse and neglect, Zuravin reached the following conclusions. Child abuse is more likely to occur in neighborhoods where there is a large percentage of vacant housing, a high number of single-family dwellings, and large numbers of families with an income within 200% of the poverty line. It was also noted that child abuse occurrences were lower in areas where mothers of children under the age of 6 were employed outside the home. All of these factors, with the exception of the income levels, indicate a low availability of individuals for support and an environment that may prohibit the formation of social networks.

SUBSTANCE ABUSE AND CHILD MALTREATMENT

The connection between substance abuse and child abuse is unclear. Substances that receive considerable attention in the literature include cocaine, especially crack cocaine (Bresnahan, Brooks, & Zuckerman, 1991; and Jacques & Snyder, 1991). The biological effects of cocaine use during pregnancy are well documented (Bresnahan et. al.) and include preterm birth, abruptio placentae, and small-for-gestational age babies in addition to placing the infant at risk for various developmental problems. Some have argued that prenatal exposure to cocaine should be considered child abuse (Horowitz, 1990), subject to the same criminal standards as parents who physically harm their already born children. Others (Gittler & McPherson, 1990) have argued that this type of prosecution discriminates against the pregnant woman (i.e., would nonpregnant cocaine users be prosecuted in the same way?).

The environment in which the crack cocaine addict exists is often wrought with violence. Cocaine-abusing women tend to have a low sense of self-esteem, and often become involved with violent men who batter and abuse them. The subculture of the drug world also is violent. Mothers may use welfare checks and food stamps, specifically targeted to providing for the family, to buy drugs, leaving the children with little food and often poor shelter. Living in these conditions predisposes children to both abuse and neglect.

Many substance-abusing mothers desperately need treatment; however, they are reluctant to seek treatment for fear of losing their children. Traditional treatment programs are often patterned to meet the needs of male addicts who are generally alone. Women, on the other hand, are frequently heads of households with several children. These women are unique and require a unique treatment program that takes place within the context of the family (Finkelstein, Duncan, Derman, & Smeltz, 1980).

SUMMARY

This chapter has reviewed current literature relevant to child abuse and its contributing factors. The incidence of child abuse has shown a 55% increase from 1980 to 1985 (NACHRI, 1989). Factors that may bias the determination of an actual number of children abused include variations in reporting criteria from state to state, individual biases, and study sample parameters. Child abuse is a complex phenomenon with many hypothesized causative factors. Retrospective studies have identified that the most frequent perpetrator in cases of child abuse and neglect is the mother, and in cases of fatal child abuse is the mother's boyfriend. Although it has been stated that child abuse is universal, studies have indicated that it occurs with greater frequency in poor populations.

The historical background of child maltreatment is long-standing and evolving with its definition. Theoretical frameworks that seek to explain child abuse and neglect include the mental illness model, environmental stress model, resilience model, and several social-psychological models. A nursing model has been proposed as a framework for nursing theory development and research.

Characteristics of abusive parents include low self-esteem, ineffective stress-coping strategies, tendency toward aggressive behavior, low impulse control, and a high degree of hostility. In addition, parents who abused their children reported a low degree of social support. Parent characteristics that are linked to a low degree of social support include low self-esteem, shyness, low degree of assertiveness, and low degree of emotional control.

Aside from the obvious physical health deviations that abused children suffer, they also demonstrate a higher frequency of childhood illness, more frequent somatic complaints, decreased readiness to learn, decreased psychological well-being, and decreased attachment than nonabused children. It has been demonstrated that if abused children are removed from the abusive environment, that they can "catch up" on both physical and developmental areas.

Theories of causation and empirical validation through research contribute to nursing knowledge of child abuse and neglect. The next step is the incorporation of this new knowledge into nursing practice. Theory and research are thus the basis for the direct application of care to children and families experiencing violence.

REFERENCES

Aber, J. L., & Allen, J. P. (1987). Effect of maltreatment on young children's socioemotional development: An attachment theory perspective. *Developmental Psychology*, 23(3), 406-414.

Adamakos, H., Ryan, K., Ullman, D. G., Pascoe, J., Diaz, R., & Chessare, J. (1986). Maternal social support as a predictor of mother-child stress and stimulation. *Child Abuse and Neglect*, 10, 463-470.

Ammerman, R. T. (1990). Etiological models of child maltreatment: A behavioral perspective. *Behavior Modification*, 14, 230-254.

Ammerman, R. T., Van Hasselt, V. B., & Hersen, M. (1988). Maltreatment of handicapped children: A critical review. *Journal of Family Violence*, 3, 53-72.

Aries, P. (1962). *Centuries of childhood: A social history of family life* (R. Baldick, Trans.). New York: Random House.

Azar, S. T., Robinson, R. R., Hekimian, E., & Twentyman, C. T. (1984). Unrealistic expectations and problem-solving ability in maltreating and comparison mothers. *Journal of Consulting and Clinical Psychology*, 52, 687-691.

Bandura, A. (1974). Behavior theory and the models of man. *American Psychologist*, 29, 859-870.

Belsky, J. (1980). Child maltreatment: An ecological integration. *American Psychologist*, 35, 320-35.

Berger, A. (1980). The child abusing family. *The American Journal of Family Therapy*, 8, 52-68.

Blumberg, M. L. (1980). The abusing mother—criminal, psychopath, or victim of circumstances? *American Journal of Psychotherapy, 34,* 350-358.

Bolton, F. G., & Laner, R. H. (1986). Children rearing children: A study of reportedly maltreating younger adolescents. *Journal of Family Violence, 1,* 181-196.

Bremner, R. H. (Ed.). (1970). *Children and youth in America: A documentary history* (Vols. 1-2). Cambridge, MA: Harvard University Press.

Bresnahan, K., Brooks, C., & Zuckerman, B. (1991). Prenatal cocaine use: Impact on infants and mothers. *Pediatric Nursing, 17*(2), 123-129.

Bronfenbrenner, U. (1979). *The ecology of human development.* Cambridge, MA: Harvard University Press.

Caffey, J. (1946). Multiple fractures in the long bones of infants suffering from chronic subdural hematoma. *American Journal of Roentgenology, 56,* 163-173.

Caplan, P. J., & Dinardo, L. (1986). Is there a relationship between child abuse and learning disability? *Canadian Journal of Behavioral Science, 18,* 337-380.

Child Protection Law (1974). Child Abuse and Treatment Act (PL-93237). Lansing, MI: Department of Social Services.

Child Protection Law, P.A. 1975, No. 238 Eff. Oct 1. Department of Social Services Publication, 3 (rev. 10-75), Lansing, MI.

Claussen, A. H., & Crittenden, P. M. (1991). Physical and psychological maltreatment: Relations among types of maltreatment. *Child Abuse and Neglect, 15,* 5-18.

Cobb, S. (1976). Social support as a moderator of life stress. *Psychosomatic Medicine, 38,* 300-314.

Conger, R. D., Burgess, R. L., & Barrett, C. (1979). Child abuse related to life change and perceptions of illness: Some preliminary findings. *The Family Coordinator, 28,* 73-78.

Corey, E. J., Miller, C. L., & Widlak, F. W. (1975). Factors contributing to child abuse. *Nursing Research, 24,* 293-95.

Crittenden, P. M. (1988). Distorted patterns of relationship in maltreating families: The role of internal representation models. *Journal of Reproductive and Infant Psychology, 6,* 183-199.

Dietrich, D., Berkowitz, L., Kadushin, A., & McGloin, J. (1990). Some factors influencing abusers justification of their child abuse. *Child Abuse and Neglect, 14,* 337-345.

Dukes, R. & Kean, R. B. (1989). An experimental study of gender and situation in the perception and reportage of child abuse. *Child Abuse and Neglect, 13,* 351-360.

Dumas, J. E. (1984). Child, adult-interactional and socioeconomic setting events as predictors of parent training outcome. *Education and Treatment of Children, 7,* 351-364.

Egbuonu, L., & Starfield, B. (1982). Child health and social status. *Pediatrics, 69,* 550-557.

Egeland, B., Jacobvitz, D., & Sroufe, L. A. (1988). Breaking the cycle of abuse: Relationship predictors. *Child Development, 59,* 1080-1088.

Elder, G. (1977). Family history and the life course. *Journal of Family History, 2*(4), 279-304.

Elliott, F. A. (1988). Neurological factors. In V. B. Van Hasselt, R. L. Morrison, A. S. Bellack, & M. Hersen (Eds.), *Handbook of family violence* (pp. 359-382). New York: Plenum.

Elmer, E. (1977). Follow-up study of traumatized children. *Pediatrics, 59,* 273-279.

Estroff, T. W., Herrera, C., Gaines, R., Shaffer, D., Gould, M., & Green, A. H. (1984). Maternal psychopathology and perception of child behavior in psychiatrically referred and child maltreatment families. *Journal of the American Academy of Child Psychiatry, 23,* 649-652.

Evans, A. L. (1981). *Personality characteristics and discipline attitudes of child abusing mothers.* Saratoga, NY: Century Twenty-One.

Farrington, K. (1986). The application of stress theory to the study of family violence: Principles, problems, and prospects. *Journal of Family Violence, 1,* 131-147.

Finkelhor, D., Gelles, R. J., Hotaling, G. T., & Straus, M. A. (Eds.). (1983). *The dark side of families: Current family violence research.* Beverly Hills: Sage.

Finkelstein, N., Duncan, S., Derman, L., & Smeltz, J. (1980). *Getting sober, getting well: A treatment guide for caregivers who work with women.* Cambridge, MA: Women's Alcoholism Program of CASPAR.

Frey, M. S. (1985). *An ecological framework for examining the relationship between social support, family health, and child health in families with a diabetic child.* Paper presented at the Beatrice Paulucci Symposium, Michigan State University, East Lansing, MI.

Friedrich, W. N., & Boriskin, J. A. (1976). The role of the child in abuse: A review of the literature. *American Journal of Orthopsychiatry, 46,* 580-590.

Gaines, R., Sandgrund, S., Green, A. H., & Power, E. (1978). Etiological factors in child maltreatment: A multivariate study of abusing, neglecting and normal mothers. *Journal of Abnormal Psychology, 87,* 531-540.

Garbarino, J. (1977). The human ecology of child maltreatment: A conceptual model for research. *Journal of Marriage and the Family, 39,* 721-735.

Garbarino, J., & Gillian, G. (1980). *Understanding abusive families.* Toronto: Lexington.

Garmezy, N. (1983). Stressors of childhood. In N. Garmezy (Ed.), *Stress, coping, and development in children* (pp. 43-84). New York: McGraw-Hill.

Gaudin, J. M., & Pollane, L. (1983). Social networks, stress and child abuse. *Children and Youth Services Review, 5,* 91-102.

Gelles, R. J. (1972). *The violent home.* Beverly Hills: Sage.

Gelles, R. J. (1980). Violence in the family: A review of research in the seventies. *Journal of Marriage and the Family, 42,* 873-885.

Gelles, R. J. (1987). The family and its role in abuse of children. *Psychiatric Annals, 17,* 229-232.

Gelles, R. J., & Harrop, J. W. (1989). Violence, battering and psychological distress among women. *Journal of Interpersonal Violence, 4*, 400-420.

Gelles, R. J., & Straus, M. A. (1979). Violence in the American Family. *Journal of Social Issues, 35*, 20-35.

George, C., & Main, M. (1979). Social interactions of young abused children: Approach, avoidance, and aggression. *Child Development, 50*, 306-318.

Gil, D. G. (1970). *Violence against children.* Cambridge, MA: Harvard University Press.

Gil, D. G. (1976). Primary prevention of child abuse: A philosophical and political issue. *Psychiatric Opinion, 13*, 30-33.

Giovannono, J., & Billingsley, A. (1970). Child neglect among the poor. *Child Welfare, 49*, 196-204.

Gittler, J., & McPherson, M. (1990). Prenatal substance abuse. *Children Today, 19*(4), 3-7.

Goldson, E., Fitch, M. J., Wendell, T. A., & Knapp, G. (1978). Child abuse: Its relationship to birthweight, Apgar score, and developmental testing. *American Journal of Diseases of Children, 132*, 790-793.

Green, A. H. (1968). Self-destructive behavior in physically abused schizophrenic children. *Archives of General Psychiatry, 19*, 171-179.

Hamilton, L. R. (1989). Variables associated with child maltreatment and implications for prevention and treatment. *Early Child Development and Care, 42*, 31-56.

Hampton, R. L. & Newberger, E. H. (1985). Hospitals as gatekeepers: Recognition and reporting in the national incidence study of child abuse and neglect. *Report to National Center on Child Abuse and Neglect.* Children's Bureau, Administration for Children, Youth, and Families, Office of Human Development Services, U.S. Department of Health and Human Services.

Helfer, R. E. (1973). The etiology of child abuse. *Pediatrics, 51*, 777-779.

Helfer, R. E., & Kempe, C. H. (1968). *The battered child.* Chicago: University of Chicago Press.

Hoffman-Plotkin, D., & Twentyman, C. (1984). A multimodal assessment of behavioral and cognitive deficits in abused and neglected preschoolers. *Child Development, 52*, 13-30.

Horowitz, R. (1990). Perinatal substance abuse. *Children Today, 19*(4), 8-12.

Hudson, W. W., & McIntosh, S. R. (1981, November). The assessment of spouse abuse: Two quantifiable dimensions. *Journal of Marriage and the Family, 43*, 873-885.

Hunter, R., & Kilstrom, N. (1979). Breaking the cycle in abusive families. *American Journal of Psychiatry, 136*, 1320-1322.

Jacques, J. T., & Snyder, N. (1991, July). Newborn victims of addiction. *RN*, 47-53.

Jason, J., & Anderec, N. D. (1983). Fatal child abuse in Georgia: The epidemiology of severe physical child abuse. *Child Abuse and Neglect, 7*, 1-9.

Justice, B., & Justice, R. (1976). *The abusing family.* New York: Human Sciences Press.

Kaufman, J., & Zigler, E. (1987). Do abused children become abusive parents? *American Journal of Orthopsychiatry, 57*, 186-193.

Kempe, C. H., & Helfer, R. E. (Eds.) (1972). *Helping the battered child and his family.* Philadelphia: Lippincott.

Kempe, R. S., & Kempe, H. C. (1978). *Child abuse and neglect: The developing child.* Cambridge, MA: Harvard University Press.

Kempe, C. H., Silver, F., Steele, B., Droegemueller, W., & Silver, H. (1962). The battered child syndrome. *JAMA, 181*, 17-24.

Keurouac, S., Taggart, M. E., Lescop, J., & Fortim, M. F. (1987). Children's health in violent families. *Canadian Journal of Public Health, 78*, 369-373.

Kinard, E. M., & Klerman, L. B. (1980). Teenage parenting and child abuse: Are they related? *American Journal of Orthopsychiatry, 50*, 481-488.

King, J. M., & Taitz, L. S. (1985). Catch up growth following abuse. *Archives of Disease in Childhood, 60*, 1154-1163.

Klaus, M. H., & Kennell, J. (1976). *Maternal-infant bonding.* St. Louis: Mosby-Year Book.

Knitzer, J. (1977). Spare the rod and spoil the child revisited. *American Journal of Orthopsychiatry, 47*, 372-73.

Knudsen, D. D. (1988). Child maltreatment over two decades: Change or continuity? *Violence and Victims, 1*(2), 129-144.

Korbin, J. E. (1977). Anthropological contributions to the study of child abuse. *Child Abuse and Neglect, 1*, 7-24.

Korbin, J. E. (1979). A cross-cultural perspective on the role of the community in child abuse and neglect. *Child Abuse and Neglect, 3*, 9-18.

Korbin, J. E. (1991). Cross-cultural perspectives and research directions for the 21st century. *Child Abuse and Neglect, 15*, 67-77.

Kugler, K. E., & Hansson, R. O. (1988). Relational competence and social support among parents at risk of child abuse. *Family Relations, 37*, 328-332.

Lazoritz, S. (1990). Whatever happened to Mary Ellen? *Child Abuse and Neglect, 14*, 143-149.

Levinson, D. (1989). *Family violence in cross-cultural perspective.* Newbury Park, CA: Sage.

Long, K. A. (1986). Cultural considerations in the assessment and treatment of intrafamilial abuse. *American Journal of Orthopsychiatry, 56*, (1), 131-136.

Lubchenco, L. O. (1980). Routine neonatal circumcision: A surgical anachronism. *Clinical Obstetrics and Gynecology, 23*, 135-140.

Lynch, M. A. (1985). Child abuse before Kempe: An historical literature review. *Child Abuse and Neglect, 9*, 7-15.

Maden, M. F., & Wrench, D. F. (1977). Significant findings in child abuse research. *Victimology: An International Journal, 2*, 196-213.

Martin, M. J., & Waters, J. (1982, May). Familial correlates of selected types of child abuse and neglect. *Journal of Marriage and the Family, 44,* 267-276.

Mash, E. J., Johnston, C., & Kovitz, K. (1983). A comparison of the mother-child interactions of physically abused and nonabused children during play and task situations. *Journal of Clinical Child Psychology, 12,* 337-346.

McClelland, D. (1973). Testing for competence rather than intelligence. *American Psychologist, 28,* 1-14.

Millor, G. K. (1981). Theoretical framework for nursing research in child abuse and neglect. *Nursing Research, 30,* 78-83.

Milner, J. S. (1988). An ego-strength scale for the Child Abuse Potential Inventory. *Journal of Family Violence, 3,* 151-162.

Morse, A. E., Hyde, J. N., Newberger, E. H., & Reed, R. B. (1977). Environmental correlates of pediatric social illness: Preventive implications of an advocacy approach. *American Journal of Public Health, 67,* 612-615.

Mrazek, P. J., & Mrazek, D. A. (1987). Resilience in child maltreatment victims: A conceptual exploration. *Child Abuse and Neglect, 11,* 357-366.

National Association of Children's Hospitals and Related Institutions (NACHRI). (1989). *Profile of child health in the United States.* Washington, DC: NACHRI publications.

National Center on Child Abuse and Neglect. (1988). *Study of National Incidence and Prevalence of Child Abuse and Neglect: 1988.* (Contract No. 105-85-1702). Washington, DC: U.S. Department of Health and Human Services.

Newberger, E. H., & Bourne, R. (1978) The medicalization and legalization of child abuse. *American Journal of Orthopsychiatry, 48,* 593-607.

Ney, P. G. (1987). Does verbal abuse leave deeper scars: A study of children and parents. *American Journal of Psychiatry, 32,* 371-378.

Nkpa, N. K. (1980). Victimization of babies in Nigerian urban centers. *Victimology, 5,* (2-4), 251-262.

Oates, R. K., Forrest, D., & Peacock, A. (1985). Mothers of abused children. *Clinical Pediatrics, 24,* (1), 9-13.

Panter, B. M. (1977). Lithium in the treatment of a child abuser. *American Journal of Psychiatry, 134,* 1436-1437.

Parke, R., & Collmer, C. W. (1975). Child abuse: An interdisciplinary analysis. In E. M. Hetherington (Ed.), *Review of child development research* (Vol. 5). Chicago: University of Chicago Press.

Pelton, L. H. (1979). Interpreting family violence data. *American Journal of Orthopsychiatry, 49,* 372-374.

Radbill, S. X. (1980). Children in a world of violence: A history of child abuse. In C. H. Kempe & R. E. Helfer, (Eds.), *The battered child* (3rd ed.) (pp 3-20). Chicago: University of Chicago Press.

Seagull, E. A. (1987). Social support and child maltreatment: A review of the evidence. *Child Abuse and Neglect, 11,* 41-52.

Schinde, S. P., Schilling, R. F., Barth R. P., Gilchrist, L. D., & Maxwell, J. S. (1986). Stress management intervention to prevent family violence. *Journal of Family Violence, 1,* 13-26.

Sherrod, K. B., O'Connor, S., Vietze, P. M., Altemeier, W. A. (1984). Child health and maltreatment. *Child Development, 5,* 1174-1183.

Showers, J., Apolo, J., Thomas, J., & Beavers, S. (1985). Fatal child abuse: A two-decade review. *Pediatric Emergency Care, 1*(2), 66-70.

Steele, S. (1986). Nonorganic failure to thrive: A pediatric social illness. *Issues in Comprehensive Pediatric Nursing, 9,* 47-58.

Steinmetz, S. K. (1977). The use of force for resolving family conflict: The training ground for abuse. *Family Coordinator, 26,* 19-26.

Straus, M. A. (1980). Stress and child abuse. In C. H. Kempe & R. E. Helfer, (Eds.), *The battered child* (3rd ed.). Chicago: University of Chicago Press.

Straus, M. A. (1974). Forward. In R. J. Gelles, *The violent home: A study of physical aggression between husbands and wives* (pp. 13-17). Beverly Hills: Sage.

Straus, M. A., & Gelles, R. J. (1986). Societal change and change in family violence from 1975 to 1985 as revealed by two national surveys. *Journal of Marriage and the Family, 48,* 465-479.

Straus, M. A., & Gelles, R. J. (Eds.). (1990). *Physical violence in American families: risk factors and adaptations in 8,145 families.* New Brunswick, NJ: Transaction.

Straus, M. A., Gelles, R. J., & Steinmetz, S. K. (1980). *Behind closed doors: Violence in the American family.* Garden City, NY: Doubleday.

Susman, E. J., Trinkett, P. K., Lannotti, R. J., Hollenbeck, B. E., & Zahn-Waxler, C. (1985). Child-rearing patterns in depressed, abusive and normal mothers. *American Journal of Orthopsychiatry, 55,* (2), 237-251.

Trinkett, P. K., Aber, J. L., Carlson, V., & Cicchetti, D. (1991). Relationships of socioeconomic status to the etiology & development sequelae of physical child abuse. *Developmental Psychology, 27,* 148-158.

Ulbrich, P., & Huber, J. (1981). Observing parental violence: Distribution and effects. *Journal of Marriage and the Family, 43,* 623-631.

Vaughn-Switzer, J. (1986). Reporting child abuse. *The American Journal of Nursing, 86*(6), 663-664.

Vondra, J. I., & Toth, S. L. (1989). Ecological perspectives on child maltreatment: Research and intervention. *Early Child Development and Care, 42,* 11-29.

von Koss Krowchuk, H. (1989). Child abuser stereotypes: Consensus among clinicians. *Applied Nursing Research, 2*(1), 35-39.

Wagatsuma, H. (1981). Child abandonment and infanticide: A Japanese case. In J. E. Korbin (Ed.), *Child abuse and neglect* (pp. 120-132). Berkeley: University of California Press.

Watters, J., Parry, R., Caplan, P. J., & Bates, R. (1986). A comparison of child abuse and child neglect. *Canadian Journal of Behavioral Science, 18,* 449-459.

Wauchope, B., & Straus, M. (1990). Age, gender and class differences in physical punishment and physical abuse of American children. In M. Straus & R. J. Gelles (Eds.), *Physical violence in American families: Risk factors and adaptations in 8,145 families* (pp. 133-148). New Brunswick, NJ: Transaction.

Witt, D. D. (1987). A conflict theory of family violence. *Journal of Family Violence, 2,* 291-301.

Wolfe, D. A. (1987). *Child abuse: Implications for child development and psychopathology.* Newbury Park, CA: Sage.

Zuravin, S. J. (1988a). Child maltreatment and teenage first births: A relationship mediated by chronic sociodemographic stress? *American Journal of Orthopsychiatry, 58,* 91-103.

Zuravin, S. J. (1988b). Fertility patterns: Their relationship to child physical abuse and child neglect. *Journal of Marriage and Family, 50,* 983-993.

Zuravin, S. J. (1989). The ecology of child abused and neglect: Review of the literature and presentation of data. *Violence and Victims, 4,* 101-120.

CHAPTER

3

Abuse of Female Partners

Jacquelyn Campbell *and* Nancy Fishwick

Abuse of female partners began to receive public attention in the 1970s, largely through the efforts of grass-roots women's groups. Scholarly attention to this significant social and health problem has increased dramatically over the past two decades. The theoretical formulations that have been advanced to explain the phenomenon are related to coexisting theories of violence, family functioning, and women's status in society. This chapter uses results of research of wife abuse to suggest a theoretical base for nursing research and practice with battered women. Abuse of female partners is examined as a significant health problem of vital concern to nursing. The historical roots and traditional and contemporary theoretical approaches to the phenomenon are analyzed, and the concept of machismo is described as a theoretical construct providing gender-related insight into the abuse of women. Finally, the explanatory frameworks that

suggest the reasons for continuation of battering relationships are critically examined.

PARAMETERS OF ABUSE
Nature of the Problem

Abuse of female partners is a significant health problem that encompasses a wide range of behaviors and diverse adult intimate relationships. The abuse directed to a woman may be predominantly a harmful physical, psychological, or sexual behavior. However, abuse is more likely to entail a complex web of behaviors that include physical battery, verbal threats or intimidating gestures of assault, verbal denigration, forced sexual activity, social isolation, and economic deprivation (Okun, 1986; Pagelow, 1981; Walker, 1979, 1984). The majority of research on the nature of abusive adult intimate relationships has focused on physical assault, and, more recently, rape in the context of marriage (Campbell, 1989a; Campbell, 1989b; Finkelhor & Yllo, 1983; Pagelow, 1988; Russell, 1990; Shields & Hanneke, 1983). Therefore, for the purposes of this chapter, *wife abuse* is defined as deliberate and repeated physical aggression or sexual assault inflicted on a woman by a man with whom she has or has had an intimate relationship (Campbell, 1989a). Abuse is thus a pattern, not a single incident, and the man and woman are not necessarily married. The phrase "abuse of female partners" most accurately reflects the pattern of abusive behavior and the nature of the relationship between the perpetrator and target of abuse. For convenience, the terms "wife abuse" and "battered woman" will also be used.

Wife Abuse, Not Spouse Abuse

An important conceptual problem addressed in this chapter is the deliberate choice of the term *abuse of female partners*, or, more loosely, *wife abuse*, rather than *spouse abuse*. The terms "spouse abuse," "conjugal violence," and "domestic violence" imply that abuse directed from women to men is equal in nature to abuse directed from men to women (Berk, Berk, Loseke, & Rauma, 1983; Saunders, 1986). Women may, indeed, use physical violence in self-defense or retaliation against the perpetrator, or in "mutual combat," but the injuries inflicted are less severe than those they receive (Pagelow, 1981; Saunders, 1986; Walker, 1989; Walker & Browne, 1985). Although it is true that husband battering does occur, the preponderance of evidence suggests that the incidence is very low. This controversial issue surfaced from the research findings of Steinmetz (1977, 1977-78), who contends that husband abuse is nearly as prevalent as wife abuse, and coined the term "battered husband syndrome" (Steinmetz, 1977, 1977-78; Steinmetz & Lucca, 1988). Critical analysis of the research methods used by Steinmetz revealed the danger of relying on simple counts of physical acts between intimate partners to discern the nature of the problem. Taking the behaviors out of context obscured the fact that women rarely *initiated* an attack of severe violence unless they thought they or their children were in imminent

danger of great harm (Saunders, 1988). The majority of women who did engage in physical assault on their partners did so in self-defense or "fighting back," and the methods used, such as slapping, pushing, throwing objects, or hitting, were not likely to cause injury.

It is undoubtedly true that there are husbands who are abused by wives. It is also a fact that some couples are equally assaultive toward each other. However, the consensus of most experts on battering is that the type of repetitive, prolonged, serious assault involving severe injury, done intentionally with minimal provocation, and in the interest of coercive control, that constitutes actual abuse, is almost exclusively reserved for women (Dobash & Dobash, 1979).

Abuse is not restricted to heterosexual relationships. Battering in lesbian and gay relationships has recently been described in the literature and in public forums on domestic violence (Lobel, 1986; Renzetti, 1989). The fundamental dynamic of an individual using violence to exert power and maintain control over their intimate partner may be similar in abusive heterosexual and homosexual relationships (NiCarthy, 1986). However, the theoretical and empirical studies conducted with heterosexual couples cannot be assumed to translate directly to the experiences of homosexual couples. Because virtually all available literature reports focus on male-to-female violence, this chapter is confined to abuse in heterosexual relationships. Nurses should be aware of the possibility of abuse within homosexual relationships in the clinical practice setting.

Scope of the Problem

To determine the incidence of abuse of female partners, most authors have relied on physical abuse as the criterion for estimation of incidence. Incidence estimates of severe and repeated battering range from 10% to 50% of the heterosexual couples in the United States (Russell, 1990; Straus & Gelles, 1986). The estimates found in the literature vary widely because abuse is difficult to uncover. Investigators have had to use indirect measures, such as the number of wife abuse claims handled by family courts

(O'Brien, 1971), the number of domestic disturbance calls reported to police departments (Dobash
& Dobash, 1979), or the number of battered women
using public social agencies. Perhaps the most systematic and accurate indication of the amount of
violence against wives is derived from two national,
representative sample surveys of family violence
done by Straus et al. (Straus, Gelles, & Steinmetz,
1988; Straus & Gelles, 1986). The first survey, based
on self-reports from 2,143 individual family members, showed that 3.8% of the women in the sample, or one of 26 American wives, are beaten by
their husbands every year (Straus, et al.). Similar
percentages were found in the second national survey conducted 10 years later that involved a larger
sample (Straus & Gelles). These results indicate that
at least 1.8 million wives are abused per year in this
country alone. Estimates from other nations indicate equally widespread and serious incidence
(Chester & Streather, 1972; Heffner, 1977-78; Russell
& Van de Ven, 1976). To make the numbers more
meaningful, a nurse should remember that it is
likely that approximately one in every ten women
who are in intimate heterosexual relationships, *encountered in any health care setting,* is a victim of abuse
by her male partner (Sampselle, 1991).

Significance as a Health Problem

Battering by an intimate partner may be the single
most common cause of injury to women nationally,
occurring more often than auto accidents, muggings, and rape combined (Stark & Flitcraft, 1988).
In a review of records of 481 women who sought
treatment in a hospital emergency room during 1
month, Stark, Flitcraft, and Frazier (1979) found
10% who had definitely been battered at least once,
15% who had trauma histories indicative of partner
assault, and another 16% with injuries suggestive of
abuse. The physical health problems that women
may experience as a direct consequence of abuse
include bruises, lacerations, abrasions, fractured
bones, head injuries leading to loss of consciousness, and internal abdominal injuries (Dobash &
Dobash, 1979; Drake, 1982; Okun, 1986; Pagelow,
1981; Walker, 1984). Less extreme, but equally debilitating are the long-term health sequelae of
chronic pain and disability from repeated physical
damage, stress-related problems of depression and
anxiety, and the damaging coping behaviors of alcohol and drug abuse (Jaffe, Wolfe, Wilson, & Zak,
1986; Stark & Flitcraft, 1988; Walker, 1984).

In examining abuse of female partners as a serious health problem, the emotional effects on the
women, not only of the violence itself but also of the
psychological abuse typically inflicted on these
women, must also be considered. Some authors
have included emotional or psychological dimensions in their formal definitions of abusive behavior,
and several accept the woman defining herself as
abused, regardless of the consequences. Forms of
psychological abuse certainly exist, which would be
potential precursors to physical violence and therefore in need of nursing intervention, but this analysis is limited to abuse resulting in physical injury.
Emotional abuse is considered a sign of family dysfunction and is examined as such in Chapter 8.

Abuse and Homicide
Homicide of women

One of the most frightening aspects of abuse of female partners is its connection with homicide of
women. The level of danger for women in abusive
relationships is verified by U.S. Crime Report data
that one third of all female homicide victims were
murdered by a husband or boyfriend (Federal Bureau of Investigation, 1986). Research suggests that
wife abuse was a significant antecedent factor in
these homicides (Bourdouris, 1971; Russell, 1990).
As Walker (1979) states, "homicide between man and
woman is not a 'crime of passion' but rather the end
result of unchecked, long-standing violence" (p. 27).

The most direct relationship between wife abuse
and homicide of women was found in a study by
Gregory (1976), who learned that the majority of
husbands who killed their wives in England and
Wales between 1957 and 1968 had previously assaulted them. A later study of homicide in England
and Wales revealed that 58% of the female victims
were married to or sexually intimate with their killers (Dobash & Dobash, 1979).

Research in the United States supports the relationship between wife abuse and murder of women. A nursing research study conducted by Campbell (1981) used a retrospective analysis of the police files of murdered women and women who perpetrated homicide in Dayton, Ohio. The findings of this study cannot be generalized, but they follow the tradition of several epidemiological investigations of homicide in various urban areas to identify possible factors affecting inner-city homicide. The most significant finding of the study was that, between 1975 and 1979, 71.9% of the intersex killing between husbands and wives, boyfriends and girlfriends, or estranged intimate relationships, involved a prior history of wife abuse. Of the 28 women who were killed by a man in an intimate relationship, 18 (64.3%) had been abused by that man. In these cases, the battering was reported to the police by family members or friends and neighbors when they were interviewed after the crime. Unless the police asked, the information was usually not offered, and the police frequently neither inquired nor did they always interview someone who might have known of abuse between the couple. Thus the 64.3% figure may be an underestimation.

Battered women themselves are acutely aware that they are in danger of being killed. It is estimated that women are at greatest risk of being murdered when they take deliberate action to sever a dangerously abusive relationship (Browne, 1987; Okun, 1986). Women frequently remain in the relationship because of the realistic fear of life-threatening consequences, but their fear has not always been treated as valid by the public (Roy, 1977). The Dayton data show that 30% of the female homicide victims from 1974 to 1979 who were killed by a husband or boyfriend, had divorced, separated from, or broken up with the man who later murdered them. Several other cases involved women who were trying to end the relationship (Campbell, 1981). Makman (1978) theorizes that violent men are often dependent on control of their female partners for continued self-esteem and that actual or threatened loss of the partner by separation or divorce may lead to "paranoia," increasing the danger of further violence and murder. Elbow (1977) asserts,

"The abusive husband in formal or common law marriages is strongly opposed to his wife's terminating the relationship to the extent of threatening to kill her, and in some instances, carrying out the threat" (p. 515).

Homicide of the abuser

Nationwide, approximately 2,000 women are incarcerated for murdering their batterers (Grossfeld, 1991). Women do not usually kill; they perpetrate 14% of the homicides in the United States (Browne & Williams, 1989). When women do kill, it often involves a male partner and is done in self-defense. However, as Gillespie (1989) describes in her thorough treatise on justifiable homicide, women who have killed their batterers traditionally have been charged with first- or second-degree murder or a reduced charge of manslaughter, or they have had to plead temporary insanity. Because the battered woman's lethal act is often temporally removed from assaults directed at her, she usually could not claim self-defense as the motive for her action. Legally, self-defense requires the reasonable belief of imminent danger of death or serious injury and that the action taken was a reasonable response to perceived danger rather than an overreaction (Gillespie). Fortunately, many courts have recently broadened the definition of self-defense in response to the circumstances of battered women. Despite intense public and legal controversy, governors in several states have granted clemency to battered women currently serving prison sentences, because their actions are now considered justifiable (Grossfeld, 1991).

To learn more about women's circumstances before they killed their batterers, Browne (1987) interviewed 42 women who were facing murder or attempted murder charges in the death or serious injury of their mates. Their accounts of their relationships were then compared with accounts of women who were in abusive relationships but had not taken lethal action. Several important differences became apparent. The men who had been killed had a history of frequent intoxication, abused prescription and street drugs, had extensive police records for a variety of criminal offenses, had often threatened to kill someone, and had abused their own children significantly more than the men in the nonhomicide group. Furthermore, the women who were charged with murder had sustained significantly more severe injury and been injured more often, including frequent rapes, than women whose abusive partners were still living. Browne also found that, over the years of the relationship, the women had, indeed, made many attempts to obtain outside intervention for the violence directed at them; the responses received from the police and legal system were ineffective. Browne concluded that women who murder their abusers have become trapped in a seemingly inescapable spiral of escalating violence against them, desperately fear for their lives and the lives of their children, and therefore take lethal action for survival. A smaller nursing study of 12 women incarcerated for killing their batterers supported most of Browne's conclusions, with the exception that the women did not note an escalation in the frequency or severity of the physical or sexual abuse directed at them before murdering the batterer (Foster, Veale, & Fogel, 1989).

Interface of Wife Abuse and Nursing

Despite the prevalence of wife abuse and its serious health consequences, women in abusive relationships are often undetected in the health care setting. In the study of 481 women entering a hospital emergency room, physicians had identified 14 battered women (2.8%), although an additional 72 women (16%) had injuries deemed as indicative of abuse by the investigators (Stark et al., 1979). In a later review of 3,676 medical records of women seen for injuries in an urban emergency room, clinicians identified only one in 35 battered women, even though scrutiny of the records indicated that 19% of the injured women had a history of abuse (Stark & Flitcraft, 1988).

The psychological consequences of living in an abusive relationship often lead women to seek help from mental health services. Hilberman and Munson (1977-78) noted that one half of all women referred by the medical staff of a rural health clinic for psychiatric evaluation were found to be victims of marital violence. The history of violence was known to the referring physician in only four of the 60 cases, although most of the women and their children received ongoing medical care at the clinic. Other investigators point out that women's experiences of psychological and sexual abuse are likely to manifest themselves as symptoms of depression, anxiety, and other psychological disorders, thus incurring mental illness labels and psychopharmacological treatment rather than attention to the underlying problem of abuse (Rosewater, 1988; Stark et al., 1979). This is substantiated by findings that abused women are more likely than nonabused women to leave an emergency room with prescriptions for pain killers and tranquilizers (Stark et al., 1979) and by survey findings that 18% of women in shelters brought psychoactive prescription medications with them (Okun, 1986). Women's suicide attempts are another alarming manifestation of abuse that may come to the attention of mental health nurses. Stark et al. (1981) estimate that 26% of all female suicide attempts during the year of their hospital research were associated with battering relationships. By their calculation, women in abusive relationships experience a relative risk of attempted suicide that is 4.8 times higher than nonbattered women.

The widespread incidence of battering during pregnancy suggests another important area where wife abuse can be identified and attended to by nurses. Prenatal clinics, private obstetrical offices, childbirth education classes, and inpatient postpartum services are all places where nurses can be alert for women who have been abused by their partners. Walker's (1984) research with 403 battered women found a high incidence of battering with each pregnancy; 59% reported battering in the first pregnancy, 63% during the second, and 55% during the third. Drake's (1982) pilot exploratory study revealed that the 11 women who had ever been pregnant had all been beaten during the pregnancy. In a recent random sample of 290 healthy pregnant women, 8% reported battering during the current pregnancy and 15% reported battering that predated the current pregnancy (Helton, McFarlane, & Anderson, 1987a). It is ironic that prenatal care routinely includes close monitoring for physiological disorders, some of which are very rare, in the interest of healthy outcomes for mothers and infants, yet does not routinely include screening for physical abuse from the woman's partner. The nursing research program of Helton, Bullock, Anderson, and McFarlane has been pivotal in attracting the attention of the March of Dimes and the Centers for Disease Control to the need for further research and interventions to alleviate battering during pregnancy (Bullock, McFarlane, Bateman, & Miller, 1989; Helton, 1987; Helton, McFarlane, & Anderson, 1987b).

In community health settings, nurses are in key positions to identify and address abuse toward women by virtue of their acceptance in clients' homes and long-term involvement with families and communities. In such settings, wife abuse may easily be revealed if the nurse is alert to the possibility and gently asks opening questions. Most battered women welcome the opportunity to discuss their experiences if they are questioned in a nonjudgmental manner and are in a safe and private environment. Fortunately, as nurses become increasingly aware of the problem, they are taking active roles in both identifying and providing services for battered women in the practice setting or in shelters for battered women and their children (Campbell, 1986; Campbell & Humphreys, 1987; Hollenkamp & Attala, 1986).

HISTORICAL PERSPECTIVE

Abuse of female partners is not a new problem in society. Abuse of women has deep historical roots and continues to be condoned and even legally sanctioned in many societies. Dobash and Dobash (1979) place such abuse in its historical context as a form of behavior that has

> . . . existed for centuries as an acceptable, and, indeed, a desirable part of a patriarchal family system within a patriarchal society, and much of the ideology and many of the institutional arrangements which supported the patriarchy through the subordination, domination and control of women are still reflected in our culture and our social institutions. (p. 31)

From several excellent historical studies of wife abuse, a brief synopsis is presented to increase understanding of current violence against women and the traditional responses of social institutions.

The Bible provides the earliest prescription for physical punishment of wives. Deuteronomy 22:13-21 gives a law condemning brides to death by stoning if unable to prove virginity (Davidson, 1977). In early Rome, husbands and fathers could legally beat or put women to death for many reasons, but especially for adultery or suspected infidelity, reflecting "not so much thwarted love but loss of control and damage to a possession" (Dobash & Dobash, 1979, p. 37). Jesus was more egalitarian in his thinking, but the sexist statements of Saint Paul set the tone for the Christian church. Constantine, the emperor and religious leader of the Byzantine branch of Christianity, set the example for treatment of wives by putting his own young wife to death by scalding (Davidson, 1977). By medieval times, the widespread nature of wifebeating had been documented in several ways. According to Spanish law, a woman who committed adultery could be killed with impunity. In France, female sexual infidelity was punishable by beating, as was disobedience. Italian men punished unfaithful women with severe flogging and exile for 3 years (Dobash & Dobash, 1979). A medieval theological manual refers to the necessity of men beating their wives "for correction," according to church doctrine. A Catholic abbé decried the common cruelty to and murder of the wives of prominent Christian men (Davidson, 1977).

Dobash and Dobash explain that the medieval "age of chivalry" was actually an attitude based on the ideal of female chastity before marriage and subsequent fidelity that were important aspects of male property rights and outward signs of the master maintaining control. This glorification of women as asexual, weak adornments actually contributed to their subjugation and was associated with the use of male force in rescues and tournaments. The close of the Middle Ages saw the rise of the nuclear family as well as the development of modern states and the beginning of capitalism, all of which eroded the position of women and strengthened the authority of men. In sixteenth-century England there was a campaign in support of the nuclear family and loyalty to husband and the king, who was trying to consolidate his power. Allegiance to fathers and husbands was equated with loyalty to the king and God (Dobash & Dobash, 1979).

Effects of Capitalism and Protestantism

Capitalism and Protestantism rose together. The basic unit of production moved outside the family, and for the first time wages were paid for work on a regular basis. Wives became separated from production and exchange. Because domestic work received no wages, it became devalued. The Protestant religion idealized marriage and equated wifely obedience with moral duty. The head of the household gained much of the power that formerly belonged to priests (Dobash & Dobash, 1979). Martin Luther is considered less misogynistic than most of the men in his time, but even he equated female autonomy with the woman's role and admitted to boxing his wife's ear when she got "saucy" (Davidson, 1977). John Knox insisted that the "natural" subordination of women was ordained by God. Wifebeating was discouraged by the Protestant theologians, but the husbands' right to do so was acknowledged and the practice was widespread (Dobash & Dobash, 1979). As May (1978) explains, "children, property, earning, and even the wife's conscience belonged to the husband" (p. 38). During the seventeenth, eighteenth, and nineteenth centuries in the Western world, there was little objection to the husband using force provided it did not exceed certain limits. The wife could be beaten if she "caused jealousy, was lazy, unwilling to work in the fields, became drunk, spent too much money, or neglected the house" (May, 1978, p. 138). The prevailing perception that women's position was privileged and protected was therefore in direct opposition to women's reality.

While the Reformation set the tone in the rest of Europe, Napoleon influenced France, Holland, Italy, and sections of Switzerland and Germany. He thought of wives as "fickle, defenseless, mindless beings, tending toward Eve-like evil" and deserving

of punishment for misdeeds as "causing" bankruptcy or criminality in her husband (Davidson, 1977, pp. 14-16). He is quoted as saying to the Council of State:

> The husband must possess the absolute power and right to say to his wife: "Madam, you shall not go out, you shall not go to the theatre, you shall not receive such and such a person; for the children you bear shall be mine." (Davidson, 1977, p. 15)

The common saying of the times was, "Women, like walnut trees, should be beaten every day" (Davidson, 1977, p. 14). German husbands had a duty to beat their wives for misdemeanors during this period; they were subject to fine if they did not. In France, King Humbert IV declared, "Every inhabitant of Villefranche has the right to beat his wife, providing death does not ensue" (Janssen-Jurreit, 1982, pp. 225-26).

British common law in the eighteenth century also established the legal right of a man to use force with his wife to ensure that she fulfilled her wifely obligations, "the consummation of marriage, cohabitation, conjugal rights, sexual fidelity and general obedience and respect for his wishes" (Dobash & Dobash, 1979, pp. 14, 74). John Stuart Mill petitioned Parliament to end the brutal treatment of British wives in 1869. The legal changes that followed were directed not toward eliminating the practice of wifebeating but toward limiting the amount of damage that was being done. The nineteenth century in England was also marked by more tolerance of conjugal violence in the lower classes while more chivalry was expected by the upper classes (May, 1978).

Historical Influence Today

In our own country, founded on the equal rights of *men,* not of women, John Adams rejected his wife's plea for better treatment of women in the new government. Sir William Blackstone's interpretation of English law, which upheld the husband's right to employ moderate chastisement in response to improper wifely behavior, was used as a model for American law. In 1824, the state of Mississippi legalized wifebeating, and, in 1886, a proposed law for punishment of wifebeating husbands was defeated in Pennsylvania. North Carolina passed the first law against wifebeating, but the court pronounced that it did not intend to hear cases unless there was permanent damage or danger to life (Davidson, 1977). As late as 1915, a London police magistrate reaffirmed that wives could be beaten at home legally as long as the stick used was no bigger than the man's thumb ("the rule of thumb" from a 1782 judge's proclamation) (Dobash & Dobash, 1979; May, 1978). Clearly, the law has condoned violence to wives for centuries. The influences of the history of wifebeating remain today, not only in the behavior of husbands but also in the attitudes of the courts, police, and society. The conclusion of Dobash and Dobash (1979) is an appropriate summary:

> The ideologies and institutions that made such treatment both possible and justifiable have survived, albeit somewhat altered from century to century, and have been woven into the fabric of our culture and are thriving today. (p. 31)

THEORETICAL FRAMEWORKS

Wife abuse was barely recognized, and certainly not carefully studied, until the 1970s. Scholarly attention to the issue has increased exponentially in the past decade as public funds have been allocated for research, education, treatment services, and prevention programs. Diverse and competing theories from the social and health sciences have been offered to explain the social structures, cultural traditions, and personal behaviors that create and perpetuate abuse and violence. However, the relatively scarce current empirical work, is often inadequate in design and inconsistent in findings. One of the primary purposes of the early research was to establish the widespread prevalence of the problem and to explode the myth that wifebeating is confined to a few pathologically exceptional individuals. This goal has been achieved through large national surveys and smaller descriptive studies. In addition, descriptive studies have been helpful in identifying factors associated with abuse of female partners. However, few studies have used statistically sophis-

ticated analysis or nonabused comparison groups, and little has been done to formulate or empirically test explanatory theories of wife abuse. Therefore theory development and testing regarding abuse of female partners is in its infancy.

The literature on the causes of wife abuse reflects the diverse disciplinary perspectives addressing the problem. As with the literature on violence in general, there are viewpoints that emphasize the psychological, sociological, and biological determinants of abuse. In addition, there is a feminist body of literature that critically analyzes the patriarchal roots of the phenomenon as well as the theoretical formulations and research regarding wife abuse. The literature also reflects many commendable attempts to integrate these viewpoints and resist the temptation to rely on simplistic, single-cause formulations.

Theories of Causation
Traditional psychiatric viewpoints

Studies of wife abuse before the 1970s were generally from the field of psychiatry and tended to focus on the individual psychopathology of the abuser and his victim. Traditionally, the intrapsychic basis of battering was assumed to be related to masochism. The underlying assumptions include ideas that the battered woman enjoys abuse and deliberately provokes attacks because of her need to suffer (Martin, 1976). For example, in response to 12 case studies, a group of psychiatrists concluded, "We see the husband's aggressive behavior as freeing masochistic needs of the wife and to be necessary for the wife's (and the couple's) equilibrium" (Snell, Rosenwald, & Robey, 1964, p. 110). Such studies generally used small samples, often drawn from already diagnosed mentally ill populations, and are biased by adherence to the Freudian conceptualization that all women have masochistic tendencies. In contrast, reports published after 1970 conclude that wife abusers and their victims are no more likely to be diagnosed as mentally ill than the rest of the population and dismiss the myth of female masochism (Renvoize, 1978).

Despite the overwhelming rejection of masochism as a causative factor in wife abuse, some vestiges of the theory remain in the research literature and popular press. Shainess (1979) redefines masochists as women who do not enjoy suffering, but do employ an "all pervasive cognitive style" of submission and self-destruction that makes them more vulnerable to violence (pp. 174, 188).

Another vestige of the masochism myth is revealed when authors overemphasize the role of the woman in provoking abuse. On the basis of 23 cases of men in custody for murdering or assaulting their wives, Faulk (1974) concluded that nine of the wives were so "demanding" that the husband finally "exploded" and attacked her, implying that *her* behavior was the problem. It is morally impossible to justify murdering, attempting to murder, or harming someone because of excessive verbal demands. As Walker (1979) states, "By perpetuating the belief that it is rational to blame the victim for her abuse, we ultimately excuse men for the crime" (p. 15). The lenient sentences that Faulk's offenders received reflect this belief; their lack of previous offenses and the circumstances of their crimes led the "court to a sympathetic approach" (p. 183).

A separate viewpoint of psychiatric literature is represented by Bach and Wyden (1969), who maintain that fighting between married couples is necessary for true intimacy. They prefer verbal conflict and advocative rules to keep the fights fair but assert, "We believe that the exchange of spanks, blows and slaps between consenting adults is more civilized than the camouflaged or silent hostilities of ostensibly well-behaved fight-evaders . . . " (pp. 1, 111). In contrast to this view, there is substantial evidence from studies of abused wives showing that physical attack is often preceded by verbal arguments; that spouses who scream also tend to use violent means of conflict resolution; that, as the level of verbal aggression increases, the level of physical aggression increases even more rapidly; and that physical abuse, once begun, escalates over time (Dobash & Dobash, 1979; Steinmetz, 1977; Walker, 1984). Bach and Wyden operate from a catharsis belief that the wife abuse literature has tended to disprove, adding to the weight of evidence against it from other studies reviewed in Chapter 2.

The role of alcohol and other drugs

Alcohol and drug abuse of the perpetrator. Alcohol abuse has consistently been noted in connection with wife abuse, but has not been proved as an actual cause. As chemical abuse and addiction continue to spiral in the United States, concern is also raised about violence associated with cocaine and other illicit drugs. Hotaling and Sugarman's (1986) analysis of 52 case-comparison studies led them to conclude that alcohol usage was a consistent risk marker for men's use of violence against female partners. Kantor and Straus' (1987) analysis of data from the National Family Violence Survey of 6,002 households found that excessive drinking is associated with higher rates of wife abuse, but alcohol was *not* used immediately before an assault in 76% of the cases of husband-to-wife violence. A study by Van Hasselt, Morrison and Bellack (1985) revealed that men who physically abused their wives had significantly stronger evidence of alcoholism when compared with two groups of nonviolent couples. Similarly, as a counselor for men who batter their partners, Okun (1986) estimated that 64% of the 119 abusive men in his study were active problem drinkers. Although alcohol use and violence are correlated in several studies, the investigators point out that alcohol is only one factor among many that *interact* to create abuse of female partners.

The methods of gathering and reporting the data on alcohol and drug usage vary considerably, leaving many questions unanswered. Is the batterer always drunk when he is abusive? Conversely, is he always abusive when drunk? Is alcohol or drug abuse a problem in other facets of his life, or is it limited to his interactions with his partner? Is the batterer intoxicated when he becomes abusive, or has he had only a few drinks? Until more of these questions are answered, the role of alcohol and other drugs in abuse of female partners will remain unclear.

Alcohol is commonly believed to have a biochemically "disinhibiting effect," whereby a person's usual voluntary behavioral constraints are temporarily removed, and may result in aggressive behavior. Other theorists speculate that intoxicated behavior is, to some extent, learned. Individuals are excused and forgiven for violent behavior that occurs while drinking; drinking thus provides a "grace period" when one may behave in ways that would be unacceptable if sober (Gayford, 1979; Gelles, 1974; Kantor & Straus, 1987). Gelles notes that alcohol can provide an "excuse in advance," since alcoholism is regarded as an illness in our society, and behavior under the influence is seen as uncharacteristic and uncontrollable (Gelles, 1974). Walker (1979) found that for the problem drinkers described by her sample of battered women, "Drinking seemed to give them a sense of power," which was then demonstrated by violence (p. 24). Downey and Howell (1976) conclude that men who batter women may drink *in order to* carry out violence. In summary, a correlation between alcohol abuse and wife battering has been established that is similar to the connections between alcohol and violence in general described in Chapter 1. Alcohol as a *cause* of wife abuse has been neither claimed nor demonstrated, and explanations for the phenomenon vary considerably.

Alcohol and drug abuse of the victim. Research on wife abuse rarely includes information on the woman's use of alcohol and other drugs. Available data suggest that alcohol is infrequently abused by battered wives (Hotaling & Sugarman, 1986; Kantor & Straus, 1987; Van Hasselt et al., 1985). However, living with abuse and becoming dependent on alcohol and other drugs are intertwined problems for many women. Counselors who work with women in chemical dependency programs are beginning to realize that chemically dependent women are at high risk for relationship abuse and are likely to have abuse and violence in their backgrounds (Ladwig & Andersen, 1989; Woodhouse, 1990). In a similar fashion, those who work with battered women are aware that the use and abuse of alcohol and drugs is one way of coping with the abusive relationship and with society's lack of response to her circumstances. Experiential insights are supported by research that correlates women's experiences of violence with chemical dependency. Review of the medical records of injured women in an emergency room suggested that indicators of physical battery preceded documentation of alcohol use in 15% of

the women (Stark et al., 1979). Using a life history approach with 25 women in a chemical dependency program, more than half the women reported past rapes, incest, child abuse, or domestic violence, and most had experienced the violence before their addictions. The women stated that they had been medicating their pain and feelings of fear and worthlessness (Woodhouse, 1990). Clearly, programs for chemically dependent women and battered women must competently address both problems.

Socialization for abuse

Social learning and/or situational stress or frustration factors are often emphasized as the key components that lead to wife abuse. Murray Straus and his colleagues at the Family Research Laboratory at the University of New Hampshire have developed a multifactorial system that recognizes the societal background of a high level of violence in our culture, the sexist organization of the society and its family system, and cultural norms legitimizing violence against family members (Hotaling & Straus, 1980; Straus, 1979; Yllo & Straus, 1990). With this background of societal influences, Straus points out that the family is inherently at high risk for violent interaction by virtue of the great amount of time family members spend interacting; the broad range of activities over which conflict can occur; the intensity of emotional involvement of the members; the involuntary nature of family membership; the infringement of family members on each other's personal space, time, and life-styles; and the assumption of family members that they have the right to try to change each other's behavior (Straus, 1980). Within these societal and familial contexts, Straus and others believe that people can be socialized to use violence for conflict resolution. Children learn this by observing parental violence, experiencing physical punishment, seeing their parents tolerate sibling fighting, and, if boys, being taught to value violence. This socialization teaches the association of love with violence and justifies the use of physical force as a morally correct means of solving disputes.

Abusive behaviors learned in childhood. Much theoretical and empirical attention has focused on the idea that men's abuse of women is behavior learned in childhood—a notion derived from social-learning theory. The hypothesis states that boys who are reared in violent homes learn to use aggression to cope with a variety of negative feelings; this leads to long-term consequences of becoming an abusive parent or spouse, or developing other criminally abusive behaviors in adulthood. In Roy's (1977) sample of violent husbands, 81.1% were reported to have been victims of child abuse or had parents who used violence with each other. In a study of 57 families, all patterns of conflict resolution repeated themselves for at least three generations with a consistent degree of violence (Steinmetz, 1977). In Walker's (1984) large sample, battering was reported in 81% of the abusive men's childhood homes, compared with only 24% of the homes of nonbattering male partners. Other samples show variations from 27% to 59% of abusive men having witnessed and/or experienced violence in their homes as children (Carlson, 1977; Dobash & Dobash, 1979; Gayford, 1979). Okun's (1986) work with 119 abusive men revealed that men who had, as children, witnessed abuse between their parents, and men who had been physically abused in childhood committed significantly more assaults on their wives than men who were raised in nonviolent homes. Furthermore, men who had grown up with both experiences of witnessing and receiving abuse committed even more severe assaults on their partners.

Confidence in the research findings regarding men's childhood experiences with abuse is seriously limited for several reasons. First, information about the batterer's childhood experiences relies on the accuracy of his memory and on his perceptions of what constitutes abusive behaviors. Second, much of the available information on men who batter their female partners has been obtained indirectly through interviews with the woman who has been abused. Research samples that include the batterer have relied on men in therapeutic groups or treatment programs, many of whom are under court order to attend the program and therefore may not be forthcoming with information that could prolong their program (Fagan, Stewart, & Hansen, 1983). Finally, the descriptive statistics of specific populations with these studies cannot be used to demonstrate cause and effect. In a thorough analysis of the literature, Widom (1989) concluded that there is little empirical support for the linear notion of the intergenerational transmission of violence. The long-term outcomes of early childhood experiences with aggression may reflect the interaction of many as yet unidentified factors.

Another aspect of learning suspected to promote abuse of women is the influence of television and other entertainment media. The most attractive men on television, or the most favored cartoon characters, epitomize cultural stereotypes of masculinity, dominance in their heterosexual relationships, and use of violence with impunity. Most television husbands control their families, and some programs convey the effectiveness of verbal abuse. Aggression, or the threat of aggression, is shown as an effective way to achieve power, success, and control. Beaulieu (1978) thinks that this "important, insidious and pervasive impact" of television that fosters "norms, values and attitudes which favor violence" is an important factor in family violence (pp. 60-62).

Gender differences in learning. Some authors have also linked social-learning theory to the women's role as victim. Gelles theorizes that the more frequently a woman was hit by her parents, the more vulnerable she is to being a victim of marital violence (Gelles, 1974, 1976). The mechanism supposedly at work is that a woman learns to be a victim by prior conditioning (Shainess, 1979). Unfortunately, this theory echoes the masochism myth in a slightly different form—because women have learned to be victims, they somehow precipitate abuse from their partners and accept their further victimization. Gelles' (1976) findings support this view to some degree; in his sample of 80 families, women who observed spousal violence in the family of origin were more likely to be victims of violence in their family of procreation. Parker and Schumacker's (1977) controlled pilot study of 50 women (20 battered and 30 nonbattered women) found a positive correlation between the woman's mother being a victim of abuse and the probability that the woman would be battered by her husband. In Walker's (1984) sample of 403 battered women, battering was reported in 67% of the women's childhood homes. In addition, 48% of the women reported being victims of sexual abuse as children.

Contradictory evidence, however, abounds in available research. For example, Carroll (1977), using a control group of nonviolent couples, was surprised to note that daughters who received less physical punishment from their fathers were *more* likely to report that violence was a problem in their current conjugal relationship than those women who had been subjected to a greater amount of punishment in their childhood. Only 29% of the abused wives studied by Dobash and Dobash (1979) reported any violence at all in their childhood homes. Okun's (1986) record review of 300 women in a battered women's shelter showed no difference in the prevalence of past childhood violence compared with American women in general.

In all these studies, the level of childhood violence was significantly higher for the abusers than for the victims. Approximately one fourth of the battered women in Pagelow's (1981) study saw their mothers being beaten by their fathers, whereas more than half of their batterers had observed such behavior. The men were also punished significantly more often and severely than the women (19% of the women were severely victimized as children versus 48% of their spouses). By using a small control group of nonbattered women, Star (1978) found that 35% of the battered women came from homes where they experienced or witnessed violence, whereas 50% of the control group had similar experiences. The situation for the violent husbands was clearly the opposite; 55% observed beating or had been abused, whereas only 17% of the nonviolent men had abuse in their childhood backgrounds. The preponderance of evidence thus seems to indicate that social-learning theory potentially offers explanatory value for the behavior of abusive men, but does not consistently account for women's experiences in abusive intimate adult relationships.

Family stress

Social scientists also emphasize situational and societal stressors as causative factors in abuse of female partners. Steinmetz (1977) points out that the

family has to absorb emotional tension from both external and internal sources. This approach echoes the frustration leading to aggression theory on general violence. This is thought to be especially important in the context of the family since, "In general, people tend to take out their frustration on those to whom they are closest" (Shainess, 1977, p. 112). Central to this argument is the idea that poverty or low social status creates excessive stress in the family. As Carlson (1977) states, "Sources of family violence are complex structural circumstances creating environmental stresses that are distributed unevenly across the social structure" (pp. 456, 458). Her sample of 101 cases of abusive families included 29% unemployed males and 37% earning less than $9,000 per year. Only 7.6% of the battering husbands were in professional occupations. Using data from the 1975 National Family Violence Survey, Straus (1990) found that, although educational level had little influence on a man's use of violence against his wife, men of lower socioeconomic status were significantly more violent toward their wives than were men of adequate financial means. Gayford (1979) concludes that wifebeaters have a low frustration tolerance. Because they have seen crises solved with aggression and violence, they respond to stress and frustration from outside the home with violence within the home, especially if inhibitions are lowered by alcohol.

Other data tend to contradict these findings. For example, Flynn (1977) found no relationship to socioeconomic status in his review of police records on familial assaults, but he did find the majority of his families to be under stress of some kind. Montgomery County, Maryland, one of the nation's wealthiest suburbs, reported a high incidence of verified assaults on wives (Langley & Levy, 1977). During the same period in 1974, Norwalk, Connecticut, a middle-class community, and Harlem, New York, had an approximately equal incidence (per 100,000 population) of wife abuse reported to police (Barden & Barden, 1976). Nearly 70% of 119 abusive men in counseling were employed (Okun, 1986). Many of the women in Walker's (1984) research reported that income was not a problem; however, the abusive man had extravagant spending binges, leaving the woman to manage the household with little money. Hotaling and Sugarman's (1986) research literature analysis confirms that income level, educational level, occupational level, or race do not discriminate assaultive husbands from nonassaultive husbands. Although many studies do not reflect this, the skewed information is likely related to the fact that battered women with financial resources are unlikely to be available for research participation. Women with financial means are less likely to report abuse to the police, to resort to battered women's shelters, from which most research samples are drawn, or to use public social service agencies. Another problem with citing poverty and/or unemployment as the main stressor leading to wife abuse is its failure to account for the preponderance of males who are doing the battering when the wife in such a situation would be equally frustrated or stressed.

The theory is better supported and made more explanatory when linked to the male's prescribed role in society. The possibility of wife abuse being related to the woman surpassing the man in terms of education, occupation, and/or income is suggested by several authors (Carlson, 1977; Prescott & Letko, 1977). As Langley and Levy (1977) state, "Many wifebeaters regard themselves as inadequate in some aspect of the prescribed male role in our society" (p. 53). Another way to describe the same mechanism is to consider the husband's use of violence as compensation for his lack of resources (financial, educational, occupational) needed to maintain his assumed dominant role in the family and in the culture. O'Brien's (1971) study of 150 middle- and working-class applicants for divorce showed that more of the abusing husbands were underachievers in their work role in terms of education or satisfaction with their job than those who were nonviolent. Gelles (1974) found a higher level of abuse when the wife's job was of higher status than the husband's, when the husband's occupational status was lower than the neighbors', and when unemployment was a threat in the man's job.

Other stressors that have been suggested as contributors to wife abuse include the husband's poor verbal skills, social isolation of the family resulting in decreased social support, pregnancy and other family developmental crises, differing religions or lack of family religion, and chronic health problems that drain economic and personal resources (Gelles, 1974). When social scientists link stress to social-learning theory and the norms and values regarding violence and marital relationships in our culture, they have identified a potentially important group of factors predisposing toward wife abuse. However, conclusions cannot be drawn from the mainly anecdotal evidence or from the relatively small statistical relationships that are available. The other primary criticism of this viewpoint is its lack of parsimony and terms of emphasis, not faulty reasoning. Although such researchers as Steinmetz and Straus mention "the male dominance and machismo values and norms which form a subtle but powerful part of our sexual and family system," they fail to see this as perhaps the underlying causative factor (Steinmetz & Straus, 1974, p. 20).

Cultural support for wife abuse

There is widespread cultural support for wife abuse. Collusion between cultural norms and abuse of female partners is reflected in several surveys of public attitudes toward assault of women. In a national, representative 1968 poll of 1,176 American adults, one fifth approved of "slapping one's spouse on appropriate occasions" (Stark & McEvoy, 1970). In a primarily male sample of college students and middle-class businessmen, 62% thought that violence would be justified if the spouse was involved in extramarital sex (Whitehurst, 1971). The majority of 1,626 men questioned about their perceptions of sanctions for wife assault believed that men could, indeed, physically abuse their wives with impunity; adverse consequences in terms of social condemnation or legal penalty were perceived as minimal (Carmody & Williams, 1987). Such tolerant attitudes are not limited to men. A cross-sectional survey of 422 adult women found that nearly 19% of the sample accepted the idea that a wife may deserve a beating if she flirts with other men, has an affair with another man, becomes drunk, or nags (Gentemann, 1984). Of a national sample of married people, 27.6% thought that slapping a spouse was necessary, normal, or good (Dibble & Straus, 1980). These authors warn the reader that consistency between attitudes and behavior cannot be taken for granted according to their research.

More specific and behavioral, but less generalizable, evidence for the presence of socioculture attitudes supporting wife abuse is demonstrated in two laboratory studies. In one study, Straus (1976) gave student subjects a description of an assault of a woman by a man that resulted in her losing consciousness. If the subjects were told the couple was married, they suggested a significantly less severe punishment for the man than if they were described as "going together." In another laboratory study, a staged physical attack on a female by a male resulted in 65% of the subjects intervening when they had been led to believe the pair were strangers versus only 19% intervening when they thought the couple was married (Shotland & Straw, 1976). Those authors concluded: "If bystanders, and, one would guess, society do not regard wife beating seriously, this act cannot be controlled" (pp. 992, 999). In real life, 21 of Rounsaville's (1978) sample of 31 battered women (68%) had been beaten in public, but only one received any help from strangers.

Wife abuse can also be viewed in the context of behavior that is thought to be appropriate for the male sex in general. The National Commission on the Causes of Violence found that proving masculinity in our culture may require "frequent rehearsals of toughness" and the exploitation of women (Davidson, 1977). As Whitehurst (1974) states, "When all other sources of masculine identity fail, men can always rely on being 'tough' as a sign of manhood" (p. 78). Men who assault their wives live up to cultural prescriptions that are valued in Western society: aggressiveness, male dominance, and female subordination (Dobash & Dobash, 1977-78).

Lester's (1980) cross-cultural study of wife abuse found that wifebeating was significantly more common in societies where the status of women was rated as inferior. In a similar study of primitive societies, Masumura (1979) found wife abuse significantly correlated with other forms of violence, such as warfare, personal crime, and feuding. Extensive analysis of the Human Relations Area Files of 90

preliterate and peasant societies led Levinson (1989) to conclude that the incidence and frequency of wifebeating is greatest in societies in which men control the family wealth, adults engage in violent conflict resolution, men hold domestic authority, and divorce is restricted for women. Unfortunately, Levinson's reliance on cultural information in the preexisting data bank limits confidence in the conclusions. To avoid the methodological biases and information gaps inherent in data banks, Campbell (1985) compared ethnographies of 11 societies written by women researchers who used women as their primary informants. Although cross-cultural patterns were not discerned, culturally specific forms of wife abuse and the cultural norms that may precipitate wife abuse were illuminated.

Carroll (1980) has argued that the elements of a culture tend to be interdependent, that norms of male dominance (as in the Mexican-American culture) and prescriptions against challenging that dominance are consistent with high rates of battering, and that equality and conflict resolution through verbal dialogue supports nonviolence between spouses (as in the Jewish-American culture). These "informal and ideological controls" can become so deeply embedded that they appear natural (Marsden, 1978, p. 116). In a survey of attribution of blame for wifebeating in a written vignette, 23.7% of 338 respondents said the wife was equally to blame for violence against her that was unprovoked or that came after a "heated verbal argument"; 3.3% said she was predominantly or totally to blame (Kalmuss, 1979). Within the context of marriage or other forms of adult intimate relationships, there is clearly both overt and covert cultural support for violence against women.

HISTORICAL FORMS OF VIOLENCE AGAINST WOMEN

It is important to view wife abuse in a wider perspective. A crucial aspect of the cultural support for beating women is derived from the historical and contemporary context of the many forms of violence against women that operate to maintain the patriarchal structure of most societies. Patriarchy can be defined as "any kind of group organization in which males hold dominant power and determine what part females shall and shall not play, and in which capabilities assigned to women are relegated generally to the mystical and aesthetic and excluded from the practical and political realms" (Rich, 1979, p. 78). As Sandelowski (1980) asserts, "women are immobilized by and imprisoned within the fear of violence" (p. 204). Isolated acts of wife abuse do not keep our society sexist, but when the acts are multiplied and coupled with the frightening incidence of rape, homicide of women, and genital mutilation, combined with the historical precedents of suttee, witchburning, footbinding, mutilating surgery, and female infanticide, patriarchy's power can be seen to be based ultimately on violence.

Witchburning is the earliest well-documented form of violence against women. "Tens of thousands of female peasant lay healers and midwives were burned as witches" in Europe and America from the 1500s to the 1700s (Dreifus, 1977, p. xxi). Feminist analysis of this practice has revealed that the main crime of the women involved was a lack of submission to the stereotyped role of the subservient medieval woman. During the same period, the practice of suttee, or inclusion of the widow and concubines in the male's funeral pyre, was being performed in India. The women were often drugged or coerced to the pyre. Even when she was not forced, the widow knew that her alternatives to death on the pyre consisted of prostitution or a life of servitude and starvation with her husband's relatives. Cultural beliefs held the widow to blame for the man's death, if not during her present life, then in her past ones. The Chinese custom of footbinding was forced by male insistence that women were not attractive unless their feet were tiny stumps caused by years of excruciatingly painful breaking of the bones and binding. As a result, women were forced to be absolutely dependent on men, since they could take only a few tottering steps without assistance. In the late nineteenth century Western medicine used the surgical procedures of clitoridectomy, oophorectomy, and hysterectomy to "cure" masturbation, insanity, deviation from the "proper" female role, heightened sexual appetites, and rebellion

against husband or father (Daly, 1978). Radical feminists argue that contemporary medical practices of superfluous hysterectomies, unnecessarily mutilating surgery for breast cancer, the use of the Dalkon Shield intrauterine contraceptive device and diethylstilbestrol (DES), and the coercive sterilization of impoverished or mentally retarded women are evidence of continued violence against women by male-dominated medicine.

CONTEMPORARY FORMS OF VIOLENCE AGAINST WOMEN

Female infanticide, homicide of women, and genital mutilation are three forms of violence directed at females that are rooted in history and continue today. They are found in their most blatant forms in societies that rigidly adhere to male dominance. Janssen-Jurreit (1982) points out that because of the higher life expectancy of females, the proportion of women should be higher in relation to men; however, world statistics show only a 49:50 female-to-male ratio. That proportion is lowest in Arab and Islamic countries. Western countries show a higher male infant mortality rate, whereas Arab and Islamic nations, as well as India, have a significantly higher female infant mortality rate. The statistics seem to indicate "negligent care of female newborns" at the very least. India and the Arabic and Islamic nations also practice the killing of adult women with frightening regularity. Without punishment, men can kill wives and daughters for "public embarrassment," especially "habitual disobedience" and for having illegitimate children in contemporary India (Driver, 1971). In rural Arabic villages a woman who has had sex before marriage is such a stigma to the family that they are obliged to kill her, even if she has been raped (Janssen-Jurreit, 1982; Malik & Salvi, 1976).

Genital mutilation is a widespread form of female destruction practiced in much of East, West, and Central Africa and in parts of the Middle East. The mutilation can take the form of removal of the tip of the clitoris, complete clitoridectomy, or excision of all of the external genitalia except the labia majora and may be accompanied by infibulation, the closure of the wound by sewing with catgut or using thorns, leaving a small opening for urination and menstrual flow. Infibulation involves opening the aperture further for intercourse and childbirth and resewing at the husband's command. The practices are often carried out without anesthesia, with crude instruments, and with no regard for prevention of infection; complications are rampant (Hosken, 1977-78). In Egypt the majority of girls between age 8 and 10 have a clitoridectomy performed. In these cultures such practices are considered necessary for a woman to be marriageable; without marriage, a woman is considered worthless (Janssen-Jurreit, 1982).

A form of violence against women most in the realm of public awareness is rape. Dworkin (1976) states: "Rape is no excess, no aberration, no accident, no mistake—it embodies sexuality as the culture defines it" (p. 46). Rape takes many forms: sexual abuse of children, gang rape, forced intercourse with wives, sexual torture of female prisoners, intercourse with therapists, bride capture and group rape as a puberty rite, as well as the more identified form as sexual assault on a female by an unknown male (Brownmiller, 1975). Rape is "an exercise of domination and the infliction of degradation upon the victim" and serves to restrict the independence of women and remind them of their vulnerability, thereby keeping them subjugated across all patriarchal societies (Schram, 1978, p. 78).

Rape is a crime of violence, not sex. The recent increases of rape, assault, and murder in the United States all follow the same upward curve. The characteristics of rapists have been found to closely resemble those of other violent offenders (Lewis, 1977). A study of 133 convicted rapists in Massachusetts found that power or anger motives were dominant in all their acts of rape; sexuality was being used to express the emotions (Groth, 1977). From their extensive work with rape victims and research of the issue Burgess and Holmstrom (1979) conclude, "Although different patterns of rape are apparent, they *all* have a common motivational basis: power" (p. 28).

A final form of violence against women is physical aggression in dating situations. Several recent studies have documented an alarming rate of violence between couples on today's college campuses. Approximately one in four college women have been victims of rape or attempted rape, and 57% of those rapes occurred on dates (Koss, Gidycz, & Wisniewski, 1987; Levy, 1991; Warshaw, 1988). Such violence against women has special ramifications in the understanding of wife abuse. It has been noted that battered women frequently were assaulted by their mates before marrying or living with them. Researchers have speculated that, since the women knew of probable abuse beforehand and entered a permanent relationship regardless of the abuse, they must be accepting of abuse. If premarital violence is as common as these recent studies suggest, it can be understood why women would conclude that such behavior is relatively common and should be tolerated. As with other forms of violence against women, society becomes inured to its occurrence. Without careful study and constant reminders, society accepts incidents as inevitable, not to be questioned, not to be decried. The myths and silences that surround such practices serve to keep women quiet about them, while the underlying fear that they engender successfully keeps patriarchy intact.

A SYNTHESIZING CONCEPTUAL FRAMEWORK: MACHISMO

From the study of violence in general and specifically wife abuse, Campbell has concluded that there is a conceptual framework that can be distinguished that has previously been embedded within other theoretical formulations. The concept of machismo or compulsive masculinity can be found in psychological, sociological, and anthropological literature on violence and is also mentioned in much of the literature on wife abuse. It can be used as a unifying concept from which to view both wifebeating and violence against women. This section examines explanations for the occurrence of machismo, delineates characteristics associated with it, briefly describes some of the general violence literature as it relates to machismo, and explains the association of machismo with wife abuse.

Origins and Associated Characteristics

Parsons, Cohen, and Miller first linked a machismo-like concept to violence. They postulated that boys seldom see their fathers and therefore have trouble making a masculine definition, but have incorporated some of the feminine characteristics of their mothers. When the boys come under social pressure to establish their own masculine identity, they reject their own feminine natures and overemphasize the traditional male values of toughness and hardness and may commit deviant acts "as a public pronouncement" that they are "real men" (Gibbons, 1970; Miller, 1958).

Psychoanalytical literature attributed compulsive masculinity to dominating mothers, but in reality, as Whiting (1965) states, "an individual identifies with that person who is perceived as controlling those resources that he wants" (p. 126). Relegation of all or most early child care to females does result in first identification with mothers, but when boys realize (after the first 2 to 3 years) that the world is obviously dominated by males, they try to change allegiance totally, leading to inner conflict. Anthropological data from Whiting and Mead document the problems in primitive societies and polygynous cultures when fathers are completely separated from women and children, and a more violent society results from compulsive masculinity (Mead, 1949; Whiting, 1965). In our own country, lower-economic class white fathers have the least role in child-rearing. Lower-economic class black males also have less of a role than middle-class fathers, but the pattern of men excluding themselves from child care predominates over all groups (Houtan, 1970). All boys feel they need to prove their masculinity to some extent and reject feminine characteristics that they recognize within themselves because they see that this is not what "wins" in the patriarchal world. Even for boys from female-headed households, television, family relationships with other adult males, and a look at the "street" provide models of tough masculine behavior (Nobels, 1978).

Tiger (1969) postulated that a proclivity for male bonding is innate, and that machismo-type behavior originates from this instinct. We can reject the idea of such an instinct by cross-cultural data indi-cating that such behavior is not universal. However, Tiger makes some interesting observations in his study of all-male groups. When they are connected with initiations and secret societies in primitive cultures, they become a factor in the breaking of ties with mothers and in maintaining dominance over and social distance from females. All-male groups in any culture tend to facilitate the expression of aggression and provide group standards for maleness, such as bravery and toughness. It is easy to apply these concepts to inner-city gangs, motorcycle gangs, Ku Klux Klan, the military, etc.

However, male bonding can only be regarded as a manifestation of machismo, not as a cause. Anthropologists, feminists, and psychoanalysts have all noted the more or less unconscious fear and envy men have of women because of their unique and awesome ability to bear children (Lederer, 1968; Mead, 1949; Chester, 1978). In peaceful, primitive cultures this female power is glorified and women are given rightful respect for it, but in patriarchal societies, female power has been denied and denigrated. In patriarchy there is a basic ambivalence toward women, originating in "uterus envy" and compounded by guilt, denial, displacement, projection, and rationalization (Lederer, 1968; Weimer, 1978). This helps to explain some of the roots of violence against women, including wife abuse.

Socialization for machismo

The training for the male role starts early. More stringent demands are made and enforced more harshly on boys than on girls at an early age. Rohner (1972) found boys age 2 to 6 already more aggressive in 71% of the societies in a cross-cultural study, but there were great differences in the amount of that aggression, depending on how the children were raised. Hartley (1974) found kindergarten boys already restricting their interests and activities to those traditionally labeled masculine, whereas girls took another 5 or more years to limit their activities to those labeled feminine. Male school and peer group activities are explicitly organized around struggle, and boys are encouraged to hunt, fish, fight, and play war games with their fathers (Tolson, 1977). Boys at age 8 and 11 were found to be saying "they have to be able to fight in case a bully comes along," and they are expected "to be noisy" and "to get into trouble more than girls" (Hartley, 1974, p. 10).

Violence can be viewed "as a clandestine masculine ideal in Western culture" (Toby, 1966, p. 19). Male heroes are "Rambo" types and playboys, both of whom treat women with disdain. The ideal male wields authority, especially over women, has unlimited sexual prowess, is invulnerable, has competition as his guiding principle, never discloses emotion, is tough and brave, has great power, is adept at one-upmanship, can always fight victoriously if he needs to, and doesn't need anyone (Balswick & Peck, 1971; Fasteau, 1974). This is, of course, an impossible standard and creates anxiety in men because of their inability to reach it.

Characteristics of machismo

Many characteristics have been cited as representative of machismo behavior. Whiting (1965) identifies "a preoccupation with physical strength and athletic prowess, or attempts to demonstrate daring and valor or behavior that is violent and aggressive" (p. 127). Thrill-seeking behavior, inability to express emotions, independence, egotism, and support of the military have been noted by other authors (Balswick & Peck, 1971; Greenburg, 1977; Lewis, 1971; Toplin, 1975). Sexist attitudes are inherent in machismo and are demonstrated by the valuing of sexual virility, the treatment of women as commodities and conquest objects, the insistence on female subjugation, the inability to cooperate with women, and the adherence to the "unwritten law" that female sexual infidelity must be avenged (Bromberg, 1961; Coser, 1966; MacDonald, 1961; Miller, 1958; Sherwood & McGrath, 1976; Tedeschi, 1977; Toplin, 1975). The danger of machismo to women is illustrated in this quote from McCormack (1978): "Machismo is an attitude of male pride in sexual virility, a form of narcissism, that condones the sexual use and abuse of women, and, in the extreme, violence as a dimension of sexual gratification and instrumental to sexual goals" (p. 545). Therefore machismo can be defined as the male attitudes and behavior arising from and supported by the patriar-

chal social structure that express sexism and male ownership of women, glorify violence, emphasize virility, and despise gentleness and the expression of any emotions except anger and rage.

Further relationships of machismo and violence

There is considerable evidence of linkages between machismo attitudes and violent behavior. One of the additional characteristics of machismo behavior is owning and/or carrying a gun (Toplin, 1975; Wright & Marston, 1974). In a multistate sample of 1,504 American men and women, the most significant correlation with gun ownership was the approval of and willingness to use violence. Having been a victim of violent crime showed no correlation with gun ownership, suggesting that other variables, such as machismo, are more important than realistic fear (Williams & McGrath, 1978). Handguns cannot be considered as a cause of violence; however, guns in the home, ostensibly kept for defense, are sometimes used impulsively in the heat of an argument, without death being intended by the perpetrator.

Many other indicators link violence with machismo. Two of the countries with the highest homicide rates in the world, Columbia and Mexico, also have strong machismo ethics (Weimer, 1978). The highest rates of homicide in the United States are found in the deep South (Mississippi, Alabama, and Louisiana) and in the West (Texas, New Mexico, and Nevada), both areas characterized by exaggerated machismo. These six states have an average homicide rate of 13.6 per 100,000 population, which is almost four times greater than the rate in all of New England, an area that less idealizes rugged masculinity (Webster, 1989). Arizona, Texas, and Mississippi also have the highest number of guns per capita, whereas New England and the Eastern United States have approximately one half the percentage of households owning guns than the South and the West (Clark, 1970). Clinard and Abbott, when determining the differences between two slum areas in Kampala, Uganda, found that the area characterized by fewer negative attitudes toward fighting, and by more prostitution and wifebeating, was also the area of the greatly higher crime rate (Clinard & Abbott, 1973). Sipes (1973) found that cultures exhibiting a great deal of warlike activity were significantly more likely to engage in combative sports activities. Both Hepburn (1971) and Erlanger (1974) concluded from separate reviews of empirical research concerned with the subculture of violence theory that a "subculture of masculinity" better explains the evidence.

Machismo and murder

Several studies of murderers have noted machismo characteristics. Ruotolo (1975) described only four male murderers, but noticed that they all "confused gentleness with weakness" (p. 16). Maletzky (1973) examined 22 male subjects with long histories of violent behavior. They exhibited a variety of other characteristics, but all "appeared hypermasculine" (Maletzky, 1973, pp. 179–80). Bach-Y-Rita's (1971) group of 117 male inpatients whose chief complaint was explosive violent behavior also showed a variety of incidence of neurological symptoms, but were "generally outwardly hypermasculine and intent on physically defending their masculinity against other men" (p. 1,477). In psychiatric exams of 367 men accused of murder in Scotland, Gillies (1976) found evidence of tolerance of brutality, drunkenness, wifebeating, robbery, murder, and rape; 101 of these men had killed women.

Machismo and aggressive behavior

A series of laboratory experiments also show the connection between aggressiveness and machismo characteristics. Perry and Perry (1974) found that aggressive boys are likely to perceive signs of suffering as indications of success of their aggression. They found that when a victim did not express pain, these boys became very hostile and gave increasingly intensive shocks. Taylor and Smith (1974) found that male students exhibiting traditionally dominant attitudes toward women also showed more aggressive behavior toward both males and females. Using electronically measured pillow clubs, Young et al. (1975) showed that young men favoring subordinate status for women were less aggressive toward female opponents when the women were passive and only defended themselves. However, when the females attacked, the traditionalists increased significantly the intensity of the blows, much more so than the egalitarian males (Young et al., 1975). In another study dogmatism (measuring authoritarianism) was related to aggression and hostility for males, but only to hostility in females (Heyman, 1977). Although caution must be exercised in applying laboratory data on aggression to real life, these studies support the association of various characteristics of machismo with aggression in males.

Machismo and culture

Machismo is present to some extent in most men, but its outward display is more prevalent in males in lower socioeconomic groups. There is also empirical evidence for the idea that machismo is especially evident in the United States in black males (Ten Houten, 1970). Black gang members were more likely to rate images of sexual virility, approval of pimping (objectification of females), and defense of a fighting or tough reputation higher than middle- or lower-class black or white teenaged boys (Gordon et al., 1963). As Wallace (1978) points out, machismo attitudes in black men are not a result of racial characteristics or the family heritage of slavery; they resulted from the systematic degradation of black men (and equally so, black women) by white racist society, which was revolted against by black men in the 1960s with an image of strength and violence. Along with this image came sexism, which was in part an adoption of white male patriarchal values (it works for them), partially a result of encouragement for this sentiment by white racists, and somewhat a scapegoating mechanism. "Black macho" has been fostered by the continuing powerlessness of the black male.

Curtis (1975) has developed a theory to explain the prevalence of criminal violence in poor black young men. He first identifies subcultural values of the majority of people who are black and poor. They are different from the values of the dominant culture (which includes middle-class blacks), but they do not include violence. However, there is a group of poor black males who hold different and opposing values to the dominant culture that Curtis identifies as a violent contraculture. These men have found it impossible to express the characteristics of the ideal male through economic or occupational roles, and rather than accepting their fate or turning hostility inward through mental illness or drug addiction, they have accepted attitudes that foster violence. These include an "emphasis on physical prowess and toughness," on "sexual prowess and exploitation . . . on shrewdness and manipulativeness," and on "thrill seeking and change." These can be identified as machismo values. Curtis also conceptualizes that the high rate of intermale black violence further reflects the acceptance of a violent resolution of conflict, the prevalence of jealousy, a "brittle sensitivity," and the abundance of gun carrying by these men (pp. 12, 23-24, 29-30, 50-52).

Machismo is also widespread in middle-class white society; the images of women being sexually and physically abused in pornography, on record albums and music videos, in fashion magazines, and on billboards are rampant (Gayford, 1978; Landon, 1977-78). Seven of ten American men think it is a good idea for their sons to engage in fistfights (Stark & McEvoy, 1970). Machismo is not a characteristic of only poor black men, but it is often more directly expressed in that culture because white, racist patriarchal society has rendered these men powerless except on the street and in their own homes. This can at least partially explain both the high rate of black male violence in the ghetto and also the higher rate of black female homicide victims than that of white female victims (Lercher, 1979; Straus et al., 1988).

Machismo can thus be substantially linked to violence in our culture and cross-culturally. Machismo attitudes are often strongest where other forms of violence against women are the most violent and patriarchy, the strongest. The machismo ethic is similar to the "honor code" of many Arab and other Mediterranean cultures, wherein the woman is defined as property, and the man must defend that property with violence if necessary toward other men and/or toward the woman (Loizos, 1978). One of the forms that this violence may take is wife abuse; the male who holds strong machismo values usually considers it his right to beat his wife.

Machismo and Abuse

The nature of the patriarchal system and resulting sexist machismo attitudes toward women, especially female partners, is deeply embedded in our culture and can be argued to be the root cause of wife abuse. Dobash and Dobash (1979) express the idea in the following phrase: " . . . the legacy of the patriarchy continues to generate the conditions and relationships that lead to a husband's use of force against his wife" (p. 9). The other contributing factors previously reviewed can be understood within this context. Alcohol can be seen as a disinhibiting agent that weakens the social prescription against doing physical harm to women, at least in certain situations. Intoxication can then be used as a convenient excuse for battering a woman since our society teaches that such behavior is less reprehensible when the perpetrator is under the influence. Alcohol, therefore, can give a man the courage, the excuse, and the convenient loss of social veneer necessary to behaviorally express his need for power and macho attitudes.

Social learning, wife abuse, and machismo

Machismo also fits into social-learning theory and the idea that stressors and/or frustration may result in wife abuse. The patriarchal family arrangement clarifies that the man may appropriately express his frustration toward his wife. Steinmetz and Straus (1974) point out that husbands who hit wives are "carrying out a role model learned from parents and brought into play when social stresses become intolerable" (p. 7). Actually, the model is the one learned from the father, an identification with the aggressor. In Gayford's (1979) study, 41.6% of the abusive husbands saw their father being violent, whereas only 6.9% experienced a violent mother. Carroll (1977) also found only male sex linkages, between violent fathers and battering sons, in the intergenerational transmission of violence. Dobash and Dobash (1979) further explain social learning when they state, "Thus, all men see themselves as controllers of women, and because they are socialized into the use of violence, they are (all) potential aggressors against their wives" (p. 22).

Television is also replete with male heroes using

violence to achieve goals without negative consequences. In a survey of programming from 1967 to 1975, it was found that the "good" guys were most likely to be the killers. Women were the most often killed, and the heroes treated women with disdain (Garbner & Gross, 1976). Even the commercials show male authority (Welch, 1979). Children's books (including classroom texts) and movies display the same theme (Rickel & Grant, 1979).

Machismo and powerlessness

Goode (1971) relates family violence to the theoretical framework of social systems and social stratification. According to Goode, the family is a power system like all other social units, which "all rest to some degree on force and its threat" to operate. Goode indicates four ways by which people succumb to authority: (1) force and its threat (power), (2) economic variables, (3) prestige or respect, and (4) likability, attractiveness, friendship, or love. Within the marital relationship, males use a combination of these factors to preserve dominance. The threat of force is used more frequently than, and in conjunction with, actual violence (Gelles, 1974). Physical abuse occurs more often, according to Goode, when the other three persuasive mechanisms fail or when the male feels his authority is threatened. Thus battering behavior is more likely to appear when the man's control and therefore his macho pride are challenged by the woman's job, pregnancy, or the possibility of infidelity, and when the man feels insecure about his own power from other means. As Storr (1978) states: "It is the insecure and inadequate who most easily feel threatened and who resort to violence as a primitive way of restoring dominance" (pp. 2-8).

The man who feels any sort of inadequacy or powerlessness in the male world is most likely to use force and violence where he can, in the home and in his neighborhood. Bednarik (1970) finds modern men generally in a crisis of masculinity. Only a few men actually achieve dominance in work and economically, and their traditional male role in the home is being threatened. He describes the symptoms of this crisis as "impotent anger," demonstrated by outbursts of blind rage and mysterious

acts of violence, and the transfer of women into a sexual commodity. The lower-class male is the least powerful man and the farthest from the ideal in society and is therefore likely to be more overt in his machismo and violent behavior. Tolson (1977) notes that working-class masculinity is characterized by an "impulsive, aggressive style" more so than middle-class masculinity. Normal masculinity in the lower class is a threatening demeanor and "drunken violence is the last line of defense" (pp. 28, 30). The lower-class male is more likely to *insist* on his "conjugal right" to authority in the home, and violence is used when his power seems to be slipping (Komavovsky, 1964; Tolson, 1977). The data on unemployment, poverty, lack of skills, and lower levels of education in many battering men illustrate this mechanism. It has also been suggested that the high incidence of child abuse or excessive physical punishment in the background of many wifebeaters has contributed to a sense of inadequacy and problems in identification with the father in these men, which is later expressed as compulsive masculinity (Lystaad, 1975). Violence against wives usually has aspects of enforcing or reasserting the control of one particular man in a relationship, and it thereby reinforces the whole of patriarchy. Most wife abusers are staunch supporters of the traditional male role of dominance and authority, and their behavior is designed to perpetuate that role both at home and in society (Walker, 1979). As Davidson (1978) notes, the wifebeater intends to cause injury and pain and assumes that there will be no retaliation from male-oriented society. She finds three common attitudes in most wife abusers: (1) the behavior is acceptable and/or justified, (2) the man is unsure of the reason for the battering, except that it is a continuation of a ritual, (3) there is a lack of guilt and shame and a mystification that the law should object to the violent behavior.

Asserting control through abuse

The controlling nature of wife abuse is shown in many ways. The wifebeaters' justifications are often trivial. For example, Martin (1976) cites these cases: a woman broke the egg yolk when frying her husband's breakfast, another wife wore her hair in a ponytail, and a third served a casserole instead of fresh meat. As Martin points out, these are only excuses, not reasons for beatings. Several authors have noted that wife abuse is not always preceded by verbal argument or conflict at all (Dobash & Dobash, 1979; Walker, 1979, 1984). Walker found that "it is not uncommon for the batterer to wake the woman out of a deep sleep to begin his assault." She also states that "although these women did or said things to make the batterer angry, it was obvious he would have beaten her anyway" (Walker, 1979, pp. 14, 61).

Hilberman and Munson (1977-78) drew the following conclusion from their interviews: "Violence erupted in any situation in which the husband did not immediately get his way." They also found that the majority of the men in their sample were "making active and successful efforts to keep their wives ignorant and isolated" and therefore more submissive (pp. 461-62). In Gelles' (1974) study, many of the men tried to control their wives' activities by restricting or trying to restrict their access to the car and/or money. If the wife rebelled or disobeyed, a beating resulted, as a last means of controlling his wife's behavior.

Dobash and Dobash (1979) found that the courtship phase of the abusive marriage was characterized by increasing isolation of the woman and increasing possessiveness of her by the man. The few incidents of battering during courtship (experienced by 23% of the women) were sparked by issues of male possession and authority. After marriage, most of any remaining independent social activity by the wife swiftly ended, while the man retained his habits of going out with his friends. The first beating usually occurred within the first 6 months of marriage, showing the husband's attempt to establish complete control early.

When a woman is married in a patriarchy, her primary responsibilities become child-rearing, domestic labor, and "personal and psychic service" to her mate. The household responsibilities are seen as a service to the person in authority, the husband, and how well they are done is a symbol of "commitment and subservience" (Dobash & Dobash, 1979). This helps to explain the often trivial nature

of the incident preceding battering; it is often over performance of a small household chore. If performed poorly or reluctantly in the perception of the man, it is a symbol of some spark of rebellion against his total dominance. Such revolt must be quelled swiftly, with force if necessary, and such force has great symbolic meaning for the future.

Returning to Goode's (1971) basic premises, other characteristics of wife abuse can be explored. To use the third and fourth means of influence, prestige or love, a husband needs to be verbally persuasive. Several authors have listed poor communication skills as a factor predisposing men to abuse (Gelles, 1974; Symonds, 1978). Goode postulates that lower-class males may have fewer verbal skills, as well as less prestige and decreased economic resources, and they therefore have to rely more frequently on brute power to maintain their position in the family. He contrasts this with the middle-class male, whom Goode characterizes in the following way: "The greater the other resources an individual can command, the more force he can muster, but the less he will actually deploy or use force in an overt manner" (p. 628). Goode further notes that the middle-class male has been taught to avoid the use of force by his childhood training. Whitehurst (1971) maintains that the only difference according to class is in terms of degree and frequency; the issue is still control and dominance. The middle-class husband is more likely to hit his wife only once at a time and then regain his control as he considers the consequences to his position if he were known as a batterer. Yet even one blow is a powerful symbol of force and authority. As Stark et al. (1979) describe, the most probable interpretation of these characteristics of wifebeating is that "Complex social factors may determine whether and in what combination physical, ideological, political, and economic force will be used to control women . . ." (p. 481).

Jealousy and machismo

Jealousy, noted by most authors as a major cause of the wifebeater's behavior, and also a major cause of husbands killing wives, is most logically viewed within the context of the husband's effort to maintain control over his wife and his machismo attitude. One of the dictionary definitions of jealous is "zealous in guarding." Ownership is implied. Because women are considered the possession of a husband, real or imagined sexual infidelity is the gravest threat to male dominance. Of 100 abused women in Gayford's (1979) sample, 66 cited their husband's jealousy as the main cause of abuse, although only 17 had ever actually been unfaithful in comparison with 44 of the husbands. The beaten wives in Walker's (1979) study "almost universally reported irrational jealousy" shown by the males (p. 114). Campbell's (1981) research on 28 homicides of women in intimate relationships revealed that male jealousy was the major cause cited in 64.3% of the killings; male dominance issues sparked another 17.9%. Whitehurst (1971) concluded from his study of 100 court cases: "At the core of nearly all the cases involving physical violence, the husband responded out of frustration at being unable to control his wife, often accusing her of being a whore or having an affair with another male, usually without justification" (p. 77). In a review of all wife abuse literature, Brandon (1976) found that jealousy was second only to alcohol in frequency when causes of wifebeating were enumerated. Renvoize (1978) emphasizes the connection between jealousy and dominance when she states, "The jealousy so often manifested by battering husbands may be one aspect of the need for one partner to have complete power over the other" (p. 34).

Other aspects of jealousy connected with wife abuse have also been discovered. Walker (1979) finds that the "batterer's need to possess his woman totally" often causes her to leave or lose her job. The man becomes jealous of her work relationships, even when she feels her home role is most important, lets him control all her earnings, and tries hard to convince him that he is still head of the family. Other authors have also noted that the abusive husband is threatened when the wife wants to get a job (Prescott & Letko, 1977). Battering men also frequently limit the wife's visits with even female friends and relatives (Rounsaville, 1978).

The frequent wifebeating that occurs when the woman is pregnant may also express jealousy and possessiveness more than anything else; a child can divert some of a wife's attention and loyalty away from the husband (Dobash & Dobash, 1979). Walker (1979) found that most of the women she interviewed reported more severe and more frequent violence during pregnancy and, importantly, during the child's early infancy. She also concludes that this phenomenon is directly related to the husband's possessiveness. These forms of jealousy, cited so often as a cause of wife abuse in and of themselves, are seen from a machismo viewpoint as part of the larger, overall cause of the patriarchal system and its substrates: the need for male dominance and sexism.

Sexual relationships as an outgrowth of machismo

The machismo attitudes of wifebeaters are also shown in their sexual relationships with their wives. Martin (1976) notes that these men see conquest as an integral part of sex. Several samples have shown sexual abuse as a part of the pattern of victimization (Campbell, 1989b; Finkelhor & Yllo, 1983, Prescott & Letko, 1977; Russell, 1990). Stark et al. (1979) felt that the deliberate, sexual nature of wife abuse is shown in the predominance of injuries to the face, chest, breast, and abdomen. Walker (1979, 1984) found that the majority of abusive men in her sample used sex as an act of aggression; many had mutilated their wives sexually, some forced their wives into extraordinary sex practices, and most of the women felt as if they had been raped at least once during the marriage. Walker (1979) also notes that the violence and brutality in the sexual relationship seem to escalate over time. Other researchers have noted that when the wife refuses sex, it becomes a provocation to the husband (Renvoize, 1978). This can be viewed as part of the need for sexual dominance in the machismo syndrome, and when seen in the context of the frequent sexual abuse, refusal of sex seems to be a reasonable action on the part of the wives.

In summary, the concept of machismo can be seen to link a proposed root of wife abuse, the patriarchal system, with the behaviors of violent men, and wife abusers. Data from mainly descriptive studies have been used to document that wifebeaters are frequently virulently possessive and desperately try to maintain control over their wives. Richards (1991) found that a sample of young women reported that their battering male partners had significantly more of the machismo characteristics described here than did their nonbattering partner. In addition, Symonds (1979) reports that the largest group of wife abusers can be categorized by a machismo attitude, little guilt, a violent character structure, and a pathological need for control. These men have learned that it is appropriate to use physical aggression and to direct that force against their wives. Stress and threats to macho pride may spark such expressions of violence; alcohol may facilitate it. There is cultural support and historical precedent from patriarchal society to batter women, especially for men in the lower socioeconomic class and certain cultures where machismo is more widespread. Machismo cannot be said to be a direct cause of wife abuse, but it is a useful concept in understanding the phenomenon.

THEORETICAL FRAMEWORKS EXPLAINING CONTINUATION

One of the most difficult dynamics of wife abuse for professionals and the general public to understand is why a battered wife would stay with her spouse, sometimes for many years. The question has been addressed from many perspectives, and several theoretical frameworks have been advanced, although none has a substantial body of supportive empirical work. Advocates for battered women have pointed out that the question to be answered is not "Why does she stay?" but instead, "Why do so many men beat their wives?" and "What is preventing her from leaving?"

This section of the chapter examines the existing theoretical formulations under three major headings: (1) societal responses to victims, (2) psychological responses of abused women, and (3) coping with abusive relationships.

An important caveat to remember is that there are undoubtedly many women who *do*, in fact, extricate themselves from relationships at the onset of abuse, or soon after. However, because most research has drawn samples from women in shelters or women seeking other kinds of help for prolonged abuse, our knowledge of women who quickly break free is very limited. At least two studies now indicate that the majority of battered women do leave or manage to end the abuse but the process may take many years (Campbell, 1992; Okun, 1986). Therefore the theoretical and empirical work accomplished to date is more useful in understanding the responses of women who endure abuse over a longer period of time.

Sociocultural Perspectives

Sociocultural explanations of the perpetuation of violence against female partners focus on society's explicit and implicit rules that legitimize violence under certain circumstances. Straus (1980) maintains that American social structures contain a cultural norm that permits physical violence within marriage. According to this view, women remain in abusive relationships because of the social barriers that keep them there. Family, friends, and neighbors are reluctant to become involved in families' "private business." Official "helping" agencies, such as the police, the court system, clergy, professional counselors, and health care professionals, all perpetuate the sanctity of the family and are unresponsive to battered women's needs.

The police would ordinarily be the first agency called when assault occurs and are thought to have the power to protect a citizen from further harm from an attacker. However, police do not always respond when they receive a call from a woman abused by her partner or from neighbors calling on her behalf. When they do respond, they are frequently ineffective in ending the abuse beyond the time of their physical presence. Consequently, after a few disappointing responses, battered women seldom call the police because they anticipate little help and fear retaliation after they leave (Kantor & Straus, 1990). The 136 formerly battered women in Bowker's (1983) research on the help-seeking strategies of battered women rated the police as the *least* helpful of the formal sources of help they had sought. Police arrested the batterer in just 15% of the reported incidents; instead, they had the batterer "cool down" and urged reconciliation of the couple. Even more distressing is the fact that some police officers "laughed and joked with the husband" and told the wife that she deserved the beating (p. 88). Because of recent efforts of police officials this grim picture is beginning to change in some parts of the country. The relationship of wife abuse and the police is further explored in Chapter 12. The courts have also traditionally been of little help to abused women. The problems in the legal system and recent changes in the laws are examined in Chapter 14.

Clergy are often consulted for advice on how to resolve an abusive relationship. In Prescott and Letko's (1977) sample, of 10 women who contacted a minister or priest for advice, only one found him or her helpful (Prescott & Letko, 1977). The women in Bowker's (1983) research rated the clergy as the most conservative advice-givers of the formal sources of help they had turned to. Clergy tended to hold the woman responsible for the abuse *and* held her responsible for making amends and keeping the family together. It is disappointing that this potentially crucial source of support and advocacy for battered women has not been helpful. The traditional response of clergy is being challenged by educational initiatives for clergy to better prepare them to respond effectively to crime victims, including battered women (Spiritual Dimension in Victim Services, 1990).

As discussed earlier in this chapter, health care professionals have also been unhelpful to battered women. Although the health care encounter is a potentially useful resource for women in abusive relationships, research indicates that, for a variety of reasons, health professionals do not identify or attend to abuse, even if it is disclosed or suspected. The poor response of health professionals to abused women has been attributed to three factors: (1) strict adherence to the biomedical model of care delivery that focuses on diagnosis of a biological pathological condition, (2) personal negative attitudes and beliefs toward women in abusive relationships that are reflective of the general public, and (3) lack of professional education related to abuse of female partners (Helton et al., 1987b; Kurz, 1987, Rose & Saun-

ders, 1986; Stark et al., 1979). Efforts to improve the response of health care systems to the needs of abused women are underway throughout the country through educational programs and the establishment of clinical protocols (Helton, 1987; Stark et al., 1981). Nursing care of the woman being abused by her partner is covered in depth in Chapter 9.

Social Resources

Gelles (1974, 1976) was one of the first sociologists to seek an answer to the question "Why would a woman who has been physically abused by a man remain with him?" Gelles hypothesized that a woman with few resources consequently has fewer alternatives to an abusive marriage, thus she is "trapped" in the marriage and reluctant to seek outside intervention. Interviews conducted with 80 couples (40 couples experiencing husband-to-wife violence and 40 nonviolent neighboring couples) led Gelles to conclude that the greater the severity and frequency of the violence, and if the woman held a job, the more likely she was to seek outside intervention. Employment outside the home was thought to be crucial not only for the woman's economic independence from her partner, but also because the employed woman was less socially isolated than one who is confined to the home, and thus had access to informal support and accurate information. However, this finding was not supported by Okun's (1986) review of 300 shelter records of battered women; women who were employed outside the home were no more likely than full-time homemakers to terminate the abusive relationship.

If, in spite of her terror and despair, in spite of the knowledge that the courts and police are unlikely to protect her from further retaliation, and in spite of the unfairness that the battered woman must relinquish her home and belongings in the interest of safety for herself and her children, she finds the courage to pack up and leave with her children, where is the battered woman supposed to go? The consensus of the chief circuit judges in Florida was that abused wives stay in the relationship because there are no viable alternatives (Kutum,

1977). The research of Strube and Barbour (1984) with 251 women seeking help for domestic violence supported the conclusion that women who perceived that they had nowhere else to go, were not employed outside the home, and were experiencing financial hardship were less likely to leave an abusive relationship. Housing authorities have not viewed battered women who have fled their homes for safety as technically "homeless," and therefore do not always provide public housing or assistance in obtaining shelter (McCabe, 1977). Furthermore, in most urban areas, safe, affordable housing for single female-headed families is scarce.

Social networks

The formerly battered women in Bowker's (1983) study reported mixed responses from the family and friends they turned to for help and advice. Their disclosures and requests for help were often met with disbelief or the feeling that their stories and perceived danger were exaggerated, or they were urged to remain in the relationship and work harder to make it succeed. Women fortunate enough to be given support and temporary shelter by family or friends expressed concern that they may be jeopardizing the safety of their helpers. Over time, family and friends often became discouraged and would eventually cut ties with women who returned to the batterer after temporary separations. Hypothesizing that the availability of social support would mediate the effects of abuse on women's psychological health, Mitchell and Hodson (1983) learned that, as violence grew more severe for the 60 battered women in their study, friends were less likely to respond favorably to requests for assistance. In direct contrast, the in-depth interviews and social network analysis conducted by Hoff (1990) with nine battered women in an emergency shelter and 25 members of their natural social networks revealed that, with one exception, the battered women felt supported by their close family and friends. Although the network members were often limited in their ability to offer tangible aid, they strongly disapproved of the violence directed at the women and were willing to help in any way they could.

Since the women's movement brought wife abuse to the public eye in the 1970s, shelters for battered women and their children have been created worldwide. Although shelter programs are the first to acknowledge that shelters alone are not the solution to wife abuse, they do provide crucial sanctuary where a woman's physical and emotional wounds may heal, support can be gained from women who are currently in, or have successfully resolved, abusive relationships, and accurate information can be obtained to make difficult decisions about the future. Unfortunately, there are not enough shelters to meet the demand. Many communities, particularly in rural areas, do not have shelters for battered women and their children, and funding to maintain existing shelters is scarce. Statistics kept by the National Coalition Against Domestic Violence reveal that, in urban areas, of every 10 requests for shelter, 7 women must be turned away (1992).

Societal myths

It is interesting to note some of the mechanisms that may operate in society to perpetuate the unhelpful response to women seeking to end the abuse from their partners. As Symonds (1975) notes, "There seems to be a marked reluctance and resistance to accept the innocence" of all victims of violence (pp. 19–22). Most people's response, generated by the need to have rational explanations for horrible occurrences, is to imply that victims could have somehow avoided their misfortune. Without such rationalizations, there are feelings of vulnerability that, if the victim is not somehow to blame, then the same thing may happen to them. There is also the irrational fear of some kind of contamination, and the tendency to put the victim out of sight and out of mind (Janoff-Bulman & Frieze, 1983; Ryan, 1971). Myths have therefore arisen that blame the victim and/or "explain away" the facts and thus avoid the real issues—that society as a whole, and each individual member in that society, must be held accountable for perpetuating abuse of female partners.

Some of the common myths embedded in society are that women are masochistic and ask for abuse, that battered women are mentally ill, that abused wives are free to leave at any time, and that these women deserve to be beaten because of some personality flaw or inappropriate behavior (King & Ryan, 1989; Walker, 1979). Women are encouraged to internalize these myths, and, indeed, the battered women in Walker's research sample believed all the myths of wifebeating (Walker, 1979, 1984). The notion that battered women could simply choose to leave the abusive relationship is particularly naive. This myth is based on the assumption that leaving the relationship will end the violence, which is often not true. Despite divorce or separation from abusive partners, women are often pursued, harassed, threatened, and assaulted by the estranged abuser (Browne, 1987; Okun, 1986). Erroneous myths have influenced the behavior of the police, the courts, and many of the helping professionals who then perpetuate the abused women's entrapment. Walker (1979) has also identified prejudicial myths that are prevalent in other areas of violence against women: rape, incest, pornography, prostitution, sexual harassment at the workplace, and sexual activity between women clients and male psychotherapists. When taken in conjunction with the commonly held false beliefs about wife abuse, these myths prevent women from feeling the full outrage about their persecution. These myths emphasize the woman's part in her own victimization and thereby mask the blame of the abusers and society.

Psychological Perspectives

Learned helplessness

Walker (1979, 1984) has analyzed the psychological and behavioral responses of battered women in terms of Seligman's theory of "learned helplessness." This phenomenon was first seen in dogs, but it has been replicated in humans in experimental laboratory settings and is described as the behavior that results when an "organism has learned that outcomes are uncontrollable by his responses and is seriously debilitated by that knowledge" (Maier & Seligman, 1976, pp. 4, 7). When taught that a painful experience occurs randomly and regardless of

anything done to avoid or stop it, a person or animal becomes less motivated to try measures to end the pain; has trouble learning that responding controls outcomes generally; and exhibits anxiety, depression, and dependence (Maier & Seligman, 1976). Wife abuse usually also occurs randomly, regardless of the victim's attempts to avoid or stop it.

When applied to battered women, learned helplessness theory suggests that repeated battering leads to the development of a cognitive perception that the woman is unable to resolve her current life situation. "Once women are operating from a belief of helplessness, the perception becomes reality, and they become passive, submissive, and helpless" (Walker, 1979, p. 47). The resulting sense of helplessness leads to feelings of depression and anxiety, which in turn reduces problem-solving ability and motivation, resulting in an inability to leave the relationship (Walker, 1984). Walker's in-depth study with 403 women in abusive relationships suggested that learned helplessness theory was useful in understanding the response of *some* women to abuse (Walker, 1984). The women in Walker's sample were significantly depressed, but, contrary to predictions, did not view themselves as not having control over the abusive events, and did not show evidence of poor self-esteem. Furthermore, rather than becoming more passive and immobilized over time, the women's help-seeking seemed to increase with increasing frequency and severity of violence.

Walker's cycle theory of violence

Walker has also identified a "cycle theory of violence" from her extensive interviews with battered women (Walker, 1979, 1984). The first phase, the "tension-building phase," is characterized by an escalation of tension with verbal abuse and minor battering incidents. The woman engages in placating behavior, trying desperately to avoid serious incidents. Her feelings of helplessness and fear escalate as the incidents worsen over time. This phase may last for weeks or even years, until the tension has mounted to the breaking point. Phase two, "the acute battering incident," is the outbreak of serious violence that may last from 2 to 24 hours. The woman is powerless to affect the outcome of the second phase and can only try to protect herself and her children. In the third phase, the aftermath, the man is contrite and loving, and promises to reform. This phase reinforces the woman's hope that the beatings will end. Unfortunately, the cycle almost always repeats itself. Over time, the third phase occurs less often, leaving the woman trapped between the preoutburst tension and the battering episodes.

Empirical tests of Walker's cycle of violence theory lend inconsistent support for the three phases. From detailed descriptions of past battering incidents, 65% of Walker's sample gave evidence of a tension-building phase before the battering and 58% gave evidence of loving contrition after the battering (Walker, 1984). Conversely, Dobash and Dobash (1984) used similar research methods with 109 battered women, but did not find support for Walker's third phase of the cycle of violence; only 14% of the batterers apologized after the worst incident of assault. In a smaller study, Painter and Dutton (1985) found unpredictable male behavior after men violently attacked their female partners. Nevertheless, Walker's cycle of violence theory has been accepted by lay and professional helpers as a plausible explanation for the behavior of abused women. The cycle description often appears in recent protocol material for professional education and in community education efforts by women's groups.

Problem-solving abilities

Several investigations have focused on the problem-solving abilities of battered women, guided by the assumption that learned helplessness creates a cognitive deficit that interferes with the ability to perceive, generate, and evaluate solutions to problems. For example, Claerhout, Elder, and James (1982) concluded that battered women generated fewer total solutions, fewer effective solutions, and more avoidant solutions than nonbattered women in response to vignettes depicting husband-to-wife violence. However, conclusions in this and other studies (Launius & Jensen, 1987; Launius & Lindquist, 1988) have failed to acknowledge the battered women's frame of reference; that is, battered women know from their firsthand experience that an

"avoidant" response, or no response, is the optimum choice for immediate survival.

Grief model

The learned helplessness model has been compared with a model of grief to explain women's responses to battering (Campbell, 1989a). Although explanations based on learned helplessness dominated the literature on battered women, Campbell speculated that women's responses to abusive relationships were similar to the normative resolution process of personal loss and grief that accompanies the dissolution of any valued intimate relationship. The depression experienced by battered women may be a normative response to the anticipated termination of the relationship, and the temporary separations and reunions with the abusive partner are comparable to the reconciliations of any troubled marriage or significant relationship. With this reasoning, Campbell compared the responses of 97 battered women with the responses of 96 women who were in troubled, but nonviolent relationships. Although analysis found both theoretical models nearly equal in explanatory power, several important differences between the groups were evident. Battered women were, indeed, more severely depressed than women in troubled, but nonviolent, relationships, lending support to the contention that depression is a *result* of abuse rather than a predisposing factor. Battered women also experienced more frequent and severe physical symptoms of stress and grief than the nonbattered women. Despite their aversive circumstances and depression, the battered women had thought of or tried significantly *more* solutions to their relationship problems than had women in troubled, but nonviolent, relationships, which attests to the strengths and creativity of women trying to end abuse in a relationship.

Survivor model

The dominant learned helplessness model has also been challenged by a model of survival in which battered women are viewed as active survivors rather than helpless victims (Gondolf & Fisher, 1988; Hoff, 1990; Kelly, 1988). In an extensive review of data from 6,612 records from 50 battered women's shelters in Texas using sophisticated statistical model testing techniques, the authors found evidence that battered women persistently sought help in ending the abuse directed at them. Help-seeking efforts seemed to increase when the batterer's level of violence increased, particularly when the batterer engaged in more antisocial or criminal behavior in general. The inadequate response of social agencies to the needs of battered women led the authors to conclude that "learned helplessness" is more prevalent in existing formal helping systems, which are overwhelmed with the needs of battered women and limited in their ability to respond. The authors suggest that, rather than maintain a narrow focus on how to effectively "treat" battered women, helping agencies must first "treat" themselves in terms of strengthening their advocacy role for women and removing the barriers that have kept them trapped in abusive relationships.

Coercive control model

A compelling theoretical analogy between the techniques of Chinese Communist thought reform of the late 1940s and 1950s and contemporary abuse of female partners has been drawn by Okun (1986), who defines coercive control as:

> . . . a controller who takes enormous power—usually through confinement or isolation—over a victim he seeks to control by demanding compliance and violently enforcing that demand. The captive victim is made very dependent upon the controller; in fact, usually the controller will have the power to dictate whether or not the victim survives. (p. 113)

The battered woman's situation resembles that of a prisoner subjected to thought reform in many ways. The battered woman is subjected to beatings and other physical abuse, verbal abuse, death threats, restriction of activity to the point of imprisonment, and the induction of false confessions to infidelity or other fabricated behaviors, while the batterer portrays himself as being above reproach and justified in his treatment. Just as the purpose of thought reform is to produce a psychological breakdown in the prisoner, so too does battering of women reduce them to compliance with the batterer's demands (Okun, 1986).

Similar analogies have been drawn between the responses of women in abusive relationships and people who have survived hostage situations. A theory of "traumatic bonding" compared women's responses to abusive partners with responses of hostages in which the victim may develop loyalty to the captor (Painter & Dutton, 1985). Similarly, the Stockholm syndrome has been proposed as an explanation for the behavior of battered women who minimize their abuse, remain in the abusive relationship, and often publicly defend their batterers and reject the aid of intervenors (Graham, Rawlings, & Rimini, 1988). Traumatic bonding and the Stockholm syndrome are thought to be operative when there is a substantial imbalance of power between the captor and the hostage, or the abusive man and the abused women. The captor uses death threats, physical force and assault, imprisonment, and intermittent kindness, or at least nonabusive behavior, to control the hostage. Women hostages have the additional fear of rape from their captors. Women's responses to an abusive relationship can thus be viewed as a normative process of adaptation for survival.

Self-esteem

Many authors have noted the low self-esteem of women in abusive relationships, although the evidence of low self-esteem is inconsistent. Women with low self-esteem are thought to be vulnerable to abuse and more tolerant in permitting the abuse to continue. However, because research measures of self-esteem are only known while women are in the midst of an abusive relationship and on leaving the relationship, no cause-and-effect relationship can be stated. An erosion of self-esteem is understandable considering how women in patriarchy are traditionally taught to define their sense of self-worth in terms of their domestic work and family service. Walker (1984) was surprised to learn that the battered women in her sample perceived themselves as stronger, more independent, and more liberal in their views of sex roles than other women. However, the women viewed their partners as holding more rigid, traditional views of male and female roles. Pagelow (1981) also expected that women with "traditional ideology" of gender roles would be more likely to remain in abusive relationships. Data from 350 battered women did not support that expectation, however; whether they had liberal or conservative views did not seem to be related to the length of the abusive relationship. Both battered and nonbattered women in Campbell's (1989a) sample scored significantly lower than established norms for self-concept, again indicating that the difference is more likely related to reasons other than the battering.

Other psychological responses to abuse

Walker and other authors have noted several different psychological mechanisms that may influence a woman's response to abuse and leave her less able to escape the situation. The realistic fear of further injury and death has already been explored in relation to homicide. Of the battered women in Walker's sample, 92% believed that their batterer could or would kill them (Walker, 1984).

The extreme fear of battered women may interact with low self-esteem to create a state of "paralyzing terror." Hilberman and Munson (1977-78) described this reaction as one of unending stress, chronic apprehension of doom, overwhelming passivity, and a pervasive sense of hopelessness. Symonds (1975) has likened this state to the reaction of victims after natural disasters or war-caused catastrophes when they become paralyzed by terror or mental confusion and exhibit passivity and apathy. She also compares the abused woman to victims of other violent crimes, who have been noted to show shock and denial, appeasing behavior, and/or depression, withdrawal, and guilt. In such an emotional state, the woman is likely to turn her natural retaliatory aggression inward and blame herself. She knows that retaliation will bring worse punishment (Dobash & Dobash, 1979; Hilberman & Munson, 1977-78). As previously mentioned, it is common for abused women to make suicidal attempts or gestures and to feel guilty (Stark & Flitcraft, 1988).

Coping with Abuse

As appreciation of the complex nature and patriarchal sociocultural context of abusive relationships has grown, and the easy answers have been dis-

carded, several investigators have focused on the nature of the experience from the women's perspective and on the coping strategies used by women to maintain some semblance of well-being for themselves and their children. An important unifying theme in recent research is that women's responses to abuse reflect a dynamic process that evolves according to the nature of the abuse, their interpretations of the abuse and the relationship as a whole, as well as the pragmatic consequences of remaining in or severing the relationship.

One way in which women cope with abuse in their relationships appears to be through rationalization of their experiences. Through a participant-observation study that included interviews with 120 women in shelters, Ferraro and Johnson (1983) identified six ways in which women rationalize the abuse as being justifiable. One rationalization entailed an "appeal to the salvation ethic," in which the woman believes the batterer's recovery is dependent on her ability to solve his problems. The man's abusive behavior is excusable, from the woman's perspective, because of a lifetime of rejection and misunderstanding by others; the woman feels challenged to remain steadfast and reliable for his needs. "Denial of the victimizer" serves as another rationalization. The violence is believed to be a response to a temporary stressful condition, such as unemployment or alcoholism, and the violence will end when the condition changes. Women may also deny or minimize the violence and injuries, at least in the early stages of battering. Denial of the violence protects the belief that the relationship is healthy and that the violent episode was a minor aberration. Women may also "deny their victimization" altogether because they believe the abuse was justified punishment for some failure on their part. A fifth rationalization entails "denial of options," in which women do not choose options available to them because emotionally they are convinced of their inability to survive without their partners. A final powerful rationalization discussed by Ferraro and Johnson is that of an "appeal to higher loyalties," which reflects patriarchal religious and cultural traditions that sanctify the family and insist on women's submission to their husbands. As long as women rationalize their abusive experiences, change seems unlikely. However, when previously-rationalized violence is reinterpreted as dangerous and unjustified, battered women do, indeed, seek alternatives. Catalysts for change include a sudden increase in the violence, deterioration of the emotional bond with the partner, despair that the situation will not improve, increased visibility of the violence (either occurring in front of witnesses or leaving visible injuries), knowledge of new resources such as shelters, and commentary from people outside the relationship who define it as abusive and unjustified.

The research of Landenburger (1989) explored the personal meaning of abusive experiences, the process of self-evaluation of the abusive relationship, and the influence of personal meaning on the choices made by women in abusive relationships. Core themes were discerned from interviews with 30 women recruited from the community who were currently in, or recently had left, abusive relationships. Women described four phases of binding, enduring, disengaging, and recovering through which they progressively pass as changes occur in the meaning ascribed to the abuse, to interactions with her abusive partner, and to her self. During the binding phase, when the relationship is new and loving, women respond to abuse with redoubled efforts to make the relationship work and to prevent future abuse. Logical, creative strategies are used to appease the abusive partner. Over time, the futility of her problem-solving efforts becomes apparent and the woman begins to question the durability of the relationship. In the second phase, or time of enduring, a woman tolerates the abuse because of the positive aspects of the relationship and because she feels at least partially responsible for the abuse. Although a woman may tentatively seek outside help at this time, she does not openly disclose her circumstances to others for fear of the consequences to her safety and to her partner's social status. The phase of disengaging involves the woman labeling her situation as being abusive and herself as undeserving of abusive treatment. A breaking point may be reached when women realize their danger, as well as the knowledge that they might attempt to kill the abuser. As women struggle with independent living and safety concerns,

they may leave and return to the abusive relationship several times. After a time of readjustment, and successfully overcoming the many barriers that could trap her in the abusive relationship, the woman may enter a phase of recovery in which she remains separated from the abuser. An important point for nurses and other helpers to realize is that, from the woman's perspective, the abuse was just one aspect of a whole relationship that may still have some positive elements in it—the woman wants to end the abuse, but wants to maintain the good aspects of the relationship.

The process of entrapment and recovery from an abusive relationship explicated by Landenburger also emerged in a smaller qualitative study with 10 battered women (Mills, 1985). As women separated from the abusive relationship, taking on the negative identity of "victim" or the positive identity of "survivor" seemed related to women's outlook for their future success.

SUMMARY

Abuse of female partners is a health problem of considerable magnitude with much potential for nursing intervention. Even though its significance is just beginning to be realized, the historical roots of abuse of female partners reveal that the problem is not new. In considering the theoretical frameworks advanced to explain its causes, the roles of intrapsychic factors, alcohol, stress, socialization for abuse, and cultural support have been examined. Wife abuse was also placed in the broader perspective of violence against women in general. The concept of machismo is important in explaining the behavior of abusive men. It has been proposed that the social organization of patriarchy, from which arise the historical roots of wife abuse, cultural support for the phenomenon, and machismo, may be said to set the stage for stress to precipitate violence against wives in men who have learned abusive behavior. The formulations that propose explanations for the continuation of abusive behavior in a relationship, for societal responses, and for psychological factors were also explored. The theoretical frameworks that have been examined provide the basis for nursing care of battered women, but further research is needed in all the areas examined, as well as research to further elucidate the relationships between abuse of female partners and the wider problem of violence in society.

REFERENCES

Bach, G. R., & Wyden, P. (1969). *The intimate enemy.* New York: William Morrow.

Bach-Y-Rita, G. (1971). Episodic dyscontrol: A study of 130 violent patients. *American Journal of Psychiatry, 127,* 1473-1478.

Balswick, J. O., & Peck, C. (1971). The inexpressive male: A tragedy of American society. *Family Coordinator, 20,* 364.

Barden, C., & Barden, J. (1976, June). The battered wife syndrome. *Viva,* 79-81, 108-110.

Beaulieu, L. (1978). Media, violence, and the family. In J. M. Eekelaar & S. Katz (Eds.), *Family violence* (pp. 60-62). Toronto: Butterworth.

Bednarik, K. (1970). *The male in crisis.* New York: Alfred A. Knopf.

Berk, R. A., Berk, S. F., Loseke, D. R., & Rauma, D. (1983). Mutual combat and other family violence myths. In D. Finkelhor, R. J. Gelles, G. T. Hotaling, & M. A. Straus (Eds.), *The dark side of families: Current family violence research* (pp. 197-212). Beverly Hills: Sage.

Bourdouris, J. (1971). Homicide in the family. *Journal of Marriage and the Family, 33,* 667-676.

Bowker, L. H. (1983). *Beating wife-beating.* Lexington, MA: Lexington Books.

Brandon, S. (1976). Physical violence in the family: An overview. In M. Borland (Ed.), *Violence in the family* (pp. 1-24). Atlantic Highlands, NJ: Humanities Press.

Bromberg, W. (1961). *The mold of murder.* New York: Grune & Stratton.

Browne, A. (1987). *When battered women kill.* New York: Free Press.

Browne, A., & Williams, K. R. (1989). Resource availability for women at risk and partner homicide. *Law and Society Review, 23,* 75-94.

Brownmiller, S. (1975). *Against our will: Men, women, and rape.* New York: Bantam Books.

Bullock, L., McFarlane, J., Bateman, L. H., & Miller, V. (1989). The prevalence and characteristics of battered women in a primary care setting. *Nurse Practitioner, 14*(6), 47-56.

Burgess, A., & Holmstrom, L. (1979). *Rape: Crisis and recovering.* Bowie, MD: Robert J. Brady.

Campbell, J. C. (1981). Misogyny and homicide of women. *Advances in Nursing Science, 3*(2), 67-85.

Campbell, J. C. (1985). Beating of wives: A cross-cultural perspective. *Victimology, 10*(1-4), 174-185.

Campbell, J. C. (1986). A survivor group for battered women. *Advances in Nursing Science, 8*(2), 13-20.

Campbell, J. C. (1989a). A test of two explanatory models of women's responses to battering. *Nursing Research, 38*(1), 18-24.

Campbell, J. C. (1989b). Women's responses to sexual abuse in intimate relationships. *Health Care for Women International, 8,* 335-347.

Campbell, J. C. (1992). *Relationship status of battered women over time.* Unpublished manuscript.

Campbell, J. C., & Humphreys, J. (1987). Providing health care in shelters. *Response, 10*(1), 21-24.

Carlson, B. (1977). Battered women and their assailants. *Social Work, 22,* 455-465.

Carmody, D. C., & Williams, K. R. (1987). Wife assault and perceptions of sanctions. *Violence and Victims, 2*(1), 25-38.

Carroll, J. C. (1977). The intergenerational transmission of family violence. *Aggressive Behavior, 3*(3), 289-299.

Carroll, J. C. (1980). Cultural-consistency theory of family violence in Mexican-American and Jewish-ethnic groups. In M. A. Straus & G. T. Hotaling (Eds.), *The social causes of husband-to-wife violence* (pp. 68-81). Minneapolis: University of Minnesota Press.

Chester, P. (1978). *About men.* New York: Simon & Schuster.

Chester, R., & Streather, J. (1972). Cruelty in English divorce: Some empirical findings. *Journal of Marriage and the Family, 34,* 706-710.

Claerhout, S., Elder, J., & Janes, C. (1982). Problem-solving skills of battered women. *American Journal of Community Psychology, 10*(5), 605-612.

Clark, R. (1970). *Crime in America.* New York: Simon & Schuster.

Clinard, M., & Abbott, D. (1973). *Crime in developing countries.* New York: John Wiley & Sons.

Coser, L. (1966). Some social functions of violence. *Annals of the American Academy of Political and Social Science, 364,* 11.

Curtis, L. A. (1975). *Violence, race, and culture.* Lexington, MA: D. C. Heath & Co.

Daly, M. (1978). *Gyn/Ecology: The metaethics of radical feminism.* Boston: Beacon Press.

Davidson, T. (1977). Wifebeating: A recurring phenomenon throughout history. In M. Roy (Ed.), *Battered women* (pp. 2-23). New York: Van Nostrand.

Davidson, T. (1978). *Conjugal crime: Understanding and changing the wifebeating problem.* New York: Hawthorn Books.

Dibble, U., & Straus, M. (1980). Some social structural determinants of inconsistency between attitudes and behavior. *Journal of Marriage and the Family, 42,* 73, 79.

Dobash, R. E., & Dobash, R. P. (1977-78). Wives: The "appropriate" victims of marital violence. *Victimology: An International Journal, 2*(3-4), 426-442.

Dobash, R. E., & Dobash, R. P. (1979). *Violence against wives.* New York: Free Press.

Dobash, R. E., & Dobash, R. P. (1984). The nature and antecedants of violent events. *British Journal of Criminology, 23*(3), 269-288.

Downey, J., & Howell, J. (1976). *Wife battering.* Vancouver: United Way of Greater Vancouver.

Drake, V. K. (1982). Battered women: A health care problem in disguise. *Image, 14*(2), 40-47.

Dreifus, C. (Ed.) (1977). *Seizing our bodies.* New York: Vintage Books.

Driver, E. D. (1971). Interaction and criminal homicide in India. *Social Forces, 60,* 155-156.

Dworkin, A. (1976). *Our blood: Prophecies and discourses on sexual politics.* New York: Harper & Row.

Elbow, M. (1977). Theoretical considerations of violent marriages. *Social Casework, 58,* 515-526.

Erlanger, H. S. (1974). The empirical status of the subculture of violence thesis. *Social Problems, 22,* 289.

Fagan, J. A., Stewart, D. K., & Hansen, K. V. (1983). Violent men or violent husbands? Background factors and situational correlates. In D. Finkelhor, R. J. Gelles, G. T. Hotaling, & M. A. Straus (Eds.), *The dark side of families: Current family violence research* (pp. 49-67). Beverly Hills: Sage.

Fasteau, M. (1974). *The male machine.* New York: McGraw-Hill.

Faulk, M. (1974). Men who assault their wives. *Medicine, Science, and the Law, 14,* 180-183.

Federal Bureau of Investigation (1986). *Uniform crime reports for the United States.* Washington, DC: U.S. Department of Justice.

Ferraro, K. J., & Johnson, J. M. (1983). How women experience battering: The process of victimization. *Social Problems, 30*(3), 325-339.

Finkelhor, D., & Yllo, K. (1983). Rape in marriage: A sociological view. In D. Finkelhor, R. J. Gelles, G. T. Hotaling, & M. A. Straus (Eds.), *The dark side of families: Current family violence research* (pp. 119-130). Beverly Hills: Sage.

Flynn, J. (1977). Recent findings related to wife abuse. *Social Casework, 63,* 13-20.

Foster, L. A., Veale, C. M., & Fogel, C. I. (1989). Factors present when battered women kill. *Issues in Mental Health Nursing, 10,* 273-284.

Garbner, G., & Gross, L. (1976). Living with television: The violence profile. *Journal of Communications, 26,* 189, 190.

Gayford, J. J. (1978). Sex magazines. *Medicine, Science, and the Law, 18,* 48.

Gayford, J. J. (1979). The aetiology of repeated serious physical assaults by husbands on wives. *Medicine, Science, and the Law, 19,* 19-24.

Gelles, R. J. (1974). *The violent home.* Newbury Park, CA: Sage.

Gelles, R. J. (1976). Abused wives: Why do they stay? *Journal of Marriage and the Family, 38*(3), 659-668.

Gentemann, K. M. (1984). Wife beating: Attitudes of a nonclinical population. *Victimology, 9,* 101-119.

Gibbons, D. C. (1970). *Delinquent behavior.* Englewood Cliffs, NJ: Prentice Hall.

Gillespie, C. K. (1989). *Justifiable homicide.* Columbus: Ohio State University Press.

Gillies, H. (1976). Homicide in the west of Scotland. *British Journal of Psychology, 28,* 116.

Gondolf, E. W., & Fisher, E. R. (1988). *Battered women as survivors: An alternative to learned helplessness.* Lexington, MA: Lexington Books.

Goode, W. (1971). Force and violence in the family. *Journal of Marriage and the Family, 33*(4), 624-636.

Gordon, R. et al. (1963). Values and gang delinquency: A study of street corner groups. *American Journal of Sociology, 69,* 123.

Graham, D., Rawlings, E., & Rimini, N. (1988). Survivors of terror: Battered women, hostages, and the Stockholm Syndrome. In K. Yllo & M. Bograd (Eds.), *Feminist perspectives on wife abuse* (pp. 217-233). Newbury Park, CA: Sage.

Greenberg, P. (1977). The thrill seekers. *Human Behavior, 6,* 16-23.

Gregory, M. (1976). Battered wives. In M. Borland (Ed.), *Violence in the family* (pp. 107-128). Atlantic Highlands, NJ: Humanities Press.

Grossfeld, S. (1991, September 2). "Safer" and in jail: Women who kill their batterers. *Boston Globe,* pp. 1, 12, 13.

Groth, A. N. (1977). Rape: Power, anger, and sexuality. *American Journal of Psychiatry, 134,* 1239-1243.

Hartley, R. E. (1974). Sex-role pressure and the socialization of the male child. In J. H. Pleck & J. Sawyer (Eds.), *Men and masculinity.* Englewood Cliffs, NJ: Prentice-Hall.

Heffner, S. (1977-78). Wife abuse in West Germany. *Victimology, 2,* 472-476.

Helton, A. (1987). *Protocol of care for the battered woman.* White Plains, NY: March of Dimes Birth Defects Foundation.

Helton, A., McFarlane, J., & Anderson, E. (1987a). Battered and pregnant: A prevalence study. *American Journal of Public Health, 77*(10), 1337-1339.

Helton, A., McFarlane, J., & Anderson, E. (1987b). Prevention of battering during pregnancy: Focus on behavioral change. *Public Health Nursing, 4*(3), 166-174.

Hepburn, J. (1971). Subcultures, violence, and the subculture of violence: An old rut or a new road. *Criminology, 9,* 93.

Heyman, S. (1977). Dogmatism, hostility, aggression, and gender roles. *Journal of Clinical Psychology, 33,* 695.

Hilberman, E., & Munson, K. (1977-78). Sixty battered women. *Victimology, 2,* 460-470.

Hoff, L. A. (1990). *Battered women as survivors.* New York: Routledge.

Hollenkamp, M., & Attala, J. (1986). Meeting health needs in a crisis shelter: A challenge to nurses in the community. *Journal of Community Health Nursing, 3*(4), 201-209.

Hosken, F. P. (1977-78). Female circumcision in Africa. *Victimology, 2,* 487-498.

Hotaling, G. T., & Straus, M. A. (1980). Culture, social organization, and irony in the study of family violence. In M. A. Straus & G. T. Hotaling (Eds.), *The social causes of husband-wife violence* (pp. 3-22). Minneapolis: University of Minnesota Press.

Hotaling, G. T., & Sugarman, D. B. (1986). An analysis of risk markers in husband to wife violence: The current state of knowledge. *Violence and Victims, 1*(2), 101-124.

Jaffe, P., Wolfe, D. A., Wilson, S., & Zak, L. (1986). Emotional and physical health problems of battered women. *Canadian Journal of Psychiatry, 31,* 625-629.

Janoff-Bulman, R., & Frieze, I. H. (1983). A theoretical perspective for understanding reactions to victimization. *Journal of Social Issues, 39*(2), 1-17.

Janssen-Jurreit, M. (1982). *Sexism: The male monopoly on history and thought* (V. Moberg, Trans.). New York: Farrar, Straus & Giroux.

Kalmuss, D. (1979). The attribution of responsibility in a wife-abuse context. *Victimology, 4,* 286.

Kantor, G. K., & Straus, M. A. (1987). The "drunken bum" theory of wife beating. *Social Problems, 34*(3), 213-230.

Kantor, G. K., & Straus, M. A. (1990). Response of victims and police to assaults on wives. In M. A. Straus & R. J. Gelles (Eds.), *Physical violence in American families* (pp. 473-487). New Brunswick, NJ: Transaction.

Kelly, L. (1988). How women define their experiences of violence. In K. Yllo & M. Bograd (Eds.), *Feminist perspectives on wife abuse* (pp. 114-132). Beverly Hills: Sage.

King, M. C., & Ryan, J. (1989). Abused women: Dispelling myths and encouraging intervention. *Nurse Practitioner, 14*(5), 47-58.

Komavovsky, M. (1964). *Blue collar marriage.* New York: Vintage Books.

Koss, M. P., Gidycz, C. A., & Wisniewski, N. (1987). The scope of rape: Incidence and prevalence of sexual aggression and victimization in a national sample of higher education students. *Journal of Consulting and Clinical Psychology, 55*(2), 162-170.

Kurz, D. (1987). Emergency department responses to battered women: Resistance to medicalization. *Social Problems, 34*(1), 69-81.

Kutum, B. (1977). Legislative needs and solutions. In M. Roy (Ed.), *Battered women* (pp. 277-287). New York: Van Nostrand.

Ladwig, G. B., & Andersen, M. D. (1989). Substance abuse in women: Relationship between chemical dependency of women and past reports of physical and/or sexual abuse. *The International Journal of the Addictions, 24*(8), 739-754.

Landenburger, K. (1989). A process of entrapment in and recovery from an abusive relationship. *Issues in Mental Health Nursing, 10,* 209-227.

Landon, J. (1977-78). Images of violence against women. *Victimology, 2,* 510.

Langley, R., & Levy, R. (1977). *Wifebeating: The silent crisis.* New York: E. P. Dutton.

Launius, M., & Jensen, B. (1987). Interpersonal problem-solving skills in battered, counseling, and control women. *Journal of Family Violence, 2*(2), 151-162.

Launius, M., & Lindquist, C. (1988). Learned helplessness, external locus of control, and passivity in battered women. *Journal of Interpersonal Violence, 3*(3), 307-318.

Lederer, W. (1968). *The fear of women.* New York: Harcourt Brace Jovanovich.

Letcher, M. (1979). Black women and homicide. In H. M. Rose (Ed.), *Lethal aspects of urban violence* (pp. 83-90). Lexington, MA: Lexington Books.

Lester, D. (1980). A cross-cultural study of wife abuse. *Aggressive Behavior, 6,* 361-364.

Levinson, D. (1989). *Family violence in cross cultural perspective.* Newbury Park, CA: Sage.

Levy, B. (Ed.) (1991). *Dating violence.* Seattle: Seal Press.

Lewis, D. O. (1977). Juvenile male sexual assaulters. *American Journal of Psychiatry, 136,* 1194-1196.

Lewis, R. A. (1971). Socialization into national violence: Familial correlates of hawkish attitudes toward war. *Journal of Marriage and the Family, 33,* 702.

Lobel, K. (Ed.) (1986). *Naming the violence.* Seattle: Seal Press.

Loizos, M. (1978). Violence and the family: Some Mediterranean examples. In J. P. Martin (Ed.), *Violence and the family* (pp. 183-195). Chichester: John Wiley & Sons.

Lystaad, M. H. (1975). Violence at home. *American Journal of Orthopsychiatry, 45,* 339.

MacDonald, J. (1961). *The murderer and his victim.* Springfield, IL: Charles C. Thomas.

McCabe, S. (1977). A note on the reports of the select committees on violence in marriage and violence in the family. *British Journal of Criminology, 17,* 283.

McCormack, T. (1978). Machismo in media research: A critical review of research on violence and pornography. *Social Problems, 25,* 545.

Maier, S., & Seligman, M. (1976). Learned helplessness: Theory and evidence. *Journal of Experimental Psychology, 105,* 3-46.

Makman, R. (1978). Some clinical aspects of interspousal violence. In J. M. Eekelaar & Katz, S. N. (Eds.), *Family violence.* Toronto: Butterworth.

Maletzky, B. M. (1973). The episodic dyscontrol syndrome. *Diseases of the Nervous System, 34,* 179-180.

Malik, M. O. A., & Salvi, O. (1976). A profile of homicide in the Sudan. *Forensic Science, 7,* 141-150.

Marsden, D. (1978). Sociological perspectives on family violence. In J. P. Martin (Ed.), *Violence and the family* (pp. 103-133). Chichester: John Wiley & Sons.

Martin, D. (1976). *Battered wives.* San Francisco: Glide Publications.

Masumura, W. T. (1979). Wife abuse and other forms of aggression. *Victimology, 4,* 52.

May, M. (1978). Violence in the family: An historical perspective. In J. P. Martin (Ed.), *Violence and the family* (pp. 135-163). Chichester: John Wiley & Sons.

Mead, M. (1949). *Male and female.* New York: William Morrow.

Miller, W. (1958). Lower class culture as a generation milieu of gang delinquency. *Journal of Social Issues, 14,* 5-19.

Mills, T. (1985). The assault on the self: Stages in coping with battering husbands. *Qualitative Sociology, 8*(2), 103-123.

Mitchell, R. E., & Hodson, C. A. (1983). Coping with domestic violence: Social support and psychological health among battered women. *American Journal of Community Psychology, 11*(6), 629-654.

National Coalition Against Domestic Violence (1992). *Statistical bulletin.* Denver: NCADV.

NiCarthy, G. (1986). *Getting free: A handbook for women in abusive relationships.* Seattle: Seal Press.

Nobels, W. (1978). Toward an empirical and theoretical framework for defining black families. *Journal of Marriage and the Family, 40,* 687.

O'Brien, J. E. (1971). Violence in divorce prone families. *Journal of Marriage and the Family, 33*(4), 692-698.

Okun, L. (1986). *Woman abuse: Facts replacing myths.* Albany: State University of New York.

Pagelow, M. D. (1981). *Woman-battering: Victims and their experiences.* Beverly Hills: Sage.

Pagelow, M. D. (1988). Marital rape. In V. B. Van Hasselt, R. L. Morrison, A. S. Bellack, & M. Hersen (Eds.), *Handbook of family violence* (pp. 207-232). New York: Plenum Press.

Painter, S. L., & Dutton, D. (1985). Patterns of emotional bonding in women: Traumatic bonding. *International Journal of Women's Studies, 8*(4), 363-375.

Parker, B., & Schumacker, D. N. (1977). The battered wife syndrome and violence in the nuclear family of origin: A controlled pilot study. *American Journal of Public Health, 67*(8), 760-761.

Perry, D. G., & Perry, L. C. (1974). Denial of suffering in the victim as a stimulant to violence in aggressive boys. *Child Development, 45,* 55, 60.

Prescott, S., & Letko, C. (1977). Battered women: A social psychological perspective. In M. Roy (Ed.), *Battered women.* New York: Van Nostrand.

Renvoize, J. (1978). *Web of violence.* London: Routledge & Kegan Paul.

Renzetti, C. (1989). Building a second closet: Third party responses to victims of lesbian partner abuse. *Family Relations, 38,* 157-163.

Rich, A. (1979). *On lies, secrets, and silence.* New York: W. W. Norton.

Richards, J. A. (1991). Battering in a population of adolescent females. *Journal of American Academy of Nurse Practitioners, 3,* 180-185.

Rickel, A., & Grant, L. (1979). Sex role stereotypes in the mass media and schools: Five consistent themes. *International Journal of Women's Studies, 2,* 164-179.

Rohner, R. P. (1972). Sex differences in aggression. *Ethos, 4,* 57-72.

Rose, K, & Saunders, D. G. (1986). Nurses' and physicians' attitudes about women abuse: The effects of gender and professional role. *Health Care for Women International, 7,* 427-438.

Rosewater, L. B. (1988). Battered or schizophrenic? Psychological tests can't tell. In K. Yllo & M. Bograd (Eds.), *Feminist perspectives on wife abuse* (pp. 200-216). Beverly Hills: Sage.

Rounsaville, B. J. (1978). Theories in marital violence: Evidence from a study of battered women. *Victimology, 3,* 11-31.

Roy, M. (1977). A research project probing a cross-section of battered wives. In M. Roy (Ed.), *Battered women* (pp. 3-16). New York: Van Nostrand.

Ruotolo, A. K. (1975). Neurotic pride and homicide. *American Journal of Psychoanalysis, 35,* 16.

Russell, D. (1990). *Rape in marriage.* Bloomington, IN: Indiana University Press.

Russell, D., & Van de Ven, N. (1976). *Crimes against women.* Millbrae, CA: Les Femmes.

Ryan, W. (1971). *Blaming the victim.* New York: Vintage Books.

Sampselle, C. M. (1991). The role of nursing in preventing violence against women. *Journal of Obstetrical and Gynecological Nursing, 20*(6), 481-487.

Sandelowski, M. (1980). *Women, health and choice.* Englewood Cliffs, NJ: Prentice Hall.

Saunders, D. G. (1986). When battered women use violence: Husband-abuse or self-defense? *Violence and Victims, 1*(1), 47-60.

Saunders, D. G. (1988). Wife abuse, husband abuse, or mutual combat? In K. Yllo & M. Bograd (Eds.), *Feminist perspectives on wife abuse* (pp. 90-113). Beverly Hills: Sage.

Schram, D. (1978). Rape. In J. R. Chapman & M. Gates (Eds.), *The victimization of women* (pp. 53-79). Beverly Hills: Sage.

Shainess, N. (1977). Psychological aspects of wifebeating. In M. Roy (Ed.), *Battered women* (pp. 72-96). New York: Van Nostrand Reinhold.

Shainess, N. (1979). Vulnerability to violence: Masochism as process. *American Journal of Psychotherapy, 33,* 174-189.

Sherwood, J. W., & McGrath J.H., III. (1976). Why people own guns. *Journal of Communications, 26,* 613.

Shields, N. M., & Hanneke, C. R. (1983). Battered women's reactions to marital rape. In D. Finkelhor, R. J. Gelles, G. T. Hotaling, & M. A. Straus (Eds.), *The dark side of families: Current family violence research* (pp. 132-148). Beverly Hills: Sage.

Shotland, L. R., & Straw, M. K. (1976). Bystander response when a man attacks a woman. *Journal of Personality and Social Psychology, 34*, 992, 999.

Sipes, R. G. (1973). War, sports, and aggression: An empirical test of two rival theories. *American Anthropologist, 75*, 71.

Snell, J. E., Rosenwald, R. J., & Robey, A. (1964). The wife-beater's wife. *Archives of General Psychiatry, 11*, 107-112.

The Spiritual Dimension in Victim Services (1990). *Clergy in-service training manual.* Sacramento, CA: Spiritual Dimension in Victim Services.

Star, B. (1978). Comparing battered and non-battered women. *Victimology, 3*(1-2), 32-44.

Stark, E., & Flitcraft, A. (1988). Violence among intimates: An epidemiologic review. In. V. B. Van Hasselt, R. L. Morrison, A. S. Bellack, & M. Hersen (Eds.), *Handbook of family violence* (pp. 293-317). New York: Plenum Press.

Stark, E., Flitcraft, A., & Frazier, W. (1979). Medicine and patriachal violence: The social construction of a "private" event. *International Journal of Health Services, 9*, 461-493.

Stark, E., Flitcraft, A., Zuckerman, D., Grey, A., Robison, J., & Frazier, W. (1981). *Wife abuse in the medical setting.* Rockville, MD: National Clearinghouse on Domestic Violence.

Stark, R., & McEvoy, J. (1970, November). Middle-class violence. *Psychology Today, 4*, 52-56, 110-112.

Steinmetz, S. K. (1977). *The cycle of violence: Assertive, aggressive and abusive family interaction.* New York: Praeger.

Steinmetz, S. K. (1977-78). The battered husband syndrome. *Victimology, 2*, 499-502.

Steinmetz, S. K., & Lucca, J. S. (1988). Husband battering. In V. B. Van Hasselt, R. L. Morrison, A. S. Bellack, & M. Hersen (Eds.), *Handbook of family violence* (pp. 233-246). New York: Plenum.

Steinmetz, S. K., & Straus, M. A. (Eds.) (1974). *Violence in the family.* New York: Harper & Row.

Storr, A. (1978). Introduction. In J. M. Eekelaar & S. Katz (Eds.), *Family violence.* Toronto: Butterworth.

Straus, M. (1976). Sexual inequality, cultural norms, and wifebeating. *Victimology, 1*, 62.

Straus, M. A. (1979). A sociological perspective on the prevention and treatment of wifebeating. *Nursing Dimensions, 7*(1), 45-63.

Straus, M. A. (1980). Wife-beating: How common and why? In M. A. Straus & G. T. Hotaling (Eds.), *The social causes of husband-wife violence* (pp. 23-38). Minneapolis: University of Minnesota Press.

Straus, M. (1990). Social stress and marital violence in a national sample of American families. In M. A. Straus & R. J. Gelles (Eds.), *Physical violence in American families* (pp. 181-201). New Brunswick, NJ: Transaction.

Straus, M. A., & Gelles, R. J. (1986). Societal change and change in family violence from 1975 to 1985 as revealed by two national surveys. *Journal of Marriage and the Family, 48*, 465-479.

Straus, M. A., Gelles, R. J., & Steinmetz, S. K. (1988). *Behind closed doors: Violence in the American family.* Newbury Park, CA: Sage.

Strube, M. J., & Barbour, L. S. (1984). Factors related to the decision to leave an abusive relationship. *Journal of Marriage and the Family, 45*, 837-844.

Symonds, A. (1979). Violence against women: The myth of masochism. *American Journal of Psychotherapy, 33*, 161-173.

Symonds, M. (1975). Victims of violence: Psychological effects and after-effects. *American Journal of Psychoanalysis, 35*, 19-22.

Symonds, M. (1978). The psychodynamics of violence-prone marriages. *American Journal of Psychotherapy, 38*, 219.

Taylor, S. P. & Smith, I. (1974). Aggression as a function of sex of victim and males' attitude toward female. *Psychological Reports, 35*, 1096-1097.

Tedeschi, J. T. (1977). Aggression and the use of coercive power. *Journal of Social Issues, 33*, 114.

Ten Houten, W. D. (1970). The black family: Myth and reality. *Psychiatry, 33*, 145-173.

Tiger, L. (1969). *Men in groups.* New York: Random House.

Toby, J. (1966). Violence and the masculine ideal. *American Academy of Political and Social Science, 364*, 19.

Tolson, A. (1977). *The limits of masculinity.* New York: Harper & Row.

Toplin, R. B. (1975). *Unchallenged violence.* Westport, CT: Greenwood Press.

Van Hasselt, V. B., Morrison, R. L., & Bellack, A. S. (1985). Alcohol use in wife abusers and their spouses. *Addictive Behaviors, 10*, 127-135.

Walker, L. E. (1979). *The battered woman.* New York: Harper & Row.

Walker, L. E. (1984). *The battered woman syndrome.* New York: Springer.

Walker, L. E. (1989). Psychology and violence against women. *American Psychologist, 44*(4), 695-702.

Walker, L. E., & Browne, A. (1985). Gender and victimization by intimates. *Journal of Personality, 53*(2), 179-195.

Wallace, M. (1978). *Black macho and the myth of the superwoman.* New York: Dial Press.

Warshaw, R. (1988). *I never called it rape.* New York: Harper & Row.

Webster, W. H. (1989). *Uniform crime reports.* Washington, DC: U.S. Department of Justice.

Weimer, J. M. (1978). The mother, the macho, and the state. *International Journal of Women's Studies, 1*, 73.

Welch, R. L. (1979). Subtle sex-role cues in children's commercials. *Journal of Communications, 29*, 207.

Whitehurst, R. (1971). Violence potential in extramarital sexual responses. *Journal of Marriage and the Family, 11*, 688.

Whitehurst, R. (1974). Violence in husband wife interaction. In Steinmetz, S. K., & Straus, M. A. (Eds.), *Violence in the family.* New York: Harper & Row.

Whiting, B. (1965). Sex identity conflict and physical violence: A comparative study. *American Anthropologist, 67,* 126.

Widom, C. S. (1989). Does violence beget violence? A critical examination of the literature. Psychological Bulletin, *106*(1), 3-28.

Williams, J. S., & McGrath, J. (1978). A social profile of urban gun owners. In J. A. Lonciardi & A. E. Pottieger (Eds.), *Violent Crime.* Beverly Hills: Sage.

Woodhouse, L. D. (1990). An exploratory study of the use of life history methods to determine treatment needs for female substance abusers. *Response, 13*(3), 12-15.

Wright, J. D., & Marston, L. L. (1974). The ownership of the means of destruction: Weapons in the U.S. *Social Problems, 23,* 101.

Yllo, K. A., & Straus, M. A. (1990). Patriarchy and violence against wives: The impact of structural and normative factors. In M. A. Straus & R. J. Gelles (Eds.), *Physical violence in American families* (pp. 383-399). New Brunswick, NJ: Transaction.

Young, D. M. et al. (1975). Is chivalry dead? *Journal of Communications, 25,* 63.

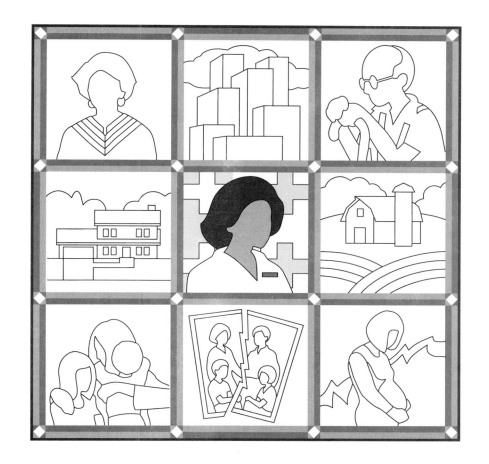

PART

II

Theory and Application

C H A P T E R

4

Children of Battered Women

Janice Humphreys

"Shelter"
big old house
creaks and moans
til mothers come
and children's sounds
fill its empty rooms
little families
with shattered dreams
and broken hearts
run from daddy's fist
to this
a shelter home
refuge from
sweet love
gone amiss
                    Susan Venters*

C hildren of battered women are exposed to family violence during their growth years, the time when they are learning about themselves, relationships, and the world around them. Children of battered women experience the world as a place where adults in intimate relationships hurt each other and sometimes other people around them. Children who live in homes where women are subject to beatings see families as places where women are subordinate to men, and where men assert their power with their fists. Until recently little has been written about the children of battered women and even less research has been reported on the consequences of growing up in such circumstances. This chapter reviews the literature on the children of battered women. Information on the estimated number of children exposed to abuse of their mothers, theories and models that attempt to explain children's experiences, the characteristics of these children, and proposed nursing care are presented. As with other research of family violence, knowledge of children of battered women has its limitations. Nevertheless, a growing awareness of the problems and strengths of the children of battered women is manifest. Insight into this literature can provide an initial step toward understanding the needs for nursing exhibited by these children and families.

SCOPE OF THE PROBLEM

The last two decades have been associated with increasingly frequent reports in both the scholarly and

---

*Reprinted from *Every Twelve Seconds*, compiled by Susan Venters (Hillsboro, Oregon: Shelter, 1981) by permission of the author.

lay literature of family violence. Although these articles have highlighted the problem of family violence, the literature has focused primarily on abuse of children, adult women, and elders in that order. Not surprisingly, the children of battered women have received much less attention. Unlike children or adults who are directly subject to the shocking violence reported in the media, children of battered women are less well-recognized survivors of family violence. Children of battered women have only received attention when they too, generally inadvertently, became injured during a violent episode. The nature of their experience is less visible, perhaps more insidious than others who are directly abused on a regular basis. The extent of the scope and impact of family violence on the children of battered women has only recently been examined.

Estimates vary on the number of children exposed to battered women, their mothers. Davidson (1978) reported that children were present in 41% of the domestic disturbances in which police intervened. Wasileski, Callaghan-Chaffee, and Chaffee (1982) reported that in their study of spouse abuse in military homes (N = 60), two thirds had children and 45% reported that their children witnessed the abuse. Carlson (1984) estimates (based on an average of two children in 55% of violent households) that at least 3.3 million children in the United States between the ages of 3 and 17 years are at risk of exposure to parental violence every year.

In a national representative sample of adults in households (N = 3,520) surveyed by telephone in 1985, Straus and Gelles (1986) found a rate of overall violence of 113 per 1,000 couples and of "wife beating" (severe violence) of 30 per 1,000 couples. Given a population of approximately 54 million couples in the U.S. in 1985, this figure represents approximately 1,620,000 women beaten each year by their male partners. If Carlson's (1984) estimate of 55% is applied to these figures, it can be estimated that 1,782,000 children were exposed to the battering of their mothers. Although Straus and Gelles discuss the relative decrease in the reported incidence of battering in this 1985 study compared with their 1975 study and limited their sampling to households with telephones, the decrease was not statis-

tically significant and suggests that violence against women and the effect on their children continues as a serious problem in the United States.

Relationship to Other Types of Abuse

The impact on children of observing abuse of their mothers is unclear. Research has described even young children's sensitivities to conflict and distress in their homes (Cummings, Pellegrini, Notarius, & Cummings, 1989). Furthermore, interviews with children often reveal that children were much more aware of the violence in the home than parents believed.

Several authors have stated that children who come from violent homes are likely to experience violence in future relationships. Kalmuss (1984) used survey data from adults and found that observing aggression and violence between parents was more strongly related to involvement in severe marital violence than was being a victim of abuse during adolescence. Early research on violence in dating relationships also correlates with childhood exposure to violence between parents (Breslin, Riggs, O'Leary & Arias, 1990). Furthermore, the problem of marital violence in adulthood increased dramatically when, as children or adolescents, respondents had experienced both types of family violence (Carlson, 1990; Davis & Carlson, 1987; Kalmuss, 1984). The majority of batterers have witnessed this behavior in their families of origin, and the rate of wifebeating is dramatically higher for sons of batterers compared with sons of nonviolent fathers (Straus, Gelles, & Steinmetz, 1980). However, not all sons who grew up in violent homes become batterers; in fact, many siblings of batterers may live peacefully in nonviolent marriages (Dobash & Dobash, 1979). Stark and Flitcraft (1988) advocate that the conclusion that violence in childhood produces violence in adult life is erroneous. In a reexamination of the data from the random 1980 study (Straus et al., 1980), Stark and Flitcraft conclude that although boys who experienced violence as children were disproportionately violent as adults, 90% of all children from violent homes and 80% from homes described as "most violent" did not subsequently abuse their wives. Kaufman and Zigler (1987) state that no more than 30% of those who experienced or witnessed violence as children are currently abusive, an estimate that Stark and Flitcraft believe is too high. Nevertheless, a history of violence in the family of origin can seriously affect children, but exposure to violence does not automatically result in serious behavioral problems and a certainty of violence in future relationships.

Many authors have also noted a significant overlap between abuse of women and child abuse. The risk of exposure to abuse begins before the child is born. There is a growing awareness that pregnancy itself may trigger battering and/or significantly increase its severity. See Chapter 6 for a more detailed discussion of the dynamics of the phenomenon.

Jouriles, Barling, and O'Leary (1987) reported that interspousal aggression was highly associated with parental aggression directed toward children. The researchers also noted that parental reports of parent-child aggression were more strongly linked to child behavior problems than parental reports of interspousal aggression.

McKibben, De Vos, and Newberger (1989) examined emergency room hospital records of children identified as abused and a matched comparison group. From record review alone, almost 60% of the mothers could also be diagnosed as abused. For children who both observe their mothers being abused and who are abused themselves the consequences have been reported to be traumatic (Jaffe, Wolfe, Wilson, & Zak, 1986), especially for young children (Hughes, 1988). In a feminist analysis of mothers of child abuse victims, Stark and Flitcraft (1988) conclude that battering is the most common context for child abuse, and that the battering male is the typical child abuser.

THEORIES/MODELS

Theories and models of children's responses to abuse of their mothers have only recently been described in the literature. Nevertheless, they provide a framework for greater understanding and suggest areas in need of research.

Children who are exposed to wife abuse may be at increased risk of developing adjustment problems. This vulnerability may be the result of several interrelated factors, including their exposure to violent role models, their experience of the discord that accompanies wife abuse, the lack of physically and emotionally available caregivers, and/or the fear that their mothers or they may be physically injured (Rosenbaum & O'Leary, 1981).

Aversion Theory

Emery (1989) encourages theory development that is multicausal to better explain the diversity of children's responses to family violence. While analyzing the literature on child abuse, he suggests that other factors associated with abuse (e.g., general family disruption) may account for disturbances in children's psychological adjustment.

Emery (1989) proposes a three-component model of children's reactions to parental conflict "wherein (a) the conflict serves as an aversive event that creates distress in the child, (b) the child reacts emotionally or instrumentally in attempt to alleviate the distress, and (c) the child's actions that reduce the conflict are likely to be maintained because of the function they serve for the child and for the family as a whole" (p. 325). Emery theorizes that children experience distress when they observe violent conflict between adults. Research of children as young as 12 months has reported that children manifest distress (crying to increased aggression) when in the presence of conflict not directed at them. Secondary to their emotional distress, children are thought to respond either emotionally or instrumentally to the adult violence. Emery categorizes children's response strategies as differing on the basis of how direct the strategy is, how powerful the child is in the family, and whether the child remains neutral or allies with one parent or the other (1989, p. 325). The third component of Emery's model considers the function of children's actions in response to adult violence. He suggests that within the family system, children act in various ways that can decrease the violence and thus diminish the distress the children experience. He suggests distraction (e.g., describing the events of the school day) and scapegoating (e.g., becoming the focus of adult attention) as two ways children can function to stop battering of their mothers. He identifies that responses that are maladaptive to children may serve a useful purpose within the violent family system.

Emery states that his model is in the early stages of development; nevertheless, he contributes several important aspects to the theoretical basis of children's responses to battering of their mothers. Emery proposes that children are important elements within the family system and suggests that family functioning is a result of interchange within and outside of the family itself. He recognizes that children are very aware of conflict between adults, a conclusion that is often not fully realized by parents. Children experience distress when they become aware of adult conflict, experience emotional and/or instrumental responses, and in turn act on those responses. Emery, however, fails to consider

developmental state as influencing children's cognitive functioning and emotional development. He further fails to mention that although children may act to diminish their own internal emotional distress, they may also be strongly motivated to protect their parents, most often mothers. His references to scapegoating suggest a negative intent on the part of children responding in this fashion. A more positive label might be protecting since research with children of battered women has found that this is often the actual intent (Humphreys, 1989).

Stress and Coping Theory

Jaffe, Wolfe, and Wilson (1990) propose a model that attempts to explain the links between wife abuse and children's developmental problems (Figure 4-1). Their model interrelates what they term wife abuse with maternal stress and coping, and children's stress and coping responses. They pro-

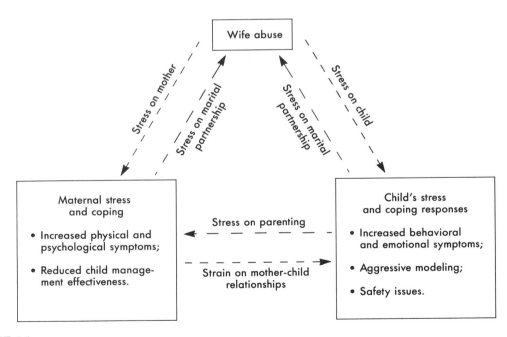

FIGURE 4-1

The links between wife abuse and children's developmental disorders. (Copyright © 1990, Sage. Reproduced with permission from *Children of battered women* by P. G. Jaffe, D. A. Wolfe, & S. K. Wilson, p. 64.)

pose that each of these three factors places stress on each other, stress on their interrelationships, and thus results in detrimental consequences for both mothers and children. Within their model, abused mothers experience physical and psychological symptoms, resulting in reduced child management effectiveness; therefore, children demonstrate increased behavioral and emotional symptoms, are exposed to aggressive modeling, and sometimes are directly endangered by the violence directed at their mothers. This model is noteworthy for several reasons. First, it delineates that children are directly affected by the violence they observe inflicted on their mothers (intergenerational transmission theory), as well as indirectly affected via the changes that occur within the caretaking environment (family disruption theory). They acknowledge that the specific type of stressor may not be as critical to children's adaptation as the amount of stressors and the children's perceptions of them. Second, their model acknowledges the role of mothers to mediate, to a degree, the effects of violence on children. Finally, it incorporates children's responses to abuse of their mothers as having both a direct and indirect effect on the violence. Although acknowledging the coping and adaptation of children in response to the abuse of their mothers, Jaffe et al. also recognize that the long-term consequences of childhood exposure to violence can be variable and significant.

A growing body of empirical evidence lends support to the work of Jaffe et al. Not surprisingly, several investigations have documented that battered women experience more distress and disorganization than women who are not battered (Christopoulos et al., 1987). In a 1985 study Wolfe, Jaffe, Wilson, and Zak reported that children who experienced clinically significant behavioral problems were more likely to have been exposed to a higher frequency and intensity of physical violence, and their mothers reported more negative life events over the previous year than the mothers of children who were adjusted. The investigators confirmed that the impact of witnessing abuse was partially mediated by factors associated with maternal stress. These findings support the direct (high frequency and inten-

sity) and indirect (lack of maternal coping) effects of battering of their mothers on children. In a retrospective study of college students' experiences with family violence, Resick and Reese (1986) report that violent families were characterized by a dominance hierarchy, open expression of anger, conflictual interactions, and a lack of organization. These findings support the hypotheses that violent families provide aggressive modeling for children (direct effects) and concurrent family disorganization that indirectly affects children. Jaffe et al. are to be commended for their program of research that methodically addresses each aspect of their model.

Posttraumatic Stress Theory

Silvern and Kaersvang (1989) suggest that observing violence between parents itself rather than the combination of violence and family disruption traumatizes children, affecting them like other victims of posttraumatic disorders. They propose that exposure to battering of their mothers is a traumatic event for children. They further suggest that trauma can result from perceived endangerment, even if no physical harm actually occurs. Within this framework, trauma within the family relationship is especially disturbing since families rely on a sense of trust between members, which is shattered by violence. When children observe violence they experience fragmentation of self, and fragmented, uninterpreted images of the event. Normal psychological tasks require that survivors come to understand the event, establish meaning and their personal emotions so that the trauma can be experienced as past. Survivors of trauma may experience difficulties in this process. These difficulties manifest in children of battered mothers as the various problems described by researchers (see later section in this chapter).

In support of their theory Silvern and Kaersvang (1989) suggest that social-learning theory predicts gender-based differences in children's responses to the abuse of their mothers. Yet research to date has offered inconsistent findings related to children's gender. Recently Jouriles, Murphy, and O'Leary (1989) found that in 87 couples requesting marital therapy, marital aggression did contribute unique variance to each child-problem subscale (conduct disorders, personality disorder, inadequacy-immaturity) as measured by the Behavior Problems Checklist. When marital discord, child's age, child's sex, and marital discord and child's sex interaction were controlled for, physical aggression between spouses still contributed unique variance to the prediction of child behavior problems. Although these findings are limited in their generalizability, they do offer support for the significant contribution that the trauma of violence between parents can have on some children.

Silvern and Kaersvang (1989) clearly state that their interest lies in "shock trauma" and pathogenic processes, not the cumulative trauma of living in a violent household. Their theory, although potentially explanatory in dealings with some children, may lack the scope necessary to deal with all children of battered women over time. Nevertheless, their hypotheses do suggest interventions for some children of battered women, especially during the immediate crisis phase.

CHARACTERISTICS AND CONTRIBUTING FACTORS

Compared with literature on child abuse and abuse of women, there are few published reports about the children of battered women, a fact that has been recognized (Giles-Sims, 1985; Hershorn & Rosenbaum, 1984). This is particularly disturbing because many articles reported intervention programs with the children of battered women (Alessi & Hearn, 1984; Gentry & Eaddy, 1982; Hughes, 1981, 1982; Hughes & Barad, 1983).

The literature on children of battered women generally has examined the pathology or difficulties (Hughes & Barad 1983; Levine, 1975; Westra & Martin, 1981) of these children or focused on their observations of violence between adults (Davidson, 1978; Layzer, Goodson, & deLange, 1986; Ulbrich & Huber, 1981). Early research reported some gender-related differences (Forsstrom-Cohen & Rosenbaum, 1985; Hershorn & Rosenbaum, 1985; Hinchey & Gavelek, 1982; Porter & O'Leary, 1980), but the significance of this variable remains uncertain.

The body of knowledge about children of battered women is still developing, and thus the overall picture of their experience remains unclear. This section describes the current data about the children of battered women to develop a better understanding of their experience, their potential and actual problems, and their strengths. Particular attention is given to the increasing evidence on factors that can mediate the effects of family violence on children, and on the worries and caring behaviors of children on behalf of their mothers. This literature is applied to the development of nursing care to children of battered women in a subsequent section.

Early studies on shelters for battered women began to identify the needs of children who accompanied their mothers to safety. At least 70% of all battered women seeking shelter have children who accompany them, and 17% of the women bring three or more children (MacLeod, 1989). Earliest reports were from battered women's shelters where children were observed to demonstrate a variety of responses to the crises. These reports described a variety of stress-related symptoms presented by children residents.

Children's responses to witnessing their father assault their mother have been reported to vary according to their age, gender, stage of development, and role in the family. Many other factors may play a role, such as the extent and frequency of the violence, mothers' response to the violence, repeated separations and moves, economic and social disadvantage, and special needs that a child may have independent of the violence. Some authors have equated children's responses to the abuse of their mothers as consistent with those of children who have been exposed to other types of trauma (Silvern & Kaersvang, 1989). Emery (1982) concluded that children in homes that have interparental conflict are at greater risk than children from intact or broken homes that are relatively conflict-free. He also suggested that both the amount and type of interparental conflict to which children are exposed are important determinants of the effect of conflict on the children. In this section children's responses to the battering of their mothers are examined according to commonly reported classifications of those re-

---

> ### Cognitive and Emotional Responses of Children of Battered Mothers
>
> **Early research**
>
> 1. Decreased verbal and quantitative abilities
> 2. Increased anxiety, low self-esteem
> 3. Decreased empathic abilities
> 4. Increased aggression (males), impaired cognitive, verbal, and motor abilities
>
> **Later research**
>
> 1. Higher levels of internalizing and overcontrolled problem behaviors
> 2. Increased anxiety
> 3. Withdrawn and suicidal behavior
> 4. Higher internalizing (anxiety, social withdrawal, depression) and externalizing (aggression, hyperactivity, conduct problems)
> 5. Concerns about potential and actual (e.g., mothers' health, battering) hazards to their mothers

sponses. These are cognitive and emotional responses, and behavioral responses, including caring behaviors. Attention is also focused on the long-term consequences of witnessing spouse abuse and the role of factors that can mediate those consequences.

Cognitive and Emotional Responses

Much of the research on children of battered women has described them as demonstrating a variety of cognitive and emotional responses. The research findings to date have been somewhat contradictory; this may be partially related to limitations in the methodology used (see the box above).

Early research suggested that the children of battered women demonstrated a wide variety of difficulties. These include: truancy, bullying, disturbed sleeping patterns, excessive screaming, clinging behaviors, failure to thrive, vomiting and diarrhea, headaches, bedwetting, speech disorders, and cognitive difficulties, including decreased verbal and quantitative abilities (Hilberman & Munson, 1978). However, this and other studies (Giles-Sims, 1985;

Hershorn & Rosenbaum, 1985) are limited because they interviewed only the mothers and did not evaluate the children directly, an approach that has been identified as problematic (Porter & O'Leary, 1980). Other studies have reported that children of battered women experienced increased anxiety, low self-esteem (Hughes & Barad, 1983), and lacked empathic abilities (Hinchey & Gavelek, 1982). However, these studies were also limited by the small clinical samples and/or the lack of comparison groups. They did, however, recognize in the literature children who had previously been unstudied.

Other research has provided additional, although not necessarily clearer, descriptions of these children. Westra and Martin (1981) reported that the children of battered women showed more aggression, at least in males, than other children; and demonstrated impaired cognitive, verbal, and motor abilities when compared with standardized norms. Hershorn and Rosenbaum (1985) reported that both the children of abused mothers and nonviolent, but conflicted mothers differed significantly from children coming from households where marital satisfaction was reported.

Some investigators have found significantly higher levels of internalizing and overcontrolled problem behaviors among shelter children (Hughes, 1988). Other authors have noted that some children of battered women experience high degrees of anxiety (Alessi & Hearn, 1984), are withdrawn, and are suicidal (Hughes, 1986; Pfeffer, 1985).

In a study of children's (ages 6-16) adjustment, Wolfe, Zak, Wilson, and Jaffe (1986) interviewed mothers (half from shelters and half from the community) about experiences with violence, maternal responses, and family stability. They reported that when children's internalizing (e.g., anxiety, depression, somatic symptoms) and externalizing (e.g., aggressiveness, disobedience) behavioral problems were predicted on the basis of the amount and severity of wife abuse, and level of maternal stress, 19% of the variance was explained. The researchers concluded that both degree of experience with violence as well as the mother's reaction to the violence significantly influence children's responses.

Although Christopoulos et al. (1987) reported that 40 children in a battered women's shelter demonstrated above-expected scores on both the internalizing (e.g., anxiety, social withdrawal, depression) and externalizing (e.g., aggression, hyperactivity, conduct problems) subscales of the Child Behavior Checklist (adult's perception of child behavior problems), boys in the community comparison group also obtained elevated scores on the internalizing subscale. They conclude that the shared experience of low socioeconomic background may be the most significant factor contributing to the children's elevated internalizing subscale scores.

Recently Humphreys (1991) conducted a study that sought to describe the phenomenon of dependent care directed toward the prevention of hazards in mothers and their children who experience family violence. Conceptualized within Orem's (1985) framework, Humphreys proposed that in families where violence is a frequent occurrence, mothers and their children experience worries and their protective caring behaviors (dependent care) can provide valuable assistance in the prevention of actual and/or potential hazards to life, health, and well-being. Elaboration of Humphreys' work in this section is limited to the worries of children of battered women.

Using qualitative research methods and analyses and paying particular attention to credibility, transferability, dependability, and confirmability of the data as described by Lincoln and Guba (1985), Humphreys interviewed a convenience sample of 50 children who resided in five battered women's shelters (two urban, three suburban) in Southeastern Michigan. The child interview guide consisted of general questions about child-identified worries or fears about their mothers. Reports of worrisome situations were elicited, allowing children to describe their own life experiences. In addition, demographic data were collected from both children and their mothers (e.g., age, developmental state, life experience, sociocultural orientation, health, available resources).

Although a comparison group of children not in battered women's shelters was unavailable (this is a limitation of the research), the worries of children of battered mothers are not surprising. Two patterns

(types) of worries were identified. One consisted of potential hazards to mothers and the other was characterized by actual hazards to mothers.

The potential hazards pattern was composed of two categories of responses by children about worries they experienced regarding hazards that could or might happen. Children's worries seemed to suggest that their awareness of the potential danger to their mothers existed, but had not actually occurred. The nature of these worries also was vague at times, as might be expected with children in general. Frequently children's expressed worry for their mothers also seemed to contain overtones of fear of abandonment, a common childhood fear.

The second category of responses was characterized by children's expressed worry about anger as a potential hazard. At times the source of anger was the abusive adult male. At other times the source of anger was the mother and directed at an outside party; sometimes the source of anger was the child herself.

The actual hazard pattern was composed of two categories of responses by children about worries they experienced regarding health hazards to their mothers. In the first category, children's worries suggested that the danger to their mothers was known and existed. These worries were much more specific than those of the potential hazard pattern and reflected explicit concerns about mothers' health. Not surprisingly, the greatest number (50%) of worries for children on behalf of their mothers concerned battering. The violence inflicted on their mothers was the most-mentioned source of worry for all the children.

The last category was composed of seven responses that reflected worries about mothers, but were *not* associated with battering. These children voiced concerns about their mothers' health in very specific areas. Several children mentioned being worried about their pregnant mothers. Other concerns combined general and specific (not pregnancy-related) worries.

Humphreys (1991) also found that there were no significant differences in the types of worries expressed by children of battered women based on selected demographic factors. This finding is somewhat surprising and intriguing. Several of these fac-

<table>
<tr><td>

Behavioral Responses of Children of Battered Women

1. Truancy, bullying, disturbed sleeping patterns, excessive screaming, clinging behaviors, failure to thrive, vomiting and diarrhea, headaches, bedwetting, speech disorders
2. Child management problems, school problems, and lack of positive peer relations
3. Fewer interests and social activities and lower school performance
4. More behavioral problems and less social competence
5. No increase in behavioral problems
6. Inconsistent gender differences in aggressive behavior
7. A variety of caring behaviors on behalf of their mothers

</td></tr>
</table>

tors have consistently been noted as influencing the kinds of worries children report (gender, age). Humphreys concluded that, unlike the rather global worries that other researchers have described, factors that influence global worries do not affect concerns that children experience in relation to their mothers to the same extent. Furthermore, because of their exposure to violence, children experience more worries about violence, and these, too, are less influenced by demographic factors. She proposed that children at battered women's shelters may experience different worries about their mothers than other children and that their concerns are less influenced by demographic factors than children who have not experienced family violence.

Behavioral Responses

Much of the research on children of battered women has described them as demonstrating a variety of behavioral problems. Jaffe et al. (1990) note behavioral disturbances often are associated with child management problems, school problems, and lack of positive peer relations. The box above summarizes these behavioral responses.

The research findings to date are often limited by methodological considerations. For example, Webster-

Stratton and Hammond (1988) found that maternal depression, a frequent concurrent problem for battered women, led to negative perceptions of children, and then to increased commands and criticisms. Although others have posed that child conduct problems were the consequence of such maternal behavior, Webster-Stratton and Hammond report that in their research, as measured by an observer, there were no differences in conduct between children of depressed and nondepressed mothers. Investigations that limit their assessments of children to interviews with their battered and possibly depressed mothers may obtain significantly biased results. Nevertheless, children of battered women have been reported to experience developmental and behavioral difficulties that have frequently manifested differently in males and females. These findings are presented below.

In a study of battered women's shelter residents, former residents, and women who never experienced violence, Wolfe, et al. (1986) found that although children recently exposed to family violence had fewer interests and social activities and lower school performance, they were not significantly inclined to have behavioral problems. In fact, although former shelter residents and their children obtained the highest scores on the Family Disadvantage Index, these mothers and children had no more behavioral or emotional symptoms than the nonviolent community sample.

Gender differences

Wolfe et al. (1985) reported that male children of battered women demonstrated more behavioral problems and less social competence than nonbattered children in a control group. Christopoulos et al. (1987) compared 40 children from shelters and 40 children from the community. They found that the former did *not* demonstrate more behavior problems than the latter, and that boys did *not* act more aggressively, and that girls did *not* act more like victims than their nonshelter counterparts. Other research results have found no significant differences in children based on gender (Jouriles et al., 1987). Davis and Carlson (1987) reported that although many of the children demonstrated difficulties, in their study girls manifested more aggressive behavior. In another study (Carlson, 1990) of adolescents who observed battering of their mothers, males were found more likely to run away, to report suicidal thoughts, and somewhat more likely to hit their mothers compared with nonobservers. In the same study, female adolescents' behavior and well-being were unrelated to witnessing violence against their mothers.

The significance of these research findings regarding children of battered women is unclear. However, there appears to be some evidence that violence in the family is detrimental to many children under certain circumstances (Emery, 1982). In addition, the findings indicate that a child's gender and age, the frequency and severity of battering to the mother, and the mother's response may influence the child's reaction to family violence.

Caring behaviors. In one of the first and most influential books on battered women, Martin (1976) described how her own 8-year-old grandchild was shaken by the violence he observed directed at his mother. Nevertheless, he became quite interested in developing strategies that he might use in future similar situations.

A small but significant group of nursing research reports addressed the caring behaviors of children for their battered mothers (Humphreys, 1989, 1990; Monsma, 1984; Westra, 1984; Westra & Martin, 1981). At least one non-nurse researcher has suggested that the relationship between battered women and their children is a fertile area for study (Emery, 1982).

Westra (1984; Westra & Martin, 1981), a nurse-researcher, sought to describe the children of women who experienced family violence. Her sample consisted of 20 subjects obtained from three shelters for battered women in metropolitan Denver. To minimize the effect of acclimation to a new environment on subject responses, only children who had been in the shelter for more than 4 days were included in the study. Although Westra's primary focus was on the development of the children she studied, she also included the Preschool Behavior Questionnaire as a measure of behavior. Limitations of Westra's research include the small sample and the absence of a comparison group. Neverthe-

less, she did report some interesting findings with regard to the behavior of the children toward their mothers.

Her research on children at a battered women's shelter reported a variety of strategies used by the children to protect their mothers: "Some try to appease the offender and in some cases offer themselves as the victim. Others may try to protect the victim" (Westra, 1984, p. 319). This was particularly noteworthy since Westra's sample of children was composed of preschool and young school-age children.

Another study provides more insight into children's thoughts when their mothers are battered. Monsma (1984), also a nurse, conducted a qualitative study of the perceptions and interpretations of wife abuse by the children of victims. She conducted in-depth, semistructured interviews with 12 children, 6 boys and 6 girls, between the ages of 8 and 12. She analyzed these interviews using content analysis and identified three major themes: (1) the destructiveness of the abuser during an assault on the child's mother, (2) the child's self-preservation strategies, and (3) the child protecting the real and imagined mother. Monsma reported that the children developed deliberate, creative ways of protecting their mothers. These caring behaviors often required the child's monitoring the situation and anticipating the actual hazard to prevent the assault. "Thad, a 10-year-old boy, claimed he knew when his mom was getting into trouble and so he and his siblings would try to prevent the assault on her" (p. 41). At other times the hazard of being battered could not be prevented; the child and/or children might then seek to protect the mother by direct and/or indirect intervention. One method identified by several of the children as a mechanism for protecting their mothers was to call the police.

> Five children, three boys and two girls, mentioned they had called the police to stop an assault. This often involved the teamwork of siblings. Joan, for example, was a 10-year-old with four siblings. She told the researcher about various times when "Dee [her 13-year-old sister] would tell us to call the police. Lee [her 12-year-old brother] would stay home to help her and I would run to the corner to call the police" (p. 41).

Humphreys' (1989) research on the worries of children of battered women also described children's behavioral responses to those fears (dependent care). Qualitative analysis revealed that children of battered women demonstrate creative, deliberate, and diverse caring behaviors. Patterns of children's dependent care were protection and supporting. Protection, the largest group of caring behaviors, was characterized by direct, immediate, and often ongoing actions. The mechanism of intervention varied with the circumstance, involving physical action, verbal action, or both. Often children directly intervened on behalf of their mothers to try to protect them, even if it placed them in jeopardy. Examples of their interventions follow. "I tried to break it up, I yanked him off her, after I called Tom (adult's nonabusive male friend)" (p.115); "I tried to get in the room where she was (being beaten)" (p.115); or "I could hear him in there beating on her. I started to cry. I heard Momma say 'She's awake.' He said 'No she's not.' So I cried louder" (p.115). The chief concern by the children was to take immediate action to protect their mothers with only occasional concern about the future.

Supporting, the other pattern of caring actions reported by Humphreys, consisted of behaviors wherein the children helped their mothers through some instrumental assistance in the immediate home or area. Examples of these are: "If my Mom had an appointment, I'd watch (little sisters)"; or "I try to help her in the house or take care of the kids so she can rest" (p. 118). The intent of this type of caring behavior seems to be to alleviate the general burden to the children's mothers and to offer support. The nature of these actions also served to enhance the relationship between battered mother and child, a relationship that may mediate the long-term effects of the violence on the child.

Although children of battered women have been found to be aware of parental conflict, and take protective and supportive actions on their behalf, the long-term consequences of growing up in violent homes cannot be viewed as somehow beneficial to children. Much of the literature on children of battered women has examined the serious consequences for many children of witnessing and possibly directly experiencing family violence. However, there is, growing evidence describing the strengths and resourcefulness of children of battered women. Nursing knowledge of children's strengths, risks, and mediating factors suggest appropriate areas for intervention.

Developmental differences

Some of the earliest research on children of battered women addressed concerns about their potential for developmental delays. This research was generally built on earlier work reporting that abused children experienced significantly more developmental problems compared with nonabused children. Previously cited research has also described the disruptive nature of violent homes; this too was believed to affect children's developmental development.

In a study of 20 children (aged 2½ to 8 years) in battered women's shelters, Westra and Martin (1981) found several areas of developmental delay. Subjects demonstrated impaired cognitive abilities, delays in verbal development, and poorer motor abilities than a standardized population. There was no comparison group and the researchers questioned the reliability of their findings given the crisis often associated with admission into a women's shelter. Nevertheless, they directly examined the children with standardized instruments and procedures (neurological examination by physician) and concluded that violence that is not directed at children can still be detrimental to children.

Resilience and Other Factors

Initially it would seem that growing up in a violent home would be devastating to children, yet many children see their mothers battered on a regular basis and later have successful relationships. Attention has only recently been directed to children of battered women who do not develop clinical pathological conditions. See the box on p. 118 for a list of resilience factors.

Jouriles et al. (1989) note that 50% of the children in one study and approximately 70% in several others (Milner & Gold, 1986; Wolfe, et al., 1985) from maritally aggressive homes did *not* show evidence

---

Resilience Factors of Children of Battered Women

1. A particularly warm relationship with one parent, foster parent, adult, or caring friend
2. Temperament—flexibility of response, a positive mood, positive sense of self, active
3. Personality—cooperative, nonaggressive
4. Cognitive style—reflectiveness, not impulsive
5. Family warmth—protective, praising, close
6. Family support—assistance with problems and school
7. Family organization—orderliness or roles and home, rule setting
8. Mothers' style of coping and compensating for absent fathers
9. Extensive social support and supportive environment—external support from peers, significant adults, school system
10. Sense of identification with community
11. Families with fewer ambivalent feelings about their children
12. Healthy children
13. Fewer life stressors
14. Open expressions of anger
15. Parents abused by only one parent
16. Parent involved in an emotional supportive relationship with their partner
17. Parents resolved not to repeat pattern of abuse with their own children

---

of problems at clinical levels, suggesting that for at least some children negative factors in their homes environments (violence and disorder) did not adversely affect them in clinically recognizable ways. Several authors (Emery, 1982; Milner, Robertson, & Rogers, 1990) have concluded that a particularly warm relationship with one parent, adult, or caring friend can mitigate, but not eliminate, the effects of marital turmoil on children.

Garmezy (1983) has examined the role of resilience and other factors in children's responses to stressful life events. He defines these factors as "attributes of persons, environments, situations, and events that appear to temper predictions of psychopathology based upon an individual's at-risk status" (Garmezy, 1981, p. 73). His review of the literature consistently identifies a constellation of three factors that seem to mediate the effects of even chronic stress on children. They are: (1) dispositional attributes in the child, (2) family milieu, and (3) supportive environment. Garmezy does not report specifically on children of battered women, but his conclusions may reasonably be applied to them.

Dispositional attributes refer to a child's temper-

ament (e.g., flexibility of response, a positive mood, positive sense of self, active), personality (e.g., cooperative, nonaggressive), and cognitive style (e.g., reflectiveness, not impulsive). Family milieu refers to family warmth (e.g., protective, praising, close), support (e.g., assistance with problems and school), and organization (e.g., orderliness of roles and home, rule setting). It is important to note that "an intact family was *not* an identifiable consistent correlate" (Garmezy, 1983, p. 75). According to Garmezy, there was a striking lack of any consistent evidence in the studies reviewed that father absence had an adverse effect on children. What did have a powerful positive effect were the mothers' styles of coping with and compensating for absent fathers. Finally, supportive environment refers to external support (e.g., from peers, significant adults, school system) and a sense of identification with the community. "Significant adults provided for the children a representation of their efficacy and ability to exert control in the midst of upheaval" (Garmezy, 1981, p. 76). According to Garmezy, in multiple studies using different methods with various groups these factors have been shown to mediate the detrimental effects of stressful life even on children. Knowledge of these factors offers suggestions for nursing practice with battered women and their children.

In a critical review of the literature on intergenerational transmission, Kaufman and Zigler (1987) conclude that the experience of family violence as a child does not necessarily result in later abuse of one's own children. These findings have significance for nursing practice with battered women and their children. Kaufman and Zigler concluded that although methodological variations in the current research limit the integration of findings, certain factors do appear to influence the effects of family violence on children. To summarize those factors, parents whose families of origin were violent, but who did not subsequently experience abuse with their children were characterized as follows:

1. They had more extensive social supports (Hunter & Kilstrom, 1979).
2. They had fewer ambivalent feelings about their children (Hunter & Kilstrom, 1979).
3. Their children were healthier (Hunter & Kilstrom, 1979) or they reported fewer life stressors (Egeland, Jacobvitz, & Sroufe, 1988).
4. They were more openly angry about their earlier abuse and better able to give detailed accounts of those experiences (Hunter & Kilstrom, 1979; Egeland, Jacobvitz, & Sroufe, 1988).
5. They were more likely to have been abused by only one of their parents (Hunter & Kilstrom, 1979).
6. They were more likely to report a supportive relationship with one parent (Hunter & Kilstrom, 1979)/foster parent (Egeland, et al.).
7. They were more likely to be involved in an emotionally supportive relationship with their partner (Egeland, et al.).
8. They resolved not to repeat the pattern of abuse with their own children (Egeland et al.).

Kaufman and Zigler concluded that a history of abuse does not automatically mean that a child will become an abusive adult. Rather, there are multiple determinants of future abuse (e.g., history of abuse, poverty, stress, lack of support). When there is a history of abuse, the presence of significant positive relationships with one or more persons (support) can mediate the detrimental effects of family violence.

Assessment

Every client should be assessed for family violence. Throughout this text data have been presented that document the pervasiveness of family violence. Too often abuse in families remains unrecognized even when the evidence is obvious. In review of charts of children identified as abused and a matched comparison group (not abused) McKibben et al. (1989) noted that many (59.4%) of the mothers also could be diagnosed as battered. Particularly disheartening was the finding that 16% of the mothers in the comparison group were battered as well.

Nurses should assess every client for family violence, just as they assess for other potential or actual health problems. The indicators of potential or actual wife abuse from both health history and physical examination listed in Chapter 9 can be used to identify battered women (see Table 9–1 and 9–2). Even if clients deny exposure to family violence, the nonjudgmental approach of nurses indicates that violence is an acceptable topic to discuss. Furthermore, nurses who inquire of all clients "Has anyone ever hurt you?" "Has anyone ever forced you to do something that made you uncomfortable?" "How are conflicts resolved at your house?" "How do decisions get made at your house?" or similar appropriate questions educate clients that problems in these areas are important. The nurse who never assesses for family violence is likely to never "see" it in the clients she or he serves. Unfortunately, the violence will still be "unseen" nevertheless.

McKibben et al. (1989) recommend the wider use of family violence protocols in adults and pediatric health care settings. "The systematic collection of data and engagement of protective interventions should include both children and their mothers" (p. 532). Mothers should be assessed for their perceptions of the children's involvement in and reactions to family violence. Assuming that the mothers

---

Interventions

Primary prevention

1. Prevention of battering of women and abuse of children
2. Decreased societal tolerance for violence (within families and without)
3. Family life classes in schools that provide experience with child-rearing and adult relationship dilemmas
4. Big Brothers and Big Sisters programs
5. Education in schools on family violence and violence in dating relationships
6. Nonviolent conflict resolution programs for children

Secondary prevention

1. Development and implementation of protocols to routinely identify, treat, and refer survivors of family violence
2. Programs for women and children at battered women's shelters
   a. Developmentally appropriate support and encouragement to discuss worries and concerns
   b. Health screening for women and children on entry
   c. Crisis intervention
   d. Academic programs for shelter children
   e. Structured, developmentally appropriate daily programs for children
   f. Therapy and counseling as needed
   g. Parent-child programs that enhance child-rearing
   h. Follow-up to evaluate the effectiveness of programs and services

Tertiary prevention

1. Public health or visiting nurse referrals for rehabilitation services
2. Support and services to assist in marital and/or child custody disputes

---

themselves are not so emotionally wrought and depressed that they are unable to experience the needs of their children, mothers still may be unaware of children's perception of parental conflict. They may also lack knowledge of children's responses to conflict.

Intervention

Interventions with children of battered women cover a broad spectrum. The nurse is concerned about the inadvertently injured child of a battered woman as well as the adolescent who has questions about violence in adult relationships. The following discussion describes general areas of intervention according to the level of prevention. Particular attention is given to children in battered women's shelters because this group is the most obvious and

the most studied. The box above summarizes primary and secondary interventions.

Primary prevention

Primary prevention includes all interventions that prevent battering of women and the primary prevention strategies discussed for child abuse (see Chapter 8). Prevention of woman abuse is discussed at length in Chapter 9, and readers are referred to those earlier sections in the text. Primary prevention includes child and family health promotion activities with both well and "at-risk" populations. The type of nursing intervention at this level varies with the location and nature of practice.

Societal interventions. All types of abuse of family members occur in a society that condones violence within the context of the family. Implicit and explicit approval for the use of violence contributes to its occurrence within families. Therefore interventions at the societal level that diminish tolerance for violence serve as primary prevention for all types of violence. When violence against family members is no longer tolerated under any circumstances (including corporal punishment as discipline for children), much will have been accomplished toward diminishing the incidence of violence of all kinds.

In a retrospective study of the social climate in students' homes (N = 144), Resick and Reese (1986) reported that violent and nonaggressive households differed. Homes in which battering of mothers occurred were characterized as hierarchical (patriarchical), openly aggressive, conflictive, and disorganized. Nonviolent families were characterized by spontaneous expression of feelings and problems, shared pleasurable activities and goals, and emphasized personal rights and freedoms. In previous discussion of Garmezy's (1983) review of the literature on resilience, similar factors were noted to mediate the effects of stressful life events on children. It is imperative that all who have the opportunity to influence children and families teach styles of interaction and conflict resolution techniques that will enhance rather than impede development.

Family life classes in schools provide school-age children and adolescents with opportunities to experiment with various child-rearing and adult relationship dilemmas under the supervision of experienced nurses, counselors, and teachers. Involvement of parents in such programs further allows parents themselves to become more knowledgeable and to guide their children toward greater understanding on the difficulties of adult relationships and parenting within real life settings.

Programs such as Big Brothers and Big Sisters can assist children to develop significant, supportive relationships outside their immediate families. When children lack frequent contact with one parent, most often fathers, Big Brothers and Big Sisters can provide positive experiences and role modeling that can enhance children's resilience to potential and actual stressors.

Education. Educational programs at all school levels should address family violence. Schools play an important role in educating children about violence

and reinforcing values that contribute to its end. In setting objectives for improving the health of the nation, The Surgeon General of the United States has recognized the serious consequences of family violence (Public Health Service, 1990). To decrease the overall occurrence of violence within the nation the following objective was developed: "Increase to at least 50 percent the proportion of elementary and secondary schools that teach nonviolent conflict resolution skills, preferably as part of a quality school health education" (p. 101).

My Family and Me: Violence Free is a domestic violence prevention curriculum for kindergarten through third grades and fourth through sixth grades (Petersen & Gamache, 1988). The purpose of this curriculum is the primary prevention of family violence. "However, by helping children to identify abusive actions, the curriculum can also promote early intervention with students who are being physically abused or are witnessing violence in their homes" (Minnesota Coalition for Battered Women). Under the guidance of their teachers, the curriculum helps children gain a sense of their own uniqueness and worth, learn assertiveness skills for nonviolent conflict resolution, and develop a personal safety plan to use in violent emergency situations.

Children need to learn that violence is only one way, albeit unacceptable, of dealing with anger, and that other means are also available. Helping children confront and deal with their own anger and see that alternatives to violence are available can be addressed individually and in groups.

Some schools have peer patrol programs that offer nonviolent ways to resolve conflicts. At one Oak Park, Michigan elementary school, the STOP (Students Talk Out Problems) program specially trains fourth- and fifth-grade students in conflict resolution (Kovanis, 1990). These red-vested patrols team up during lunchtime and after school to stop fights and arguments. The principal reports one fourth the number of fights of previous years, and being on the STOP squad has now become a status symbol. Such creative approaches help children at home and away learn nonviolent conflict resolution tactics.

Ever-increasing reports of violence in dating relationships further support the need for education in schools (Breslin et al., 1990). Adolescents need to learn that even though they may have observed violence against women in their homes, battering is not a necessary part of intimate relationships. Classroom discussions with nurses and/or teachers and peers can be particularly influential with adolescents.

There has been little research on education and primary prevention programs on violence with children. A notable exception is the work of Nibert, Cooper, Ford, Fitch, and Robinson (1989). These researchers report that even preschool children are able to learn basic prevention concepts for concrete, threatening situations. In an investigation of young children's short-term acquisition and program-specific application of prevention concepts, Nibert et al. studied 116 children aged 3 to 5 years at two socially diverse sites. Although the researchers did not address battering of women, they did study young children's abilities to learn basic prevention in four threatening situations (e.g., threatened by bully, stranger lure, stranger abduction, abuse by a known adult). The investigators state that future research is needed to determine if young children can retain and generalize prevention information. If so, instruction in prevention techniques in the studied threatening situations may also be relevant to helping children protect themselves in nonstudied situations (e.g., battering of mothers, sibling abuse). The underlying belief is relevant to discussion of children of battered women, namely, that children are more vulnerable to abuse if they are unaware of their rights and basic abuse prevention strategies. The research of Nibert et al. is presented briefly in the following discussion.

The Child Assault Prevention (CAP) Project Preschool Model has been used with elementary school children in Columbus, Ohio since 1978. The purpose of this research was to determine the capacity for young children to acquire basic and concrete prevention strategies. The research was especially noteworthy in the following areas:

1. It required both verbal responses and behavioral responses in children who sometimes lack verbal skills.

2. It required that children provide the response for a fictional boy/girl (e.g., Chris) in a storybook scenario and for themselves.
3. The threatening situations were unambiguous.
4. The methodology incorporated both pretests and posttests (1 week later).

The investigators note that because children remember information does not necessarily mean that they have *learned* from the instruction.

Within the CAP project children were instructed on basic prevention strategies over 3 days, with 20-minute workshops each day, and informal post-workshop discussions. "The program instructs children on how to handle abusive situations by peers, increases their awareness of prevention of stranger abduction and assault, and supplies them with information to increase their resistance to physical and sexual abuse" (Nibert et al., 1989, p. 15). Children are taught to use assertiveness skills, to physically move away from the abusive situation, to use a self-defense yell, to use physical resistance techniques in the abduction situation, and to tell trusted adults. The researchers found that even though they studied two socially diverse groups of children (middle-income, private preschool and Head Start program), children gave appropriate responses at levels of statistical significance pretest to posttest on three of the four scenarios. Children at both sites had the most difficulty with items pertaining to being threatened by a bully. Although the tendency was reduced at the time of posttest, children continued to say that they would hit or injure the bully in some manner, a strategy that places the children themselves in jeopardy of injury. However, the findings do indicate that even young children have substantial ability to learn basic prevention strategies when they are presented in clear and concrete context. Furthermore, the children's responses to the bully scenario allow for further discussion of appropriate use of physical responses as a defensive strategy compared with the unnecessary use of aggression and violence (Nybert et al., 1989).

Secondary prevention

When children are exposed to the abuse of their mothers, nursing interventions are termed "secondary prevention." The goals of secondary prevention are early diagnosis and intervention to prevent recurrence. Battering has already occurred at the level of secondary prevention. Nursing interventions are aimed at limiting the impact of battering of mothers on their children.

Service and protection objectives have been established by the Surgeon General to facilitate early identification and treatment of family violence. These include the following objective: "Extend protocols for routinely identifying, treating, and properly referring suicide attempters, victims of sexual assault, and victims of spouse, elder, and child abuse to at least 90 percent of hospital emergency departments" (Public Health Service, 1990, p. 101). Nurses clearly have an important role in developing and implementing such protocols.

Direct interventions with children of battered women depend on the timing of the encounter, age and response of the child, and family circumstances. Even children in battered women's shelters require different interventions. If the child is returning to the violent home, interventions may need to focus on the most basic safety needs. If the family is relocating, the nurse may have the opportunity to help the mother and child to learn new ways of living and responding. Interventions that address a variety of potential times and experiences are presented below.

Nursing research indicates that children of battered women have worries and need reassurance. Battered women use a variety of strategies to stop abuse; not the least of these is the temporary removal of their children and themselves from the violent home. Children of battered women need reassurance that their mothers will not leave them, too (Westra & Martin, 1981).

Children of battered women, like all children, need to express their worries and concerns. Nurses need to ask children of battered women about their worries or fears. With information about the children's worries regarding their mothers, nurses can help them deal with their expressed concerns. Nurses need to give information to these children, but they also need to help the children of battered women work through their feelings.

Adolescents who seek independence and self-control may need help to identify those worries

about their mothers that they cannot control. Nurses can assist adolescents to problem solve about worries that can reasonably be affected. Nurses also can help children, with their permission, share their worries with their mothers. The sharing process itself can be therapeutic for both battered women and their children. Lentz (1985) suggests that questioning about "being afraid" and "being worried" obtained very different responses from young children. In practice, nurses may want to asked both "Are you ever worried for your mother?" and "Are you ever afraid for your mother?"

With the children's permission, nurses can help children and mothers talk about the events in the home. Mothers frequently are unaware of the children's experiences and perceptions during violent events. Discussions can address real and/or perceived responsibilities during the events and any feeling of blame children may experience.

Battered women's shelters. Although there is some variability, battered women's shelters are generally emergency shelters for women and their children. Women and children are provided temporary safe haven within a communal shelter setting. Battered women and their children are allowed to stay at the shelter for a relatively short period of time (usually a maximum of 30 days), during which they are assisted in assessing their situation, gaining knowledge and insight on family violence, and obtaining social services. Battered women and their children may leave the shelter to move in with family, friends, or their own new residence. Many women and their children also return to their homes with the hope and belief that their leaving and their new information and insight will help to stop the violence. Battered women's shelters provide mothers and children safety, information, and opportunities for a short time. Many shelters also offer nonresidential group counseling and other services.

The services provided by battered women's shelters to children vary greatly. Because of limited resources, many shelters are only able to provide child care services, instead using their scant funds to assist mothers with counseling, social, and potential relocation services. Ideally, services should be available for children of battered women as well, but assisting mothers to cope with recent crises also benefits their children.

There has been increased attention to children's needs while in shelters. In fact, even with limited funds some battered women's shelters have always offered specialized services to children. Nurses involved with shelters can contribute to those services or can assist in their development when such services are unavailable. As with every practice setting, certain aspects constrain practice. Characteristics of battered women and their children in shelters are as follows:

1. The population is transient. Families are there for varying lengths of time (a few days to several months).
2. The age range of the children is wide (infants to teenagers). This results in a variety of developmental stages.
3. The availability of shelter staff to provide services is often limited. This is related to fiscal constraints, time limitations and/or lack of expertise.
4. An appropriate place to provide services/ treatment is often hard to find. Privacy, space, and accessibility must be considered (Alessi & Hearn, 1984, p. 53).

Many articles describe shelter services for children of battered women. Unfortunately, the majority of the programs do not include an evaluation component to measure the effects of their programs on children of battered women. Although the programs are to be commended for attending to the needs of children and in response developing specialized services, the lack of rigorous evaluation limits the significance of their programs and the future development and enhancement of all programs. Current reports of and recommendations for children's services in battered women's shelters are discussed.

If the battered women's shelter is to be a positive experience for children, then immediate activities must be engaged to make the children as welcome and comfortable as possible when they enter the environment (deLange, 1986). Children should be shown around the shelter and introduced to play areas and other children. An individual assessment of each child should be conducted to identify his or her experience and responses (Carlson, 1984).

Layzer et al. (1986) recommend that all children admitted to battered women's shelters have access to health screening and treatment. Nursing involvement is an obvious benefit and can provide an excellent opportunity for nursing student clinical experiences (Urbancic, Campbell, & Humphreys, manuscript submitted). As with all children, children in shelters have the regular need for health screening. Mothers also have needs for feedback on their children's growth, development, state of health, and anticipatory guidance. Clinical experience with battered women and their children in shelters has revealed many more commonalities to the provision of maternal-child care in these and other settings than might be expected. In addition, children of battered women may have difficulties that are unique to their experience. Some children have been physically injured in the attack on their mothers immediately preceding admission to the shelter. These traumatic injuries require the same attention as any other injury, with particular attention to preventing infection, maintaining alignment with fractures, and facilitating suture removal.

Gross and Rosenberg (1987) have described the role of shelters as an underrecognized source of communicable disease transmission. Of the 73 full-time government-funded shelters they surveyed in five geographic regions in 15 states, only 5% (4/73) employed health care workers. In contrast, outbreaks of diarrheal illness involving more than 10 persons were reported by 12% (9/73) of shelter directors. Gross and Rosenberg recommend that even basic hygienic practices, such as strict handwashing and identification and grouping of sick clients, may significantly reduce the transmission of a variety of communicable diseases. Experience has indicated that nurses can easily provide advice and assistance in establishing shelter guidelines in these areas. Mothers and staff usually are happy to comply since they have had limited experience with communal living in large numbers. Nursing colleagues in public health setting are obvious resources in matters of communicable disease prevention procedures.

Many children experience a variety of stress-related symptoms during their stays at shelters. Children may return to behaviors such as bedwetting, thumb-sucking, and bottle feeding that previously had been abandoned. Clinical experience has also revealed that many children no longer demonstrate stress-related problems after admission to the shelter. Nurses can assess children's stress and coping and discuss them with mothers. Mothers frequently lack knowledge of children's behaviors and are reassured to know that they are normal and generally disappear without attention once order has been established.

Battered women's shelters with children's services usually offer some structured programs to children. The form of these programs varies greatly, according to literature reports. They generally include all or part of the following components: crisis intervention activities, academic program, daily program, therapy/counseling, parent-child program, advocacy program. These components are not mutually exclusive. Various approaches to these components have been reported and are presented in the following discussion.

Crisis intervention. According to Jaffe et al. (1990), the difficulties that children often face as an accompaniment to family violence may be further exacerbated for those children who are brought to shelters for victims of domestic violence. Children in shelters are likely to have experienced a complete disruption in their social support systems, particularly with their school, friends, neighborhood, and usually the significant adult male in their lives.

In an early study of 12 children (six males, six females), Hughes and Barad (1983) found significant differences in (pretest, posttest) levels of anxiety after an average stay of 21 days in a shelter. The researchers studied several characteristics (e.g., self-esteem, behavior, anxiety) and reported surprise that no other significant differences were obtained. Furthermore, at the time of discharge from the shelter, the average children's anxiety score fell almost one standard deviation below the normative mean. They attribute the decrease in children's anxiety to the therapeutic environment of the battered women's shelter.

Jaffe et al. (1990) have identified what they term "subtle symptoms" in children of battered women. They indicate that three areas require careful investigation, especially in children who do not demonstrate pronounced reactions to observations of abuse. They categorize these areas as follows: (1) responses and attitudes about conflict resolution, (2) assigning responsibility for violence, and (3) knowledge and skills in dealing with violence incidents. Jaffe et al. suggest that children often experience violence in ways that are not always apparent. Within the category of responses and attitudes, they describe children who concluded that violent conflict resolution was acceptable behavior, children who learn to rationalize the violence, and children who blame their mothers for causing the violence. Other children assigned blame for the violence to their fathers, but pursued strategies for resolution of the violence (e.g., poisoning father) that were clearly desperate. Some children accepted an exaggerated sense of responsibility for the violence in their family. This response was reported as typical of many young children. Finally, Jaffe et al. were surprised to report that children often failed to have even basic knowledge and skills to handle emergency situations. Children in their research did not have knowledge and skills of community services and other resources to assist them with crises associated with violence at home.

Silvern and Kaersvang (1989) concluded that adults were readier, in regard to children, to leave "well enough alone." Adults were too easy to accept children's responses that "Nothing was wrong." Although it is true that children, as with adults, must be allowed the opportunity to share their feelings in their own way and time, frequent responses of "not bothered" by events leading to admission to shelters must be investigated. It is not helpful to assume that upsetting events are best left undisclosed. Nurses can used their therapeutic communication techniques to help children express themselves and their experiences.

Academic program. Children in battered women's shelters for safety (fathers may attempt to find them through school attendance) and other reasons (teasing or harassment by peers) frequently are unable to attend their regular schools. Some shelters send children to local schools where the circumstances of children's attendance are understood.

Kates and Pepler (1989) describe a reception classroom for children at emergency shelters in Canada that was specifically developed to meet the needs of children of battered women. The primary object of the reception classroom program was to meet the academic, social, and emotional needs of children of battered women. The classroom is located within a host school, but operates independently. The classroom is staffed by a special education teacher and a child care worker. The intent is to provide a high staff-to-child ratio in a comfortable, nonstigmatizing surrounding (other children of battered women), and to extend support to mothers as well. The program generally serves children age 3 to 12 years and the average length of stay is 10 days. As children are ready they interact with other children at the school, not in the reception classroom.

The reception classroom program includes several components: academic, social, emotional. The academic component attempts to maintain continuity in the children's education by assessing and addressing their academic needs. The authors acknowledge that for many children their academic delays are linked to an inability to concentrate, related to household turmoil rather than lack of intellectual capacity.

The academic needs of children receive priority in the reception classroom. However, assessment of social and emotional needs provides guidelines to the education of children in the special program. Children are assessed informally, in group discussions, and can expect on-the-spot counseling. Social skills training is offered to children 6 to 12 years of age, and close contact is maintained with mothers in the shelters.

Although the reception classroom builds on existing knowledge of the needs of children of battered women (Kates & Pepler cite the excellent work of Jaffe et al. throughout), anecdotal data included in the report are the only means of evaluating the program. Kates and Pepler state that greater research is needed on specialized programs for children of battered women.

School nurses can make important contributions to specialized academic programs for children of battered women. Previously discussed approaches that encourage children and mothers to disclose their worries and fears help children in school settings as well. Often nurses who are initially approached with some physical problem will be sought out in the future for other less tangible difficulties after they have been perceived as helpful by children. School nurses also can help teachers and other staff members understand why children sometimes return to the security of habits (i.e., thumb-sucking, special toys, nail biting) during times of stress. Nursing assessments of some children's physical complaints (stomach pains, etc.) can serve to reassure everyone that the problem can be "cured" with attention, quiet time, and reassurance rather than a visit to the emergency room.

Daily program. There is great variability in the routine daily programs for children in shelters. Generally they are structured to the extent that a similar schedule is followed most weekdays. At a minimum routine child care in shelters allows mothers to attend to the many obligations associated with obtaining social services, hunting for an apartment, and finding employment. For children in women's shelters, structured time and activities provide organization and security in strange environments. If sufficiently qualified staff are available, routine play sessions can be used for additional educational and therapeutic group sessions that enhance individual counseling.

It is important for children of battered women to be exposed to adults, both female and male, who respect each other and work together. Early in the women's shelter movement, men were rarely seen inside shelters. Fortunately, many male staff and volunteers now provide positive role models for children.

Therapy/counseling. Children need to talk about their experiences and their feelings. Children of battered women may blame themselves for the violence in their homes, especially if abusive episodes were associated with parental conflicts over child-rearing. This perception is not totally unfounded. "Sex and money are widely believed to be the issues which cause the most trouble. But our data show that neither of these provoked the most violence. Rather, it is conflict over the children that is most likely to lead a couple to blows" (Straus et al., 1980).

Children may also perceive that they are responsible for the decision to leave the home, to return, and to get a divorce. As Elbow (1982) notes, what appears to be an egocentric perception by children of battered women may be reality. The best interests of children are frequently central to battered women's decisions about the future. A mother may stay in an abusive relationship because she believes that her children will benefit from the ongoing presence of an adult male. A battered woman may also decide to finally leave an abusive situation because of the impact the violence is having on her children. In either case, children may feel responsible, not just for themselves, but for the entire family.

Children may have spent an inordinate amount of time trying to be "good" to prevent future episodes of violence. For example, one child described past episodes of violence against his mother that began when his father returned home and found toys in the living room. In an effort to prevent future episodes of battering of his mother, he convinced his younger sister to play with him in the bedroom closet. That way all the toys would be confined to the closet and the home would appear tidy "like Daddy likes it."

If children have intervened in attempts to stop violence between adults, they may have a false sense of confidence in their abilities to keep batterers from abusing again. If successful in the past at stopping abuse, children may feel personal failure if subsequent interventions were unsuccessful.

Many authors have described the valuable role of therapy for children. In one of the earliest reports on children's services in battered women's shelters, Hughes (1982) recommends that therapy and counseling vary from Big Brother/Sister recreational-type approaches to longer-term, more intensive contacts that closely resemble traditional psychotherapy. The type of intervention depends on the ages and needs of the children. Jaffe, Wilson, and Wolfe (1986) recommend that interventions be sensitive to children's developmental levels and needs, and focus

on children's attitudes about aggression and family behavior. They and others (Grusznski, Brink, & Edleson, 1988) suggest that children learn basic skills in resolving interpersonal problems. Hughes advocates individual counseling along with peer, sibling, or family groups. Rhodes and Zelman (1986) report success with multifamily groups. Their reports suggest that when specific problems (i.e., substance abuse) affected children and mothers, special counseling with others with similar concerns should be devoted to those problems. Elbow (1982) notes that play therapy was a useful approach to helping children express their feelings.

Parent-child program. Some shelters are able to provide services to battered women that help them to enhance their relationships with their children and, if necessary, learn nonviolent methods of child-rearing. Shelters do not allow the use of violent conflict resolution tactics, including corporal punishment, by anyone. For some mothers this necessitates learning different ways of disciplining their children. Many mothers have heard of "time out" strategies for disciplining children, but using these methods can be much more difficult. Nurses can take an active role in helping mothers learn different approaches to discipline, considering the most appropriate approach for their children and circumstances, and role-modeling the use of the different strategies. Interventions with mothers in shelters have been shown to reduce subsequent episodes of violence directed toward children (Giles-Sims, 1985).

Armstrong (1986) describes a formal curriculum presented at a shelter in five weekly sessions, each 2 hours in duration. The purpose is to provide new information and reinforcement to mothers. The program focuses on increasing the mothers' competence in several areas: interpersonal skills (communication, self-control, through the introduction of stress management techniques), empathy (through understanding developmental issues and learning to view situations from a child's perspective), parenting skills (through the introduction of practical guidelines on discipline and supervision), and relationship building (through learning the language of encouragement as well as how to "enjoy" time spent with one's children) (Armstrong, 1986). Use of a group format for such sessions has been reported by many to help mothers gain insight, support, and ideas from other women with similar experiences.

Advocacy program. Finally, battered women and their children need follow-up services after they leave shelters. Frequently the funds for such services are even more meager than for the shelter themselves. According to Layzer et al. (1986), of the six demonstration projects funded by the National Center on Child Abuse and Neglect, five continued after the initial funding year. Of those five, only one was funded to provide follow-up services to women and children who left the shelter. Whether initial proposals included follow-up services is unknown. However, battered women and their children need the knowledge of and access to community services even after discharge from shelters. Nurses can provide information and make appropriate referrals.

Tertiary prevention

Ideally, battering of women is never allowed to progress to this stage of intervention; however, this is often the case. Tertiary prevention is required when children of battered women have experienced irreversible effects from the violence. The goal of tertiary prevention is rehabilitation of the children to the maximum level of functioning possible with the limitations of disabilities.

When physical injuries have resulted in disability, women and their children may be eligible for additional social services. Referrals to public health and visiting nurse agencies can secure follow-up for those who are eligible.

Although the majority of children of battered women are unlikely to be abused themselves, research suggests that approximately 30% of children are abused. Nurses and others who assist battered women and their children should continually assess for child abuse and work closely with Child Protective Services to ensure early identification of suspected abuse and neglect. As Cummings and Mooney (1988) point out, child protective service workers and battered women's advocates often find themselves at odds while trying to work with families. Both groups share an interest in stopping violence, yet their perspectives and approaches are frequently in conflict. Nurses are in an excellent position to collaborate with both groups of professionals, all working toward the common goal.

Children of battered women are often victimized by prolonged legal disputes regarding which parent should have custody after separation or reasonable visitation. The legal battle is a prolonged affair, involving years of threats and conflicts, which many of the children discover continues long after the separation and any court decisions.

Even before separation, many battered women are threatened with the fact that their husbands will seek custody of the children if the women decide to leave. Often this threat will be a central issue in keeping a woman prisoner in her own home for fear of this and other consequences (NiCarthy, 1982). Women who feel most vulnerable in these circumstances are those who believe that because their husbands have never directly abused the children, the husbands have a good opportunity to be awarded custody. Many such women describe their husbands as better suited for the court battle because of the husbands' ability to "charm and con selected important people for short-term interactions" required by this process (Walker & Edwall, 1987, p.128).

Several authors have suggested that battered women's anxiety about legal proceedings is well founded, in light of a strong bias by many judges about the father's right to his children (Chesler, 1986; Walker, 1989). In her book titled *Mothers on trial: The battle for children and custody,* Chesler (1986) indicated that nearly two thirds of the women she interviewed felt "legally or judicially battered" by the process they had to endure in seeking custody of their children. The fathers in Chesler's descriptions were often uninvolved parents and abusive men. This abuse was not considered a relevant factor in the cases reported.

Evaluation

At the point of evaluation in the nursing process the nurse reviews what changes have occurred, based on the identified goals. The nurse must be realistic yet hopeful in her evaluation of children of battered women. Evaluation is not the final step in working with children from violent families but an ongoing process.

SUMMARY

Children of battered women are at risk for a variety of emotional, cognitive, and behavioral difficulties. However, research has described the important, mediating effects on children of even one positive relationship with a significant person. Nurses should be aware of family violence and assess *every* client and family for this problem. Early identification and intervention can stem detrimental effects and help individuals and families toward recovery.

REFERENCES

Alessi, J. J., & Hearn, K. (1984). Group treatment of children in shelters for battered women. In A. R. Roberts (Ed.), *Battered women and their families* (pp. 49-61). New York: Springer.

Armstrong, D. T. (1986). Shelter-based parenting services: A skill-building process. *Children Today, 15*(2), 16-20.

Breslin, F. C., Riggs, D. S., O'Leary, K. D., & Arias, I. (1990). Family precursors: Expected and actual consequences of dating aggression. *Journal of Interpersonal Violence, 5,* 247-258.

Carlson, B. E. (1984). Children's observations of interparental violence. In A. R. Roberts (Ed.), *Battered women and their families: Intervention strategies and treatment programs* (pp. 147-167). New York: Springer.

Carlson, B. E. (1990). Adolescent observers of marital violence. *Journal of Family Violence, 5,* 285-299.

Chesler, P. (1986). *Mothers on trial: The battle for children and custody.* Seattle: Seal Press.

Christopoulos, C., Cohn, D. A., Shaw, D. S., Joyce,. S., Sullivan-Hanson, J., Kraft, S. P., & Emery. R. (1987). Children of abused women: I. Adjustment at time of shelter residence. *Journal of Marriage and the Family, 49,* 611-619.

Cummings, J. S., Pellegrini, D. S., Notarius, C. I., & Cummings E. M. (1989). Children's responses to angry adult behavior as a function of marital distress and history of interparent hostility. *Child Development, 60,* 1035-1043.

Cummings, N., & Mooney, A. (1988). Child protective workers and battered women's advocates: A strategy for family violence intervention. *Response, 11*(2), 4-9.

Davidson, T. (1978). *Conjugal crime: Understanding and changing the wife-beating pattern.* New York: Ballantine.

Davis, L. V., & Carlson, B. E. (1987). Observation of spouse abuse: What happens to the children? *Journal of Interpersonal Violence, 2,* 278-291.

deLange, C. (1986). The Family Place Children's Therapeutic Program. *Children Today, 15*(2), 12-15.

Dobash, R. E., & Dobash, R. (1979). *Violence against wives: A case against the patriarchy.* New York: Free Press.

Egeland, B., Jacobvitz, D., & Sroufe, L. A. (1988). Breaking the cycle of abuse: Relationship predictors. *Child Development, 59,* 1080-1088.

Elbow, M. (1982). Children of violent marriages: The forgotten victims. *Social Casework, 63,* 465-471.

Emery, R. E. (1982). Interparental conflict and the children of discord and divorce. *Psychological Bulletin, 92,* 310-330.

Emery, R. E. (1989). Family violence. *American Psychologist, 44,* 321-328.

Forsstrom-Cohen, B., & Rosenbaum, A. (1985). The effects of parental marital violence on young adults: An exploratory investigation. *Journal of Marriage and the Family, 47,* 467-472.

Garmezy, N. (1981). Children under stress: Perspectives on antecedents and correlates of vulnerability and resistance to psychopathology. In A. I. Rabin, J. Arnoff, A. M. Barclay, & R. A. Zucker (Eds.), *Further explorations in personality* (pp. 70-81). New York: Wiley Interscience.

Garmezy, N. (1983). Stressors of childhood. In N. Garmezy (Ed.), *Stress, coping, and development in children* (pp. 43-84). New York: McGraw-Hill.

Gentry, C. E., & Eaddy, V. B. (1982). Treatment of children in spouse abusive families. *Victimology: An International Journal, 5,* 240-250.

Giles-Sims, J. (1985). A longitudinal study of battered children of battered wives. *Family Relations, 34,* 205-210.

Gross, T. P., & Rosenberg, M. L. (1987). Shelters for battered women and their children: An under-recognized source of communicable disease transmission. *American Journal of Public Health, 77,* 1198-1201.

Grusznski, R. J., Brink, J. C., & Edleson, J. L. (1988). Support and education groups for children of battered women. *Child Welfare, 67,* 431-445.

Hershorn, M., & Rosenbaum, A A. (1984). Children of marital violence: A closer look at the unintended victims. *American Journal of Orthopsychiatry, 55,* 260-266.

Hilberman, E., & Munson, K. (1978). Sixty battered women. *Victimology: An International Journal, 2,* 460-470.

Hinchey, F. S., & Gavelek, J. R. (1982). Empathic responding in children of battered mothers. *Child Abuse and Neglect, 6,* 395-401.

Hughes, H. M. (1981). Advocacy for children of domestic violence: Helping battered women with non-sexist childrearing. *Victimology: An International Journal 6,* 262-271.

Hughes, H. M. (1982). Brief interventions with children in a battered women's shelter: A model preventive program. *Family Relations, 31,* 495-502.

Hughes, H. M. (1986). Research with children in shelters: Implications for clinical services. *Children Today, 15*(2), 21-25.

Hughes, H. M. (1988). Psychological and behavioral correlates of family violence in child witnesses and victims. *American Journal of Orthopsychiatry, 58,* 77-90.

Hughes, H. M., & Barad, S. J. (1983). Changes in the psychological functioning of children in a battered women's shelter: A pilot study. *Victimology: An International Journal, 7*(1-4), 60-68.

Humphreys, J. (1989). Dependent-care directed toward the prevention of hazards to life, health, and well-being in mothers and children who experience family violence (Doctoral dissertation, Wayne State University, Detroit, MI, unpublished).

Humphreys, J. (1990). Dependent-care directed toward the prevention of hazards to life, health, and well-being in mothers and children who experience family violence. *MAINlines, 11*(1), 6-7.

Humphreys, J. (1991). Children of battered women: Worries about their mothers. *Pediatric Nursing, 17,* 342-345.

Hunter, R., & Kilstrom, N. (1979). Breaking the cycle in abusive families. *American Journal of Psychiatry, 136,* 1320-1322.

Jaffe, P., Wilson, S., & Wolfe, D. A. (1986). Promoting changes in attitudes and understanding of conflict resolution among child witnesses of family violence. *Canadian Journal of Behavioral Science, 18,* 356-366.

Jaffe, P. G., Wolfe, D. A., & Wilson, S. K. (1990). *Children of battered women.* Newbury Park, CA: Sage.

Jaffe, P. G., Wolfe, D. A., Wilson, S. K., & Zak, L. (1986). Family violence and child adjustment: A comparative analysis of girls' and boys' behavioral symptoms. *American Journal of Psychiatry, 143,* 74-77.

Jouriles, E. N., Barling, J., & O'Leary K. D. (1987). Predicting child behavior problems in maritally violent families. *Journal of Abnormal Child Psychology, 15,* 165-173.

Jouriles, E. N., Murphy, C. M., & O'Leary, K. D. (1989). Interspousal aggression, marital discord, and child problems. *Journal of Consulting and Clinical Psychology, 57,* 453-455.

Kalmuss, D. (1984). The intergenerational transmission of marital aggression. *Journal of Marriage and the Family, 46,* 11-19.

Kates, M., & Pepler, D. (1989). A reception classroom for children of battered women in emergency shelters. *Canada's Mental Health, 37*(3), 7-10.

Kaufman, J., & Zigler, E. (1987). Do abused children become abusive parents? *American Journal of Orthopsychiatry, 57,* 186-193.

Kovanis, G. (1990, October 19). Young peacemakers: Students are schooled in settling conflicts without help of adults. *Detroit Free Press,* pp. 1A, 15A.

Layzer, J. I., Goodson, B. D., & deLange, C. (1986). Children in shelters. *Children Today, 15*(2), 5-11.

Lentz, K. (1985). Fears and worries of young children as expressed in a contextual play setting. *Journal of Child Psychology and Psychiatry, 26,* 981-987.

Levine, M. B. (1975). Interparental violence and its effect on the children: A study of 50 families in general practice. *Medicine, Science, and the Law, 15*(3), 172-176.

Lincoln, Y. S., & Guba, E. G. (1985) *Naturalistic inquiry.* Beverly Hills: Sage.

MacLeod, L. (1989). *Wife battering and the web of hope: Progress, dilemmas, and visions of prevention.* Ottawa: Health & Welfare Canada.

Martin, D. (1976). *Battered wives.* San Francisco: Glide.

McKibben, L., De Vos, E., & Newberger, E. H. (1989). Victimization of mothers of abused children: A controlled study. *Pediatrics, 84,* 531-535.

Milner, J. S., & Gold, R. G. (1986). Screening spouse abusers for child abuse potential. *Journal of Clinical Psychology, 42,* 169-172.

Milner, J. S., Robertson, K. R., & Rogers, D. L. (1990). Childhood history of abuse and adult child abuse potential. *Journal of Family Violence, 5,* 15-34.

Minnesota Coalition for Battered Women. *My family and me: Violence free.* (Available from The Minnesota Coalition for Battered Women, Hamline Park Plaza, Suite 201, 570 Asbury St., St. Paul, MN 55104).

Monsma, J. (1984). *The children of battered women: Perceptions and interpretations of wife abuse* (Unpublished manuscript, Wayne State University, Detroit, MI).

Nibert, D., Cooper, S., Ford, J., Fitch, L. K., & Robinson, J. (1989). The ability of young children to learn abuse prevention. *Response, 12*(4), 14-20.

NiCarthy, G. (1982). *Getting free: A handbook for women in abusive relationships* (2nd ed.). Seattle: Seal Press.

Orem, D.E. (1985). *Nursing: Concepts of practice.* (3rd ed.). New York: McGraw-Hill.

Petersen, K., & Gamache, D. (1988). Family and me: Violence free: A domestic violence prevention curriculum. St. Paul: Minnesota Coalition for Battered Women.

Pfeffer, C. R. (1985). Self-destructive behavior in children and adolescents. *Psychiatric Clinics of North America, 8,* 215-226.

Porter, B., & O'Leary, K. D. (1980). Marital discord and childhood behavior problems. *Journal of Abnormal Psychology, 8,* 287-295.

Public Health Service. (1990). *Healthy people 2000: National health promotion and disease prevention objectives* (DHHS Publication No. PHS 91-50213). Washington, DC: U.S. Government Printing Office.

Resick, P. A., & Reese, D. (1986). Perception of family social climate and physical aggression in the home. *Journal of Family Violence, 1,* 71-83.

Rhodes, R. M., & Zelman, A. B. (1986). An ongoing multifamily group in a women's shelter. *American Journal of Orthopsychiatry, 56,* 120-130.

Rosenbaum, A., & O'Leary, K. D. (1981). Children: The unintended victims of marital violence. *American Journal of Orthopsychiatry, 51,* 692-699.

Silvern, L., & Kaersvang, L. (1989). The traumatized children of violent marriages. *Child Welfare, 68,* 421-436.

Stark, E., & Flitcraft, A. H. (1988). Women and children at risk: A feminist perspective on child abuse. *International Journal of Health Services, 18,* 97-118.

Straus, M. A., & Gelles, R. J. (1986). Societal change and change in family violence from 1975 to 1985 as revealed by two national surveys. *Journal of Marriage and the Family, 48,* 465-479.

Straus, M. A., Gelles, R. J., & Steinmetz, S. K. (1980). *Behind closed doors: A survey of family violence in America.* New York: Doubleday.

Ulbrich, P., & Huber, H. (1981). Observing parental violence: Distribution and effects. *Journal of Marriage and the Family, 43,* 623-631.

Urbancic, J., Campbell, J. C., & Humphreys, J. (1991). *Getting into the swamp: Caring for the battered woman.* Manuscript submitted for publication.

Walker, L. E. (1989). Psychology and violence against women. *American Psychologist, 44,* 695-702.

Walker, L. E., & Edwall, G. E. (1987). Domestic violence and determination of visitation and custody in divorce. In D. J. Sonkin (Ed.), *Domestic violence on trial: Psychological and legal dimensions of family violence* (pp. 127-152). New York: Springer.

Wasileski, M., Callaghan-Chaffee, M. E., & Chaffee, R. B. (1982). Spousal violence in military homes: An initial survey. *Military Medicine, 147,* 761-765.

Webster-Stratton, C., & Hammond, M. (1988). Maternal depression and its relationship to life stress, perceptions of child behavior problems, parenting behaviors and child conduct problems. *Journal of Abnormal Child Psychology, 16,* 299-315.

Westra, B. (1984). Nursing care of children of violent families. In J. C. Campbell, & J. Humphreys, *Nursing care of victims of family violence* (pp. 315-339). Reston, VA: Reston.

Westra, B., & Martin, H. P. (1981). Children of battered women. *Maternal-Child Nursing Journal, 10,* 41-54.

Wolfe, D. A., Jaffe, P., Wilson, S. K., & Zak, L. (1985). Children of battered women: The relation of child behavior to family violence and maternal stress. *Journal of Consulting and Clinical Psychology, 53,* 657-665.

Wolfe, D. A., Zak, L., Wilson, S., & Jaffe, P. (1986). Child witnesses to violence between parents: Critical issues in behavioral and social adjustment. *Journal of Abnormal Child Psychology, 14,* 95-104.

5 *Intrafamilial Sexual Abuse*

Joan C. Urbancic

I n recent years, intrafamilial sexual abuse (incest) has received much attention on television, in films, and through celebrity disclosures of childhood incestual abuse. Despite the heightened public awareness of incest and its traumatic aftereffects, it basically remains a hidden problem of great magnitude that affects all strata of society.

The majority of children never disclose their abuse, and the experiences of those who do disclose often involve blame or disbelief by those from whom they seek protection. As adults, survivors of incest continue to experience blame, disbelief and/or minimization of their experiences. When they seek treatment as adults, survivors frequently must try multiple therapists before they are successful in finding one who is helpful in resolving their childhood sexual trauma.

Although nurses are frequently in key positions to identify and provide therapeutic involvement

with adult and child victims, they are often uncomfortable and reluctant to confront the issue. This reluctance may be interpreted to mean the subject must not be broached, thereby reinforcing the guilt, shame, and self-blame of the victim.

Before nurses can effectively engage in therapeutic involvement with adult and/or child victims of incest, they must become aware of their own attitudes about incest and also increase their knowledge about this serious mental health problem. Such preparation may enable nurses to change negative or ambivalent attitudes about incest, thereby facilitating self-disclosure by children and adults who have had incest experiences. By encouraging self-disclosure and resolution of the incest conflict, the nurse may provide the stimulus for recovery and healing of the incest trauma.

This chapter provides an overview of incest in terms of historical and theoretical perspectives, short- and long-term effects, treatment modalities, and nursing interventions.

DEFINITION OF INCEST

The traditional definition of incest has been "sexual intercourse between relatives too close to marry." Today much broader definitions are being used by clinicians and researchers. Redefinition is necessary because intercourse with a female child is usually difficult before the child reaches puberty, but other types of sexual activities do occur that can leave the child feeling betrayed, exploited, and guilt-ridden.

The definition of childhood incest used in this chapter is as follows: any type of exploitative sexual experience between relatives or surrogate relatives before the victim reaches 18 years of age. Exploitation involves a variety of behaviors that the adult uses with the child for sexual gratification. Behaviors may include disrobing, nudity, masturbation, fondling, digital penetration, and anal, oral, or vaginal penetration. Surrogate relatives include stepfathers, mothers' boyfriends, and close family friends who may assume caretaker roles.

The definition assumes a power imbalance between the child and the offender so that the child or adolescent is unable to give true consent because of physical, cognitive, and psychological immaturity. This is the case even though the child may believe she consented. Courtois (1988) states that children submit rather than consent. Consequently, it is widely accepted that the child is always a "victim" in incestuous relationships because children are never in a position to give informed consent. The adult always assumes a power position and pressures or forces the child in various ways to cooperate. These pressures as perceived by the child may be fear of punishment, rejection, or abandonment by the adult, as well as promises of material goods and special favors or privileges. Because "children are children," it is natural for them to seek what is pleasurable. It is the adult who is always responsible and the adult who must nurture, protect, set limits on inappropriate behaviors, and teach age-appropriate behaviors to the child.

Although it may seem clear that the adult is always the responsible person, earlier research reported seductive behaviors and active participation by the children (Bender & Blau, 1937; Henderson, 1972). Current investigators and clinicians maintain that flirtatious behavior is an attempt for nurturance, not sexual gratification. If the child is seductive, it is because she has been taught that sexual contact is an effective means to gain attention, affection, and special favors.

Because the sexual activity usually begins with fondling and rarely involves violence, it may be pleasurable and sexually stimulating for the child. Finch (1973) maintains that all children are "polymorphous perverse," which means they have the potential for enjoying a variety of sexual activities that they are "taught." For the adult survivor who believes that she voluntarily participated in the incest, issues of guilt, shame, and self-blame may be intensified.

The most typical pattern of incestuous activity involves a gradual escalation of sexual activity over time. If the incest has continued for years, it is common to progress to oral sex, mutual masturbation, and even vaginal intercourse. It is the pressure on the child to cooperate and to maintain the relationship that is the most crucial issue to assess in incest experiences. Many children have severe guilt, feelings of helplessness, and shame, but they continue to maintain the secrecy because of domination by the adult and fear that disclosure will lead to punishment, greater shame, rejection, and disbelief by the social network. Although a variety of psychological and physical symptoms are likely to develop when the incestuous relationship becomes protracted, the majority of children fail to self-disclose.

Courtois (1988) states that although it is widely accepted that cross-generational incest should be defined as abusive, it is less clear when making a determination about same-age peers. Russell (1986) used an age differential of 5 years to qualify sexual activity between siblings as abusive. However, clinical practice and research (Urbancic, 1992) has identified frequent cases of females who were coerced into sexual activity by brothers of similar age to the victim. According to Courtois, "incest can be considered nonabusive when it occurs between brothers, sisters, cousins, or other relatives who are age peers when it is mutually desired and without coercion" (p. 20). Therefore coercion rather than age appears to be the most important consideration in the determination of whether sexual activity between siblings is abusive.

Male children are also the victims of childhood sexual abuse, and the caseloads of therapists are beginning to support the belief that male child sexual abuse is underreported and more prevalent than statistics indicate. Nevertheless, research (Russell, 1986) indicates that female children are sexually abused more frequently than male children, and most of the literature relates to the female child victim. For that reason, the female rather than the male pronoun will be used throughout this chapter. Because sexual abuse is a criminal offense with mandatory reporting, the perpetrator will most commonly be referred to as the "offender" and the object of his abuse as the "victim." Since the majority of offenders are male, the pronoun "he" will be used when discussing the offender.

Many researchers use the broader term *childhood sexual abuse* and do not distinguish between the incest and sexual abuse. The reasoning seems to be that all childhood sexual abuse is traumatic, and because the majority of cases of sexual abuse occurs between family and/or close friends, most qualify as incestuous. Therefore when childhood sexual abuse is discussed, it is understood that most cases are incestuous.

It is important to note that intrafamilial abuse (incest) has a greater potential for trauma than extrafamilial abuse because the child may experience a sense of betrayal by a trusted caretaker, greater frequency and duration of abuse, denial by caretakers, and the imposition of secrecy, which precludes the possibility of social support that the extrafamilial abuse victim is more likely to receive.

PREVALENCE OF INCEST

Incest is a phenomenon that occurs more frequently than society recognizes, and the incidence appears to be increasing each year. Some argue that the increasing incidence is related to a growing awareness by the public and skillful assessment by professionals. However, a counterargument points to the weakening of the family in terms of divorce, stepfamilies, and single families. Studies (Finkelhor, 1979; Russell, 1986) indicate that stepfathers are eight times more likely to abuse their stepdaughters, use force, and engage in more protracted and severe abuse than biological fathers. These studies support the belief that because biological fathers generally have more involvement in the early socialization of their daughters than stepfathers, they have stronger parent-child bonding, which is a strong deterrent to incest.

In addition to the weakening of parent-child bonding, another important factor contributing to the increasing incidence of childhood sexual abuse is the deterioration of sexual mores and the widespread acceptance of "sexual liberation" for everyone. Television, movies, and videos promote "doing whatever feels good," and females are depicted as seductive or insatiable sexual objects. Although condoms are crucial for promoting "safe sex" in the age of AIDS, the possibility that sometimes abstinence is the "safest sex" is rarely a consideration in a society that values individualism and unfettered sexual gratification more than self-discipline and responsibility.

Although there is agreement that reports of incest are increasing, incidence and prevalence studies (Finkelhor, 1986; Russell, 1986; Wyatt & Powell, 1988) for childhood incest have reported a wide range of figures, primarily because of the differences in definition and methodology. The most valid study in terms of sample and methodology appears to be Russell's (1986) large study (N = 953) of a randomly selected sample of women from the San Francisco area. Russell identified 16% of the sample as being sexually abused by a relative before the age of 18; 4.5% of the victims in the sexually abused subsample were abused by their fathers. Wyatt's (1985) random sample study of 248 women supported Russell's findings.

Jacobson and Herald (1990) reported a prevalence of one in six males and one in five females who disclosed a history of major childhood sexual abuse on admission to a psychiatric inpatient setting. In addition, 56% of those who had been abused had not disclosed this abuse to previous therapists. Other studies have identified a much higher incidence. Craine, Henson, Colliver, and MacLean (1988) reported 51% of a sample of 105 female state hospital patients as having disclosed a sexual abusive history in childhood or adolescence. Before the study, 57% of the sexually abused sample had never been identified as such. Rieker and Carmen (1986) reported that 43% of their sample of patients in a psychiatric hospital had histories of physical or sexual abuse. Of these abused patients, 48% were sexually abused.

It is unclear why such a high prevalence of sexual abuse exists among psychiatric patients. Craine et al. (1988) postulate that the victims may come from highly dysfunctional families and it is this experience that forms the core of their mental health problems. Although it is true that many victims come from severely dysfunctional families, others come from families that do not appear overtly dysfunctional. An alternate explanation is that the sexual abuse itself is frequently the core problem. A reluctance by mental health professionals to accept that childhood sexual abuse can be a core factor in adult mental health illness reflects the continuing adherence to Freudian Oedipal theory in which the victim is blamed and the abuse is minimized.

Because of the multiple and converging studies of childhood sexual abuse in recent years, several risk factors for abuse have been identified. Female children are at greater risk and have been studied more frequently than males. This has probably caused an impression that male child abuse is unusual when the opposite is true. Studies indicate that the most vulnerable age for sexual abuse is between 10 and 11 years. Despite many studies, no evidence exists to indicate that childhood sexual abuse is more common among lower socioeconomic groups or between black and white populations.

Children who live with a stepfather are at risk, especially if the mother is employed outside the home. In addition, children from socially isolated, dysfunctional, or abusive families are at risk. Unavailability of parents and families in which parents were abused are other risk factors.

HISTORICAL AND THEORETICAL PERSPECTIVES

Various anthropological theories have been presented to explain the universal taboo against incest. Some anthropologists explain the origin of prohibition against incest in terms of the need for kinship ties that are necessary for survival and are maintained through exogamy (Levi-Strauss, 1949). Psychological anthropologists view the prohibition as necessary to prevent dysfunction and chaos in family roles (Whiting, 1963). Other anthropologists maintain that there are genetic contraindications to incest (Fox, 1983).

Shepher (1983), who researched sexual behavior of children who grew up in the kibbutz, espouses a sociobiological view of incest and maintains that a negative imprinting or sexual indifference occurs among young people who are raised together. According to Shepher, the avoidance of incest occurs first (inhibition), and the coercion and intellectual understanding (prohibition) occurs later. Although a universal prohibition against incest exists, Courtois (1988) claims that a growing body of research suggests that incest "has been embedded in and covertly allowed in most cultures, while being overtly and publicly decried and denied" (p. 7).

Although the theme of incest has been prevalent in art and literature since ancient times, research has not been extensive until the last 15 years. Earlier research focused primarily on the characteristics of the offender and the family dynamics. Few studies examined the effects of incest on the child, and those that did were limited by sample size, control, and methodology.

Nevertheless, the earlier studies claimed that trauma to the child (usually a female) was rare, and researchers reported that the younger partner often initiated and enjoyed the incestuous relationship. In addition to the belief of questionable trauma, many clinicians did not think incest was a significant issue because of its rare occurrence. As late as 1972, the prominent psychiatrist Henderson insisted that incest was an uncommon event and therefore of little concern.

Freud was among the early writers who explored the cause of incest. In letters to Wilhelm Fliess from 1887 to 1902 (published in 1954), Freud discussed the development of his concepts on infantile sexuality and neurosis. He was amazed by the frequency of incestuous experiences reported by his female patients. Because Freud was unable to accept the possible reality of such reports among respectable families, he believed the reports were the result of the fantasies of hysterical females. Freud's work in this area culminated in his Oedipal theory, which places the responsibility for incestuous feelings on the child.

Most psychiatrists interpreted Freud's work on hysteria to mean that childhood seduction was rare and that female patients had fantasized and desired the incestual experience. This interpretation was erroneous because Freud (1954) reported that many of his female patients actually had been molested as children. Nevertheless, many writers claim that it was Freud's theory that established the groundwork for the disregard of children's reports of sexual molestation and for the focus on their supposed fantasies and seductive behavior rather than on irresponsible adults who exploit the innocence and trust of the child to satisfy their own emotional needs. Freud's views continue to have a powerful impact on mental health professionals, as shown by the disbelief and discomfort that many professionals feel when confronted by disclosures of incest by clients (Courtois, 1988; Russell, 1986; Wyatt & Powell, 1988).

Feminists have been extremely critical of Freudian theory and maintained that the Oedipal theory has intensified the trauma of incest by denying the experiences and blaming the victims rather than placing the blame on the irresponsible adults. Feminists (Herman, 1981; Rush, 1980; Russell, 1986) have viewed incest and family violence as extreme manifestations of the imbalance of power between men and women. Within this view, females are socialized to be devalued sexual objects.

Burgess, Groth, Holstrom, and Sgroi (1978) espoused a sexual abuse model for incest and claimed

that this is appropriate because in the majority of cases of sexual abuse, the offender is a family member or someone well-known to the child. The model espoused by Burgess et al. maintained that the child is always a "victim" in incestuous relationships because children are never in a position to give informed consent since they lack cognitive, psychological, and physical maturity.

Many frameworks have been presented to explain the traumatic effects of childhood sexual abuse. Burgess, a nurse researcher, has worked with members of other disciplines to develop a cognitive model of sexual abuse (Burgess, Hartman, Wolbert, & Grant, 1987). This framework, known as the Information Processing of Trauma model (IPT), is based on research that found that cognitive-behavioral responses to traumatic events are based on informational processing. If a traumatic experience has appropriate processing, it will become neutralized, resolved, and stored in distant memory. When traumatic experiences are not resolved, they remain in active memory or are defended by cognitive mechanisms. This cognitive mechanism is a process termed trauma encapsulation, and it is viewed as the basis for posttraumatic stress disorder by Burgess et al.

Trauma encapsulation (Burgess et al., 1987) is an effort by the child victim to function in daily life while protecting herself from the painful memory of the traumatic event. A number of cognitive defenses are used to achieve this protection including dissociation, repression, splitting, suppression, and compartmentalization. Because the sexual offender demands secrecy, the child is forced to develop defenses to prevent disclosure, and development proceeds for the child under the profound burden of trauma encapsulation. According to Burgess et al., childhood sexual abuse experiences result in long-term effects of low self-worth, self-blame, a lack of self-efficacy, self-fragmentation, dissociations, and self-destructive behaviors.

Carmen and Rieker's Psychosocial Model of the Victim-to-Patient (1989) also focuses on the cognitive aspects of sexual abuse. These researchers claim that three cognitive strategies are involved in defending self from the abuse: denial, changing the affective response to the abuse, and changing the meaning of the abuse. These three processes form the basis for the damaged self. "In a sense, the victim's survival is dependent on adjusting to a psychotic world where abusive behavior is acceptable but telling the truth about it is sinful" (p. 434). Carmen and Rieker claim that when the victim is denied the experience of knowing and remembering, assigning meaning, and responding affectively to the sexual abuse, a process called defensive exclusion occurs. This process is similar to the process of trauma encapsulation (Burgess et al., 1987) because both models explain that victims attempt to cope by using defense mechanisms such as denial, repression, disassociation, and compartmentalization to decontextualize their traumatic experiences. Thus the defenses that originally were adaptive for the victims eventually become the core of their mental health problems.

Figley (1985) and Van der Kolk (1987) claimed that incest trauma can be considered as posttraumatic stress disorder (PTSD), and many incest survivors reveal symptoms that fulfill the DSM-III criteria for PTSD. Van der Kolk identified the following characteristics in the person with PTSD: fixation on the trauma, dissociation or reenactment of the trauma, loss of capacity to modulate anxiety and aggression, helplessness, loss of control, and future vulnerability. Van der Kolk also identified six factors that affect the severity of the trauma response: severity of the stressor, genetic predisposition, developmental phase, social support, prior traumatization, and preexisting personality factors.

Some researchers of incest have maintained that explaining incest trauma as a form of PTSD is incomplete as a theory to explain the traumatic effects of the incest experience. These researchers (Briere & Runtz, 1988) have identified many characteristics in women who have been sexually abused as children that cannot be neatly subsumed within PTSD. Women in their sample reported behaviors such as dissociation, suicide attempts, revictimization, distorted beliefs about self, and substance abuse, which all fall outside the affective realm focus of PTSD. The research of Kilpatrick, Amick-McMullan, Best, Burke, and Saunders (1986) with a sample of 126 women who reported childhood sexual abuse found only 10% of women who qualified as currently having PTSD and 36% who qualified as experiencing PTSD at one time. These researchers drew attention to factors that are unique to incest: the repeated incest experiences by a trusted adult, the pressure to maintain secrecy, and the fact that the victim has no one to turn to for support or assistance. Thus with incest the trauma is compounded because of repeated and ongoing trauma and because of the sense of betrayal, abandonment, and powerlessness.

Finkelhor and Browne (1986) rejected the PTSD explanation in favor of their own model, which consists of four trauma-causing factors called traumagenic dynamics. Finkelhor and Browne maintained that some of these four factors occur in all types of psychologically traumatic situations, but it is only in the incest experience that all four occur together. The four factors are the following:

1. "*Traumatic sexualization* refers to a process in which a child's sexuality (including both sexual feelings and sexual attitudes) is shaped in a developmentally inappropriate and interpersonally dysfunctional fashion as a result of the sexual abuse" (p. 181). Some of the ways that traumatic sexualization can occur are: (1) rewarding the child for the sexual behavior, which in turn teaches the child that sexual behavior can be used as a means to meet one's needs; (2) placing distorted importance to particular parts of a child's anatomy; (3) providing distorted information to the child about sexuality; (4) experiencing frightening memories of the sexual activity. Finkelhor and Browne have claimed that children with incest experiences develop inappropriate repertoires of sexual behavior, are confused about sexual self-concepts, and have unusual emotional associations to sexual activities.

2. "*Betrayal* refers to the dynamic in which children discover that someone on whom they are vitally dependent has caused them harm" (p. 182). The child may experience betrayal by the actions of the abuser, as well as from the nonoffending parent and other adults to whom they seek protection.

3. *"Powerlessness*—or what might also be called 'disempowerment,' the dynamic of rendering the victim powerless—refers to the process in which the child's will, desires and sense of efficacy are continually contravened" (p. 183). Powerlessness occurs when a child is repeatedly used sexually against her will and is unable to disclose the activity because of a fear of the consequences.

4. *"Stigmatization*, the final dynamic, refers to the negative connotations—for example, badness, shame and guilt—that are communicated to the child about the experiences and that then become incorporated into the child's self-image" (p. 184). The stigmatization may develop during the abuse itself or after disclosure when adults react with shock, horror, and blame of the child.

According to Finkelhor (1986), the four traumagenic dynamics account for the primary sources of trauma of child sexual abuse. The categories are best viewed as broad clusterings of negative influences with a common theme. Finkelhor further elaborates the four dynamics by identifying both psychological impact and behavioral manifestations of each dynamic.

Finkelhor's model and the models of Burgess et al. (1987) and Carmen and Rieker (1989) have not been subjected to empirical testing. However, all the models are based on data derived from research, and all three address cognitive, social, behavioral, and psychological aspects of childhood sexual abuse on some level.

FAMILY CHARACTERISTICS

Weinberg (1955) identified two types of incestuous families. The first was the "ingrown or endogamous" family, which was unable to establish relationships outside the family. The second family type involved the very free family in which sexual activity was not a private behavior. Later studies confirmed Weinberg's classification but identified the endogamous family as the commonly reported type (Cormeier, Kennedy, & Sangowicz, 1962; Lustig, Dresser, Spellmen, & Murray, 1966).

Today the incestuous family is still viewed most typically as endogamous or enmeshed. These families are characterized by relatively closed boundaries to the outside world and a lack of boundaries within the family. Because they are physically, socially, and psychologically isolated from outsiders, they become excessively dependent on each other for satisfaction of physical, social, and psychological needs. Courtois (1988) notes that despite the fact that these family members are excessively dependent on each other, emotional and physical deprivation prevails. Thus the only source of love and affection for the children in these families may be through sexual contact.

Role reversals also are common in the enmeshed family. Gelinas (1983) identified a fairly common pattern of role reversal behavior among women with histories of childhood incest that she calls "parentification." This phenomenon is characterized by the sexually abused child in the family (often the oldest daughter) functioning as a parent. In addition to functioning as a parent, the child internalizes the role and its responsibilities so that her own identity develops around the caretaking of others to the exclusion of her own needs.

Despite the identification of a common family pattern, Finkelhor (1986) cautions that incest is a highly complex phenomenon that cannot be reduced to simplistic causality. It must be emphasized that each family has its own set of unique circumstances and consequences.

CHARACTERISTICS OF OFFENDERS

Research on child sexual offenders is still in its infancy, evidenced by the fact that the majority of studies recruit subjects (adult males) from the criminal justice system. These subjects involve a small percentage of the total number of child sexual abusers. In Russell's study (1986), only 2% of the incest offenders were reported to the police. Among the offenders that are reported only a few are apprehended and proceed to trial. The even smaller number convicted probably represents the most flagrant and repetitive sexual offenders (Finkelhor, 1986). Therefore it is clear that samples from the criminal justice system are not representative of offenders.

More research is needed to develop primary prevention sexual abuse programs, to identify people at risk for offending, and to predict the likelihood of identified offenders repeating their sexual abuse.

In addition to samples culled from the criminal justice system, the studies usually represent male offenders in father-daughter relationships. Therefore in the following discussion the offenders are referred to as males and the victims, as daughters.

Weinberg (1955) was one of the earliest researchers of child sexual offenders within the criminal justice system. In addition to the description of two primary incestuous family types, Weinberg discussed three personality types of incestuous father figures. The first was a psychopathic personality type who engaged in indiscriminate promiscuity. The second type involved the socially immature male who exhibited a pedophilic orientation, and the third type was described as introverted. In their work with 112 incestuous families, Justice and Justice (1979) described the same types, but they referred to the introverted group as "symbiotic" and added a fourth heterogeneous category called "other." According to Justice and Justice, the symbiotic type accounted for 80% to 85% of all abusers.

Justice and Justice (1979) described the symbiotic abuser as a male who was raised in a dysfunctional, emotionally deprived family. These researchers further categorized the symbiotic abuser into four subgroups based on the way that the abuser attempts to satisfy his unmet needs for love and closeness through sex. Because the daughters are starved for affection and attention, they usually submit without the need for force. The subgroups are introverted, rationalizing, tyrannical, and alcoholic.

1. The *symbiotic introvert* is characterized by the emotionally needy, isolated male who is married and dependent on his family to meet his insatiable psychological needs. Externally he may appear to be a model father and husband, but he has great difficulty achieving closeness to anyone outside his own family, is easily stressed by his work responsibilities, and believes the family's responsibility is to meet his unmet needs. Thus a sexual relationship with his daughter is an entitlement as father of the household.

2. The *symbiotic rationalizer* uses a variety of reasons why sexual activity with his daughter is appropriate. He views himself as her rightful protector, teacher, and lover. Therefore he must initiate and teach her about sex so that she can be liberated and enjoy healthy sexual activity with her father, who is the person most concerned with her welfare. The daughter is his rightful property to use as he pleases.

3. The *symbiotic tyrant* is characterized by his brutal dominance of his family, who fear him and go to great lengths to avoid his anger. The tyrant does not hesitate to use physical force to have his sexual needs met by his daughter. Females are sexual objects, and he models these expectations to his sons, who may be physically abused by him.

4. The *symbiotic alcoholic* type comprises 10% to 15% of the males who commit incest. Alcohol allows the male to become disinhibited about sexually abusing his daughter. If confronted later, this abuser blames the alcohol for his behavior rather than accepting the fact that the alcohol was used to give him the courage to abuse.

According to the Justice and Justice classification, the second main sexual abuse personality type is the psychopath who is without any guilt, remorse, or concern for anyone. The psychopath may be promiscuous and will have sex with any or all partners in or outside of the family, including his sons and daughters. Sex is used for physical stimulation and excitement rather than for satisfaction of love and closeness.

The third type is the pedophiliac incest offender. Justice and Justice claim this type of father-daughter incest offender is rare because they are too immature and inadequate to marry. When they are married, they usually confine themselves to younger daughters and do not progress past fondling and kissing.

The last type of incest offenders represents a mixed group, consisting of a small percentage of psychotic offenders and a larger group of rural, isolated people for whom incest may be culturally sanctioned.

Groth (1978) also described offenders. His classification is a simple but commonly used one. According to Groth, offenders are either fixated or regressed pedophiliacs. The fixated child offender has a primary and enduring attraction to children. This attraction does not engender any guilt or shame for them. Groth views these offenders as addicted to children, even though they can still have adult relations.

The regressed offender is characterized by a male who initially prefers adults but because of some crisis begins to focus on children. Because such persons' traditional values and beliefs are suspended, they have the potential for feeling distressed and remorseful over their abusive behavior. Incest offenders are usually in this category.

Groth also classifies offenders according to whether they use pressure or actual force with children. The sex-pressure offender uses enticement or entrapment to involve the child and is usually the offender who has some concern for the child. Thus he exploits his position of trust and affection with the child to satisfy his own needs for physical contact and affection. The goal is not sexual satisfaction but love and acceptance.

The sex-force offender's goal is sex, not nurturance, and he resorts to whatever means is necessary to achieve his goal. This offender has no emotional bond with the child nor any feelings of distress or remorse over the abusive behavior. Instead, he achieves a sense of power and satisfaction by controlling the child. Only a small number of offenders gain pleasure from sadistically hurting the child.

Russell (1986) and other feminists reject the claim by some researchers that incest is concerned with power, control, aggressive impulses, and dependency rather than sexual desire. Indeed, some reports (Freund, McKnight, Langevin, & Cibiri, 1972; Quinsey, 1977) have indicated that male sex offenders have a stronger erotic response to children than normal males, and even normal males demonstrated an erotic response to children, particularly female children. Russell viewed these studies as support for her belief that incest does involve sexuality.

In my practice a variety of motives are given by offenders for abusive behaviors. Some offenders are quite candid about their sexual attraction to children. They describe children in highly erotic terms such as soft, smooth, and innocent. Groth's classification of the fixated versus regressed offender may not always be appropriate. For some offenders a broad, deviant sexual pattern exists that surpasses attraction to children. Their behavior may be more likely described as sexual addiction because it involves intense and compulsive use of pornography, masturbation, sexual fantasy, and sex with anyone who is available. Although offenders offer a variety of reasons for their abusive behavior, it is clear that the reasons are complex and multifactorial. Many theories that were presented have never been tested empirically and others, only minimally. Therefore more research is needed before any can be accepted.

One critical point must be emphasized about all possible theoretical explanations for child sexual abuse. Regardless of the cause, the offender makes a conscious decision to abuse the child, and the responsibility for the abuse is always his (or hers) despite circumstances. A discussion of four necessary preconditions for child sexual abuse to occur elucidates this claim (Finkelhor, 1986):

> (1) The offender must have the motivation to sexually abuse, (2) the offender must overcome internal inhibitions against abusing, (3) the offender must overcome external obstacles against abusing, and (4) the offender must overcome resistance by the child. To "explain" sexual abuse fully, one must account for the presence of all four of these preconditions. (pp. 86-87)

FEMALE SEX OFFENDERS

There are few reports specifically on female offenders; however, there is consensus that the majority of sexual abuse is conducted by males and the majority of victims are females. Finkelhor (1986) claims that 95% of female child abuse and 80% of male child abuse involve male offenders. Even when female offenders are identified, it is often at the instigation of male partners. In Russell's (1986) probability sample of 930 women in the community, only 10 cases of incestuous abuse by females were identified. These 10 cases comprised 5% of the incest offenders in

TABLE 5-1
Female Offenders and Their Frequencies

FEMALE OFFENDERS	FREQUENCIES
Mothers	7
Grandmothers	3
Aunts	3
Sisters	3
Total female offenders	16 = 6.6% of all offenders
Total offenders = 243	

Russell's study and provided strong support for the argument that female child abuse by adult females represents only a small portion of the total abuse cases. In addition to the infrequency of female offenders, abuse that was perpetrated by females was less severe (Finkelhor, 1986; Russell, 1986).

In Urbancic's (1992) convenience sample of 147 female incest survivors, 6.6% (n=16) of the total offenders (N=243) were women. All 16 of the female offenders were part of a multiple family abuse system and none acted in isolation. Of the cases with female offenders, 13 involved an abusing father or stepfather. Urbancic's research supports Finkelhor's claim (1984) that when women sexually abuse children, it is usually at the instigation of male family members. Table 5-1 displays the various female offenders and their frequencies in Urbancic's study.

Some writers claim that adult females abuse male children more frequently than females, and because these activities are hidden they are seriously underreported. Since Russell's study (1986) involved abused females only, no inferences can be made about male child abuse from her work. However, if females do abuse males more frequently, it should be reported in self-reported surveys such as Finkelhor (1984) conducted with college students; this has not occurred. Both Finkelhor and Russell assert that no evidence exists to support the claim that adult females commonly abuse male children rather than females.

TREATMENT GOALS FOR CHILD SEX OFFENDERS

The basic treatment goals for offenders are:

1. To accept full responsibility for the abuse and make this known to the victim
2. To become cognitively and affectively aware of the destructive effects of the incest on the victim and her family
3. To reduce deviant arousal patterns to prevent future abuse
4. To develop adaptive methods of coping with anger, stress, loneliness, and depression
5. To develop satisfying interpersonal skills with adults
6. To learn parenting skills and principles of normal child growth and development

THE CHILD VICTIM IN THE INCESTUOUS FAMILY

The child victim in the incestuous family is usually the oldest daughter, with the average age of approximately 10 years. The majority of incest appears between the ages of 10 to 13. In Russell's study (1986), 11% occurred before age 5, 19% between 6 and 9 years, 41% between 10 and 13 years, and 29% after 14 years. It is not uncommon to find infants and toddlers who have been sexually abused. Early sexual abuse rarely involves attempts at vaginal intercourse but oral penetration is not unusual. Only recently has it become evident that almost all gonorrhea in childhood must be regarded as an indication of sexual abuse. In 44 of 45 children (ages 1 to 9 years), gonorrhea was contracted through sexual activity with a relative (Jaffe, Dynneson, & Ten Bensel, 1975). Unless the child contracts the disease during birth, sexual abuse must be assumed in cases of sexually transmitted diseases in children.

The relationship between age and degree of incest trauma is not clear—different studies have reported conflicting results (Courtois, 1988; Finkelhor, 1986; Peters, 1988; Russell, 1986). However, younger victims may repress their incest experiences to a greater degree and therefore have no recall until later years when severe stress breaks down the repression barriers.

The incestuous relationship may extend over a period of many years; the average length of time is approximately 3 years. It is common for the severity of incest to increase as the incestuous activity continues over the years. Most typically it begins with fondling and gradually evolves into oral sex and vaginal intercourse.

Few incestuous relationships involve violence or force, although coercion is usually present. Although earlier studies reported seductive behaviors and active participation by the daughters (Bender & Blau, 1937; Henderson, 1972; Weiss, Roger, Darwin, & Dutton, 1955), it is generally accepted that flirtatious behavior is a reflection of the child's search for nurturance, not sexual gratification. It is the neglect the child suffers that causes the appearance of cooperation, but in reality the child is demonstrating a desperate craving for affection and attention.

It is normal and healthy for a young female to practice her female wiles on her father, and regardless of her behavior, she needs controls and limits set by the adults in the family. Parents have the roles of teachers and protectors, not exploiters, and although all parents may experience some sexual feelings toward their children at times, it is the incestuous parent who acts on those feelings.

The majority of child incest victims never disclose, but some are able to extricate themselves from the situation in a variety of ways. If the child is able to escape the abuse, often the next daughter is forced to assume the servicing of the offender's needs. Sometimes it is the victimization of a younger sibling that motivates the oldest daughter to disclose the incestuous activity.

Cessation from the sexual abuse may occur when the daughter becomes older and more able to assert herself in some way that protects her from further abuse. If she begins dating, it is often an issue that leads to serious conflict with the father since it may engender jealousy in the father and a sense of competitiveness with the boyfriend. The escalating tension and anger may result in acting out behavior in terms of drug use and sexual promiscuity. It is not unusual for the victim to accuse the offender of sexual abuse during a heated family argument over her delinquent behavior. Subsequently, the mother may join the father in accusing the daughter of lying about the abuse and claim the motivation for the lies was revenge on the father for setting limits on the daughter's delinquent behavior.

At other times the daughter may choose to disclose the incest to a friend or teacher, who then reports the abuse to protective services. Running away from home is another frequent way of coping with the sexual abuse; therefore, anyone working with run-away teenagers should carefully assess for a history of sexual abuse.

MOTHERS AS NONOFFENDING PARENTS

Many investigators insist that the key to the incestuous family is the mother. She has been described as rejecting and dominating of both husband and daughter. Although the mother sometimes may be physically or mentally incapacitated, researchers (Henderson, 1972; Justice & Justice, 1979) report that she foists the mother-wife role on her daughter and expects the daughter to provide nurturance for her also.

These researchers also maintain that the role reversal of mother and daughter is instrumental in keeping the dysfunctional family together because the father's needs are satisfied, the mother is relieved of her responsibilities, and the daughter assumes a position of power with many payoffs. Some even suggest that the father and daughter unite to gain revenge on the rejecting mother.

However, other researchers contest the theory that places all the responsibility and blame on the mother (Herman, 1981; Rush, 1980). They maintain the mother is often depressed or physically incapacitated and therefore unable to care for herself or her family. Although the mother-blaming theory may be correct in some instances, it is unreasonable to assume that the mother consciously or unconsciously arranges and encourages the father-daughter relationship. It is argued that some mothers often tolerate physical abuse, humiliation, and poverty because of their social and economic status.

In Herman and Hirschman's study (1977), the daughters viewed their mothers as weak and downtrodden and unable to provide protection for anyone. Thus mothers are accused of being dependent or dominating, frigid or promiscuous, rejecting or domineering. Whatever language is used, they are frequently blamed for the incest instead of the offender.

In families where the mother possesses power, incest is less likely to occur. This phenomenon can be explained by Finkelhor's (1986) disinhibition factor; that is, if the father believes that the child will disclose to the mother and that the mother will take steps against the offender, then internal inhibitions against the incest will be strengthened rather than weakened, and incest is less likely to occur.

Because the literature on incest focuses on the victim and the offender, almost nothing is empirically known about the mother's perspective of the incestuous situation. In clinical practice a variety of mother-daughter scenarios are commonly presented. In clinical samples, only a small percentage of children disclose the abuse to their mothers and receive immediate, unquestioning support and protection from her.

Other mothers are confused and do not know whom to believe, especially when they trust and love the offender and he vehemently denies the incest charges. If the women believes that her husband loves her and that the marriage has been successful, the revelation of an incestuous relationship between her spouse and daughter can be overwhelming and profoundly distressing. The world becomes unpredictable and insane. No one can be trusted. Nothing makes sense. Her husband has betrayed her for a younger woman, and this younger woman is her own daughter. It is much *less devastating* to believe that it did not happen.

In the writer's clinical practice, many mothers come to therapy groups feeling angry, confused, and ambivalent, but they gradually believe their daughters, understand the dynamics of the situation, place the blame and responsibility on the offender, and accept that they must learn how to protect their children to prevent future abuse. For many mothers, belief of her victimized daughter usually

involves a crisis, followed by a process of working through feelings of shock, disbelief, ambivalence, acceptance, and eventually strong support for the daughter. However, as the mother grapples with her own pain and guilt, she also must address her daughter's pain. The daughter will be experiencing the trauma of abuse and rage and blame toward the mother for not believing and protecting her. It is not unusual for the daughter to place more blame and anger on the mother than on the offender.

If social service agencies do not follow the mother closely for a long enough period, they may only remember the mothers while they were in denial and shock and not appreciate acceptance as a gradual process. Certainly some mothers consistently deny their daughters' claims of sexual abuse and join with their husbands to accuse the daughter of lying. As noted earlier, sexually abused female adolescents frequently act out their anger and helplessness by resorting to drug use, being promiscuous, and running away from home. Because the daughter has a history of delinquent behavior, sometimes the parents claim the daughter is accusing the father of abuse to seek revenge for the limits he has set on her behavior. To relatives and friends, both parents may appear as conscientious caretakers who are being victimized by their own daughter. Mothers reinforce this victimization role by trying to convince others that the daughter is a "bad seed." They make statements such as "she began to lie as soon as she started to speak" or "she made trouble for me from the day she was born."

In other incestuous situations the abuse has continued for many years, multiple cues existed, and the daughter claimed that she told her mother; nevertheless, the mother did not intervene to protect the daughter or to stop the abuse. Once the abuse has been disclosed (usually to someone outside the immediate family or after the daughter is an adult), the mother may believe her daughter and become devastated by the knowledge of the abuse. However, many mothers vehemently deny any awareness of the abuse, just as they deny that the daughters gave them any hints about the existence of the abuse. Sauzier (1989) found that when children tried to disclose to their mothers, they gave such vague and indirect hints that the message was not really conveyed. The mothers who understood the hints had to ask many questions before the child actually disclosed.

Sauzier (1989) also reported that mothers were overwhelmingly the most common confidante for children who had been sexually victimized. Sauzier viewed this as a refutation that mothers instigate the abuse or are in collusion with the offender.

It is still difficult to explain the broad lack of support by so many mothers even when considering daughters' vague disclosures. Another explanation for the mother's denial may relate to the fact that many mothers are themselves victims of childhood incest. It is well established that women who were child victims of sexual abuse frequently fail to protect their own daughters from abuse. Some clinicians have suggested that the mother's denial and failure to protect may be the result of the unconscious coping mechanism of dissociation. Each time any cue in the environment threatens to trigger memories of her own abuse, the mother psychologically (unconsciously) separates herself from the threat (Dolan, 1991; Fredrickson, 1991; Giaretto, 1989). Dissociation would explain the lack of response or acknowledgment by the mother of her daughter's attempt to disclose. These researchers maintain that offenders, nonoffending parents, and child victims all use dissociation to some degree to cope with abuse.

REPEATED GENERATIONAL PATTERNS IN THE INCESTUOUS FAMILY

Many researchers have claimed that incestuous behaviors become repetitive generational patterns. Young girls who are abused may grow up to become adults who fail to protect their own children. Summit (1989) reports that 90% of mothers who seek help for child abuse have a history of being sexually abused as children. Other researchers report that these women often choose cruel and neglecting husbands because they view themselves as immoral and undeserving.

Because of their lack of self-esteem, unresolved anger, and sense of powerlessness, such women have difficulty maintaining healthy interpersonal relationships and are unable to protect themselves or their children. But it is vitally important to understand that although a person has been victimized as a child, it does not mean that she or he will inevitably fail to protect or become a victimizer as an adult. Statistics of mothers who fail to protect their children and of fathers who abuse their children are drawn from sexual abuse treatment programs and do not represent all men and women who have been sexually abused as children. The majority of people who have been abused do *not* grow up to be abusers. It is critical that adults with childhood incest experiences understand that they are not doomed to revictimize others.

EFFECTS OF INCEST
Short-Term Effects of Incest

Despite the influence of Freudian theory, the last 15 years have seen a wealth of both clinical and research articles and books that have supported the belief that the occurrence of childhood incest is increasing and has both short- and long-term traumatic effects. These studies were stimulated by the feminist movement and have identified a variety of short-term effects of incest in children as well as long-term effects in adult women. Because incest is multidetermined, the degree of damage depends on many variables. Unfortunately, many studies of childhood incest have not used standardized measures, adequate sample size and comparison groups, and have based their studies on clinical populations. The studies described in this chapter are generally those with stricter methodologies such as control groups, standardized measures, and probability samples of adequate size. Intrafamilial versus extrafamilial sexual abuse is not always distinguished. However, as previously noted, most childhood sexual abuse involves incestuous relationships if the broader definition of incest is used.

Most researchers appear to agree that serious effects are not inevitable, particularly if the child and family are given support and treatment. Sometimes it is believed that the effects of discovery with consequent stressful legal involvement are more traumatic than the actual incest experience, particularly if the child is removed from the home or the father is incarcerated. The child may feel guilty and may interpret removal from the home as punishment. She also may blame herself for the destruction of the family if the father is removed.

Some researchers have concentrated on documenting the short-term effects of incest on young children. They report a pattern of behavior that includes premature sexual behavior such as open masturbation, frequent exposure of genitalia, and a tendency to become involved sexually with other children. These erotic behaviors present a problem in placement and maintenance in foster care facilities. Nightmares, encopresis, enuresis, anorexia, school phobias, learning problems, genitourinary problems, and depression also are commonly seen. Infants and very young children may have reddened and swollen genitalia, sleep and eating disturbances, as well as changes in activity levels (Browne & Finkelhor, 1986; Tufts' New England Medical Center, 1984).

Adolescent incest victims tend to have many of the same problems and additional ones such as teenage pregnancy, promiscuity, truancy, running away from home, drug and alcohol abuse, eating disorders, self-mutilation, panic attacks, suicide attempts, and depression.

The conflicting role of child and lover is extremely difficult to fulfill. Sometimes it also entails the role of being a physical caretaker. Such demands on the child create confusion and interfere with the normal developmental tasks of childhood and adolescence. It typically causes rage and resentment toward authority figures as well. As previously noted, the daughter may feel deep anger and resentment toward the father figure, but she may harbor even deeper anger toward her mother for not protecting her. In addition to feeling betrayed by her father (or other surrogate male) and mother, she also may feel betrayed when she seeks professional assistance because of the blame, disbelief, or unconcern she may encounter.

It is unclear whether the effects of incest are more serious in the adolescent or younger child. Some studies have indicated a trend for abuse of younger children to be more traumatic than in older children, but these trends have not been statistically significant.

Long-Term Effects of Childhood Incest

Many studies have been conducted with samples of college students and control groups to compare the long-term effects of childhood sexual abuse. These studies found that sexually abused women demonstrated more depression, anxiety, and substance abuse than nonabused women. In a community health study with a random selection of 387 women (Bagley & Ramsey, 1985), women in the group with childhood sexual abuse histories were more depressed, experienced more somatic anxiety, and had lower self-esteem scores than nonabused controls. Other studies with strict methodologies have found statistically significant differences in sleep disturbances, sexual problems, dissociation, chronic muscle tension, alienation, and anger, as well as suicide attempts, substance abuse, and battering as adults (Briere & Runtz, 1988; Fromuth, 1986; Sedney & Brooks, 1984; Seidner & Calhoun, 1984).

In a review of the literature, Browne and Finkelhor (1986) concluded that empirical research appears to support the clinical impression of low esteem among adult women with childhood sexual abuse experiences. Research (Briere & Runtz, 1988; Brown & Garrison, 1990; Kluft, 1990) also supported the probability that incest victims were more likely to experience sexual and physical revictimization as adults by strangers, husbands, and boyfriends. Women who experienced childhood sexual abuse also were at high risk for subsequent sexual victimization by their therapists. Russell (1986) found that between 33% to 68% (depending on definition of abuse) of the childhood sexually abused women in her probability sample were subsequently raped, as compared with 17% of women without histories of childhood sexual abuse. In addition to being physically and sexually revictimized in an adult relationship, these women were more likely to have attempted suicide in the past.

Research studies show mixed results in relating objective severity measures of incest and subjective reports of the trauma. Some studies found no significant differences in the trauma as a result of genital fondling versus intercourse. However, the majority of studies have found a significant relationship between objective severity of the incest experience and perceived trauma. Researchers have identified several factors that appear to influence the severity of incest trauma. These factors include age of onset, duration, type and frequency of activity, developmental state, available social resources, family system patterns, and the child's relationship to the offender.

Courtois' Incest History Questionnaire

Because many factors interact to influence the trauma of incest, it is difficult to objectively assess its severity. Courtois (1988) assessed the severity of incest trauma by having the incest survivor describe her perception of the effects of her incest experience on eight life domains: social, psychological, physical, sexual, familial, sense of self, and relationships with males and females.

Urbancic (1992) adapted Courtois' Incest History Questionnaire for use with a convenience sample of 147 women recruited from the community. The women responded to advertisements to participate in a study on "unwanted childhood sexual experiences." The next section describes a summary of self-report statements by the women about the effects of their childhood incest experience on the eight domains identified by Courtois.

1. *Social* (e.g., feeling isolated, different from others). The majority of women reported feeling alone, empty, and scared. Even when they knew they were popular, they still felt different. Although some were professionally successful, they reported feeling "like a fake." Others chose demeaning or destructive work such as prostitution. Many reported that since they could not discriminate among people, they felt they had to be cold, angry, and dis-

trustful to protect themselves. Some reported being so shy and backward with people that they gave up trying to develop relationships. Wanting to please others without regard for their own needs was another common response.

2. *Psychological/emotional* (e.g., not being able to feel anything or having too many emotions). Many women reported numbing and denial, or closing down of emotions that vacillated with overwhelming feelings of anger, fear, suspicion, and paranoia. Feelings of being fragile and vulnerable were also noted. For many, fear of losing control and hurting others was an important issue. Some women had a need for self-mutilation. Others reported feeling depressed, suicidal, and obsessive-compulsive. Excessive anxiety, agoraphobia, and panic attacks were also frequently noted.

   Dissociation was a common defense mechanism; several women described themselves as having multiple personality disorder and being victims of ritual abuse. Many women had totally repressed their memories of childhood sexual abuse and were overwhelmed when they began experiencing memories, feelings, dreams, and flashbacks of their abuse. The reality of their abuse was difficult to accept, and many questioned their own sanity. Many of the women resorted to alcohol and drugs to cope with their nightmares, flashbacks, anxiety, and intrusive thoughts.

3. *Physical* (e.g., feeling sick at the mention of certain activities). A variety of physical complaints were reported that directly paralleled the abuse experience. These included being nauseous whenever they felt controlled, were physically touched, or smelled sexual odors. Those women whose abuse involved vaginal or anal intercourse reported having chronic pelvic pain, frequent abortions, pain during or after intercourse, and severe pain with bowel movements. Those who experienced oral sex had symptoms such as an absent gag reflex, biting the inside of the mouth until it bled, gastrointestinal disorders, and eating disorders. A variety of somatic complaints,

such as severe headaches and insomnia, and neurological symptoms, such as physical numbness and tingling of body parts, also were reported.

4. *Sexual* (e.g., wanting sex all the time or avoiding it). Many women reported that they alternated between periods of wanting sex constantly, masturbating excessively, and being promiscuous with periods of abstinence, having no physical attraction to others, and not wanting anyone to touch them. It was common for the women to confuse sex with love, and some noted that they preferred to give sexual pleasure rather than receive it. Others used sex to achieve feelings of power and mastery by controlling all aspects of the sexual activity. Others reported being controlled by the sexual demands of the male and not being able to say "no." Some became confused about the identity of their sexual partner and experienced many flashbacks and vivid memories of their abuse when they attempted to engage in sexual activity.

5. *Familial* (within or with your family; e.g., family members got closer; parents got divorced). Family patterns varied from becoming closer to mother, father, or other relatives to becoming totally estranged from them. Some reported no change over the years as the family remained in denial. Others reported significant changes, such as a family member becoming psychotic, suicidal, or alcoholic. Some children were abused by the women's mates, whereas other women were excessively protective of their children. Some reported an inability to confide in their mothers even though they repeatedly invited confidence.

6. *Sense of self* (e.g., powerful or poor sense of self-esteem). Some women fluctuated between extremes of feeling powerful and helpless, but most tended to have poor self-esteem, deep shame, and a sense of worthlessness. For many women it was important to be in control and therefore many reported being rigid and perfectionist. Typical boundary issues were as follows: has no sense of self, lives for others, cannot make deci-

sions, and only feels worthwhile if someone is sexually attracted to them. Many women noted they do not value their lives, dislike themselves, and believe that no one could love them.

7. *Relation to men* (e.g., close or hostile). For some women relations to men were described as closer than women. These women reported more male than female friends. The responses also stated that men should always come first and always be in control. Some women dated any man who asked for a date because to be wanted sexually was to be loved. The opposite group of women reported feeling apprehensive with and very hostile toward men, viewed them as seductive, and made comments like "you can't ever trust a man" and "I feel pity for them." Many women acknowledged being afraid of intimacy and commitment, having relationships that never last, and choosing partners who are destructive or unable to be intimate.

8. *Relation to women* (e.g., close or hostile). The relationships that women described with other women covered a wide range of responses from feeling safe, close, unthreatened, and trusting to feeling apprehensive, distrusting, and hostile. Mothers were singled out as being hated. Some felt superior to other women and believed that women were jealous of them. Some women reported being neutral or passive or just beginning to develop relationships with other women. Several women stated that they do not feel feminine nor can they identify with other women because they feel like children. Several mentioned being attracted to strong women and acknowledged homosexual feelings.

Summary of Effects of Incest

The growing body of research indicates that childhood incest experiences can have serious effects on both child and adult functioning and health. However, it is important to emphasize that not all of the effects can be classified as serious and long term, and many people who have had childhood sexual experiences have recovered without formal psychotherapy and professional assistance. In Urbancic's (1992) study, when survivors of incest were asked to describe the person, event, belief, or experience that was most helpful in the healing of their childhood sexual abuse, women repeatedly identified people who were available when needed, who cared, listened, validated, and understood. Usually that person was a therapist, friend, or another survivor. Nurses are often in positions to offer such essential support to women and children who have experienced childhood incest trauma.

NURSING INTERVENTIONS
Primary Prevention

Primary prevention for childhood sexual abuse began to proliferate in the 1980s. Because abuse is increasing and most victims do not disclose or have treatment, the potential for short- and long-term effects is significant. Sexual abuse educational programs for children, parents, and professionals are the first step in eliminating the trauma of sexual abuse. Although nurses are not always in a position to present such programs, it is essential that they value the critical importance of the programs and become involved in supporting programs in their schools and communities. Nurses, as health promotion advocates, must insist that these programs balance themes of violence and abuse with those of healthy touch and intimacy.

There are many agencies and institutions that provide sexual abuse primary prevention programs for children, parents, and mental health professionals. Storybooks, coloring books, videos, and films are available for children on the topic as well as workshops that incorporate art and role-plays into primary prevention education. Developmental level and cultural background of the children are important considerations when developing or selecting materials. Past educational programs focused on the "stranger" as the abuser, but today the message contains the possibility that someone whom the child knows and trusts may try to involve them in sexually inappropriate behavior. If they are involved in such an activity, children are taught to tell someone they trust and also try to resist the of-

fender in whatever manner they are able. In addition to preventing child abuse, these programs can be helpful in preventing future victimization in children who already are abused. Improving their self-esteem and sense of control and mastery over their lives may make the difference in revictimization for many children. Durfee (1989) confirmed that improving the self-esteem of children may be the best protection for a child in preventing any kind of assault.

Programs of primary prevention for children are not enough to stem the tide of childhood sexual abuse. Parents also must be involved in the primary prevention of childhood sexual abuse. However, studies indicate that parents are not involved. In a study by Finkelhor (1984), only 29% of parents claimed to have discussions about sexual abuse with their children, although almost all warned their children about the possibility of kidnaping. Even when discussions about sexual abuse did occur, they began when the child was too old (older than 9 years), and crucial facts about sexual abuse were omitted.

Parental difficulty of addressing sexual issues with their children was consistent across all socioeconomic, religious, and educational levels. Finkelhor (1984) suggested that in addition to avoiding the sensitive topic, parents believed that their children were safe; therefore the potential for sexual abuse was not a salient issue for them. It is crucial that parents become aware of the high incidence of abuse among all socioeconomic, ethnic, and religious groups and are assisted to discuss the sensitive issue of sexual abuse with their children. Durfee (1989) claimed that lowering the anxiety of parents about sexual abuse issues may be more important than the materials that are presented.

Families with high risk for abuse such as those with stepfathers, parents with a childhood history of physical or sexual abuse, or children with developmental or emotional problems, need special and concentrated attention. Nurses who teach parenting classes should emphasize the role of both parents in the caretaking of their children. In addition to the involvement of fathers, it also may be appropriate for older siblings and other caretakers to participate because knowledge about child development, bonding, attachment, and separation are the bases for prevention of child abuse. Recent research (Parker & Parker, 1986) has strongly suggested that fathers who are involved in the early care of their children are more likely to bond with their children and are less likely to sexually abuse them. Unfortunately, too often only the mothers attend parenting classes or sexual abuse workshops. Nurses who conduct parenting classes must creatively devise methods for involving both parents as caretakers of their children.

Professionals also need special training and education about childhood sexual abuse to educate the public formally and informally and become child advocates in the prevention of abuse. Nurses must demand that content on sexual abuse be incorporated into the curricula of their nursing schools and that in-service training on the topic be conducted periodically at their places of employment.

Secondary Prevention: Interventions with the Sexually Abused Child and Her Family

All professionals must be prepared to quickly and effectively intervene whenever necessary in cases of sexual abuse. Nurses are in a special position to intervene because they have intimate and frequent interactions in a variety of settings with children, adolescents, and adults who have been sexually molested as children. But nurses cannot be effective in primary and secondary prevention efforts unless they take the responsibility to examine their own feelings and educate themselves on childhood sexual abuse.

Many nurses and other professionals are uncomfortable dealing with the issue of incest, as shown by an evasive, punitive manner and the failure to respond to child sexual abuse statutes that mandate reporting if suspicion exists. If nurses and other professionals do not assume the responsibility for identifying and reporting victims of sexual abuse, they support its proliferation. In addition, failure to invite the victim to disclose and discuss the abuse will probably lead them to interpret their secret as too terrible to discuss, and, consequently, their sense of shame, guilt, and helplessness may be aggravated.

Case finding of children who have already been abused has not been an easy task because many such children do not disclose their abuse and do not fit the typical textbook picture of the abused child. In an effort to address this problem, an interdisciplinary conference was convened in 1985 to develop criteria for the diagnosis of the "Sexually Abused Child's Disorder (SACD)." According to Corwin (1988), the purpose of this effort was "to describe the specific signs and symptoms that are specific enough that together they constitute compelling clinical substantiation that a particular child has been sexually victimized" (p. 254).

It also was planned that the criteria for diagnosing the SACD be incorporated into the revised fourth edition of the Diagnostic and Statistical Manual of the American Psychiatric Association (DSM III). However, the chairperson of the revisions of the DSM III work group refused to consider the SACD for inclusion in the appendix of the new edition because in his opinion there is no Sexually Abused Child's Disorder. Efforts continue by professional groups to have the SACD included in the DSM-IV edition of the manual. Work on the criteria also continued and it was acknowledged that change of signs and symptoms from one developmental period to another occurs, as does the degree of specificity for discriminating sexual abuse from other childhood conditions. In 1987 the fourth draft of diagnostic criteria for SACD were written and are listed in the box that follows.

Physical indications of sexual abuse

Anytime child sexual abuse is suspected, a complete physical examination should be performed. Before a child is examined for the possibility of sexual abuse, the nurse and doctor must establish trust and gain the child's cooperation to prevent further victimization through the exam. In addition, a child who is frightened and tense will most likely tighten pubococcygeal muscles so that it is difficult to evaluate the vaginal canal or hymen. It may be desirable to interview the child without the mother so that the child can feel free to express herself. Using anatomically correct dolls to elicit an abuse history can be helpful because it allows children to depersonalize

---

Criteria for the Sexually Abused Child's Disorder

(A) Displays an increased awareness of differentiated sexual behaviors as demonstrated by specific knowledge, or by emotional and behavioral reactions to direct questions about parts of the body and inquiries about actual exposure to the following:
   (1) Provocative exhibition of genitals
   (2) Sexualized kissing
   (3) Sexual fondling
   (4) Vaginal or anal stimulation or penetration
   (5) Mock intercourse
   (6) Oral copulation
   (7) Child pornography: being shown or photographed
(B) Can describe or demonstrate being subjected to any of the above sexual experiences by an adult or child at least 3 years older than the reporting child, or of any age differential when force or coercion is described.
(C) Displays one or more of the following:
   (1) Attempts during initial disclosures, to resist, minimize, deny, or to avoid recalling the sexually abusive experiences. This may be followed by intermittent denial and recantation.
   (2) History of repeated attempts to engage others in sexual behavior.
   (3) Age-excessive preoccupation with genital anatomy or related terms, or differentiated sexual behavior (A. 1-7 above), for example, excessive talking about or drawing of genitals and/or repeated sexualized play with dolls.
   (4) Overdetermined or anxious avoidance of genital anatomy or related terms.
   (5) Excessive masturbation that is significantly different from peers.
   (6) Nightmares triggered by person, place, or object or including physical movements or vocalizations that are consistent with sexually abusive experiences.
   (7) Dissociation.
   (8) Unexplained person, place, object avoidance and/or fearfulness.
   (9) Medical findings indicative of sexual victimization
(D) Onset before the age of 10.
(E) Not due to consensual peer sex play, misinterpreted physical contact, observed sexual acts, fabrication, or indoctrination.

Modified from Corwin, D.L. (1988). Early diagnosis of child sexual abuse. In G.E. Wyatt & G.J. Powell (Eds.), *Lasting effects of child sexual abuse* (pp. 258–259). Newbury Park, CA: Sage.

---

the abuse. It is critical to document the history the child relates in her exact words. The first priority in dealing with a sexually abused child is to determine if it is safe for the child to return to her home.

Since most sexual abuse does not involve activity that causes physical injury, in the majority of cases the physical findings will be normal. Nevertheless, the child should be examined for bruises on the entire body as well as evidence of trauma to the external genitalia, vagina, and rectum. Assessment of sexually transmitted diseases should always be done, and their presence is an almost certain indicator of abuse. This involves cultures of the pharynx, urethra, vagina, penis, and rectum. Gonorrhea can be misdiagnosed as vulvovaginitis, which is merely the result of poor personal hygiene (Muram & Gale, 1990).

The physical position for a child to assume during a genital examination depends on the age of the child. Children younger than 3 years may be most comfortable sitting on the mother's lap. Children older than 3 will usually cooperate and lie on an examining table if rapport has been established. Dolls can be use to demonstrate desired positions to the child. McCann (1990) recommends a combination of supine and prone positions. The supine position is used to (1) separate the labia so that the vaginal introitus is visible, and (2) retract the labia majora to examine the hymen. The knee-chest prone position is the most effective for examining the entire vaginal canal without a speculum. The knee-chest position also is the easiest way to collect deep vaginal specimens without discomfort and the use of instruments. The use of colposcopy for magnification is more common today. These instruments can be equipped with cameras that can be invaluable for documenting injuries. When the examination and history are completed, any suspicions of sexual abuse must be reported to protective services by the doctor or nurse in attendance.

Additional interventions for secondary prevention

Even when all the data strongly indicate that the child has been abused, she may deny it. A basic component of the child's denial is the amount of ambivalence that she may be experiencing. One source of ambivalence for the child is her relationship to the offender. Disclosure by the child is easier if the offender is not a close, trusted person to whom the child feels a sense of commitment or loyalty.

Another reason for the child's ambivalence may be related to the threats the offender has made regarding disclosure. These threats may provoke a variety of anxious fantasies about physical harm to herself or other family members. In addition, she may fear the breakup of the family, with the offender going to prison and the rest of the family blaming her for the breakup. The victim also may fear removal from the family and placement in a foster care setting. These fears can provide powerful motivation for not disclosing or even for later retraction. Some children might choose to sacrifice themselves rather than have their dysfunctional family destroyed, whereas others feel that the positives of their relationship with the offender outweigh the negatives of the abuse. Therefore to make sense of the child's denials, retractions, and vacillations, it is essential to consider and process all possible concerns, fears, and perceptions of the child.

Initial interventions focus on stabilizing the crisis that results from the disclosure. For nurses who are in a position to work with incestuous families, the focus of care is on the individual needs of the child,

but all family members need support. Organizations that offer groups for offenders, nonoffending parents, victims, and siblings are urgently needed for effectively treating these families. These groups are beginning to develop across the country.

Groups for nonoffending parents are essential in providing support for the mother. Initially, the mother may be so overwhelmed by the disclosure and the threatened loss of her children, spouse, and economic security that without support she may side with the offender against the daughter. In addition, support of the child by the nonoffending parent has been identified as a crucial variable in ameliorating the severity of incest (Wyatt & Mickey, 1987).

Offender participation in groups is rarely successful unless it is court mandated (Giaretto, 1989). The objectives of an offenders' group are to (1) break down the offenders' denial, (2) assist them to admit they have lost control over their lives, (3) assist them to recognize that they need external controls, and (4) have them take responsibility for their behavior. Even though the offender completes treatment, admits full responsibility for the abuse, and apologizes to his entire family, the mother and children must always be on guard for a loss of the offender's inner control and resumption of the sexual abuse by the offender. Family therapy is never appropriate until the family has reached some level of stability. It is important for nurses to be aware of community resources so that referral of the family to the appropriate agency can be made.

Crisis intervention with the incestuous family requires a direct, swift, and active approach to ensure that the abuse has ended and the child will be protected. It also requires coordination with protective services, law enforcement agencies, and counselors. Usually the offender is mandated by the court to leave the home. If there is a possibility that the offender may continue to abuse and the mother cannot or will not protect her, the child may be removed from the home. Because this approach is usually traumatic for the child, it is avoided if possible.

When addressing the needs of the sexually abused child, the nurse must realize that not all destructive effects of the abuse will be obvious immediately. Therefore a physical and psychological assessment and intervention are always necessary regardless of whether the child appears traumatized. The child's age and developmental level are determining factors in choosing the type of therapy. Usually very young children will be encouraged to express themselves through art and play therapy; these therapies are helpful for older children as well.

Group therapy for sexually abused children can be a powerful modality for assisting all children older than 3 years. The group can be effective in correcting many of the traumatic sexualization behaviors that abused children exhibit, as well as improving their sense of power and self-esteem, decreasing feelings of being stigmatized, and reestablishing a sense of trust and assertiveness with people in their world. In addition, the group can address the child's understanding for the abuse so that misconceptions about her role and the roles others played can be examined and corrected. Often the child has overwhelming guilt about the pleasurable aspects of the abuse or the fact that she sometimes initiated the interactions. Some research (Janoff-Bulman, 1986) has supported the belief that children who believed they had choices and therefore some degree of self-blame in the abuse situation may have better outcomes than those who believed they were totally helpless. Thus attributions of self-blame should be examined with the child and explained as adaptive behavior in that she made the best choice under the circumstances.

A major component of therapy is directed toward decreasing anxiety and fear related to the abuse. As the child repeatedly addresses different aspects of the abuse and learns to express her anger, sadness, and grief about them, the memories of the event gradually lose their power for negative arousal. In addition, age-appropriate sex education should be provided along with discussions of cues that indicate a situation is becoming sexually threatening.

Tertiary Prevention with the Adult Sexually Abused as a Child

When discussing the adult who has been sexually abused as a child, the word "victim" has generally been replaced by the word "survivor." Not everyone agrees with the use of the term "survivor." Russell (1986) views "survivor" as only relating to those who have experienced the most severe forms of incest, whereas "victim" has broader application and is thus more appropriate for her. For this writer, the term "survivor" is preferred and is used because of the need to focus on the process of recovery through which the person proceeds rather than thinking of herself as one who continues to be helpless, injured, or destroyed.

As with the child who has been sexually abused, nurses in a variety of settings have opportunities to assist the adult survivor of abuse. Because the survivor requires support on many different levels, nurses need not be expert therapists to be helpful. Nursing interventions with adult survivors can encompass a variety of helping techniques that can mitigate the guilt and shame of the survivor's long-kept secret, as well as the denial, minimization, and blame that she has experienced from family, friends, and other professionals.

Because incest is based on abuse of power, a demand for secrecy, betrayal of trust, and disregard for the child's needs, the potential for developing profound feelings of helplessness, shame, guilt, and confusion is significant. Therefore interventions for resolving incest trauma must focus on support to empower the victim to develop a sense of self-worth, mastery, competence, and control. For nursing interventions to be effective and empowering, they must involve collaborative effort rather than the traditional patriarchical relationship of the all-knowing professional and the unknowing client. Instead, the relationship becomes a partnership in which both nurse and client cooperate in establishing and achieving objectives to resolve the incest trauma. The nurse must support the survivor to believe and act on the belief that she is the ultimate expert on herself and therefore has the ability to make appropriate decisions for her health and well-being. In addition, the nurse and client identify and develop strategies that will build on client's strengths and increase her sense of control while supporting her to take action to change her life. The following discussion involves empowerment support interventions for nurses to use with adult survivors of incest.

The first step for the survivor is to disclose the incest to someone she trusts. The nurse, as someone to whom the survivor might choose to disclose, must support the survivor to discuss the incest whenever and however she chooses. Too often the nurse may be uncomfortable with the disclosure, and this discomfort is communicated nonverbally to the client and interpreted as a sign that she is not to discuss her incest experiences. It is crucial that the survivor feels she has permission to disclose.

In addition to supporting the survivor to control the discussion and details of the disclosure, the nurse must refrain from expressing horror, shock, or dismay since these reactions may add to the survivor's existing feelings of being alienated, different, and unworthy. Rather than asking repeated intrusive questions, basic therapeutic communication techniques are highly effective when supporting the survivor to disclose. This includes simply "being with" the survivor in silence if she chooses, reflecting on her comments, encouraging a discussion of her perception and expression of feelings, following her cues, offering to strategize with her, and considering behavioral options that might help her. In addition, the nurse can assist the survivor to recognize that self-disclosure is a strength and one that requires great courage.

Psychological support also is needed when the survivor experiences flashbacks and trances. At these times she needs reassurance about the reality of her world and the power she has to decrease these painful experiences. Survivors also need assistance in learning to constructively express feelings of anger without fear of losing control, to express needs without feeling frightened or guilty, and to come to terms with the failure of her mother or other family members to protect her. In addition, she needs encouragement to try new experiences and relationships and to set time aside for herself.

Many of the empowerment support strategies that the nurse uses with the survivor involve teaching. New behaviors such as those previously mentioned and corrections of myths and distortions about incest are taught. Because the myths and distortions have shaped and conditioned the survivor from childhood, corrective learning is a lengthy, on-going process for the survivor. Before the nurse can be helpful she must acquire the knowledge about what is myth versus fact.

The nurse will be called on repeatedly to reinforce that the adult is always the responsible party in childhood sexual abuse, but women who have derived pleasure and even sought the childhood sexual activity may become especially ashamed and guilt-ridden. Thus basic principles of normal physiology and child development are taught, and it is emphasized that children normally seek that which is rewarding, feels good, and adaptive. Understanding the concept of traumatic sexualization (Finkelhor, 1986) can be helpful to the survivor who is having difficulty forgiving herself. If the survivor has young children, she must learn how to protect her children from abuse and become more sensitive to their needs.

Weaknesses are realistically discussed and analyzed, and the survivor is recognized for her courage to address these areas. Many troublesome behaviors and habits that the survivor currently identifies are explained as being linked to the incest; although these behaviors may have been necessary and adaptive in earlier years, as an adult they no longer are helpful to the survivor and may even be destructive. Nevertheless, it is reinforced that these behaviors were creative self-care behaviors. Examples of such behaviors include hyperventilation, self-abuse, somatization, dissociation, denial, repression, and substance abuse.

New behaviors can be explored and practiced, and the survivor is able to choose strategies that she finds most appropriate for herself. Examples include assertive skills; anger control techniques; various forms of writing, such as journals, essays, and poetry; drawing; sculpting; imagery; relaxation techniques; and physical exercise. The survivor is also invited to take advantage of many books, journal articles, conferences, wilderness trips, and self-help organizations to support recovery.

The group format is generally recognized as the most helpful treatment modality for the incest survivor. Many survivors are taking advantage of self-help groups that are forming around the country. Some groups such as "Survivors of Incest Anonymous" are based on the Twelve-Step Model of Alcoholics Anonymous and have male, female, and coeducational groups. Other survivors find therapy groups fit their needs better, whereas some are unable to participate in groups until they work through basic issues with an individual therapist. Nurses who work with incest survivors must be knowledgeable about referrals for community resources and skilled therapists who offer individual and group referral for incest survivors.

SUMMARY

Reports of intrafamilial child sexual abuse are increasing. It is believed that most children and adults who have been abused do not disclose their experiences. Failure to disclose may have serious short- and long-term effects on the victim. Many aspects of the aftereffects may resemble the actual abuse. Because nurses work in a variety of settings, they have many opportunities to assist victims and their families. However, nurses cannot help these families unless they first understand their own experiences and feelings about sexual abuse. Nurses also must become knowledgeable about the dynamics of incestuous behavior and the appropriate interventions for all levels of prevention.

The ultimate nursing goal is the rehabilitation of all members of the incestuous family and reconstitution of the family, if possible. The concerned, caring, and knowledgeable nurse who is willing to listen and learn from family members and to establish collaborative goals with them, but take firm action to protect its weaker members when necessary, is a valuable resource for survivors and their families.

REFERENCES

Bagley, C., & Ramsey, R. (1985). Sexual abuse in childhood: Psychosocial outcomes and implications for social work practice. *Social Work Practice in Sexual Problems, 4*, 33-47.

Bender, L., & Blau, A. (1937). The reaction of children to sexual relations with adults. *American Journal of Orthopsychiatry, 7*. 500-518.

Briere, J., & Runtz, M. (1988). Postsexual trauma. In G. E. Wyatt & G. J. Powell (Eds.), *Lasting effects of child sexual abuse* (pp. 85-99). Newbury Park, CA: Sage.

Brown, B. E., & Garrison, C. J. (1990). Patterns of symptomatology of adult women incest survivors. *Western Journal of Nursing Research, 12*, 587-600.

Browne, A., & Finkelhor, D. (1986). Impact of child sexual abuse: A review of the literature. *Psychological Bulletin, 99*, 66-77.

Burgess, A. W., Groth, A. N.; Holstrom, L. L., & Sgroi, S. (1978) *Sexual assault of children and adolescents.* Lexington, MA: D.C. Heath.

Burgess, A., Hartman, C. R., Wolbert, W. W., & Grant, C. (1987). Child molestation: Assessing impact in multiple victims (part 1). *Archives of Psychiatric Nursing, 1*, 33-39.

Carmen, E., & Rieker, P. P. (1989). A psychosocial model of the victim-to-patient process. *Psychiatric Clinics of North America, 12*, 431-443.

Cormier, B., Kennedy, M., & Sangowicz, J. Psychodynamics of father-daughter incest. *Canadian Psychiatric Association Journal, 7*, 203-217.

Corwin, D. L. (1988). Early diagnosis of child sexual abuse. In G. E. Wyatt & G. J. Powell (Eds.), *Lasting effects of child sexual abuse* (pp. 251-269). Newbury Park, CA: Sage.

Courtois, C. (1988). *Healing the incest wound.* New York: W.W. Norton.

Craine, L. S., Henson, C. E., Colliver, J. A., & MacLean, D. (1988). Prevalence of history of sexual abuse among female psychiatric patients in a state hospital system. *Hospital and Community Psychiatry, 39*, 300-304.

Dolan, Y. M. (1991). *Resolving sexual abuse: Solution focused therapy and Eriksonian hypnosis.* New York: W.W. Norton.

Durfee, M. (1989). Prevention of child sexual abuse. *Psychiatric Clinics of North America, 12*, 445-453.

Figley, C. R. (1985). *Trauma and its wake: The study and treatment of post-traumatic stress disorder.* New York: Brunner/Mazel.

Finch, S. (1973). Adult seduction of the child: Effects on the child. *Medical Aspects of Human Sexuality, 7*, 170-185.

Finkelhor, D. (1979). *Sexually victimized children.* New York: Free Press.

Finkelhor, D. (1984). *Child sexual abuse: New theory and research.* New York: Free Press.

Finkelhor, D. (1986). *A sourcebook on child sexual abuse.* Beverly Hills: Sage.

Finkelhor, D., & Browne, A. (1986). The traumatic impact of child sexual abuse: A conceptualization. *American Journal of Orthopsychiatry, 55*, 530-541.

Fox, R. (1983). *The red lamp of incest: An enquiry into the origins of mind and society.* Notre Dame, IN: University of Notre Dame Press.

Fredrickson, R. M. (1991, October). Advanced clinical skills in the treatment of sexual abuse. Workshop held at Wayne State University, Detroit, MI.

Freund, K., McKnight, C. K., Langevin, R., & Cibiri, S. (1972). The female child as surrogate object. *Archives of Sexual Behavior, 2*, 119-133.

Freud, S. (1954). *The origins of psychoanalysis: Letters to Wilhelm Fliess, drafts and notes. 1887-1902.* New York: Basic Books.

Fromuth, M. E. (1986). The relationship of childhood sexual abuse with later psychological adjustment in a sample of college women. *Child Abuse and Neglect, 10,* 5-15.

Gelinas, D. J. (1983). The persisting negative effects of incest. *Psychiatry, 46,* 312-332.

Giaretto, H. (1989). Community-based treatment of the incest family. *Psychiatric Clinics of North America, 12,* 351-61.

Groth, N. A. (1978). Guidelines for assessment and management of the offender. In A. Burgess, N. A. Groth, L. Holstrom, & S. Sgroi (Eds.), *Sexual assault of children and adolescents* (pp. 25-42). Lexington, MA: Lexington Books.

Henderson, D. J. (1972). Incest: A synthesis of data. *Canadian Psychiatric Association Journal, 17,* 299-313.

Herman, J. (1981). *Father-daughter incest.* Cambridge, MA: Harvard University Press.

Herman, J., & Hirschman, L. (1977). Father-daughter incest. *Signs: Journal of Women in Culture and Society, 2,* 735-56.

Jaffe, A., Dynneson, L., & Ten Bensel, R. W. (1975). Sexual abuse of children. *American Journal of Diseases of Children, 129,* 689-92.

Jacobson, A., & Herald, C. (1990). The relevance of childhood sexual abuse to adult psychiatric inpatient care. *Hospital and Community Psychiatry, 41,* 154-158.

Janoff-Bulman, R. (1986). The aftermath of victimization: Rebuilding shattered assumptions. In C. Figley (Ed.), *Trauma and its wake: Study and treatment of post-traumatic stress disorder.* New York: Brunner/Mazel.

Justice, B., & Justice, R. (1979). *The broken taboo: Sex in the family.* New York: Human Sciences Press.

Kilpatrick, D. G., Amick-McMullan, A., Best, C. L., Burke, M. M., & Saunders, B. E. (1986). *Impact of child sexual abuse: Recent research findings.* Paper presented to the Fourth National Conference on the Sexual Victimization of Children, New Orleans.

Kluft, R. P. (1990). *Incest related syndromes of adult psychopathology.* Washington, DC: American Psychiatric Press.

Levi-Strauss, C. (1969). *The elementary structure of kinship.* Boston: Beacon Press.

Lustig, N., Dresser, J. W., Spellman, S. W., & Murray, T. B. (1966). Incest: A family group survival pattern. *Archives General Psychiatry, 14,* 31-40.

McCann, J. (November, 1990). How to perform a genital exam in the prepubertal girl. *Medical Aspects of Human Sexuality, 24,* 36-41.

Murram, D., & Gale, C. L. (September, 1990). Clinical assessment of the sexually abused girl. *Medical Aspects of Human Sexuality, 24,* 43-50.

Parker, H., & Parker, S. (1986). Father-daughter sexual abuse: An emerging perspective. *American Journal of Orthopsychiatry, 56,* 531-549.

Peters, S. (1988). Child sexual abuse and later psychological problems. In G. Wyatt & G. Powell (Eds.), *Lasting effects of child sexual abuse* (pp. 101-117). Beverly Hills: Sage.

Quinsey, V. L. (1977). The assessment and treatment of child molesters: A review. *Canadian Psychological Review, 18,* 204-220.

Rieker, P. P., & Carmen, E. (1986). The victim-to-patient process: The disconfirmation and transformation of abuse. *American Journal of Orthopsychiatry, 56,* 360-370.

Russell, D. (1986). *The secret trauma.* New York: Basic Books.

Rush, F. (1980). *The best kept secret: Sexual abuse of children.* Englewood Cliffs, NJ: Prentice Hall.

Sauzier, M. (1989). Disclosure of child sexual abuse. *Psychiatric Clinics of North America, 12,* 455-469.

Sedney, M. A., & Brooks, B. (1984). Factors associated with history of childhood sexual experience in a nonclinical female population. *Journal of the American Academy of Child Psychiatry, 23,* 215-218.

Seidner, M. A., & Calhoun, B. (1984, August). *Childhood sexual abuse: Factors related to differential adult adjustment.* Paper presented at the Second Annual National Family Violence Research Conference, Durham NH.

Shepher, J. (1983). *Incest: A biosocial view.* New York: Academic Press.

Summit, R. C. (1989). The centrality of victimization: Regaining the focal point of recovery for survivors of child sexual abuse. *Psychiatric Clinics of North America, 12,* 413-430.

Tufts' New England Medical Center, Division of Child Psychiatry (1984). *Sexually exploited children: Service and research project.* Final report for the Office of Juvenile Justice and Delinquency; Prevention. Washington, DC: U.S. Dept. of Justice.

Urbancic, J. C. (1992). The relationship between empowerment support, mental health self-care, incest trauma resolution, and subjective well-being. Unpublished doctoral dissertation, Detroit, Wayne State University.

Van der Kolk, B. A. (1987). *Psychological trauma.* Washington, DC: American Psychiatric Press.

Weinberg, S. K. (1955). *Incest behavior.* New York: Citadel Press.

Weiss, J., Roger, E., Darwin, M., & Dutton, C. (1955). A study of girl sex victims. *Psychiatric Quarterly, 29,* 1-27.

Whiting, B. B. (1963). *Six cultures: Studies of childrearing.* New York: John Wiley.

Wyatt, G. E. (1985). The sexual abuse of Afro-American and White-American women in childhood. *Child Abuse and Neglect, 9,* 507-519.

Wyatt, G. E., & Mickey, M. R. (1987). Ameliorating the effects of child sexual abuse: An exploratory study of support by parents and others. *Journal of Interpersonal Violence, 2,* 403-413.

Wyatt, G. E., & Powell, G. J. (1988). *Lasting effects of child sexual abuse.* Beverly Hills: Sage.

Domestic Violence and Pregnancy
Health effects and implications for nursing practice

Diane K. Bohn *and* Barbara Parker

Pregnancy is a time when friends, family, and health professionals expect a woman's partner to be particularly concerned about and attentive to her health and well-being. It is difficult to imagine that anyone, especially the father of the baby, would intentionally injure a pregnant woman, thereby jeopardizing her health and the health of the fetus. Reported numbers vary between one in twelve pregnant women (Campbell, Poland, & Waller, 1989; Helton, 1985, 1986, 1987; Helton & Snodgrass, 1987; Helton, McFarlane, & Anderson, 1987a) and one in every six women (McFarlane, Parker, Soeken, & Bullock, 1992) and one half of all battered women (Bowker, 1983; Brendtro & Bowker, 1989; Campbell, 1986; Fagen, Stewart, & Hanson, 1983; Flynn, 1977; Stacey & Schupe, 1983; Walker, 1984) are abused during pregnancy by their intimate male partners.

Trauma is the leading cause of maternal death during pregnancy (Bremer & Cassata, 1986). Follow-ing motor vehicle accidents, violent assault and suicide are the second and third leading causes of trauma death, respectively (Baker, 1982). Violence during pregnancy affects more women than hypertension, gestational diabetes, or almost any other serious antepartum complication.

The sequelae of abuse during pregnancy are not well elucidated, but may include miscarriage, preterm labor (PTL), preterm birth (PTB), low birth weight (LBW), fetal injury, and death. It is clear that violence during pregnancy poses a significant health risk for the woman and her fetus because of connections between abuse and substance use, inadequate prenatal care, as well as complicated obstetrical-gynecological histories. Abuse during pregnancy must be viewed by health professionals as a serious public health problem requiring the same vigilance currently afforded to gestational diabetes and preeclampsia.

The existence of a cause-and-effect relationship

between pregnancy and domestic violence has been questioned (Gelles, 1988). It appears, however, that in at least some cases pregnancy may precipitate the beginning or escalation of violence (Campbell, Poland, & Waller, 1989; Gayford, 1978; Helton et al., 1987a; Hillard, 1985; Hilberman & Munson, 1978; Walker, 1979). Several theories exist to explain this occurrence. In many cases, pregnancy may have little or no impact on the violence women suffer (Campbell & Oliver, 1992). They are beaten as the already existing violence continues, despite the pregnancy. For another group of women, pregnancy confers protection from ongoing violence (Fagen et al., 1983; Stacey & Schupe, 1983).

Nurses, nurse-midwives, and nurse practitioners play a crucial role in breaking the cycle of violence in the lives of the pregnant women they serve. Pregnancy may be the only time a battered woman has frequent, ongoing contact with someone capable of assisting her. The nursing process, as applied to survivors of domestic violence, includes identification, assessment, planning, intervention, and follow-up. The primary role of the nurse is that of advocate. Advocacy with the battered woman includes providing accurate information regarding abusive relationships, domestic abuse laws, resources and options, and providing ongoing emotional support regardless of the choices the battered woman makes.

PREVALENCE AND CHARACTER OF ABUSE DURING PREGNANCY

Abuse during pregnancy occurs in between 7% and 17% of all pregnancies (Amaro, Fried, Cobral, & Zuckerman, 1990; Campbell et al., 1989; Helton, 1985, 1987; Helton & Snodgrass, 1987; Helton et al., 1987a; McFarlane et al., 1992) and among approximately half of all battered women (Bowker, 1983; Brendtro & Bowker, 1989; Campbell, 1986; Fagen et al., 1983; Flynn, 1977; Stacey & Schupe, 1983; Stewart & Campbell, 1989). An additional 11% to 23% of pregnant women report a history of abuse before pregnancy (Campbell et al., 1989; Helton et al., 1987a; Hillard, 1985) and may also be at risk of violence during pregnancy.

Pregnancy or the arrival of the first child may precipitate the first episode of violence in some relationships (Gayford, 1978; Hillard, 1985). More often, the violence began before pregnancy (Helton et al., 1987a). The character of the violence may change during pregnancy, either increasing or decreasing in frequency and severity (Campbell et al., 1989; Gayford, 1978; Helton et al., 1987a; Hilberman & Munson, 1978; Hillard, 1985; Walker, 1979). Women who experience decreased or no violence during pregnancy may try to stay pregnant to avoid the abuse (Hilberman & Munson, 1978).

The abdomen becomes a more frequent site of trauma during pregnancy (Hilberman & Munson, 1978; Stark, Flitcraft, & Frazier, 1979). The breasts and genitals are also commonly attacked (Walker, 1979). Most abused pregnant women (35% to 45%) report the head or face as the most common target (Berenson, Stiglich, Wilkinson, & Anderson, 1991; McFarlane et al., 1992). Pregnant battered women are more likely to have multiple trauma sites than nonpregnant battered women (Helton & Snodgrass, 1987).

HEALTH EFFECTS OF ABUSE DURING PREGNANCY

The negative health effects of abuse during pregnancy may be direct or trauma related. Perhaps more frequently alterations in health are indirect abuse effects, resulting from stress, substance use, suicide attempts, depression, inadequate prenatal care, and complicated obstetrical and gynecological histories.

Low Birth Weight/Preterm Birth

Domestic abuse during pregnancy may be a factor in the cause of LBW and PTB. In one study (Bullock & McFarlane, 1989), significantly increased rates of LBW were found among battered women (12%) when compared with nonbattered women (6.6%). Even when seven other contributors to LBW (race, smoking, alcohol consumption, prenatal care, prior abortions, maternal complications, specific hospital) were included in the analysis, a significant abuse effect remained. Bullock and McFarlane also found a significantly increased rate of PTB (less than 37 weeks' gestation) among abused women from private hospitals (20%) when compared with those who were not abused (6.9%).

Two other studies also found decreased birth weight and gestational age among abuse survivors (Amaro et al., 1990; Campbell et al., 1989). In one study no relationship between abuse and PTB was found (Hillard, 1985).

The direct role of intentional abdominal trauma in precipitating PTB and LBW has not been established. Two abuse-focused studies provide anecdotal evidence of preterm labor (Hillard, 1985) and PTB (Hilberman & Munson, 1978) precipitated by a violent assault. Literature on unintentional trauma during pregnancy, such as that incurred in a motor vehicle accident, clearly supports abdominal trauma as a cause of PTL (Dees & Fuller, 1989; Stewart, Harding, & Davies, 1980).

Prenatal stress has been implicated in the cause of PTB (Newton, Webster, Binu, Maskrey, & Phillips, 1979) and LBW (Newton & Hunt, 1984). Certainly, women involved in relationships in which ongoing violence is present have stressful lives.

Because many factors may act or interact to influence birth weight, PTL, and PTB (National Institute of Medicine, 1985; Huddleston, 1982), it is difficult to determine the role of any one factor. However, abuse, acting directly or indirectly, should be considered in all cases of PTL, PTB, and LBW, especially when these pregnancy complications are not adequately explained by the presence of other causative factors.

Reproductive History

Men who abuse pregnant women may, through violence or coercion, exert control over the reproductive functioning of their partners. Such control may include unwanted pregnancies, not allowing or forcing the woman to have an abortion, and miscarriage resulting from a violent attack.

Some battered women report one or more pregnancies resulting from forced sexual encounters (Campbell & Alford, 1989) or their partner's refusal to practice birth control. This may account, in part, for the increased gravidity of battered versus nonbattered women noted in some studies (Campbell et al., 1989; Stark et al., 1981; Hillard, 1985). Despite increased gravidity, battered women have approximately the same number of living children as nonbattered women. This may be explained by their increased rates of abortions and miscarriages (Stark et al., 1981).

Battered women are more likely than nonbattered women to have a history of one or more elective abortions (Amaro et al., 1990; Stark et al., 1981). Abortion may be chosen by the battered woman if she believes pregnancy or the stress it creates may precipitate increased violence from her partner. She may choose abortion because she is uncertain about the future of the relationship with her partner. In one study a significantly increased number of pregnant women currently in an abusive relationship considered abortion (34%) when compared with nonabused controls (21%) (Hillard, 1985).

In some cases the abuser does not allow his partner to obtain an abortion, essentially forcing her to remain pregnant against her wishes. Alternately, a woman may be coerced into terminating a pregnancy her partner views as unwanted. Women who obtain abortions because of relationship problems are more likely to delay their abortions until the second trimester, hoping that the relationship will change (Torres & Forrest, 1988).

Battered women are also more likely than nonbattered women to have obstetrical histories complicated by one or more miscarriages (Stark et al., 1981). Although the causal role of a specific trauma event in any miscarriage is difficult to determine (Baker, 1982), there is much anecdotal evidence in the literature that implicates abuse in the cause of "spontaneous" abortion (Hilberman & Munson, 1978; Hillard, 1985; Drake, 1982). In one study of 1,000 survivors of domestic abuse, 9% of the women reported miscarriages as a result of abuse (Brendtro & Bowker 1989). In another study one woman reported being forced to drink bleach to cause an abortion (Stacey & Schupe, 1983).

In addition to the psychological and emotional damage caused by abuse-related abortions and miscarriages, these events pose both immediate and long-term health risks for the woman. Immediate risks include excessive blood loss, cervical or uterine trauma, infection, and disseminated intravascular coagulation (Hatcher et al., 1986; Whitley, 1985). Long-term risks, especially of repeated or second-trimester abortions, include cervical incompetence, PTB, LBW, and placental problems in subsequent pregnancies (Berendes, 1977; Creasy & Heron, 1981; Gonik & Creasy, 1986; Papiernik, 1984; Whitley, 1985). Women with forced pregnancies are at risk of postpartum depression and parenting difficulties.

Prenatal Care

Early and consistent prenatal care allows ongoing assessment of maternal and fetal well-being, detection of actual or potential problems, and interventions to prevent, modify, or correct pregnancy complications. Absent or inadequate prenatal care may result in suboptimal management of preexisting or pregnancy-related conditions, such as hypertension, diabetes, and infections, that could have a negative effect on pregnancy outcomes. Inadequate or absent prenatal care has also been associated with LBW and PTB (National Institute of Medicine, 1985; Placek, 1977; Scupholme, Robertson, & Kamons, 1991).

Battered women, whose pregnancies may already be at risk because of trauma or substance use, could benefit from adequate care. However, abuse survivors often do not receive adequate care (Campbell et al., 1989). They may delay entry into care and may miss scheduled appointments. In a recent study of 691 black, white, and Hispanic women, there was a statistically significant difference between abused and nonabused women's entry into prenatal care; 21% of abused women began prenatal care during the third trimester compared with 11% of nonabused women ($\chi^2 = 11.83$, df 2, p < 0.001). There were also major differences by ethnicity; black and Hispanic abused women were more likely to enter prenatal care in the third trimester compared with black and Hispanic nonabused women. There was no difference in abuse status and entry into prenatal care for white women. (McFarlane et al., 1972).

Conflicts with the father of the baby are frequently cited as one reason for delayed care among women entering prenatal care in the last month of pregnancy (Young, McMann, Bowman, & Thompson, 1989). In some cases women may delay care as they try to decide whether to continue or terminate the pregnancy. Ambivalence and denial may also play a role. In other cases their partner may prevent them from seeking care. Battered women who use or abuse substances during pregnancy may avoid prenatal care because of shame or fear of repercussions.

Women may miss appointments because their abuser will not let them go out or because he denies them access to transportation. The battered woman or her partner may decide she should miss an appointment if trauma injuries are evident. The woman may feel ashamed or guilty, or fear she could lose her children if the abuse becomes known.

Substance Use or Abuse

For many women substance use may be a way of self-medicating the pain of involvement in an abusive relationship. In a review of women's medical records, significantly increased rates of drug and alcohol use have been noted among battered women, most often beginning after the first recorded incident of abuse (Stark et al., 1979). Increased rates of substance use during pregnancy has also been noted among abuse survivors (Amaro et al., 1990; Bullock & McFarlane, 1989; Campbell et al., 1989; Hillard, 1985).

Significantly increased rates of tobacco use during pregnancy have been found among battered women compared with nonbattered women (Bullock & McFarlane, 1989; Hillard, 1985). Maternal smoking during pregnancy has been associated with LBW, PTB, intrauterine fetal demise (IUFD), premature rupture of the membranes (PROM), placenta previa and abruptio placentae, and other maternal-fetal/infant complications (Fanaroff & Martin, 1987; Meyer, 1977).

Increased rates of drug use during pregnancy among abuse survivors has also been reported (Amaro et al., 1990; Campbell et al., 1989; Hillard, 1985). Negative fetal/infant effects of maternal drug use may include LBW, PTB, congenital malformation, intrauterine growth retardation, IUFD, asphyxia, hyaline membrane disorders, abnormal behavior and state control, mental retardation, and withdrawal symptoms (Bry, 1983; Chasnoff, Burns, Burns, & Schnoll, 1986). Cocaine use may cause additional problems, including cerebral infarction and increased risk for sudden infant death syndrome (Chasnoff, 1987; Chasnoff, Bussey, Savich, & Stack, 1986; Schneider & Chasnoff, 1987). Maternal problems related to drug use during pregnancy may include miscarriage, abruptio placentae, delayed or absent prenatal care, anemia, sexually transmitted and other infectious diseases, and parenting problems (Bry, 1983; Chasnoff, 1987; Schneider & Chasnoff, 1987).

Studies that examined alcohol use during pregnancy among battered women have yielded conflicting results. Two studies found increased usage (Amaro et al., 1990; Hillard, 1985), whereas two others report decreased usage (Bullock & McFarlane, 1989; Campbell et al., 1989). Alcohol consumption during pregnancy, especially if chronic or heavy, is associated with numerous fetal/infant problems. These may include growth and mental retardation, LBW, microcephaly and behavioral, facial, limb, cardiac, genital, and neurological abnormalities (Bry, 1983; Fanaroff & Martin, 1987).

Depression and Suicidal Gestures

It is not surprising that depression and suicidal gestures are common among battered women (Amaro et al., 1990; Gayford, 1978; Hilberman & Munson, 1978; Hillard, 1985; Stark et al., 1979; Stark et al., 1981), who often feel trapped in a never-ending cycle of violence. During pregnancy depression could result in suboptimal self-care and difficulty mastering the developmental tasks of pregnancy, including bonding with the infant, and may contribute to postpartum depression. Suicidal gestures represent potential risks for women, their fetuses, and pregnancy outcomes.

In one study 84% of women abused during pregnancy reported being depressed in the immediate postpartum period (Campbell et al., 1989). Another study found that among women who attempt suicide, battered women are four times more likely to be pregnant at the time of the suicide attempt than nonbattered women (Stark et al., 1981). Depression and suicidal gestures among pregnant battered women have not been addressed elsewhere in the literature. Certainly, it may be assumed that near-lethal suicidal gestures or those that involve toxic substances or asphyxia could pose both short- and long-term health risks for women and their fetuses/infants. Depression could impair the woman's ability to parent.

Sexual Assault

Sexual assault is part of the pattern of domestic violence in many, if not most, abusive relationships (Bowker, 1983; Brendtro & Bowker, 1989; Campbell, 1986; Stacey & Schupe, 1983). Sexual assault includes rape as well as hitting, kicking, or mutilation of the breasts and genitals (Bowker, 1983; Walker, 1979). Other forms of sexual abuse reported by battered women include being forced into homosexual sex; sex with animals; prostitution; public exposure; being hit, kicked, or burned during sex; and being vaginally or rectally raped with objects (Campbell & Alford, 1989).

The prevalence and effects of sexual assault during pregnancy are not well documented. Miscarriages and stillbirths are among the problems reported by battered women who were sexually assaulted by their partners during pregnancy (Campbell & Alford, 1989). Many battered women state they were coerced into sex immediately after childbirth (Campbell & Alford, 1989; Domestic Abuse Intervention Project, 1990). One woman reported needing a dilatation and curettage because she was forced to have intercourse the day after delivery (Campbell & Alford, 1989).

There are additional potential problems that could result from sexual assault during the antepartum or immediate postpartum periods. Mutilation or blows to the breasts and genitals could result in complicated deliveries or breast-feeding problems. Forced sexual encounters in the antepartum period could conceivably stimulate PTL. Sexual intercourse in the immediate postpartum period could result in endometritis or disrupt the healing of episiotomies or lacerations.

Women with a history of sexual assault often find vaginal examinations to be painful and traumatic, requiring extreme patience and gentleness by the examiner. Women who have been battered, sexually assaulted, or both may also experience "fetal retention syndrome," in which they have difficulty allowing labor and birth to occur (Diegmann, 1991).

Sexually Transmitted Diseases

Many battered women report contracting sexually transmitted diseases (STDs) from their partners. Battered women are at increased risk of STDs because of the intermittent nature of many abusive relationships, as well as sexual assaults that occur after the relationship has been terminated. In addition, having multiple sexual partners is often part of the pattern of abuse exhibited by male batterers. Women who are forced by their partner to have sex with others are also at increased risk of STDs.

In one study of battered women, 6.5% reported STDs secondary to sexual abuse by their partner (Campbell & Alford, 1989). In another study women who had been sexually or physically assaulted just before or during pregnancy were more than twice as likely as nonvictimized women to have a history of STDs. Most of the women in this study were assumed to have been assaulted by their partners (Amaro et al., 1990).

In clinical practice the diagnosis of an STD during pregnancy is so frequently associated with emotional, physical abuse, or both that the issue should always be addressed. Women with histories of multiple, and especially recurrent, STDs are also frequently noted to have histories of abuse. Men who refuse treatment for an STD or who prevent their partner from being treated are almost always otherwise abusive.

STDs have serious health implications for pregnant women. Premature, preterm rupture of the membranes (PPROM) and subsequent PTB and chorioamnionitis may result from cervical colonization with sexually transmitted organisms such as *Chlamydia trachomatis* or *Neisseria gonorrhoeae* (Alger & Pupkin, 1986; Miller & Pastorek, 1986). The presence of an STD in the immediate postpartum period may result in endometritis and other upper genital and peritoneal infections (Varney, 1987). Primary *Herpes simplex* infection during pregnancy or active lesions at the time of delivery may have serious and often fatal consequences for the infant or result in cesarean birth. A history of STDs also places a woman at increased risk of ectopic pregnancy and infertility.

Other Health Effects

Several other health effects of abuse during pregnancy have appeared in the literature as anecdotal or case study reports. Reported health effects include fetal bruising, intraventricular hemorrhage, and neonatal death (Morey, Bigleiter, & Harris, 1981), newborn gastric ulceration and hemorrhage (Pugh, Newton, & Piercy, 1979), tibial deformity, hip dislocation, and scleral opacities (Hillard, 1985), and stillbirth (Campbell & Alford, 1989).

Blunt abdominal trauma during pregnancy can cause a variety of pregnancy complications. Reports addressing trauma during pregnancy rarely include references to intentional injuries, focusing instead on unintentional injuries, such as those caused by motor vehicle accidents. However, a domestic assault that includes a forcible kick, punch, or blow with an object to the abdomen, or the woman being pushed down stairs or into an object, could result in similar injuries. The effects of blunt abdominal trauma noted in the literature include fetal closed head injury, cardiac contusion, and broken bones including ribs, clavicle, and skull; placental damage or abruptio placentae; uterine perforation, laceration, rupture or evulsion; rupture of the bladder; amniotic fluid embolus; hemorrhage; disseminated intravascular coagulation, and PROM (Dees & Fuller, 1989; Patterson, 1984; Stauffer, 1986; Stewart, Harding, & Davies, 1980).

Bullet wounds are the most frequent cause of penetrating injury during pregnancy and often result in life-threatening damage to the woman and fetus (Stauffer, 1986). In many instances the gun is intentionally fired by the woman's partner.

Although motor vehicle accidents remain the leading cause of trauma injuries during pregnancy (Baker, 1982), it must be remembered that some abuse survivors explain their assault injuries by stating they were involved in an accident. Particularly when women delay treatment for such injuries, or when law enforcement or emergency medical personnel were not involved, the woman should be questioned about possible abuse.

The adverse health effects of abuse are not confined to those caused by trauma. Some abusers severely restrict their partner's caloric intake during pregnancy, which could result in intrauterine growth retardation and other nutrition-related problems. One woman's partner allowed her to consume only one meal a day; she was otherwise restricted to soda crackers and water. Other women may restrict their own intake to minimize abusive remarks about their weight or size. Eating disorders or poor weight gain during pregnancy should prompt abuse evaluation.

THEORIES: WHY IS THERE ABUSE DURING PREGNANCY?

To understand why some men choose to abuse their pregnant partners, this question must be posed to the abusers themselves. To date, such research has not been attempted. Few abusers have the degree of insight and willingness to discuss their violent behavior necessary to make an honest appraisal of their motives. Explanations of abuse during pregnancy are therefore derived from the subjective reports of abuse survivors and the educated speculation of researchers. The resulting theories vary widely.

The most commonly cited reason for abuse during pregnancy is jealousy. The abuser may view the fetus as a competitor for the woman's attention, or as an intruder in their relationship (Bry, 1977; Campbell, 1986; Stacey & Schupe, 1983; Walker, 1979). The man's desire for power and control over the woman may be magnified by pregnancy as the woman's attention is focused on her own health and on the developing fetus (Helton, 1985). He may

resent the woman's increased contact with friends, family, and health care providers during pregnancy (Helton & Snodgrass, 1987). Many women report the abuser's response to the pregnancy is to deny paternity and to accuse her of infidelity (Parker, 1991). In such cases the abuse may reflect sexual jealousy, a hallmark of abusive men.

Stress is another commonly cited reason for abuse during pregnancy. The stress may derive from an unwanted or unplanned pregnancy (Gelles, 1975; Roy, 1977) or marriage because of pregnancy (Bowker, 1983; Gelles, 1975). Increased gravidity may be a factor in abuse during pregnancy (Bowker, 1983; Stark et al., 1981), perhaps because yet another child is unwanted or is perceived as a financial burden. Stress and conflict may also arise from discordance between the couple's feelings regarding the pregnancy (Hillard, 1985).

Blows directed at the abdomen of a pregnant woman may represent a form of prenatal child abuse (Campbell, 1986; Gelles, 1975; Stacey & Schupe, 1983; Walker, 1979). The abuse may be a conscious or unconscious attempt to terminate the pregnancy or kill the fetus (Gelles, 1974, 1975). A number of women in one study reported abdominal beatings they believe were deliberate attempts to induce abortion because the abuser did not want the child to be born (Brendtro & Bowker, 1989).

Men who are the most violent may be more likely to abuse their partners during pregnancy. Battering during pregnancy has been correlated with increased severity and frequency of abuse (Bowker, 1983; Fagen et al., 1983) and the abuser being violent outside the home (Fagen et al., 1983). Gelles (1988) found rates of minor, severe, and overall violence to be increased in homes where the woman was pregnant, but these differences were not significant.

Other explanations for battering during pregnancy have been postulated. Gelles (1975) suggested sexual frustration might be a factor, with one or both partners experiencing decreased sexual desire during pregnancy. Gelles also states biochemical changes in the woman, causing her to be more irritable and critical and to pick on her partner, might be contributing factors. This explanation erroneously places responsibility for the man's violence on the woman.

In a more recent study Gelles (1988) disputes any relationship between abuse and pregnancy. He states the proposed relationship is spurious—a methodological artifact, resulting from an age, rather than a pregnancy effect. He believes that because abuse is most commonly experienced during a woman's childbearing years, an erroneous perception has resulted that pregnancy and abuse are related. This claim that no relationship exists has been disavowed by many experts in the area of domestic violence during pregnancy.

Although each of the foregoing explanations of abuse during pregnancy may apply in any single abuse situation, none solely explains all cases of abuse during pregnancy. In a recent study Campbell and Oliver (1992) questioned women about their perceptions of why the abuse occurred. Their replies varied; 20% reported the abuse was directed toward the baby. Another 20% believed that the abuse was pregnancy related, resulting from her feeling ill or the stress of another child. These women thought the violence was directed at them, rather than at the baby. Another group of women cited jealousy as a factor. In the majority of cases, however, abuse during pregnancy was simply the continuation of ongoing violence and was unrelated to the pregnancy itself. In another study Helton et al., (1987a) found abuse before pregnancy to be the best predictor of abuse during pregnancy, occurring in 87.5% of all cases.

Physical abuse generally does not begin in a relationship until some level of commitment exists. In some cases, that commitment is symbolized by marriage. Brendtro and Bowker (1989) reported that violence began only after marriage for nearly three fourths of the women in their study. Pregnancy may also be perceived as a symbol of real or imagined commitment. As with marriage, pregnancy may precipitate abuse simply because the abuser believes he can abuse his partner with impunity, and that the woman will not leave him because of the violence.

Abuse generally increases in severity and frequency over time (Dobash & Dobash, 1979). It is

possible that some men who do not abuse their partners during a single pregnancy have not yet established a pattern of violence, and are therefore more easily held by societal condemnation of violence toward pregnant women. Over time, as the violence becomes a more integral part of the relationship, pregnancy may no longer act as a deterrent. This may, in part, explain the increased rates of violence noted among women of greater parity (Bowker, 1983; Stark et al., 1981).

Some battered women are never beaten or experience decreased abuse when they are pregnant. The possibility that cultural orientation may influence abuse during pregnancy is currently being examined in two large national studies. Research to clarify which factors best predict and have a protective effect on abuse during pregnancy is needed.

Ultimately, it is the abuser's desire for power and control, and his belief that violence and coercion are legitimate means to achieve these ends, that prompt him to physically, sexually, or emotionally abuse his partner (DAIP, 1990). This is true both during and outside of pregnancy. It is currently unclear how pregnancy affects the abuser's use of physical force to maintain his position of control. In some cases there may be no relationship between pregnancy and abuse. How or why pregnancy affects violence against women in other situations may vary among and within abusive relationships. Further theory development to address these variations is needed.

Racial/Cultural Influences

Abuse crosses all racial boundaries. Racial and race by class differences in the prevalence, severity, and frequency of domestic abuse have been examined in previous research with inconsistent findings (Lockhart, 1987).

Racial differences in abuse during pregnancy have also been inconsistent among studies. In their study of women who experienced physical or sexual assaults just before or during pregnancy, Amaro et al. (1990) found victims were more likely to be white than North American black, and more likely to be North American black than other black or Hispanic. Similarly, two recent studies of black, white and

Hispanic women found higher rates of violence in the white populations. Berenson, Stiglich, Wilkinson, and Anderson (1991) found the prevalence of reported physical abuse was 3.5 times higher among white non-Hispanic women and 1.6 times higher than among black women. McFarlane et al. (in press) found more frequent and severe abuse during pregnancy, with almost half (48%) of abused white women reporting punches, kicks, cuts, contusions, burns, and head and internal injuries compared with 14% of Hispanic women and 29% of black women.

Helton et al. (Helton, McFarlane, & Anderson, 1987a, 1987b; Helton & Snodgrass, 1987) examined racial differences in rates of abuse and abuse during pregnancy among black, Latino, white, and other-grouped women. They concluded there were no racial differences. However, a reanalysis of their data reveals otherwise. Among blacks, whites, and others, from 40% to 50% of battered women report abuse during pregnancy. These figures are consistent with prevalence rates of abuse during pregnancy among battered women in previous research. Among Latino women, however, only 26% of battered women in this study were battered during pregnancy. Although this may reflect a greater reluctance to report abuse during pregnancy among Latino women, it may also reflect a cultural variation in the acceptance or tolerance of intentionally harming pregnant women.

IMPLICATIONS FOR NURSING PRACTICE

The goal of nursing care is to promote health. Using a holistic perspective, this includes promoting physical, emotional, and psychosocial health. Nurses, nurse-midwives, and nurse practitioners who provide care to pregnant women are aware that far more than physical well-being must be attended to to ensure an optimal pregnancy outcome. Because domestic violence impacts the lives and health of so many pregnant women, identification and assessment of and intervention with women experiencing abuse must become a routine part of prenatal care.

Before nurses can effectively assist battered women, they must examine their own beliefs and

biases. Like many people in the nonmedical community, there are nurses who believe that domestic violence is a private affair to be managed within families, and that in some instances violence against women may be justified or excused. For nurses to become effective agents in ending the cycle of violence in women's lives, they must accept two basic premises. The first premise is that domestic violence is a serious public health problem, rather than a private problem, that therefore falls within the purview of nursing. The second premise is that no woman, under any circumstances, deserves to be physically, sexually, or emotionally abused.

In addition to accepting these premises, nurses must become educated regarding the causes, characteristics, and health effects of abuse. Domestic violence, like any other specialty area or condition confronted by nurses, must be thoroughly understood before effective intervention can occur.

The nurse's tasks when dealing with battered women are to (1) identify the presence of abuse, (2) assess the nature, severity, and potential lethality of the abuse, and the impact it has had on the woman's health, (3) plan intervention strategies, (4) intervene through referrals, information sharing, and support, and (5) follow up or assess the effectiveness of interventions. Throughout the nursing process, the primary role of the nurse is that of advocate. Advocacy includes assisting the battered woman to make informed decisions by information sharing and providing continued support, regardless of the decisions and choices that are made.

Nurses often find their greatest rewards in the achievement of desired intervention outcomes. For this reason, nurses may try to "fix" things for battered women by giving advice and making elaborate arrangements to help them leave their abusers. It must be remembered that it is the abuse survivor's, not the nurses', choices and desires that must be followed. It can be very difficult and frustrating for nurses to understand and support the decisions of battered women when such decisions are contrary to their own beliefs. It is disheartening to witness the continued pain of battered women who choose to stay in abusive relationships. Effective advocacy requires understanding the difficulties involved in terminating any relationship and the knowledge that most women do eventually find a way to end the violence in their lives.

Identification

There are three methods that are useful in identifying battered women in a medical setting: chart reviews, direct questioning, and observing interaction between the woman and her partner. Chart reviews may only provide clues to past abuse (see the box that follows). Observation of the couple will probably reveal only emotional abuse. These methods must not be used to replace, but rather, should be used in conjunction with direct questioning.

There are a number of "red flag" items that may be encountered in a woman's medical record that strongly suggest abuse. These are listed in the box. In addition, references to difficulty with vaginal ex-

---

Identifying Battered Women

Chart review

- Assault, regardless of the assailant's stated identity
- Injuries inflicted by weapons
- Injuries consistent with assault that are inadequately explained
- Multiple medical visits for injuries or anxiety symptoms
- Injury or assault during pregnancy
- History of depression, drug use, or suicide attempts
- Sex-specific or disfiguring injuries, such as to the face, breasts, or genitals
- Eating disorders
- Unexplained somatic symptoms, such as back, chest, or pelvic pain, or choking sensations
- Tranquilizer or sedative use

Obstetrical/gynecological history

- Spontaneous/elective abortions
- STDs
- Sexual assault
- Late or inadequate prenatal care
- Substance use during pregnancy
- PTL or PTB
- LBW
- Unexplained fetal injuries, present at birth
- Unexplained IUFD
- Abruptio placentae
- Suicide attempts during pregnancy
- Poor weight gain during pregnancy
- Trauma injuries during pregnancy

Observations during clinic visits

- Partner is conspicuously unwilling to leave the woman's side
- Partner speaks for the woman or belittles what she says
- Partner makes derogatory comments about the woman's appearance or behavior
- Partner is oversolicitous with care providers
- Partner is emotionally absent or out of tune with the woman
- Woman is obviously afraid of her partner

aminations are frequently found in the charts of women with histories of child or adult sexual assault.

Observations of the woman and her partner during clinic visits, in childbirth classes, and during hospital stays for pregnancy complications or labor and delivery may also provide clues to the presence of abuse. Behaviors that suggest abuse are listed in the box.

Indicators of possible abuse in the woman's chart, or those noted while observing interaction between the woman and her partner, should prompt direct questions about abuse. The woman should be told what stimulated the question and why, for example, a history of preterm birth might be connected with abuse. In situations when the woman's partner is always present, it may be necessary to devise an excuse to reach her alone or to follow her into the bathroom to privately question her about abuse.

Certainly, not all survivors of domestic abuse have medical histories or partners who behave so that nurses have reason to suspect abuse. For this reason, *all* women must be assessed for abuse. This must be done by direct questioning since the majority of women will not identify themselves as abuse survivors on self-completion history forms (McFarlane, 1991). Abuse assessment should not be limited to one question in a list of previous medical conditions. Assessment of abuse should be conducted separately. Multiple abuse-focused questions should be asked because women often deny abuse with the first question, then answer positively to subsequent questions (Helton, 1985, 1987).

Clinical assessment for abuse, however, can be accomplished by a few abuse-focused questions asked in privacy and with concern for the woman. McFarlane et al. (1992) found that questions 2, 3, and 4 from the Abuse Assessment Screen described in Chapter 9 on p. 252 clearly delineated between abused and nonabused women as defined by much longer instruments developed for research (The Conflicts Tactics Scale and the Index of Spouse Abuse).

The Abuse Assessment Screen developed by the Nursing Research Consortium on Violence and Abuse (see Figure 9–1) may be useful for assessing abuse by a current partner. In obstetrical-gynecological settings, women should also be asked if they have ever been forced into sexual activities, either as a child or as an adult. Unresolved sexual assault experiences may result in women having difficulty with pelvic examinations, intercourse, and childbearing.

Some battered women may deny abuse during an initial assessment because of guilt, denial, shame, and the belief that the abuse is somehow her fault (Parker & McFarlane, 1991). Later in the woman's pregnancy, after rapport has been established with care providers, she may be more willing to reveal past or current abuse. Nurses must maintain an index of suspicion and ask additional abuse-focused questions after women's statements concerning relationship problems, or when evidence of trauma, drug use, etc. is present.

Assessment

After a woman has been identified as a survivor of domestic abuse, further assessment is needed. Assessment of the history and course of the abuse should include how long it has been occurring, the severity and frequency of the abuse, injuries and other health problems the woman believes have resulted from the abuse, and whether the abuse is escalating. When abuse episodes and resulting injuries are examined in chronological order, increasing severity and frequency may be noted.

Nonphysical and sexual abuse must also be explored. Most abusers use a number of nonviolent tactics to exert power and maintain control of the woman's thoughts, feelings, and actions. Power and control tactics include using intimidating words or gestures; abusing emotionally; isolating the woman from others; minimizing, denying, and blaming the woman for the abuse; using children as leverage; using male privilege, such as acting like the "master of the castle"; using economic abuse such as controlling her access to money; and using coercion and threats (DAIP, 1990). Knowledge of the degree of control the abuser exerts in the woman's life is useful in assessing the woman's current danger of harm and is also important when planning intervention strategies.

Assessment of the woman's current danger of serious injury or death is crucial. The Danger Assessment (see Figure 9–2) contains items believed to increase a woman's risk of homicide (Campbell, 1986). Questioning women about their perceptions of imminent danger is also useful because most abuse survivors are "tuned in" to their immediate risk of harm.

When assessing past abuse, women should be asked what resources (police, shelters, clergy, family, etc.) they have used and how helpful these individuals or organizations have been. She should be questioned regarding the use of the court system and protective orders.

All assessments must be thoroughly documented. This can be a time-consuming process, but may be helpful to the woman in future legal proceedings, as well as providing necessary communication for other health care providers involved in the woman's care. Details should be documented in the woman's own words as much as possible.

Men who abuse their partners often also abuse their children (Dobash & Dobash, 1979; Stacey & Schupe, 1983; Walker, 1979). Nurses are mandated by law to report knowledge or suspicion of child abuse to state child protection organizations. It is important for the woman to be informed of this before she reveals any information regarding abuse of her children. In the current legal system, a woman may be penalized for remaining in a relationship that poses a threat to her children. If the woman chooses to share information regarding child abuse, inform her that you must call the appropriate authorities. Encourage her to report the abuse herself because this may weigh in her favor if custody issues result.

Planning

Planning intervention strategies with survivors of domestic abuse consists of determining available options and the benefits and risks of each option. Two factors are important in this phase of the nursing process: (1) What does the woman want to

do or have happen; and (2) What is her level of current danger?

Battered women essentially have three options: (1) stay with the abuser, (2) leave for a safe place, or (3) have the abuser removed from the place of residence. In some cases, only the first two options are available. The role of the nurse in the planning phase of the nursing process is to provide the woman with the information necessary to make informed decisions.

For nurses to provide accurate information to battered women, they must become familiar with state laws concerning domestic violence, sexual assault, and protective orders, as well as what domestic violence resources are available in their community (Bohn, 1990; Parker & McFarlane, 1991). Representatives from battered women's shelters are willing to provide such education personally and often also have written material available. Although laws vary from state to state, domestic violence is illegal nationwide and can be (although it is not always) prosecuted in the same way as assault by a stranger. Many battered women are not aware of this. Marital rape is illegal in most states (Campbell & Alford, 1989), and rape outside of marriage is illegal in all.

Orders for protection have replaced unenforceable peace bonds in many states. Protective orders are court ordered directives stating that the abuser must not harass, threaten, or harm the woman (and other household members), and may also provide for temporary custody of the children as well as forcing the abuser to vacate the home or apartment. In some states, protective orders are issued in civil court, separate from any criminal charges. In other states, a woman must pursue assault charges to obtain a protective order.

Battered women's agencies and, in some cities, court advocacy services for domestic violence survivors, provide advocacy services for women who wish to pursue legal options or obtain protective orders. They will assist the woman with the necessary paperwork and will often appear in court with her.

In many cases, pressing assault charges or obtaining protective orders can be a powerful deterrent to future violence. Most often, unless the woman's partner is on probation or has had previous charges against him, he will only spend a few hours or one night in jail if arrested on assault charges. If convicted, his sentence for a first offense is generally a fine and probation. In some states, assault convictions or protective orders may force the abuser to obtain chemical dependency or male batterer's counseling sessions. Women who are aware of these options are more likely to pursue legal remedies, knowing their partner may be helped to deal with his problems.

Domestic violence organizations provide group and individual counseling for battered women and their children, and may provide counseling or educational sessions for male batterers. Battered women's shelters also provide women and children with counseling and abuse education. Shelters provide safe lodging, clothing, food, and health care access, as well as information concerning legal, economic, financial, employment, educational, and housing assistance.

The foregoing information should be provided to all battered women. Although a woman may not wish to use domestic violence services or pursue legal options at the present time, she may wish to do so in the future. Additional information regarding each of her three options should be provided.

Many if not most battered women prefer the option of staying in their current relationship if the violence would end. However, opting to stay with the abuser generally means the violence will not only continue, but will likely worsen with time. In rare cases when the abuse is infrequent, minor, or relatively new in the relationship, the woman's partner may be assisted to end the violence while the relationship remains intact. He must be willing to accept responsibility for his actions and to seek counseling. If the couple cannot talk about the violence, and if the man is unwilling to accept responsibility, the violence will most likely continue. In many cases, even when the physical abuse ends, the use of other power and control tactics continues.

When discussing leaving the abuser, abuse survivors should be informed that they may be at increased risk of serious harm or death if they leave. If

the woman has scored high on the Danger Assessment, her risk may be especially great. In extreme circumstances, battered women's shelters may help the woman relocate to another state or country.

Having the abuser removed from the home is an option available in certain circumstances. Usually the woman must obtain a protective order and request this remedy. This is generally a temporary order, and it is most likely to be granted if the woman's name is on the lease or title for the residence or if the woman is unable to enter a shelter because they are full.

Intervention

During the planning phase of the nursing process, the nurse also intervenes by providing the abuse survivor with information and by respectfully supporting the woman's decisions. Information sharing and respectful support empower women and are key elements of effective advocacy.

Throughout the process of providing information, it is appropriate for nurses to express their concerns, based on previous assessment, as long as this is done in a spirit of support rather than criticism. Gentle, sincere statements to the abuse survivor that she is a worthwhile person and does not deserve to be hurt can be very empowering. She has undoubtedly been told by her abuser that she does deserve it and may have come to believe this herself.

All battered women, regardless of their decision to leave or stay with the abuser, should be given referrals to shelters and battered women's service agencies. Many women who do not wish to use these referrals may use them in the future.

A few hospitals and clinics have in-house family violence counselors or advocates. If the abuse survivor is willing, have the advocate or counselor meet with the woman in the clinic or hospital at the time the abuse is revealed. If that is not possible, provide the woman with the advocate's phone number and encourage her to see or speak to him or her. Women who have not contacted referrals during their pregnancy may be willing to accept a visit from the advocate on the postpartum ward. Advocates from local battered women's services sometimes also visit clinics and hospitals to speak with battered women.

In hospital and clinic settings, it is often customary to refer patients with psychosocial issues to social workers, psychologists, or psychiatrists. Such referrals should never be made in place of referrals to battered women's services, and caution should be used in referring women to allied health professionals who may not have an adequate understanding of domestic violence. Referring abuse survivors to social workers, psychologists, or psychiatrists who have a poor knowledge or misunderstanding of domestic violence issues may result in further emotional damage for the woman. It is also not in the woman's best interests to unnecessarily acquire a psychiatric diagnosis (a necessary part of reimbursement for services) because this could be used against her in child custody cases.

Similar caution should be used when referring women to clergy or couples counseling. Well-meaning counselors sometimes encourage the woman to change her behavior to placate the abuser (Walker, 1984), thus reinforcing the view that the abuse is somehow her fault. Couples counseling may result in further abuse if it is attempted before the couple deals with their individual abuse issues separately. Similarly, chemical dependency counseling should not be assumed to adequately deal with abuse issues.

Further information sharing and intervention depend on the decisions made by the abuse survivor.

Plan 1: Stay with the abuser

A battered woman may choose to stay with or return to her abuser for many complex reasons. She stays or returns for many of the same reasons nonabusive but difficult relationships are maintained: financial constraints, societal and familial pressures, and because of the children. Women are less likely to leave when they are pregnant. For many women, staying in the relationship may be preferable to single parenthood, inadequate housing, and financial deprivation.

If a woman chooses to stay with her partner, help her develop an exit plan to be used if she feels in danger. She should have knowledge of where to go, phone numbers, and transportation plans. If possible, a bag with clothing, rent and utility receipts, birth certificates, toys, money, and extra car keys should be kept in a safe place. Encourage her to tell friends, family, and neighbors about the abuse so that they may be able to assist her in the future if necessary.

Encourage the abuse survivor to dial 911 if she is assaulted again. She should instruct her children to call if she is unable to do so herself. She should also be encouraged to attend battered women's support groups or to seek counseling from someone sensitive to the issue of abuse. Provide her or her partner with referrals to groups for abusive men if the partner is willing to consider this option.

Finally, assure the battered woman that she will receive continued nursing support. A woman who feels criticized for her decisions may terminate her prenatal care or seek care elsewhere, where her abuse history is not known. For the battered woman, continued nursing support may be the key to ending the violence in her life, sometime in the future.

Plan 2: Leaving

If the abuse survivor chooses to leave her abuser, she must decide where she will go and must have a clear idea of how safe she will be there. Women often choose to stay with family or friends. However, the welcome of family and friends may be short lived, and the woman may soon have to decide where to go next. Returning home to her abuser may become preferable to moving from one place to another. Or, she may be forced to return by her abuser threatening to or actually hurting her or those with whom she is staying.

The other option, although not always available, is seeking shelter at battered women's shelters or safe homes. Shelters provide a level of safety and assistance in dealing with abuse issues that most friends and family cannot. Nurses may call the shelter to inquire about available space, but shelter workers will need to talk to the abuse survivor directly. If necessary, transportation to the shelter can be arranged.

Nurses should advise women to take their children with them when they leave. If they do not, they may have great difficulty obtaining legal custody in the future. This is even more crucial if the children are also being abused by the partner. Abused children are more likely to remain in their mother's custody if she removes them from the violent situation. Shelter workers can often arrange to have children brought to the shelter from school or elsewhere.

After she leaves, discourage the woman from having any contact with her partner, including phone contact. He will often make promises to change, plead for her return, or threaten suicide if she stays away. If contact does occur, the abuser will often "sweet-talk," induce guilt, or shame the woman into returning home.

If the abuse survivor stays somewhere other than a shelter, she should have a plan of action should her partner locate her. She should consult a battered woman's advocate regarding issues such as protecting her children from being abducted by the abuser and protecting herself at work and in the home.

Nurses should discuss financial issues with the battered woman. If she and her partner share bank accounts or credit cards, he can remove the money and cancel the accounts without notifying her. It is not unusual for this to occur. The woman may also do the same if she wishes.

Plan 3: Remove the abuser from the home

The woman's partner may move out willingly or may be forced to leave by a vacate order. If he leaves, safety issues should be discussed. The woman should have all locks changed and obtain an order for protection if she has not already done so.

The abuse survivor is often the best judge of her own safety. She should plan what she would do if her partner comes to her door. She or her children should call 911 and report "some man" is at the door or trying to break in. If she reports that the man is her husband or boyfriend, police response time may be longer.

Follow-Up and Evaluation

In some cases, there will be no further contact between the nurse and the abuse survivor. This may occur if the intervention takes place on the postpartum ward, or if the woman changes location, or if she does not return to the clinic. In such cases nurses receive no feedback on their interventions. A phone call to the woman inquiring about her welfare is often welcomed.

When there is continuing contact, nurses should provide continued support and encouragement. The nurse should let the battered woman know she is still willing to discuss this issue by asking the woman how things are going. Praise her accomplishments, no matter how small. Continue to encourage her to obtain counseling or join a support group if she has not done so already.

For women who leave their abusers, there is much grieving that must be done. The woman may have lost a husband, a father for her children, perhaps her home, friends, and family. It may take time for her to work through the grief process and to begin making concrete future plans. For many women it takes years before they fully realize the impact of the abuse on their lives.

SUMMARY

Nurses encounter many abuse survivors in their clinic, hospital, and public health practices. It is important to identify battered women so that they may be assisted to end the violence in their lives. Nurses must acquire a working knowledge concerning abusive relationships, the health effects of violence against women, and the resources and options available to survivors of domestic violence, if they are to be able to intervene effectively.

Abuse during pregnancy poses an additional set of health risks for the battered woman. Her fetus may also be at risk. Because women have frequent, ongoing contact with nurses, nurse-midwives, or nurse practitioners during pregnancy, a level of rapport is often established that enhances the nurse's ability to identify and intervene with survivors of domestic abuse.

Violence against women is a serious public health problem that must be addressed by all health care professionals. Because nurses are trained in a holistic approach to health care, they are perhaps best suited to the task of providing an effective health care response to domestic violence as a public health issue. By working closely with battered women's services outside of the medical community, nurses can be an effective force in ending the violence in the lives of the women they serve.

REFERENCES

Alger, L. S., & Pupkin, M. J. (1986). Etiology of preterm premature rupture of the membranes. *Clinical Obstetrics and Gynecology, 29*(4), 758-770.

Amaro, H., Fried, L. E., Cobral, H., & Zuckerman, B. (1990). Violence during pregnancy and substance use. *American Journal of Public Health, 80*(5), 575-579.

Baker, D. P. (1982). Trauma in the pregnant patient. *Surgical Clinics of North America, 62*(2), 275-289.

Berendes, H. W. (1977). Methods of family planning and the risk of low birth weight. In D. M. Reed & F. J. Stanley (Eds.), *The epidemiology of prematurity*. Baltimore: Urban and Schwartzenberg.

Berenson, A., Stiglich, N., Wilkinson, G., & Anderson, A. (1991). Drug abuse and other risk factors for physical abuse in pregnancy among white, non-Hispanic, black, and Hispanic women. *American Journal of Obstetrics and Gynecology, 164*(6), 1491-1499.

Bohn, D. K. (1990). Domestic violence and pregnancy: Implications for practice. *Journal of Nurse-Midwifery, 35*(2), 86-98.

Bowker, L. H. (1983). *Beating wife beating*. Lexington, MA: Lexington Books.

Bremer, C., & Cassata, L. (1986). Trauma in pregnancy. *Nursing Clinics of North America, 21*, 705-716.

Brendtro, M., & Bowker, L. H. (1989). Battered women: How can nurses help? *Issues in Mental Health Nursing, 10*, 169-180.

Bry, B. H. (1983). Substance abuse in women: Etiology and prevention. *Issues in Mental Health Nursing 5*(1-4), 253-272.

Bullock, L., & McFarlane, J. (1989). The birth weight/battering connection. *American Journal of Nursing, 89*(9), 1153-1155.

Campbell, J. C. (1986). Nursing assessment for risk of homicide with battered women. *Advances in Nursing Science, 8*(4), 36-51.

Campbell, J. C., & Alford, P. (1989). The dark consequences of marital rape. *American Journal of Nursing, 89*(7), 946-949.

Campbell, J. C., & Oliver, C. (1992). *Why battering during pregnancy?* Unpublished manuscript, 1992.

Campbell, J. C., Poland, M. C., & Waller, J. B. (1989). *Effects of battery during pregnancy on prenatal care and birth weight*. Unpublished manuscript.

Chasnoff, I. J. (1987). Perinatal effects of cocaine. *Contemporary Obstetrics/Gynecology, 32*(5), 163-179.

Chasnoff, I. J., Burns, K. A., Burns, W. J., & Schnoll, S. H. (1986). Prenatal drug exposure: Effects on neonatal and infant growth and development. *Neurobehavioral Toxicology and Teratology, 8*, 357-362.

Chasnoff, I. J., Bussey, M. E., Savich, R., & Stack, C. M. (1986). Perinatal cerebral infarction and maternal cocaine use. *Journal of Pediatrics, 108*, 456-459.

Creasy, R. K., & Herron, M. A. (1981). Prevention of preterm birth. *Seminars in Perinatology, 5*(3), 295-302.

Dees, G., & Fuller, M. (1989). Blunt trauma in the pregnant patient. *Journal of Emergency Nursing, 15*(6), 495-499.

Diegmann, E. K. (1991, May). *Fetal retention syndrome: Fiction or fact?* Paper presented at the American College of Nurse-Midwives 36th annual meeting, Minneapolis, MN.

Dobash, R. E., & Dobash, R. (1979). *Violence against wives: A case against the patriarchy*. New York: Free Press.

Domestic Abuse Intervention Project (1990). *Power and control: Tactics of men who batter. An educational curriculum*. Duluth: Minnesota Program Development.

Drake, V. K. (1982). Battered women: A health care problem in disguise. *Image, 14*, 40-47.

Fagen, J., Stewart, D., & Hanson, K. (1983). Violent men or violent husbands? In D. Finklehor, R. Gelles, G. Hotaling, & M. Straus (Eds.), *The dark side of families* (pp. 49-67). Beverly Hills: Sage.

Fanaroff, A. A., & Martin, R. J. (Eds.). (1987). *Neonatal-perinatal medicine: Diseases of the fetus and infant* (4th ed.). St. Louis: Mosby–Year Book.

Flynn, J. (1977). Recent findings related to wife abuse. *Social Case Work, 58*(1), 13-20.

Gayford, J. J. (1978). Battered wives. In J. P. Martin (Ed), *Violence and the family* (pp. 19-39). New York: John Wiley & Sons.

Gelles, R. J. (1974). *The violent home: A study of physical aggression between husbands and wives*. Beverly Hills: Sage.

Gelles, R. J. (1975). Violence and pregnancy: A note on the extent of the problem and needed resources. *Family Coordinator, 24*(1), 81-86.

Gelles, R. J. (1988). Violence and pregnancy: Are pregnant women at greater risk of abuse? *Journal of Marriage and the Family, 560*, 841-847.

Gonik, B., & Creasy, R. K. (1986). Preterm labor: Its diagnosis and management. *American Journal of Obstetrics and Gynecology, 154*(1), 3-8.

Hatcher, R. A., Guest, F., Stewart, F., Stewart, G. K., Trussell, J., Cerel, S., & Cates, W. (1986). *Contraceptive technology 1986-1987*. New York: Irvington.

Helton, A. S. (1985). The pregnant battered woman. *Response, 9*(1), 22-23.

Helton, A. S. (1986). Battering during pregnancy. *American Journal of Nursing, 86,*(8), 910-913.

Helton, A. S. (1987). *Protocol of care for the battered woman.* Houston: March of Dimes Birth Defects Foundation.

Helton, A. S., McFarlane, J., & Anderson, E. T. (1987a). Battered and pregnant: A prevalence study. *American Journal of Public Health, 77*(10), 1337-1339.

Helton, A., McFarlane, J., & Anderson, E. T. (1987b). Prevention of battering during pregnancy: Focus on behavioral change. *Public Health Nursing, 4*(3), 166-174.

Helton, A. S., & Snodgrass, F. G. (1987). Battering during pregnancy: Intervention strategies. *Birth, 14*(3), 142-147.

Hilberman, E., & Munson, K. (1978). Sixty battered women. *Victimology, 2,* 460-470.

Hillard, R. J. A. (1985). Physical abuse in pregnancy. *Obstetrics and Gynecology, 66,* 185-190.

Huddleston, J. F. (1982). Preterm labor. *Clinical Obstetrics and Gynecology, 25*(1), 23-36.

Lockhart, L. L. (1987). A re-examination of the effects of race and social class on marital violence. *Journal of Marriage and the Family, 49,* 603-610.

McFarlane, J. (1991, May). *Assessing women for battering in a primary care setting: Self-report versus nurse assignment.* Paper presented at the Fourth National Nursing Conference on Violence Against Women, Detroit, MI.

McFarlane, J., Parker, B., Soeken, K., & Bullock, L. (1992) Assessing for abuse during pregnancy: Severity and frequency of injuries and associated entry into prenatal care. *Journal of the American Medical Association, 267*(23), 3176-3178.

Meyer, M. B. (1977). Effects of maternal smoking and altitude on birth weight and gestation. In D. M. Reed & F. J. Stanley (Eds.), *The epidemiology of prematurity.* Baltimore: Urban and Schwartzenberg.

Miller, J. M., & Pastorek, J. G. (1986). The microbiology of premature rupture of the membranes. *Clinical Obstetrics and Gynecology, 29*(4), 739-757.

Morey, M. A., Bigleiter, M., & Harris, D. J. (1981). Profile of a battered fetus (Letter). *Lancet, 2,* 1294-1295.

National Institute of Medicine (1985). *Preventing low birth weight.* Washington, DC: National Academy Press.

Newton, R. W., & Hunt, L. P. (1984). Psychological stress in pregnancy and its relation to low birth weight. *British Medical Journal, 288,* 1191-1194.

Newton, R. W., Webster, P. A., Binu, P. S., Maskrey, N., & Phillips, A. B. (1979). Psychosocial stress in pregnancy and its relation to the onset of premature labour. *British Medical Journal, 2,* 411-413.

Papiernik, E. (1984). Proposals for a programmed prevention policy of preterm birth. *Clinical Obstetrics and Gynecology, 27*(1), 614-35.

Parker, B. (1991, May). *Intentional injury during pregnancy.* Paper presented at the Fourth National Nursing Conference on Violence Against Women, Detroit, MI.

Parker, B., & McFarlane, J. (1991). Identifying and helping pregnant battered women. *Maternal-Child Health, 16,* 161-164.

Patterson, R. M. (1984). Trauma in pregnancy. *Clinical Obstetrics and Gynecology, 27*(1), 32-38.

Placek, P. (1977). Maternal and infant health factors associated with low infant birth weight: Findings from the 1972 national mortality survey. In D. M. Reed & F. J. Stanley (Eds.), *The epidemiology of prematurity.* Baltimore: Urban and Schwartzenberg.

Pugh, R. J., Newton, R. W., & Piercy, D. M. (1979). Fetal bleeding from gastric ulceration in the first day of life—possible association with social stress. *Archives of Diseases in Children, 84,* 146-148.

Roy, M. (1977). *Battered women: A psychological study of domestic violence.* New York: Van Nostrand Reinhold.

Schneider, J. A., & Chasnoff, I. J. (1987). Cocaine abuse during pregnancy: Its effects on infant motor development—A clinical perspective. *Topics in Acute Care Trauma Rehabilitation, 2*(1), 59-69.

Scupholme, A., Robertson, E. G., & Kamons, A. S. (1991). Barriers to prenatal care in a multiethnic urban sample. *Journal of Nurse-Midwifery, 36*(2), 111-116.

Stacey, W., & Schupe, A. (1983). *The family secret: Domestic violence in America.* Boston: Beacon Press.

Stark, A., Flitcraft, A., & Frazier, W. (1979). Medicine and patriarchal violence: The social construction of a "private" event. *International Journal of Health Services, 9*(3), 461-493.

Stark, E., Flitcraft, A. Z., Zuckerman, D., Grey, A., Robinson, J., & Frazier, W. (1981). Wife abuse in the medical setting. *Domestic Violence Monograph Series, 7*(7), 7-41.

Stauffer, D. M. (1986). The trauma patient who is pregnant. *Journal of Emergency Nursing, 12*(2), 89-93.

Stewart, E. P., & Campbell, J. C. (1989). Assessment of patterns of dangerousness with battered women. *Issues in Mental Health Nursing, 10,* 245-260.

Stewart, G. C. E., Harding, P. G. R., & Davies, E. M. (1980). Blunt abdominal trauma in pregnancy. *Canadian Medical Association Journal, 122,* 901-905.

Torres, A., & Forrest, J. D. (1988). Why do women have abortions? *Family Planning Perspectives, 20*(4), 169-176.

Varney, H. (1987). *Nurse-Midwifery* (2nd ed.). Boston: Blackwell Scientific.

Walker, L. (1979). *The battered woman.* New York: Harper & Row.

Walker, L. (1984). *The battered woman syndrome.* New York: Springer.

Whitley, N. (1985). *A manual of clinical obstetrics.* Philadelphia: J. B. Lippincott.

Young, C., McMann, J., Bowman, V., & Thompson, D. (1989). Maternal reasons for delayed prenatal care. *Nursing Research, 38,* 242-243.

CHAPTER

7 Abuse and Neglect of the Elderly in Family Settings

Mary C. Sengstock *and* Sara A. Barrett

S hould a discussion of elder abuse and neglect appear in a book on the treatment of victims of family violence? This issue is currently a matter of debate among professionals working with the elderly. In the past elder abuse has been viewed with child abuse and spouse abuse in the general category of family abuse. This situation can be shown in several ways. Textbooks on family violence tend to include elder abuse as one of the categories (Pagelow, 1984). Theoretical models are often derived from general family violence theories, focusing on such factors as the psychopathology of abusers, or on situational issues, such as general family stress or the specific stress involved in care of dependent family members (Galbraith, 1989).

From a public policy standpoint, management of elder abuse also tends to follow the model of general family abuse, making use of such procedures as mandatory reporting statutes, originally developed

for use with child abuse (Rinkle, 1989; Thobaben & Anderson, 1985). Techniques for identifying elder abuse are often borrowed from child abuse identification techniques (Sengstock & Hwalek, 1985-86). Furthermore, elder abuse is categorized as a criminal act, requiring that penalties be imposed on those responsible for the abuse (Thobaben, 1989, Quinn & Tomita, 1986).

More recently, however, some specialists who deal with the problem are beginning to suggest that elder abuse is "the wrong issue" (O'Malley, 1986). These analysts point out that much of what is termed "elder abuse" is more accurately termed "neglect," and may indeed be unintentional on the part of the so-called abuser, who may be overwhelmed by the responsibilities of caring for a dependent aged person (Douglass, 1988). Analysts who take this approach believe the problem should be viewed as mismanagement of elderly care and resist the use of the term "elder abuse," preferring to call the problem "mistreatment" (Douglass, 1988) or "inadequate care" (Callaghan, 1986).

The presence of this chapter illustrates our own characterization of elder abuse as pertinent to a discussion of family violence. However, throughout the chapter we will also review the alternative concept, as well as other theories and research related to elder abuse and neglect. Five major topics will be considered:

1. Characteristics and frequency of family abuse and neglect of the aged
2. Characteristics of abused and abuser
3. Proposed causes of elder abuse and neglect
4. Means used by agencies to identify and to serve abused and neglected elderly
5. Suggested nursing care for elderly victims

CHARACTERISTICS AND FREQUENCY OF DOMESTIC ABUSE OF THE AGED
Types of Elder Abuse

Previous research has indicated that "elder abuse" actually constitutes a variety of behaviors, all of which threaten the health, comfort, and possibly the lives of elderly people. However, the nature of the threat and its effect on aged persons' health and comfort may take different forms. Research on elder abuse has focused on a broader range of behaviors than other family abuse, including the following six major categories of abuse and neglect (Block & Sinnott, 1979; Douglass, Hickey, & Noel, 1980; Krasnow & Fleshner, 1979):

1. *Psychological or emotional neglect*—includes isolating or ignoring the elder
2. *Psychological or emotional abuse*—involves assault or the infliction of pain through verbal or emotional rather than physical means. Examples are verbal assault (screaming, yelling, berating) and threats that induce fear, but do not involve use of a weapon.
3. *Violation of personal rights*—includes acts such as forcing a person to move into a nursing home against his or her will, prohibiting him or her from marrying, or preventing free use

of the elder's own money (Krasnow & Fleshner, 1979). Violation of personal rights, together with financial abuse (listed below), are often characterized as "exploitation" of the elderly.

4. *Financial abuse*—includes the theft or misuse of an aged individual's money or property. Examples include taking money from a bank account without the elder's consent, selling a home without knowledge or permission, cashing a Social Security check and not returning the money to the recipient, etc.
5. *Physical neglect*—includes the failure to provide an aged and dependent individual with the necessities of life: food, shelter, clothing, and medical care. In fact, such neglect may be as injurious and life-threatening as a direct attack (Block & Sinnott, 1979; Lau & Kosberg, 1979). However, the major difference between direct abuse and neglect lies in the fact that neglect does not appear to involve a deliberate attempt to injure.
6. *Direct physical abuse*—includes actions that are direct attacks, are apparently deliberate, and can cause actual physical injury. Included in this category are direct physical assaults (slaps, punches, beatings, pushes, etc.), sexual assaults, as well as threats in which a weapon, such as a knife or gun, is directly involved.

Other categorizations tend to include the same types of behaviors, but may include or emphasize different types. For example, some specify sexual abuse as a separate category (Fulmer, 1989). A common distinction added to the categorization is the differentiation between "active neglect" and "passive neglect," with the former being a deliberate act, whereas the latter results from inadequate knowledge of the elder's needs or the stresses of long-term caregiving (Douglass, 1988; Wolf, Halas, Green, & McNiff, 1985–86). Regardless of the terminology, the term "elder abuse" clearly refers to a wider range of behaviors than either child abuse or spouse abuse (see also Pollick, 1987).

When compared with the other major category of

adult abuse, the term "elder abuse" includes several categories that are not part of most conceptualizations of spouse abuse. Psychological abuse and neglect, for example, are not usually considered a part of the definition of spouse abuse, which is usually confined to direct physical assault (Pagelow, 1984). Similarly, concerns about spouse abuse do not usually focus on the theft or misuse of the victim's property or the violation of the victim's rights, although both might often occur with spouse abuse. Thus a major difference between elder abuse and spouse abuse is that elder abuse tends to include a greater variety of acts against the victim.

In some ways, elder abuse appears to be more similar to child abuse than to spouse abuse, since elder abuse includes neglect, which is more appropriate to child abuse definitions than to the definition of spouse abuse (Pagelow, 1984). However, there are some major differences between elder abuse and child abuse. Reference to financial abuse of children is rare because, in contrast with the elderly, they are unlikely to have substantial amounts of money or property for others to appropriate or misuse (Quinn & Tomita, 1986). Perhaps the most significant difference between children and the elderly, however, lies in the fact that the elderly are adults and entitled to the rights of adults (Quinn & Tomita, 1986). Unless mentally impaired, they are entitled to make choices with regard to their lives and cannot be forced to alter their lifestyles without their consent. This is an important reason for distinguishing between elder abuse and child abuse because elders, unlike children, cannot simply be removed from a dangerous home situation if it is one in which they choose to remain (Quinn & Tomita, 1986).

Consequently, the first major area in which elder abuse differs from other categories of family abuse stems from the fact that categories of behavior that have been included in definitions of elder abuse are considerably broader in range than those included in either spouse or child abuse. Furthermore, there is some question regarding whether the apparently similar categories are truly equivalent; for example, neglect is a different type of behavior when directed against a child versus a dependent adult.

Frequency of Elder Abuse

Before discussing the frequency of elder abuse, it is necessary to note that the major studies on the topic present serious limitations in establishing reliable statistics. In the past, many studies have had small sample sizes (Block & Sinnott, 1979; Lau and Kosberg, 1979), and most were analyses of whatever cases the researchers were able to uncover, rather than being representative of the aged population (Sengstock & Liang, 1982; 1983). Furthermore, a widely quoted study (Douglass et al., 1980; Hickey & Douglass, 1981a, 1981b) did not examine case-related data but relied on service providers' general impressions of the nature of the problem.

These studies resulted in a number of estimates of the frequency of elder abuse. Steinmetz (1981) suggested that approximately 11% of the population might be vulnerable to elder abuse, and Block and Sinnott (1979) estimated that abuse is an actual problem for at least 4% of the elderly population. Lau and Kosberg (1979) estimated a rate of 80.58 cases of abuse per 1,000.

A recent study in Boston represents the first attempt to estimate the rate of elder abuse from a systematic sample of community-dwelling elderly (Pillemer & Finkelhor, 1988). This study, which interviewed 2,020 elderly, found a rate of 32 cases of elder abuse per 1,000. Three types of elder abuse and neglect were included: physical abuse, physical neglect, and psychological abuse. The other types listed previously—psychological neglect, violation of personal rights, and material abuse—were not included. Because some studies have suggested that financial abuse may be one of the most common types, this deficiency would substantially underestimate the number of abused elders (Sengstock & Liang, 1983). In addition, the question might be raised whether the Boston area elderly population can be considered representative of the elderly population as a whole. However, to date their figure of 32 cases per 1,000 represents the best estimate of the rate of elder abuse and neglect. Since several types of abuse have not been included, this rate should be viewed as a minimum.

Frequency of Various Abuse Types

The frequency of each type of elder abuse tends to vary in different studies. Some have found psychological abuse to be most prevalent (Block & Sinnott, 1979), whereas others have noted that physical abuse was the most common form (Lau & Kosberg, 1979). These findings might reflect the observation that agencies tend to identify forms of abuse that most closely correspond to the forms of treatment which they offer (Douglass et al., 1980; Hickey & Douglass, 1981a, 1981b; Sengstock & Barrett, 1981). Thus the finding by Block and Sinnott (1979) might reflect the fact that most professionals reporting cases of abuse to them were social workers, professionals concerned primarily with the psychological status of clients. At the same time, Lau and Kosberg's sample (1979) was derived from case records of persons who were seen at a chronic disease center for a medical malady. Consequently, this might account for the strong tendency toward physical abuse in the cases identified by their research.

Sengstock and Liang (1983), like Block and Sinnott (1979), found that psychological or emotional abuse was the most frequent type of elderly abuse, with more than 80% of cases showing some type of emotional abuse or neglect. However, this pattern should be understood in context. Several studies (Douglass et al., 1980; Hickey & Douglass, 1981a, 1981b, Lau & Kosberg, 1979; Sengstock & Liang, 1982, 1983) have found that most victims suffered from more than one form of abuse. In fact, although emotional or psychological abuse may occur independently in a few cases, it almost always is accompanied by other forms of abuse. When emotional or psychological abuse or neglect is found, service providers should investigate further because it is possible that other types of abuse may also be present.

Another frequent type of abuse is financial abuse, suffered by about one half of the cases in Sengstock and Liang's study (1983). The high prevalence of cases of financial abuse in this sample may arise, in part, from the fact that a legal aid agency reported the largest number of cases to the project. This is the type of agency that would most likely be consulted by aged persons with various financial concerns, such as the claim that someone has stolen money or misused property.

Physical abuse, neglect, or both tend to be less frequent in studies that do not directly involve health agencies. However, even in such studies their numbers are sizable; for example, Sengstock and Liang (1983) found that 20% of the victims suffered direct physical abuse, and a similar number suffered physical neglect. It is also clear that abuse or neglect rarely occurs as an isolated incident. Not only do multiple types but also multiple incidents occur (Sengstock & Liang, 1983).

The enduring character of the abuse becomes more evident when the length of time over which the abuse has occurred is considered. Reporters indicate that abuse continues over a substantial period of time (Sengstock & Liang, 1982). If it is assumed that "a long time" probably indicates at least 1 year, then apparently 60% of such victims have endured abusive family situations for a period of 1 year or longer.

Summary

Unlike other categories of domestic abuse, elder abuse tends to include more than direct physical violence. Six types of abusive behavior are commonly included. No firm generalizations can be made about the frequency of elder abuse or each specific subtype. The most accepted study suggests an overall rate of 32 cases per 1,000, but this includes only three types of abuse and excludes what may be the more frequent types.

Some studies have shown psychological abuse to be more frequent, whereas others find a prevalence of physical or financial abuse. Several studies indicated that elder abuse often involves multiple types in a single case. Elder abuse cases that have been studied also tend to involve a substantial number of separate incidents of abuse that have occurred over a considerable period of time, often lasting for months or years.

On the basis of existing data, it cannot be concluded that elder abuse is a widespread problem. The majority of the aged probably have satisfactory relationships with their children and other relatives. For those few aged who are abused, however, the abuse tends to be persistent, serious, and urgently requires attention.

CHARACTERISTICS OF ABUSED AND ABUSERS

Who is a likely victim of elder abuse? Who is most likely to be an abuser? This section discusses the demographic characteristics associated with abuse and neglect of the aged by their families. The characteristics of the victim will be considered first. For this section we rely heavily on a study in which we were involved. We will also refer to comparable data when available.

Demographic Characteristics of Victims

The reported age of elder abuse victims has varied considerably from study to study. Although some research has found the majority of victims to be very old (Block & Sinnott, 1979), others find that victims of elder abuse are more evenly divided among the elderly, from the 60s through the 80s (Sengstock & Liang, 1983). Not surprisingly, most studies have found that the majority of elder abuse victims are women (Block & Sinnott, 1979; Sengstock & Liang, 1983). Because the majority of the elderly population is female, this is to be expected. However, one study found that the *rate* of abuse of elderly males was higher than the rate of abuse of elderly females (Pillemer & Finkelhor, 1988). If this study is correct, then elderly men have a greater likelihood of being victimized, but the greater number of elderly women still results in a majority of women among elderly victims.

Most researchers have found the majority of victims to be white (Block & Sinnott, 1979). This may result, however, from a failure to include the agencies that serve blacks and other minorities among the respondents to the study. When agencies serving blacks are included, the victims are more evenly divided between blacks and whites (Sengstock & Liang, 1983). Religious preference of victims also presents an unclear picture. One study indicated that abuse was more common among Catholics (Anetzberger 1987), whereas others see more Protestant victims (Sengstock & Liang, 1983).

The socioeconomic level of victims is another enigma. For example, Block and Sinnott (1979) found that victims were evenly divided between lower and middle classes, whereas Sengstock and Liang (1983) found a majority of lower-income persons. It is easy to see why such individuals would feel dependent on their families and unable to escape the abusive situation. The wealthy are not immune to the problems of domestic abuse, however, although they may be better able to hide these problems from authorities (Steinmetz & Straus, 1974). It should also be noted that the elderly may be prone to abuse because of their financial position. Thus Wolf, Godkin & Pillemer (1984) found that, contrary to customary belief, the abusers were financially dependent on their elderly victims, who were the major source of income for their families.

The majority of the victims in the Sengstock and Liang study (1982) either lived alone or with one other person. It should be noted that living alone does not preclude the existence of abuse on the part of family members, who may abuse the aged person during visits, or subject them to neglect or isolation. One interesting pattern that appeared in the study by Sengstock and Liang was their number of contacts outside their own households. Most had family contacts, but these consisted mainly of a visit or phone call every week or less. They were less likely to have friends, but those who did tended to have closer contact with them than with their families. The picture that emerges is similar to that found by Justice and Justice (1976), in families in which child abuse was a problem. They described the abusing family as one in which the members had very limited contact outside the family, making it impossible for the members to obtain outside support in times of trouble and leaving no one to intervene if abuse occurs.

One conclusion drawn by some studies of elder abuse is that persons with some type of physical or mental disability are more likely to be abused than those who are physically strong (Block & Sinnott, 1979; Lau & Kosberg, 1979). Other studies do not corroborate this finding (Sengstock & Liang, 1982; 1983). Among the disabilities noted are some degree of emotional impairment and the inabilities to prepare food, to perform personal hygiene, or to prepare their own medicine. Also noted is that medication may itself be a means of abuse because some elders are given excessive doses of drugs by their doctors or their families to make them more manageable (Block & Sinnott, 1979).

Portrait of the Abuser

Studies of elder abuse have suggested that the abuser is most likely to be a family member of the victim, usually one of the victim's own children (Block & Sinnott, 1979; Lau & Kosberg, 1979). It has also been found that the abuser is most often 40 years of age or older (Block & Sinnott, 1979). Block and Sinnott also found that most abusers were female, a situation that may reflect the fact that women are most frequently the caretakers in constant contact with the incapacitated elderly.

According to Block and Sinnott (1979), most abusers acted because of psychological rather than economic or unknown reasons. They also found most abusers to be white, middle class, and middle-aged. This pattern contrasts with child and spouse abuse because both have been characterized as phenomena more common among the lower classes (Blumberg, 1964; Gil, 1971; Levinger, 1976; Steinmetz & Straus, 1974).

It has also been found that the abuser is more likely to be a member of the victim's household than to live elsewhere (Sengstock & Liang, 1983). The suggestion that aged persons are more likely to be abused by their own children was also borne out in the study by Sengstock and Liang (1983): one half of the abusers were the children of the victim. However, this study did not confirm the daughter as the most common abuser. Children who abused their parents were almost equally divided between sons and daughters.

Spouse abuse is not unknown among the aged, as indicated in the study by Sengstock and Liang (1983). Some experts, however, do not believe that spouse abuse should be included as a type of elder abuse, an issue discussed later (Douglass, 1988). Other abusers included grandchildren, siblings, nieces, nephews, and cousins. Sometimes the abuser is not a relative; these include friends, roomers, and landlords (Sengstock & Liang, 1983). The scenario of the abuser as somewhat advanced in age was also supported in data by Senstock and Liang. Two thirds of the abusers were 40 years of age or older, and more than one fourth were over 60, well into the category of being classified as elderly themselves (Sengstock & Liang, 1983).

One issue that should be considered is the relationship between types of abuse and the abuser. Some evidence shows that certain types of abuse are more likely to be inflicted by specific types of abusers. Thus physical abuse is more likely to be inflicted by sons; physical neglect is likely to be perpetrated either by sons or siblings (Sengstock & Liang, 1983), although differences and sample sizes are small. The abusers most likely to be involved in emotional neglect or deprivation of rights were daughters (nearly half) and sisters (one third) (Sengstock & Liang, 1983). It is interesting that no sons or unrelated persons were implicated in such cases. It might be suggested that the persons accused of emotional neglect—daughters and sisters—are persons from whom the elderly would most likely expect emotional support. This would be particularly true of daughters. Emotional support, on the other hand, is not usually thought to be the responsibility of men, so parents would not be likely to express disappointment if their sons failed to provide such support. Neither would they be likely to expect such help from unrelated persons. Hence we suggest that the prevalence of daughters and sisters in this category may be related primarily to the expectations of the elderly rather than to a different type of behavior exhibited by the alleged abusers (Sengstock, 1991).

Direct emotional abuse may be more characteristic of sons because this type of abuse includes more direct action—verbal assaults, creating fear—that many people might consider to be more appropriate masculine behavior (Sengstock, 1991). This might account for the greater representation of sons in emotional abuse than in the more passive emotional neglect. However, daughters were almost as likely to engage in direct emotional abuse as their brothers, and unrelated persons and other relatives also appeared in considerable numbers. Sons and daughters were also the most likely to engage in financial abuse, each representing about one fourth of the cases. Other relatives and unrelated persons were the next most frequent offenders (Sengstock & Liang, 1983).

Thus the data of Sengstock and Liang suggest that sons and daughters are the major perpetrators of most types of elder abuse. However, sons were noted more likely to engage in active, direct abuse. They were responsible for two thirds of the physical abuse and nearly one third of the emotional abuse. Daughters were also responsible for direct emotional abuse and were accused of the majority of indirect emotional neglect. Other relatives and unrelated persons tended to appear as suspected abusers primarily in instances of direct abuse. They were less likely to be accused of neglect, probably because the aged victims did not depend on them for help and would not recognize its absence as neglect.

PROPOSED CAUSES OF ELDER ABUSE

There are many theories explaining the existence of family violence and abuse. Theories abound that explain why parents abuse their children and husbands beat their wives. As interest in elder abuse has increased, so also have the number of theories that explain why adults abuse their aging parents. Unfortunately, most of these explanations remain at the level of untested hypotheses. Many have research to support their claims, but others are simply assertions of variables that appear to be important.

In this section we examine some of the proposed explanations for elder abuse, together with references to available research data. However, we must emphasize that none of these theories can be considered well established, accurate explanations of the problem. Certainly, no single theory yet developed is adequate to explain the existence and nature of elder abuse.

Nonetheless, such theories can provide professionals with valuable indicators of the probability of abuse. Most theories of domestic abuse have been developed from associating specific instances of known abuse with other factors in the victim's social-psychological environment. Consequently, such theories suggest the types of factors that may be related to abuse and that should be viewed as "danger signals" by nurses and other persons who work with elderly patients. Therefore, they can suggest the need for further inquiry by concerned professionals. Two categories of theories will be examined: general theories of family violence and ex-

planations of abuse relating directly to the aging process.

General Theories of Family Violence

One point that has been stressed regarding characteristics of the elderly is the continuity of personality and behavior throughout life (Back, 1976; Neugarten, Havighurst, & Tobin, 1968; Hendricks & Hendricks, 1981). Gerontologists who espouse this view emphasize the fact that most individuals exhibit a constant pattern of personality characteristics and behavior patterns from youth through middle age and into old age. Radical changes, either in personality or behavior, once one reaches old age, are rare. This theory suggests that the family problems of the aged, including potentially abusive behavior, may be similar to those of younger persons. Consequently, theories of family violence that have been useful in analyzing child and spouse abuse should be examined to determine if they apply to elderly abuse. Three types of general theories of domestic abuse are considered. These are (1) abuser-focused theories, (2) situational stress theories, and (3) theories focusing on the nature of family relationships.

Abuser-focused theories

Domestic abuse has often been explained in relation to the psychopathological state of the abuser (Gelles, 1973). In essence, these theories suggest that the abusive individual is mentally ill and that the abusive behavior is the result of this mental illness. A closely related theory associates domestic abuse with the misuse of alcohol or other substances (Gelles, 1974). This approach is often taken by persons with a serious concern about substance abuse. They suggest that persons who are alcoholics or drug addicts are highly likely to engage in abusive behavior. In contrast, some theorists suggest that the alcohol is not the basic cause of the abusive behavior, rather the abuser uses substance abuse as a "cover-up" for abusive tendencies that are already present (Gelles, 1974).

In either instance, the cause of the abuse is sought in the psychological state of the abuser. He or she is thought to be mentally ill or under the influence of alcohol or drugs, and therefore incapable of controlling behavior. This approach appears tempting because it provides an obvious factor that is responsible for the abuse and an equally obvious solution: cure the psychopathological problem and the abuse will cease.

Unfortunately, studies of domestic abuse rarely have access to independent evidence of mental illness and substance abuse. Hence it is difficult to ascertain the percentage of cases in which either or both of these factors exist. In the study by Sengstock and Liang (1982), for example, case workers were asked whether they had noted the presence of these factors in each instance of abuse reported. Workers noted the presence of mental illness, substance abuse, or both in a relatively small percentage of the cases. A combined total of only nine, or 12% of the cases, involved abusers who were alcoholics, drug abusers, or diagnosed mentally ill, and hence had a psychic state that made behavior control difficult or impossible. It appears that the psychopathological state of the abuser is responsible in relatively few cases of elder abuse.

It should be noted, however, that the failure of such causal factors to appear in studies of abuse may be related to the inability of the researchers to uncover the evidence. Either the data collection instruments may fail to elicit this information from the professional workers, or in some cases, undiagnosed mental illness, alcoholism, or drug abuse may be present and the agency workers themselves may not yet be aware of it.

Those cases of elder abuse in which mental illness or substance abuse is present appear particularly serious or difficult to control. In one instance, an alcoholic daughter subjected her recently widowed mother, who had a heart condition, to constant verbal abuse. She also depended on her mother to care for her three active children since her alcoholism had forced her to relinquish custody. Another woman was subjected to constant threats and emotional abuse by her elderly alcoholic husband. Still another woman had an alcoholic grandson who constantly stole money she had given him to pay her bills.

Even more serious abuse occurs in cases in which mental or emotional illness is present. One aged woman had been severely beaten by her schizophrenic son who lived with her. She was also deprived of the companionship of her daughter, who avoided visiting because of fear of her brother, who had beaten his sister in the past. In another case, the aged victim had evicted her emotionally ill son from her home, yet the son continued to return home, often breaking into the home while the mother was at work. The victim had sought legal assistance from a legal aid agency and the county prosecutor to protect herself from her son's abusive behavior.

In terms of providing service to victims, it appears inadvisable to rely heavily on the notion that the abuse is caused by such factors as mental illness or substance abuse. If an agency finds such problems in an instance of elder abuse, it is then imperative that these problems be treated as a part of the entire family problem. However, an assumption that such factors must be involved whenever elder abuse occurs would prevent workers from looking for other factors that could be causal variables in the majority of cases.

Such factors can be valuable to service providers since they may serve as "danger signals." Elder abuse may occur in many cases where mental illness or drug or alcohol abuse are not present, and these factors may not always lead to abuse of aged family members. Since the risk of abuse in such cases is sufficiently high, agency workers should make additional inquiries to determine the possible presence of abusive behavior. This would be necessary even if the alcoholic, drug addict, or mentally ill individual was an aged person, because such patterns can be associated with abuse in a variety of ways. The psychologically disturbed individual may abuse others, and he or she may be abused by others as a reaction to the disturbing behavior patterns. As indicated elsewhere, some elder abuse is actually elder-elder abuse. Hence aged alcoholics or drug abusers may be abusing their own aged relatives.

Situational stress theories

One of the factors frequently cited as a cause of family abuse is the prevalence of stress. Proponents of this view indicate that situational factors such as poverty, isolation, or occupational stress may cause people to abuse members of their families. Child and spouse abuse consistently occur more frequently, although not exclusively, in lower-class groups, which are presumed to experience greater stress because of economic deprivation (Blumberg, 1964; Gil, 1971; Levinger, 1976; Steinmetz & Straus, 1974).

Perhaps the primary proponent of the situational stress model was Gil (1971), who believed that there would be no child abuse if it were not for such factors as poverty or job stress. Expanding on this approach to child abuse, Justice and Justice (1976) noted that families who have a considerable number of other problems are more likely to abuse their children. In their sample of abusive parents, they found an unusually high frequency of persons who had undergone a "prolonged series of changes"—economic crises, illnesses, deaths, accidents. They emphasized that the prolonged series of stressful situations, rather than a single stressful event, promotes violence. It has also been noted that abusive families are unlikely to have social resources to call on when stressful situations occur. A high association with social isolation was found both among abusive parents (Justice & Justice, 1976) and among abused elders (Case & Lesnoff-Caravaglia, 1978).

Professionals who work with abused elders are divided in their views on the importance of life crises or situational stress factors in reference to abuse of the aged (Douglass et al., 1980; Hickey & Douglass, 1981a, 1981b). Other authorities have suggested that the problems associated with care of an aged person may create stress and promote abuse (Block & Sinnott, 1979). Such age-specific factors are discussed in a later section. In this section, we discuss some more general, non-age–related stress factors that may tend to promote elder abuse.

As indicated earlier, one theory suggests that a family is more likely to engage in abusive behavior toward their children if they have had a number of problems to deal with in a short period of time (Justice & Justice, 1976). A similar situation may possibly exist in families characterized by elder abuse. This is, abuse of the elderly may exist in families plagued with many problems, serious and otherwise. Consequently, some authorities use stress

scales to differentiate abusive from nonabusive families (Justice & Justice, 1976). In the study by Sengstock and Liang (1982), victims were asked to respond to a modified version of the Holmes and Rahe (1967) stress scale, indicating whether they or members of their families had experienced any of the 46 listed possible problems in the past year. The list included such items as death of a spouse or other family member, the existence of debts (both large and small), change in or loss of a job, changes in living arrangements, etc.

One striking characteristic of these victims was the large number of problems they or their families had experienced. Twenty percent of the interviewees stated that members of their families had experienced 20 or more of these problems in the past year. Another 30% reported having from 11 to 13 problems; 35% had from 5 to 9 problems; and only 15% had less than 5 problems. These victims' families are clearly "multiproblem" families. It is probable that the abuse of the aged person could not be corrected until the accompanying problems and tensions in the family had been alleviated. As with other types of domestic violence, treatment of the entire family and its problems is necessary (Sengstock, Barreth, & Graham, 1984).

The situational stress theory of domestic abuse has been severely criticized. It has often been noted that situational stress is inadequate in explaining child abuse because it fails to show why some families react to stress and frustration by abusing their children, while others, subjected to the same stress, do not (Justice & Justice, 1976; Spinetta & Rigler, 1972). Similarly, a stress model does not totally explain why some adults, when faced with severe family stress, would react by abusing an aged member while others would not (Steuer & Austin, 1980).

However, the stress model does call attention to the fact that outside factors must be considered in explaining the abusive behavior. Thus Justice and Justice (1976) conclude that the abuser is an individual with serious personal problems. In working with abusive parents, they contend that the problems of the abuser must be dealt with sympathetically before the relationship with the child can be rebuilt on a nonviolent basis. They further contend that the family must be dealt with as a unit, lest the abuser return to his or her abusive behavior when family problems and the interactions of other family members reassert themselves (Justice & Justice, 1976). As therapists, they attempt to provide support to the abusing parent.

Theories focusing on the nature of family relationships

Another approach to the analysis of family violence that has received considerable support is a model that views domestic abuse in the context of general family relationships. This approach suggests that a well-established pattern of violent behavior on the part of an individual need not necessarily suggest the existence of a situational or psychopathological state (Gelles, 1973). Rather, such behavior, like non-violent behavior, can be learned early in life. Evidence indicates that elderly victims, as well as the members of their families, may indeed have learned abusive behavior as an appropriate approach to solving life's problems (Sengstock & Liang, 1982).

Normative violence. It has been suggested by some authors that domestic abuse is part of a general pattern of "normative violence," in which violent behavior is accepted, even approved, as a normal part of family life. Are these victims persons who are more likely to use and approve of violent behavior, especially in family relationships? Victims were asked if they were ever punched or hit or threatened with a knife or gun (Sengstock & Liang, 1982). Responses could include the abuse reported, other family incidents, or incidents outside the family. Nearly one half of these elderly people reported that they had been punched or hit, and 10% had been threatened by another person wielding a knife. Most shocking was the fact that 35% of these aged persons had been threatened with a gun. In contrast, a study of domestic violence using a national random sample found that 10% of persons had been hit or kicked sometime during their marriages and that 4% had been threatened with a knife or gun (Straus, Gelles, & Steinmetz, 1980). Although the studies are not totally comparable, the national data do suggest that these aged victims had considerably more violence in their backgrounds. These people appeared to be part of a

"subculture of violence," and had come to accept violent action as "normative" or appropriate (Wolfgang, 1958; Wolfgang & Ferracuti, 1967).

In the first national survey of family violence, a large majority (greater than 70%) of the respondents expressed their belief that physical punishment of children was appropriate and necessary (Gelles & Straus, 1988; Straus et al., 1980). This belief may cause children to grow up with the idea that physical responses are appropriate for a larger, stronger person who has his or her will thwarted by a smaller, weaker person. It would not be surprising if child abuse victims learned that such behavior was appropriate when and if they should move into such a position in reference to their parents.

In effect, the aged parents, through their actions when their children were small, may have taught them that abusive behavior was appropriate. It was also noted that the abusive behavior is closely related to the social role that is generally associated with certain types of abusers. As noted, sons were more likely to engage in direct abuse, whereas daughters were more likely to be responsible for emotional abuse or neglectful behavior. Such differences suggest that abuse may be learned as a part of normal sex role patterns, in which men are expected to react in a direct, physical manner, and women, to react with emotional outbursts and to withhold affection and support (Sengstock, 1991). Hence the data provide some support for the learning theory of domestic abuse.

Long-standing patterns of family violence. When attitudes and behaviors that support the use of violence and force are firmly established in a family, it is likely that such violence and force will be directed toward those family members least able to defend themselves. Therefore these victims are more likely to include children or the aged. Often the most tragic cases are those showing evidence of a long-term abusive pattern in the family (Sengstock & Liang, 1982). In these cases, abusive behavior may continue for the entire duration of a marriage, or the victims of abuse may alternate between one generation and another. As Straus et al. emphasize, abusive behavior patterns are highly likely to be passed from parents to children (Straus et al., 1980). Several cases illustrate this type of pattern.

A stroke victim with partial paralysis was hospitalized following an "accident" in which she had allegedly fallen down the stairs. Actually, her husband, who had abused her for most of her married life, had pushed her down the stairs. As a child she had also been abused by her mother. In planning for her release from the hospital, the hospital staff arranged for this victim to live with her daughter instead of returning to her abusive husband. However, it was found that the daughter's husband was also abusive. Hence this family is now in its third generation of abuse and is rearing a fourth generation of young people who view abuse as a well-established and seemingly appropriate dimension of family life (see also Gesino, Smith, & Keckich, 1982).

In another case, a woman's children were removed from her custody because she had abused them. Subsequent to the removal of her children, she assumed a role in the care of her invalid father. This case was discovered when the daughter poured boiling water over her father, scalding him badly. Cases such as these suggest that the common pattern of removing a victim from an abusive situation often does little to resolve the situation. Although it may protect the specific individual victimized at a given time, it does nothing to assist the abuser in controlling his or her behavior. As a result, the abuse may simply be transferred to another likely victim: from child to aged parent, from aged parent to spouse, or perhaps to an unsuspecting friend or neighbor.

Although abuse by children seems more likely, elder abuse can also appear in marital or pseudomarital relationships (Sengstock & Liang, 1982), an issue that is not recognized by some authors (Douglass, 1988). This type of abuse may be more common when one partner is either considerably older or more infirm than the other. The example of an aged woman whose husband pushed her down the stairs has already been described.

In several cases the usual domestic violence sex roles were reversed, with the woman being the abuser and the man, the victim. In two separate cases, children removed an infirm father from the home because they saw evidence that their mother was abusing their father, either physically, emotionally, or both. In both instances the mother claimed that her children were abusing her because they had deprived her of her husband's presence in the home, yet in one instance a medical examination showed clear evidence of malnutrition in the father, whose condition improved greatly after being removed from his wife's care. A case worker reported that one of these women had stated that her husband had made her suffer for most of her life, and it was now his turn to suffer. In still a third case, the wife and children together took the husband's money and abandoned him.

Victim precipitation among the elderly. A common explanation for domestic abuse is victim precipitation: the victim "asked for it." That is, through his or her own misbehavior or goading, the victim forced the offender to take revenge. This view is found often with regard to spouse abuse (Gelles, 1974). Sengstock and Liang (1982) found evidence of this pattern in a limited number of the cases examined. Some service providers believed abuse was precipitated by the victim, at least in part, when an aged parent attempted to retain more control over his or her children than most young adults were likely to allow. In one case the mother and her abusive son had a mutually dependent relationship, which was threatened by the son's impending marriage. The abuse of the mother occurred when the mother attempted to block the marriage. In another mother-son case, the mother was an extremely religious woman who wished to convert her son. She constantly berated her son for his sins, and he responded by abusing her psychologically. In such cases, agency workers suggested that the abuse would probably not have occurred, or would not have been so severe, if the elders had not engaged in the provocative behavior. Clearly the abuse is not likely to cease unless the elderly person can be induced to give up, at least to a degree, the behavior that provokes the abuse.

Family financial issues. A considerable amount of the abuse that the Sengstock and Liang (1982) study uncovered appeared to be provoked by financial difficulties on the part of one or more members of the family. The time of death and the distribution of the decedent's property seemed to be a particularly vulnerable time for an elderly person to be victimized in this way. Abusers included siblings, spouses, grandchildren, children, and unrelated persons.

The most frequent abusers in this type of setting were still the children, however. In one instance a son was known to have taken $80,000 from his father's bank account while his widowed father was in a nursing home. The son also attempted to block his father's remarriage to protect any remaining property. Another man who spoke only Spanish was tricked into signing over his home to his son, who then mortgaged the home and forced his father to make the payments. In a third case, the abuser was a 20-year-old woman who made frequent visits to her great-grandmother; during the visits she stole the lady's bank books and emptied her great-grandmother's accounts.

In a few of these cases the family member appears to be in true financial need and therefore is tempted to take money from the aged person, who is probably seen as having little use for it. In many instances, however, such as the case of the son who had already taken $80,000 and still wanted to ensure that he would receive the rest, it is difficult to avoid the conclusion that greed motivates the actions. Observation of this factor could be an important part of the clinical assessment process. Clinical personnel should investigate the possibility of abuse in cases in which family members appear inordinately concerned about the financial assets of an elder or their possible depletion through medical expenses.

Explanations of Abuse Relating to the Aging Process

Normal family relations can by their nature be tense and stressful (Steinmetz & Straus, 1974). However, some analysts of elder abuse suggest that the nature of the aging process creates additional stress and tension in a family. Thus Block and Sinnott (1979) list five major factors related to the aging process that they believe may be possible causes of elder abuse. These five factors, as well as some manifestations of these and other factors as indicated in the literature, are described in this section.

Demographic and economic changes

There are no clear data to indicate whether the current cases of elder abuse represent either an increase or a decrease in incidence compared with such problems in the past. Current statistics concerning the frequency of elder abuse are limited; statistics on elder abuse in past decades are impossible to reconstruct. Thus it cannot be stated that elder abuse is more frequent today than in past generations.

It is suggested, however, that the demographic and economic patterns in place today promote the likelihood of elder abuse by making it increasingly difficult for adult children to provide necessary care for aged parents (Block & Sinnott, 1979). In the past, families were considerably larger, and the life expectancy of the elderly was substantially shorter. Consequently, there were several children in a family who could share the responsibilities of caring for an aged parent. Furthermore, the period of time during which an aged parent would suffer a debilitating illness and require constant care was likely to be only a few years, perhaps a decade at most.

Changes in the medical care available to the aged have greatly increased their life span, with the result that many elderly may live two or more decades during which they require constantly increasing assistance from their children. The trend toward smaller families means that this increased responsibility falls on the shoulders of fewer and fewer children. Such factors may make it difficult for even the best-intentioned children to care adequately for their aged parents (Steinmetz, 1978). The increased life span has been accomplished largely as a result of modern medicine with all of its attendant costs. In families already burdened by the high cost of living, the cost of medical care for an aged parent can "often go beyond the resources of both the elderly parent and the adult children" (Block & Sinnott, 1979, p. 53). Factors such as these probably account, in large part, for the prevalence of abuse among the aged, infirm parents (Block & Sinnott, 1979; Lau & Kosberg, 1979). Consequently, some authorities believe that elder abuse results from the absence of services to assist families in the care of their aged members (Burston, 1978).

Changes in the elderly person's life

Compounding the difficulties of care of an aged parent is the debilitating process of aging. (Block & Sinnott, 1979). Many people look forward to retirement as a time of increased freedom and opportunity. However, many factors may intervene to thwart these plans. Old age can be a time of decreasing physical and mental capacity, of increasing dependence on others, of loss of independence, and of loss of social relationships and status (Strow & MacKreth, 1977). Thus aged persons often find that the activities they were formerly able to perform for themselves—personal care, care of the home, meal preparation—are now beyond their capacity.

Social roles they formerly filled, such as caring for children or grandchildren, or holding valued positions in business or community, are no longer theirs. They may have lost valued relatives or friends through illness or death. Thus they suffer great loss of self-esteem as they see themselves becoming progressively less capable. Concurrently, they become increasingly dependent on their children, not only for personal care and assistance with normal household tasks, but also for most of their social needs. Such extreme dependency in several areas of life is often impossible for many families to handle, particularly since the increased life span may prolong this dependency for decades.

Changes in the life of the adult offspring

The increased care required by an aging parent also comes at a highly inopportune time in the lives of many adult offspring. Most caretaking offspring are in middle age, a time which is itself rife with conflict (Sengstock & Liang, 1981; 1983). Men may be facing retirement and looking forward to a more leisurely lifestyle. Children may have left the home or at least have reached an age when they no longer need constant care. Middle-aged adults often reach the point where they no longer need to obtain sitters for their children, only to discover that their mobility is now limited by the necessity of finding someone to care for an aged parent in their absence.

As Steinmetz (1978) notes, elder abuse resembles child abuse in several ways, including the factor of total dependency as well as the existence of often severe financial, emotional, and physical stress for

the caretaker. With normal child care, however, parents can usually look forward to a not-too-distant day when the child will be independent. With care of an aged parent, however, caretakers must face ever-increasing dependence for periods of indeterminable duration. There is no relief in sight. Another problem stems from the fact that the caretaking task has usually fallen to the women (Sengstock, 1991), most of whom stayed at home. In recent years, however, the increased number of women who work outside the home, particularly after their children are in school, reduces the possibility that there will be middle-aged caretakers available in the family (Block & Sinnott, 1979). This caretaking period is also likely to fall at a time when the adult offsprings are themselves aging and may be in poor health (Sengstock, 1991; Sengstock & Liang, 1983).

For many middle-aged women, the pressures of parent care may place them in a "no-win" situation. They are caught between the needs of their aged parents and in-laws and those of their husbands and children. Their husbands may demand more adult time alone; their children are reaching the difficult teen years. Conversely, their time and energies are increasingly sapped by the growing needs of their aged parents. They may often be emotionally and physically unable to cope with both.

It is tempting to criticize middle-aged offspring for being thoughtless and unloving when they resist caring for an aged parent, or even worse, when the person under their care suffers neglect or abuse. These problems in the caretakers' lives are very real, however, and the problem of elder abuse is not likely to be resolved as long as there are inadequate supports for families dealing with such stresses (Sengstock, Barrett, & Graham, 1984).

Problems of intergenerational living

Several authorities have pointed out that intergenerational living can itself create stress that may precipitate abuse (Block & Sinnott, 1979; Burston, 1978; Renvoize, 1978). Even families maintaining positive relationships may undergo severe stress by the problems of constant daily contact. Adding an additional person to a household may create problems of crowding. Adult offspring and grandchildren may be forced to give up their privacy and alter their life-styles to accommodate an aged person's needs. Often the caretaking child feels that he or she was forced into having the aged parent in the home. Power conflicts are also likely to occur, as the members of each generation, with their differing views, express conflicting opinions over household maintenance, child care, and family activities.

It is tempting to suggest that a middle-aged offspring or grandchild who would resent making such adjustments in deference to a beloved parent or grandparent is thoughtless and unfeeling. However, it must be recognized that no one can maintain a totally selfless demeanor for an extended period of time. The needs of all persons in a multigenerational household must be accommodated for such a pattern to be successful on a long-term basis. Too often the supports necessary for such accommodations are unavailable to the families who require them. Such supports might include daycare centers for the aged, provisions for short-term care to afford a family an occasional vacation, as well as financial supports for families who assume the responsibility of in-home care of the aged.

Aging and long-standing family relationships

All the factors previously mentioned can create serious difficulties even for the most loving children who are anxious to provide the best of care for their aged relatives. It must be recognized, however, that many families do not resemble the image of the loving, harmonious family (Steinmetz & Straus, 1974). We have already pointed out that some elder abuse is actually an extension into old age of abusive and violent patterns that have existed in the family for years or even generations. It is also true that families who have managed to contain their conflict within bounds in earlier periods may be unable to continue to do so when faced with the problems of old age.

Children who have never had a good relationship with their parents may be able to avoid open conflict by maintaining a degree of social distance between the generations. The constant contact required by a caretaking relationship may destroy this fragile peace; conflict and possible abuse may result.

It has also been noted that some offspring never mature to the point of accepting their parents on an adult level. They are unable to accept the new role relationship in which their parents are no longer all-powerful and are increasingly dependent on their children (Block & Sinnott, 1979). The aged parent may also be unable to accept the altered role relationship, thus the adult status of their children, and may make constant, unreasonable demands and interfere with their adult children's lives and decisions.

Such parent-adult child relationships appear most likely to be involved in elder abuse. As noted earlier, some cases of elder abuse involve spouse abuse. Cases have already been discussed that represent a continuation of an extended abusive pattern. In some instances, however, the abuse may be precipitated by problems of aging. For example, a fragile marital relationship may be unable to survive the increased contact that accompanies retirement. Couples may also find that role reversal accompanies old age. Thus a husband who is accustomed to his wife handling all household tasks may be unable to deal with her becoming an invalid. Our study uncovered one case of severe neglect that involved a frail but proud old man whose invalid wife badly needed health care assistance, but her husband insisted they could care for themselves.

Such factors may often occur with cases of neglect of the aged, since the caretakers may themselves be aged and frail. It is not unknown for 80-or 90-year-old parents to depend totally on their 60-or 70-year-old offspring, who may be incapable of performing the tasks required for the care of the parents. To accuse a 70-year-old caretaker of neglect for failing to provide the health assistance needed by a bedridden parent or spouse may be highly unreasonable. Hence nursing interventions for an aged person must be planned with assurance that the family is capable of carrying out the plans without undue stress being produced

Loneliness of the single aged as a cause of abuse

When family abuse is discussed, the usual patterns include traditional family relationships: spouses, children, or less frequently, grandchildren, siblings, nieces, and nephews. However, the majority of older persons either live alone or with a spouse (Atchley, 1991). Although most have relatives nearby to help them, some may find themselves without family on whom they can rely. Hence they may be willing to trust a friendly outsider who offers assistance, perhaps more willing than might be altogether prudent. There are many reports on the fear of crime that pervades the aged population (Midwest Research Institute, 1977; Sundeen & Mathieu, 1976). Therefore the elderly might be expected to be extremely cautious in admitting unknown persons to their homes. On occasion, however, aged persons may be less cautious, often with sad results.

In the study by Sengstock and Liang (1982), one case involved a stroke victim, who was unable to remain alone after her return from the hospital. She and her family arranged for a homemaking service agency to provide care in her home; as the cost became prohibitive, they accepted the offer of a distant relative to come into the home and provide this service at a lesser cost. Unknown to the family, the willing housekeeper was a drug addict. She was extremely abusive to the aged lady, screaming at her and refusing to assist her in going to the bathroom or the bedroom, even attacking her physically. Another aged woman took in a boarder who was presumed to be a good risk; however, she kept late hours and was loud, making it difficult for the elderly landlady to sleep. After being asked to move, she refused and the lady had to seek legal assistance to remove the boarder from the house.

Another situation that portends abuse is the lifestyle of the aged single male. Whether widowed, divorced, or never married, these men often find that their ability to attract women has drastically decreased, yet they still have the same sexual needs and desire for female companionship. As a result they often place themselves in situations in which they can easily be taken advantage of by younger women, who promise companionship and sexual favors and then abuse them, usually by stealing money. Such instances make it clear that aged persons should exercise caution before taking anyone into their home or their confidence. With family and

close friends, they are likely to have at least an inkling of the person's behavior patterns and the likelihood of risk. With strangers, they often know nothing about the risk until it is too late.

A New Question: Is It Elder Abuse or Poor Case Management?

As indicated in the introduction to this chapter, some experts question the consideration of elder abuse as a type of family violence. In contrast, they view mistreatment of the elderly as a problem in the management of their care. Their arguments are presented in three major areas, involving the types of elder abuse that have generally been included in the concept of "elder abuse," the relative frequency of each type, and the identity and intentions of the alleged "perpetrator." As discussed, the term "elder abuse" clearly refers to a wider range of behaviors than either child abuse or spouse abuse. Psychological abuse and neglect, for example, are not usually part of the definition of spouse abuse, which is usually confined to direct physical assault (Pagelow, 1984). Similarly, concerns about spouse abuse do not usually focus on the theft or misuse of the victim's property or the violation of the victim's rights, although both might occur with spouse abuse. Hence a major difference between elder abuse and spouse abuse consists of the fact that elder abuse tends to include a wider range of acts against the victim.

In some ways elder abuse appears to be more similar to child abuse than to spouse abuse, since elder abuse includes neglect, which is more appropriate to child abuse definitions (Pagelow, 1984). However, there are still some major differences between elder abuse and child abuse. Reference to financial abuse of children is rare because they, in contrast with the elderly, are unlikely to have substantial amounts of money or property for others to appropriate or misuse (Quinn & Tomita, 1986).

Perhaps the most significant difference between children and the elderly, however, lies in the fact that the elderly are adults and entitled to the rights of adults (Quinn & Tomita, 1986: 78). Unless mentally impaired, they are entitled to make choices with regard to their lives and cannot be forced to alter their lifestyles without their consent. This is an important reason for distinguishing between elder abuse and child abuse, since elders, unlike children, cannot simply be removed from a dangerous home situation if it is one in which they choose to remain (Quinn & Tomita, 1986).

Consequently, the first major area in which elder abuse differs from other categories of family abuse is that categories of behavior that have been included in definitions of elder abuse are considerably broader in range than those included in either spouse or child abuse. Furthermore, there is some question regarding whether the apparently similar categories are truly equivalent: for example, neglect is a different type of behavior when directed against a child versus a dependent adult.

Not only are the categories of abuse used with the elderly different from those used with spouse and child abuse, the relative frequency within each category is also different. As indicated previously, the major behavior associated with spouse abuse is physical assault, whereas child "abuse" can include both assault and neglect. With elder abuse, there has been considerable debate about the relative frequency of the different types of abuse; the most frequent type varies considerably from study to study (Block & Sinnott, 1979; Lau & Kosberg, 1979; Sengstock & Liang, 1983).

Those who believe that elder abuse should be viewed as a case management problem refer to several studies that indicate the major category of elder abuse to be neglect directed against a dependent elder (Douglass, 1988; Fulmer & Ashley, 1989). Consequently, they suggest that, unlike the beaten spouse or child, these elders are not injured by deliberate physical assaults but by the nondeliberate actions of inept or inadequate caregivers.

The fact that a considerable amount of elder "abuse" is actually neglect suggests the need to consider the identity and intentions of the alleged abuser. Who is the individual responsible for the alleged "abuse" of the elder? What are his/her intentions? Is the action deliberate or not? These are some of the questions with which elder abuse experts grapple.

Elder abuse experts point out that an examination of cases, particularly of elder neglect, often reveals that no single individual can be clearly identified as the "abuser." Many dependent elderly persons, particularly older women who have never married, have no close relatives to care for them (Grambs, 1989). Even in cases where there are offspring or other relatives who could provide assistance, elder care is not like child care. Although parents are required to care for their children and can be charged with neglect for failing to do so, there is still considerable debate about whether family members, even sons and daughters, should be forced to assume the care of an aged relative, and clear public policy in this area is lacking (Verma & Haviland, 1988). In addition, some elder neglect cases are actually cases of *self*-neglect (Quinn & Tomita, 1986). These are not elders living at the mercy of others, but persons who have chosen to neglect themselves—not providing themselves with sufficient food, clothing, or medicine. These cases clearly are different from both child and spouse abuse and cannot be included in a typology of "family warfare."

Even if the category of self-neglect is omitted, the alleged perpetrators of elder abuse are still considerably broader than those of child or spouse abuse. The popular image of "elder abuse" tends to assume that the adult offspring of the elder is the usual abuser (Block & Sinnott, 1979; Lau & Kosberg, 1979). As indicated, however, perpetrators may include other persons as well (Sengstock & Liang, 1983).

Some elder abuse analysts argue that only those cases of abuse or neglect that have originated in old age should be included in the category of elder abuse. For example, Douglass (1988) excludes cases of spouse abuse that have existed for many years, contending that "Husbands or wives who have been abusive through long marriages are not likely to change their behavior at age 60 or 65" (p. 3). Apparently these analysts believe that only those cases of abuse that are of recent origin are amenable to the types of remedies that can be used with elder abuse; consequently, cases that do not fit this model should be excluded from the category.

An advantage of this approach is that it excludes those cases most likely to be problematic for the theoretical model. The case management model of elder abuse is largely based on those cases that constitute neglect of a dependent elder. Cases of direct, intentional assault, or cases in which violent behavior patterns are a long-standing family norm obviously do not fit this model. Defining them out of the universe is a convenient way of reinforcing the strength of the case management model.

Finally, the intention of the alleged abuser constitutes another factor used to justify separating elder abuse from other forms of domestic abuse. Proponents argue that much elder abuse is actually neglect and beyond the control of the abuser; hence it is not really deliberate abuse. It may result from inadequate training or a physical or mental inability to provide the needed care (Douglass, 1988). In any event, they contend that it does not represent a deliberate attempt of the caregiver to injure the victim. Those who use this argument do not deal with the issue that similar factors—inadequate preparation for caregiving and the lack of a deliberate intention to injure—are often raised with regard to child abusers as well; yet child abuse continues to be considered a category of domestic abuse.

In summary, proponents of the view that elder abuse is a problem in the case management of elderly victims tend to focus on issues related to the types and frequency of abuse and on the identity and intentions of the alleged perpetrator. Elder abuse analysts who use this approach point out that elder abuse has covered a wider variety of mistreatment than either spouse abuse or child abuse, including psychological abuse and neglect, material abuse, violation of personal rights, neglect of an elder's needs, as well as the direct assault included in other categories of family violence. Furthermore, their studies indicate that neglect, rather than direct assault, is the most common type of mistreatment of the elderly.

In addition, it is noted that the elderly are not in the position of other victims of family violence. Unlike children, for whom parents can automatically be held responsible, there often is no specific party who can be held responsible for care of an elder.

Even when there is a designated caregiver who is not performing her or his duties adequately, this neglect often is not deliberate. Moreover, the individual responsible for the neglectful actions may often be the elder himself or herself.

For all of these reasons, proponents of this point of view suggest that elder abuse is a misdefined problem. They contend that it is not a category of domestic assault, but rather a problem in the management of the care of dependent elderly. These views are often offered by persons responsible for providing care or services to elderly victims of mistreatment—social workers, nurses, and analysts who research the care needs of these victims (O'Malley, 1986; Phillips, 1988).

From their point of view, it is easy to understand why they concentrate on the differences between the needs of elderly victims of neglect or poor care management and needs of the child or adult victims of direct assault. Whereas the latter may require legal assistance or police protection, the former may best be served by changing care plans or providing more adequate training and respite to the caregiver.

If proponents of the case management approach tend to focus on the most frequent types of maltreatment in cases of elder abuse, proponents of the domestic assault model of elder abuse are more likely to focus on the wide variety of mistreatment found among elders known to be victims of abuse. Focusing on the needs of the victims of passive neglect, even if it is assumed they are the most numerous of the victims of elder abuse, fails to deal with the needs of those elders who are victims of other types of elder abuse and neglect.

Proponents of the domestic violence model are also more likely to focus on the process of identifying elderly victims of abuse, a process that uses symptoms that do not always easily distinguish abuse types early in the identification process. They also emphasize that elderly victims of all types of abuse and neglect may require some of the same types of services. Among these services are those available only through agencies developed in response to the needs of family violence victims. In short, they contend that elderly abuse victims are best served if it is initially assumed that they are victims of family abuse rather than of simple errors in case management.

Obviously the pragmatic consequences of this debate are not insignificant. On its outcome rest the nature—even the existence—of services to aged victims of maltreatment, by whatever name it is called. This controversy has led one analyst to call elder abuse " . . . a dying non-issue whose time has passed" (Callaghan, 1986, p. 2). If this position prevails, then services for elderly victims are almost certain to disappear within a short time.

Needs and demands for assistance always exceed the supply, especially in today's era of budget-cutting fervor (Cravedi, 1986). Politicians have more demands for public services than they can supply. Hence they are only too ready to cut programs that can be shown to be unnecessary. This is more likely when the supposed "experts" present contradictory views (Cravedi, 1986).

Theories of Elder Abuse as Clinical Indicators

There is no clear theory that has been indisputably established as an explanation for the existence of elder abuse. The theoretical positions that have been proposed remain largely hypotheses. However, as noted earlier, these theories may serve as valuable indicators of the likelihood of abuse. Aged persons who exhibit, or whose families exhibit, any of the characteristics listed are persons whose associates or living arrangements place them in considerable danger of being abused physically or emotionally, severely neglected, or placed in a position of extreme financial disadvantage. They may need help greatly and may not know of any alternative to their present situation. Because of the greater health needs of the aged, they may have contact with nurses more than with most other professionals. The factors suggested by theories of domestic abuse provide symptoms that can help to identify those aged who may need such help.

Because the same family patterns affect young and old alike, some explanations of domestic violence in general are equally applicable to elder abuse. Hence some aged appear to be abused be-cause they have the misfortune to be associated with family members who have severe psychological or emotional problems, lending support to abuser-focused theories. The situational stress theory appears promising because a substantial number of aged abuse victims come from families that have an unusually large number of serious family problems. Support can also be found for the view that elder abuse occurs in families having a long-term, well-established behavior pattern in which violence and abuse play an accepted role.

Authorities have also noted, however, that certain social correlates of the aging process play a special role in the development of the types of family tension that may lead to elder abuse. The increased life expectancy of the aged, with its escalating years of dependency and burgeoning health care costs, places an ever-increasing burden on fewer and fewer children for a longer period of time. Such tensions often place severe stress on families already strained by crises of middle age or tenuous family ties. Steps in preventing elder abuse must recognize the legitimacy of such family needs. Proposed solutions should include the means to relieve the tensions of the caregiving family if elder abuse is to be halted or avoided.

MEANS USED BY AGENCIES IN IDENTIFYING AND SERVING ABUSED AGED

One major problem encountered in providing services to victims of elder abuse is the identification of victims. Services cannot be provided until agencies become aware of the persons in need of help. And abused elders, like other victims of family abuse, are very difficult to identify.

Most studies have suggested that abuse of the elderly is probably greatly underreported (Douglass et al., 1980; Hickey & Douglass, 1981a, 1981b). The reasons for this include both a reluctance on the part of victims to report their abuse and hesitance on the part of official agencies to invade the privacy of the home. It has been noted that victims of domestic violence are more reluctant to report their victimization than other victims. One commonly recognized reason is that people are embarrassed to admit that their own families depart from the presumed norm of family harmony and love (Gelles, 1974; Steinmetz & Straus, 1974). An admission of family violence suggests a failure in oneself for not having achieved the ideal of family harmony. Thus a battered elder may feel that he or she has failed by having raised an abusive child. Desires to maintain the family's reputation and avoid embarrassment may also serve as considerations that lead the abused person not to report the abuse to a professional (Lau & Kosberg, 1979).

Another reason for the victim's reluctance to report domestic abuse is their fear of reprisals from the abuser. Such reprisals may involve further threats of violence, loss of support, or both. Domestic abuse victims are often dependent on their abusers. As Gelles has pointed out, victims of domestic violence have "no place to go" where they can be free of the threat of further abuse (1974; p. 93). Such fears are commonly mentioned by abused wives as the reasons they do not report the abuse (Michigan Women's Commission, 1977). The fear of reprisal is also mentioned as a reason for nonreporting of elder abuse (Douglass et al., 1980; Hickey & Douglass, 1981a, 1981b). Dependence of the victim on the abuser is another factor (Block & Sinnott, 1979). It also has been pointed out that many elderly decline to report the abuse because they fear the loss of the relationship with the abuser, who may be a beloved child and perhaps their closest remaining relative (Douglass et al., 1980; Hickey & Douglass, 1981a, 1981b).

Many elderly victims are also reluctant to turn to professional agencies because they lack knowledge or have fear of the agencies themselves. Disorientation, senility, or a simple lack of knowledge concerning available services may render a victim incapable of reporting his or her abuse (Lau & Kosberg, 1979). Those victims who are aware of available resources may still resist reporting the abuse because they feel incapable of coping with the responsibilities that may ensue if they do report (Lau & Kosberg, 1979). Possible court appearances or conversations with the police can be fear-provoking experiences in themselves (Sengstock & Hwalek, 1986c).

For all of these reasons, some abuse victims are so reluctant to deal with the abuse that they refuse professional help even if it is offered (Lau & Kosberg, 1979). Hence dealing with elder abuse is a task that requires great care and tact. Block and Sinnott (1979) suggest that civil rather than criminal means are more appropriate for dealing with elder abuse. One reason is the lesser stigma that attaches to such a judgment, allowing both offender and victim to deal with the problem more easily.

This reluctance of victims to report abuse is especially serious because most agencies depend at least partially on victims' reports to identify victims. In a survey of 108 agencies, 16 of 25 agencies seeking elder abuse noted that a client report was at least one of the means by which the abusive situation was identified (Sengstock & Barrett, 1981). Others learned of the abuse through a report from another agency, including the police. Few actually observed physical symptoms such as cuts and bruises. Other means of identifying abused elders included symptoms of neglect such as malnourishment in an elder not living alone and reports from family members, neighbors, and friends. Dentists were particularly mentioned by some agencies as a source of referral.

There is great variability among agencies and workers in their ability to identify abuse. In the study by Sengstock and Liang, the largest number of cases was reported by a legal aid agency, which reported 30 cases, or nearly 40% of the total (Sengstock & Liang, 1983; Sengstock & Barrett; 1982, 1986). There are two reasons for this prevalence. First, a legal aid agency would be very likely to be consulted by persons with serious physical and/or financial abuse in an effort to deal with the problem. Second, it was quite clear that two workers in this agency were very concerned about the abuse, to the extent of rereading old case records to make accurate reports on the cases. This agency vividly illustrates the fact that agency service to elderly abuse victims is quite dependent on two factors: the nature of the agency and the interest of the individual worker.

Many agencies have developed their own techniques for the identification of elderly victims of abuse. These include clinical techniques for use in hospitals and agencies, procedures for use in state protective service departments, and measures for use in research (Sengstock & Hwalek, 1985-86, 1987; Sengstock, Hwalek, & Moshier, 1986). Early measures had numerous flaws, including the inclusion of items that measured more than one type of abuse, requiring observers to make multiple judgments, such as determining the presence of abuse as well as the deliberateness of the act and omitting some types of abuse, particularly sexual assault (Sengstock & Hwalek, 1985-86). Measures include short protocols to identify persons at risk (Hwalek & Sengstock, 1986; Neale, Hwalek, Scott, Sengstock & Stahl, 1991), as well as comprehensive measures designed to document symptoms of various types of abuse, the degree of intentionality of the abuser, and possible service needs of victims (Sengstock & Hwalek, 1986a, 1986b). The validity of such measures is still under study.

The abuse of elders confined to institutions, such as nursing homes and long-term care facilities, is also an area of concern (Select Committee, 1985). Although this is a widely discussed problem, empirical research on the subject is limited and frequently low in quality (Bragg et al., 1978-79; Himmelstein et al., 1983; Kimsey et al., 1981). Identification is a particularly critical problem with this group, because they often are fearful of retaliation if they report abuse, and they may also be unaware of their rights or physically or mentally incapable of protecting themselves (Kimsey et al., 1981). One measure has been adapted for use with this population (Sengstock & Hwalek, 1986; Sengstock, McFarland & Hwalek, 1990).

Agency Type and the Observation of Abuse

As noted earlier, there is some indication that agencies are more likely to observe abuse in the area they are accustomed to treating (Douglass et al., 1980; Hickey & Douglass, 1981a, 1981b). Physical abuse is more frequently observed by health-related agencies since they would be called on to treat the resulting injuries and are accustomed to observing such symptoms (Sengstock & Liang, 1982; 1983). Physical neglect, on the other hand, is more likely to be observed by senior service agencies, which are often called on to assist aged persons who need food, shelter, or housekeeping assistance, all of which may be related to neglect. In contrast, financial abuse and direct emotional abuse are more likely to be identified by legal aid agencies, since victims would be likely to bring such problems to an attorney. Persons who believe they have been cheated out of money or property are likely to seek a lawyer to regain what they believe is rightfully theirs. Seeking aid from an attorney also seems appropriate when the victim of verbal assault fears for his or her safety. In fact, the legal aid agencies appear to be highly promising as a mechanism for identifying elder abuse cases of all types, particularly those that involve direct action (for example, abuse as opposed to neglect). The legal aid attorney has the opportunity to interview a client and elicit information concerning all aspects of life, thus making it possible to uncover symptoms of abuse in all areas. Recognizing this, the Federal Administration of Aging has made the identification of elder abuse a priority for agencies providing legal aid to the elderly ("Elder Abuse," 1981). It is not known, however, how budget cuts will affect this or other services for abuse victims.

Identification of elder abuse victims is complicated by the fact that agencies are focused to "notice" only symptoms that characterize the problems treated by that agency. Thus hospitals are likely to observe physical abuse, but may miss psychological or financial abuse. Social agencies are more likely to observe psychological abuse and may learn of physical abuse only by reports of the victim or particularly obvious symptoms. It seems that more abuse would be uncovered if agencies that serve the aged became more aware of the symptoms of abuse other than those that their agency is used to observing.

Services Provided to Victims

Even if an abused victim decides to report the experience to some authority, it is not clear that he or she will receive any assistance in dealing with the matter. Thus Block and Sinnott found that although 95% of their sample reported their victimization, no victim received assistance (Block & Sinnott, 1979). This is similar to the pattern that appears with most domestic abuse. A tendency to "accept-and-hide" domestic violence has been encouraged by society as a whole, from friends and relatives of the violent family to official agencies. Wife abuse victims are often encouraged by their families to accept the situation (Michigan Women's Commission, 1977). Medical practitioners, who are most likely to see evidence of serious violence, often try to avoid dealing with domestic abuse, both of children (Kempe et al., 1966) and adults (Law Enforcement Assistance Administration, 1977). Police and the courts, normally the avenue of redress for the victim of criminal assault and/or civil injury, have largely ignored domestic assaults (Field & Field, 1973; Gelles, 1977; Truninger, 1971). This is due partly to the belief that such things are best left a private matter and partly to the recognition that domestic disturbance calls can be dangerous for the police (Calvert, 1974; Straus et al., 1980).

Few communities have developed special services specifically targeted at victims of elder abuse or neglect. Rather, victims tend to receive the types of services that are available to other elders in the community, although they may receive varying types of services depending on the type of abuse and other characteristics of the victims. In one study, clients who were victims of self-neglect received more services than victims of abuse or neglect by someone else (Sengstock, Hwalek, & Stahl, 1989). This suggests that service workers are still unfamiliar with direct abuse cases; consequently, they concentrate on those cases with which they are more familiar and over which they have more control.

Research has suggested a variety of services from which elderly victims of abuse or neglect could benefit. Noncriminal approaches to such domestic problems are usually recommended (Block & Sinnott, 1979). Other services recommended are in-home social work (Kinderknect, 1986); legal assistance (Sengstock & Barrett, 1986); in-patient psychiatric services (Lau, 1986); and crisis intervention, counseling, and support services for both the victim and the family (Kinney et al., 1986). However, it has also been noted that traditional counseling agencies have not dealt effectively with family violence. Marriage counselors and social workers often encourage the maintenance of family ties, even violent ones (Michigan Women's

Commission, 1977). Conflicting advice is also given. Thus some counselors encourage the open expression of aggressive feelings to vent them in appropriate channels (Steinmetz & Straus, 1974), whereas others believe that expressed hostility can generate even more aggressive feelings (Bandura & Walters, 1974; Berkowitz, 1973). Referral to other agencies for such diverse assistance is a common type of solution, but workers often cannot determine whether their assistance has improved the situation (Sengstock & Liang, 1982; 1983).

Service providers should also distinguish between services that must be provided immediately and those that should occur on a longer-term basis. The former category includes obtaining treatment for injuries and removing the victim and his/her assets from the control of the abuser (Quinn & Tomita, 1986). Experienced professionals suggest that long-term care management or monitoring is particularly useful in abuse cases, as are strategies to reduce caregiver stress; it may also be necessary to alter the living arrangements of the victim (Haviland & O'Brien, 1989; Quinn & Tomita, 1986). In general, the elderly abuse victim requires a wide variety of services, and these should be integrated into a comprehensive, unified whole (Conley, 1986; Wolf, Halas, Green & McNiff, 1985-86; Wolf, Strugnel, & Godkin, 1982).

A major complication in resolving the problem of elder abuse results from the lack of available services that may be needed by the victim. For example, police protection has been found to be unavailable to many victims (Sengstock & Hwalek, 1986c). Funding mechanisms often exclude certain types of services or make them available only after a determination of need, and some services are simply not available in many communities (Kinderknect, 1986). Service provision is often complicated by agency fragmentation (Emlet, 1984). Many service providers, trained before the recognition of the problem of elder abuse, still lack training or experience in dealing with this problem. This is especially difficult for new workers or those who handle only an occasional case of elder abuse.

In an effort to improve services to elderly victims and their families, some social and governmental agencies have developed new models for service delivery (Traxler, 1986). The value of such changes is unclear. In some instances, new models have resulted in improved services (Emlet, 1984); however, in others their initial promise has not been constant over time (Kallen, 1984). One study, of three different models of service provision for elder abuse victims found little difference in service provision based on the type of program, but suggested the variation was more related to characteristics of the victim, professional background of the worker, the type of services in which the agency specialized, or the resources more prominent in the community (Sengstock et al., 1990). Services were also found to be related to the type of abuse suffered (Sengstock, Hwalek, & Petrone, 1989).

Interest of the Individual Professional

One clear problem is the uneven quality of service provided to abuse victims by different agencies (Sengstock & Liang, 1982). Some medical institutions were quite likely to observe abuse while others avoided the problem; religious institutions were mentioned by some victims as being unsympathetic, yet some churches were quite concerned about the problem. Clearly a major factor in generating effective service for abused elders is a high degree of personal concern and interest on the part of the specific professional assigned to the case. It was not enough for the agency to have a general policy of helping abused victims because individual professionals could avoid the problem if they wished. Conversely, some providers in agencies with an apparent disinterest in the problem appeared to be among the most helpful, spending much time and effort to unravel the bureaucratic red tape impeding effective service to the abuse victims.

Hence certain professionals in an agency are more likely to develop an interest in the area of domestic abuse and to search for this problem among their clients. One might say these professionals have had their "consciousness raised" regarding the problem of domestic abuse. Consequently, they inquire about the family situation and are more likely to learn of abuse if it exists. Furthermore, agency providers in personal conversations told us that family abuse was a problem that was not likely to be uncovered easily. Rather, a substantial number of visits and a considerable rapport had to be developed with a client before most clients were willing to discuss family abuse. The professions represented by the reporters of abuse vary widely. They include legal aid attorneys, social workers, staff workers of senior centers, nurses, psychologists or counselors, and religious workers (Sengstock & Liang, 1982; 1983).

Finally, it should be mentioned that some professionals, and some agencies as well, have difficulty dealing with family abuse because of a preference for viewing the topic as a "private matter," an approach often taken with regard to child or spouse abuse. This is particularly common with elder abuse because adults are seen to have the right to make decisions on their own. Consequently, some service providers hesitate to suggest alternate living arrangements or services, fearing they will intrude into the elder's personal affairs. The result, however, is that they feel no obligation to suggest possible alternatives of which aged victims may be unaware. Therefore the abuse victim sees no alternative to accepting the abuse.

Need for Further Research and Planning

As a consequence, domestic abuse has been greatly neglected by service providers. This is true of child and spouse abuse as well as elder abuse. As Block and Sinnott (1979) point out, strategies of intervention must be developed primarily to end the abuse, but secondarily to help in establishing the physical and mental well-being of the entire family. As noted earlier, usually the abuser is also a person with severe problems that must be solved before the abuse can be stopped. For most abused elders, severance of the abusive relationship is not viewed as a desirable alternative (Douglass et al., 1980; Hickey & Douglass, 1981a, 1981b). Further research is necessary to determine the needs of aged abuse victims and the most appropriate ways to provide for them.

It has been suggested that the problems of providing care for aging family members are likely to become more severe in future years. As Block and Sinnott (1979) point out:

Decreasing fertility and mortality rates mean that there will be more older persons and fewer children available as possible caretakers. The adult child may be faced with as many as two sets of grandparents to care for as well as aging parents. (p. 93)

The emotional, physical, and financial resources of such caretaking offspring are depleted quickly, leading to resentment against the aged relatives perceived to have caused the difficulty. In such settings an increased possibility of abuse is directed against the aged requiring the care. Increased support for elders and their caretaking families is necessary if such abuse is to be avoided (Block & Sinnott, 1979).

The disagreements and conflicts between professionals and agencies concerning the definition and conceptualization of elder abuse also do considerable harm to elders and their families. As indicated earlier, these differences in conceptualization and terminology may be significant. They have consequences, not only in the manner in which the problem is viewed by researchers, but also in its perception by policy makers, who are annoyed by the absence of clear terminology and program perspectives (Callaghan, 1986). There are long-term consequences for the many competing programs that serve victims of elder abuse. If viewed as an "abuse" problem, then legal and victim assistance agencies may receive additional resources to assist elders; if viewed as a problem of "care management," then health and home service agencies can claim the need for added resources to deal with the problem. Consequently, there is likely to be considerable competition among agencies to claim expertise in the definition of the problem. This is particularly true in light of the controversy between the case management and domestic violence models of elder abuse. The status quo in social services for elderly abuse victims tends to follow a family violence model. If this model continues to prevail, it is likely that social services for aged victims will remain in much the same form as at present.

If the family violence model prevails, Adult Protective Services (APS) would continue to remain a central focus of a service plan. The likelihood of hidden abuse and the need to develop methods of identifying victims would continue to be an important part of the assistance process. Services would largely be channeled through APS, with referrals to a variety of agencies and service types, including legal assistance, police involvement, and the possibility of shelter, as well as more traditional medical and social services. The services required in each case would vary considerably, depending on the type of abuse, the identity of the abuser, the degree of intentionality, etc.

In contrast, if the care management model replaces the existing approach, drastic changes in services for the aged are likely. Adult Protective Services would be de-emphasized, since the care management model does not assume an adversarial relationship between victim and abuser. So-called abusers are actually well-meaning caregivers who will be quite willing—even anxious—to learn and adopt more effective methods of providing care. Consequently, there is no need for such programs as legal assistance, protective intervention, or temporary shelter.

Conversely, other services would be introduced or emphasized. These would largely involve services to assist caregivers in managing their roles more effectively. Examples are training programs for caregivers, in-home assistance programs to supervise the care process and monitor the patients' progress, and programs to provide respite for overburdened caregivers. Many of these services are now in short supply (Anetzberger, 1989; Cravedi, 1986).

The advantage of the case management model is obvious. The services it would emphasize are sorely needed by many elderly victims and their caregivers, particularly victims of passive neglect, on which the model is based. Because these are a major, if not *the* major category of elderly victims of abuse, the model would encourage the establishment of the most effective services to a category of victims now being inadequately served (Phillips, 1988). The disadvantage of the model is also obvious. By its unitary focus on a single type of elder abuse, albeit a common one, the model would eliminate services to elderly victims of abuse that are not included in the model of inadequate but well-meaning care. Since these victims, however few in number, may be in mortal danger and in greatest need of intervention, the omission portends dire and formidable consequences.

SUGGESTED NURSING CARE FOR ELDER ABUSE VICTIMS

As seen in this chapter, abuse of the elderly is a topic that has only recently received attention from researchers and service providers. Because of the relative "newness" of the area, research on elder abuse is limited in several respects. With one exception (Pillemer & Finkelhor, 1988), most samples are small and are purposive rather than random. All studies are exploratory in nature, concentrating on the development of hypotheses rather than on the testing of theories in existence (Phillips, 1983a). These limitations make it difficult to generate an accurate estimate of the extent and characteristics of elder abuse. Consequently, the suggestions made in this section must be viewed as tentative. It is fairly certain that the description of possible symptomatology is representative of elder abuse cases studied to date. The presented at-risk indicators may require revision, however, when more knowledge has been accumulated in this area.

Assessment

Obtaining an accurate assessment of abuse in an elderly client requires that the nurse overcome a number of formidable obstacles (Fulmer & Cahill, 1984; Phillips & Rempusheski, 1985). These include the reluctance of the victim to reveal an abusive experience; the necessity of developing a strong, trusting relationship before abuse can be identified; the absence of clearly defined symptomatology for elder abuse; the difficulty of distinguishing symptoms of elder abuse from the normal symptoms of aging; and the values held by the health care provider regarding abuse. In this section these difficulties, together with possible remedies, are discussed.

Reluctance of victims to report

The reluctance of abuse victims to report abuse and the reasons for this reluctance have been noted pre-

viously. Victims often fear retaliation from the abuser, loss of support, or loss of their relationship with loved ones. They may also feel guilt or shame if they have raised children who are abusive or have maintained close social and/or familial ties with abusive relatives. They are unwilling to admit the presence of an abusive situation to someone perceived to be an authority because they fear the possible consequences of such a report. Some elderly victims of rather severe abuse cannot admit even to themselves that a beloved relative would abuse them. Such victims are therefore incapable of reporting the abuse, since they are not really aware that abuse is occurring.

Developing trust

Such reluctance to admit abuse may be overcome if the nurse carefully develops a trusting relationship with the client. A client is not likely to admit abuse unless he or she feels that the nurse is accepting and does not present a threat to the client's well-being. Victims must believe that the nurse does not judge them for being in or remaining in an abusive situation. They must also believe that the nurse has a genuine desire to help them and will not reveal their difficulty to authorities against their will. Consequently, any aged patient with a possible vulnerability toward abuse must be approached by the nurse in a holistic and nonthreatening manner. In addition, it is preferable that the same nurse care for the patient to facilitate the development of such a relationship.

Particularly with short-term clients, it may be difficult to develop the degree of trust necessary in the nurse-client relationship to obtain an accurate patient assessment. Professionals interviewed by Sengstock and Barrett (1982) often stated that an abusive situation was not uncovered until the professional and client had established a long-term, trusting relationship. Many of the service providers expressed concern that abuse might be overlooked when the client required only short-term intervention or presented at-risk indicators that were unfamiliar to the practitioner.

This problem questions the idea that high-risk versus low-risk victim profiles can accurately assess the presence or absence of abuse, based on short-term intervention (i.e., one or two visits). Although it has been suggested that nurses initially attempt to identify high-risk victim profiles before proceeding with an in-depth assessment (Hirst & Miller, 1986), researchers focusing on the area of family violence have noted that an abuse victim may not readily offer information concerning the abuse until the latter part of a lengthy assessment (Sengstock & Barrett, 1981). Consequently, presenting factors during a short-term contact may not provide the practitioner with definitive criteria indicating the need to probe further regarding the existence of abuse.

Identification of abuse as a two-step process

Because of the difficulty of obtaining an admission of abuse, it is often the nurse's responsibility to identify a victim of elder abuse by observing presenting at-risk findings. Unfortunately, the identification of abuse is still an uncertain process. Existing procedures are still in the process of being verified (Hwalek & Sengstock, 1986; Neale et al., 1991). Although lists of indicators have been developed, there is no set of factors that can clearly identify elder abuse in the absence of other verifying evidence (Fulmer, 1989). Consequently, the identification of elderly abuse victims should be viewed as a two-step process in which at-risk individuals are first identified for special attention, and then the actual existence of abuse or neglect is verified through a more intensive examination of symptoms and case history.

Identifying at-risk elders. The first step in the identification of abused elders is distinguishing elders who are at greatest risk of being abused. In the identification of an at-risk population, the nurse should be inclusive rather than risk eliminating any possible victims. Although no measure has yet been proven successful in establishing at-risk factors, two points may be made in this regard.

First, certain characteristics of the elderly place them in a situation of extreme dependence on others. Any elder who is incapable of providing for his or her own daily needs and is dependent on another person or persons for assistance is automatically in an at-risk situation. Consequently, persons who are mentally or physically incapacitated should always

be considered at high risk, and further evaluation should take place, as described in the second step of the process. As indicated previously, *this is only an indication of risk, not abuse;* and care should be taken to ensure that a premature diagnosis of abuse not be imputed, to the embarrassment of all.

Second, elders who are fully competent and exhibit no signs of abuse should be questioned to determine whether they too may be at risk. Nurses must develop an ability to question clients about issues such as abuse or neglect in a open and accepting manner, so that the client may feel free to indicate the existence of activity about which he or she might otherwise feel embarrassment or shame. Only the nurse's accepting demeanor can indicate that she or he has heard of such cases in the past and will not be shocked by the revelation. Some techniques for such questioning can be indicated. For example, the nurse may ask an elderly client to "describe a typical day" in his or her life. In the process of describing such a day, the client may reveal that he or she is left alone for long periods or is fearful of the behaviors of other family members.

Direct questioning is also important. Clients should be directly asked if they have been struck, ridiculed, or had money stolen from them. If the nurse is open and accepting of the responses, elders will feel free to answer such questions. The "Hwalek-Sengstock Elder Abuse Screening Test" (H-S/EAST) has been developed to assist in screening elders for at-risk responses (Hwalek & Sengstock, 1986; Neale et al., 1991). This instrument is still in the process of testing and cannot be depended on as the only screening instrument, but it does provide a useful set of questions. The complete H-S/EAST consists of 15 items, with two subsets, consisting of nine and six items respectively, being tested separately. Table 7-1 provides a list of the six-item subset, together with an indication of the at-risk response for each. These items may serve as an indication of questions that might be used in interviewing elders to determine their risk for abuse or neglect.

Verification of abuse. Clients believed to be at risk should be further observed for other possible indicators of abuse. This leads to the second step in the

TABLE 7-1
Sample Questions From the Six-Item Hwalek-Sengstock Elder Abuse Screening Test (H-S/EAST)

H-S/EAST ITEM	AT-RISK RESPONSE
4. "Decisions" Who makes decisions about your life—like how you should live or where you should live?	"Someone else"
5. "Uncomfortable" Do you feel uncomfortable with anyone in your family?	"Yes"
7. "Unwanted" Do you feel that nobody wants you around?	"Yes"
10. "Being Forced" Has anyone forced you to do things you didn't want to do?	"Yes"
13. "Annoyance" Does anyone tell you that you give them too much trouble?	"Yes"
15. "Hurt/Harmed" Has anyone close to you tried to hurt you or harm you recently?	"Yes"

From Hwalek and Sengstock, 1986, p. 169; Neale et al., 1991, pp. 409, 415.

process, in which the nurse should verify the existence of abuse through the documentation of specific symptoms as well as the collection of other evidence. These characteristics can be divided into two categories: symptoms that can be determined by an examination of the patient, and characteristics that can be identified in a client's case history.

Table 7-2 lists a number of indicators that can be found in an examination of a client and that may suggest abuse. Caution must still be exercised at this point, however, since any single factor, taken as an independent entity, may not support the suspicion that the client is being victimized by family, friends, or both. For example, absence of a prosthetic device or inappropriate dress may indicate a problem in care of the elder; such a factor alone, however, does not verify the existence of abuse. Even fractures or extensive bruising, taken alone, may not be clear indicators of abuse.

Because there are no clear physical indicators of elder abuse, the nurse may often find that a victim of abuse must be identified on the basis of a configuration of symptoms, derived from the physical examination as well as the client's case history (Fulmer & Wetle, 1986; Jones, Dougherty, Scheible, & Cunningham, 1988). Hence extensive bruising or an appearance of malnourishment alone may not indicate abuse, but these findings, coupled with the nurse's observation of other indicators, such as overt antagonism between the client and family or friends, may lead to a suspicion of abuse.

Consequently, it is imperative that the nurse obtain a thorough case history of a client when abuse is a possible cause of the findings. A thorough assessment includes an overview of the physical, social, and psychological characteristics of the elder and his or her significant others, especially those on whom the supposed victim is dependent. Relevant factors in the case history are outlined in Table 7-3. Since it is recognized that this depth of information is often impossible to obtain, it is imperative that the nurse be prepared to obtain much of the assessment data from objective observations of the client and the client's family, social network, and environment.

Differentiating Abuse from the Normal Aging Process

The problem of using physical findings when assessing an elderly person for the presence of abuse deserves special attention. Although physical indicators appear to be among the most valid symptoms of abuse or neglect in the child or middle-aged person, apparent symptoms of abuse in an elderly person may in fact be related to the aging process (Ham, 1981; Sengstock & Barrett, 1981). Ham's (1981) discussion of the problems of identifying physical abuse of the elderly observes that the physiological processes that govern normal aging lead to physiological changes such as increased capillary fragility, osteoporosis, poor balance, poor vision, mental confusion, and muscu-

TABLE 7-2
Physical Examination of Elderly Persons—Indicators of Potential or Actual Elder Abuse or Neglect*

AREA OF ASSESSMENT	SYMPTOMS OF POSSIBLE ABUSE/NEGLECT
General appearance	Fearful, anxious
	Marked passivity
	Malnourished looking
	Poor hygiene
	Inappropriate dress, re: weather conditions
	Physical handicap
	Antagonism and/or detachment between elder and caregiver
Vital statistics	
Height	
Weight	Underweight
Head circumference	
Skin	Excessive or unexplainable bruises, welts, scars, possibly in various stages of healing
	Decubitus ulcers
	Burns
	Infected or untreated wound
Head	
Eyes	No prosthetic device to accommodate poor eyesight
Ears	No prosthetic device to accommodate poor hearing
Nose	
Neck	
Chest	
Abdomen	Abdominal distention
Genital/urinary	Vaginal lacerations
	Vaginal infection
	Urinary tract infection
Rectal	
Musculoskeletal	Skull/facial fractures
	Fractured femur
	Fractures of other parts of the body
Neurological	Limited motion of extremities
	Difficulty with speech
	Difficulty with swallowing

*Symptoms listed may be symptoms of normal aging. Therefore physical symptoms must be assessed in conjunction with the patient's personal history.

loskeletal stiffness. In elaborating on these physiological changes, Ham states that the elderly may be more likely to lose their balance and fall. Since they are more likely to suffer from skeletal fractures and bleed, a relatively minor fall may result in numerous fractures and extensive bruising, subdural hemato-mas, and hemorrhages that may be fatal. In addition, Ham notes that elderly clients who suffer from senile dementia may develop delusions concerning the treatment they receive from others. Thus physiological aging may generate complaints of mistreatment.

TABLE 7-3
History of Elder—Possible Indicators of Potential or Actual Elder Abuse

AREA OF ASSESSMENT	AT-RISK RESPONSES OR INDICATORS OF POSSIBLE ABUSE/NEGLECT
Primary concern/reason for visit	Historical data that conflicts with physical findings
	Acute or chronic psychological and/or physical disability
	Inability to participate independently in activities of daily living
	Inappropriate delay in bringing elder to health care facility
	Reluctance on the part of caregiver to give information on elder's condition
	Inappropriate caregiver reaction to nurse's concern (overreacts, underreacts)
Family health	
Elder	Substance abuse
	Grew up in a violent home (abused as child, spouse; abused children)
	Excessive dependence of elder on child(ren)
Child(ren) of elder	Were abused by parents as children
	Antagonistic relationship with elder
	Excessive dependence on elder
	Substance abuse
	History of violent relationship with other siblings and/or spouse
Siblings	Antagonistic relationship between siblings
	Excessive dependence of one or more siblings on another or each other
Other family members and family relations	Other history of abuse and/or neglect or violent death
Household	Violence and aggression used to resolve conflicts and solve problems
	Past history of abuse and/or neglect among family members
	Poverty
	Few or no friends or neighbors or other support systems available
	Excessive number of stressful situations encountered during a short period of time (unemployment, death of a relative or significant other, etc.)
Health history of elder	
Child	History of chronic physical and/or psychological disability
Midlife	History of chronic physical and/or psychological disability
Nutrition	History of feeding problems (GI disease, food preference idiosyncracies)
	Inappropriate food or drink
	Dietary intake that does not fit with findings
	Inadequate food or fluid intake
Drugs/medications	Drugs/medications not indicated by physical condition
	Overdose of drugs or medications (prescribed or over-the-counter)
	Medications not taken as prescribed
Personal/social	Caregiver has unrealistic expectations of elder
	Social isolation (little or no contact with friends, neighbors, or relatives; lack of outside activity)
	Substance abuse
	History of spouse abuse (as victim and/or abuser)
	History of antagonistic relationships among family members (between family members in general, including elder)
	Large age difference between elder and spouse
	Large number of family problems
	Excessive dependence on spouse, children, or significant others
Discipline	
Physical	Belief that the use of physical punishment is appropriate
	Threats with an instrument as a means to punish
	Use of an instrument to administer physical punishment
	Excessive, inappropriate, inconsistent physical punishment
	History of caregiver and/or others "losing control" and/or "hitting too hard"

TABLE 7-3 *Continued*

AREA OF ASSESSMENT	AT-RISK RESPONSES OR INDICATORS OF POSSIBLE ABUSE/NEGLECT
Emotional/violation of rights	Fear-provoking threats
	Infantilization
	Berating
	Screaming
	Forced move out of home
	Forced institutionalization
	Prohibiting marriage
	Prevention of free use of money
	Isolation
Sleep	
Elimination	
Illness	Chronic illness or handicap
	Disability requiring special treatment from caregiver and others
Operations/hospitalizations	Operations or illness that required extended and/or repeated hospitalizations
	Caregiver's refusal to have elder hospitalized
	Caregiver overanxious to have elder hospitalized
Diagnostic tests	Caregiver's refusal for further diagnostic tests
	Caregiver's overreaction or underreaction to diagnostic findings
Accidents	Repeated
	History of preceding events that do not support actual injuries
Safety	Appropriate safety precautions not taken, especially in elders known to be confused, disoriented, and/or with physical disabilities restricting mobility
Health care utilization	Infrequent
	Caregiver overanxious to have elder hospitalized
	Health care "shopping"
Review of body systems	

According to Ham (1981), all of these findings may mimic abuse; thus he warns against falsely diagnosing abuse as the cause of suspicious physical and psychological symptomatology. Although his observations may be accurate, they also mask a dangerous set of assumptions that must be avoided if aged abuse victims are to be served. Research to date on elder abuse has shown that victims are often not recognized because professionals tend to observe instances of abuse only when they are actively looking for the problem (Sengstock & Barrett, 1981). Consequently, it is imperative that professionals not dismiss prematurely the possibility of abuse when suspicious findings are present.

Results of physical examination should be assessed in conjunction with historical data that the nurse has collected on the client, as noted in Tables 7-2 and 7-3. Careful questioning by the nurse may determine such things as whether a client who complains of mistreatment is exhibiting symptoms of confusion or dementia, or is in fact expressing a valid complaint of abuse, or is actually presenting symptoms that resulted from a physical assault. Thus the importance of obtaining a thorough, objective history on elderly clients cannot be overemphasized.

Values of Health Care Providers

The beliefs of the health care provider may have a significant impact on whether an abusive situation is recognized and then treated as such. In describing the process health care providers use in identifying abuse and determining subsequent intervention strategies, Phillips and Rempusheski (1985) describe four decision outcomes. The first focuses on the resources that the caregiver possesses. For example, if the caregiver is poor, has failing health, or lacks knowledge regarding the needs of the elder, the health care provider may attribute the problem to the situation, rather than to a deliberate attempt of the caregiver to neglect the elder.

The second decision outcome considers the attributes of the elder in relation to the diagnosis of abuse. Thus if the elder is difficult to get along with or exhibits confused and combative behavior, the health care provider may attribute possible abuse symptoms to the character of the elder rather than to the behavior of the caregiver. Conversely, an elderly patient with possible abuse symptoms who is good natured and coherent may be further examined regarding the existence of abuse.

The third decision process observes that an assessment of abuse or neglect is affected by the worker's perception of caregiver effort. If the health care provider believes that the caregiver is doing his or her best to meet the elder's needs, a diagnosis of abuse is less likely to occur, even if symptoms point to its presence.

The fourth decision process refers to the relationship between the health care provider and the caregiver. A health care worker who experiences a positive relationship with the caregiver is less likely to identify abuse as the source of the elder's problems. Similarly, a poor relationship between the health care provider and the caregiver may be projected onto the relationship between the caregiver and the elder, leading to a diagnosis of abuse that may not be accurate.

Intervention

An elderly client may be reluctant to admit the existence of abuse even though a number of historical and physical findings point to its presence. It would be wise, therefore, for the nurse to proceed as if the client is at risk until abuse has been ruled out as a possible contributor to an elderly patient's problem.

This is particularly significant since the majority of states now have mandatory elder abuse laws (Gilbert, 1986). Three factors appear to be important in the development of an adequate program of intervention. These are the establishment of a strong trusting relationship with the client; maintenance of a single individual as primary care provider; and the development of a comprehensive plan that can be followed by and coordinated with all caregivers.

Trust as a major component of care

Establishing a trusting relationship appears to be the most critical component, not only in assessment, but also in the provision of adequate care to aged abuse victims. Clients, especially those who have experienced the trauma of domestic violence, are not likely to accept assistance from nurses or other outsiders unless they believe the care provider is deserving of their trust. Such trust can be fostered by the nurse's attitudes toward the elderly client. Exhibiting sympathetic concern for the client and his/her feelings, an understanding of the problems the client is experiencing, an interest in his/her well-being, and a willingness to expend effort in the client's behalf can encourage this trust. Such concern is particularly evident in the nurse's nonjudgmental demeanor. Elderly abuse victims frequently become quite defensive of their loved ones, even if they are abusive. It is crucial that the nurse allow them to maintain any defensive rationalizations that they have developed to protect their family members, even if their abusive demeanor is obvious. Abuse victims are not likely to accept care if they feel that the nurse is critical either of them or of their loved ones.

Unfortunately, the establishment of a trusting relationship is particularly difficult in elder abuse cases. This difficulty arises from two factors. One is the particular barrier to the development of a trusting relationship on the part of abuse victims. The other is the lengthy time span required for the development of trust.

It has been observed that abuse victims find it particularly difficult to establish trusting relationships (Justice & Justice, 1976). Many elder abuse victims have had little opportunity to maintain trusting relationships with others, since those who are closest to them are the same persons who abuse them. They are often unable to confide in family members other than the abuser, since such relatives may have difficulty relating both to the abuser and the victim. As a result, abused elders often lack the ability to trust and confide in anyone. The concerned nurse must overcome this barrier before a trusting relationship can be established with the victim.

Data on elder abuse also suggest that developing a trusting relationship is a time-consuming process (Sengstock & Barrett, 1981). It is often necessary for a professional to establish a long-term relationship before a victim feels sufficient trust to share confidences. Only then is the victim able to admit that abuse is present, either as the underlying problem or as an additional problem that has been overlooked. Thus intervention in cases requiring only short-term medical attention presents nurses with a particular challenge, as they strive to attain the critical characteristic of trust.

Importance of a primary care provider

The role of a primary care nurse is a critical factor, both in promoting continuity of care and in developing trust. This person must be sympathetic to the problem of abuse and be someone with whom the client is able to communicate. She or he should also be aware of assessment, supportive, and legal information regarding elder abuse (Fulmer, Street, & Carr, 1984; Hackbarth, Andreson, & Konestabo, 1989). The role of the primary care nurse can be particularly important in dealing with abuse cases since both victim and family are usually reluctant to accept outside help. Professionals who have had little contact with such persons may find them uncooperative and unwilling to accept help. The nurse who is knowledgeable about elder abuse and has established a trusting relationship with the client can act as a liaison between the victim and professionals from other areas.

An example of such intervention is the common situation in which the nurse refers a client to social services. In such a situation, the nurse should provide the social worker with a detailed history of the client, explaining why abuse is suspected and discussing all factors contributing to the abusive situation. The nurse should also prepare the client concerning this intervention and preferably be present during the social worker's initial visit. Although these measures might appear time-consuming and unnecessary under normal circumstances, in the case of the abused elder they are critical factors. Abused elders are more likely to accept outside assistance if it is encouraged and supported by a professional whom the victim already trusts.

Development of a Comprehensive Plan

The importance of a comprehensive plan cannot be overemphasized. Such interventions must be the result of an ongoing process, which is originally based on an accurate assessment of the client's condition and developed as much as possible in collaboration with the victim and family, and which undergoes constant reassessment and alteration as new observations about the client's needs become evident. Such a plan should prove to be an effective method in the establishment of a trusting relationship as well as in the provision of high-quality care to the elder abuse patient.

This plan is particularly important in cases in which only short-term care is to be provided, or in cases in which the client is to be assisted by a number of care providers. Other nurses and professionals involved in the elder's care should be fully familiarized with the plan of care for the client and should be observant of other at-risk findings that the client and situation exhibit. These observations should be continually added to the initial assessment of the client to maintain an accurate record concerning the client's overall situation.

Evaluation of Nursing Intervention

Evaluating the effectiveness of nursing intervention in elder abuse cases is another challenging problem. Particularly in cases in which nursing intervention is short term in nature, nurses may be unable to ascertain whether they had an enduring effect on the well-being of an abused elderly patient. However, the nurse may use some clues to help determine whether the assistance has been of value. These include the client's acknowledgment of the abuse; willingness of the victim, the abuser, and the family to accept outside help; and/or removal of the victim from the abusive situation.

Victim's acknowledgment of abuse

Many victims of elder abuse are reluctant to admit, even to themselves, that an abusive situation exists. Until this acknowledgment occurs, effective assistance is impossible. Hence an admission by the victim that abuse exists should be considered an important sign that the client has made progress in dealing with the abuse. Remedying an abusive situation often requires years of diligent assistance by numerous dedicated professionals. If the nurse's work leads the client to begin this process, this should be viewed as a major accomplishment.

Willingness to accept intervention

Another sign of successful nursing intervention is an observed willingness on the part of victim, abuser, or other family members to accept outside intervention and needed support services. Many contend that much elder abuse is caused by the stress of caring for an elderly, dependent relative (Block & Sinnott, 1979; Fulmer, 1989). In such cases daycare, meal services, and other assistance with activities of daily living can be of great benefit in alleviating the stress in the family and the resulting abuse as well. Hence the willingness of abuser, victim, or other family members to see a counselor, reorganize family activities, or accept daycare or housekeeping services is an indication that the abuse may be on the road to resolution.

Removal of the victim from the abusive situation

Although some elder abuse may be a problem related to caregiving, other cases are the result of a long-standing pattern of abuse in the lives of the victims and their families. In such situations, it is unlikely that even long-term nursing intervention will have a substantial impact on the abusive pattern. In long-term abusive patterns, the only likely solution is the separation of the abuser and the

abused. In these cases, separating the victim's living situation from that of the abuser should be seen as a positive step. Examples would be moving the victim to a nursing home or a senior citizens' residence. Placement with another relative may not be a positive step in a habitually abusive family because such families tend to foster abuse in all members, and the victim may simply move from one problematic situation to another.

Prospects for the future

Abuse of the elderly has been neglected by both professionals and the public. Although there has been a dramatic increase in the attention to this problem in the past decade, many service providers are still unable to deal with elder abuse in an adequate manner. Existing research provides some basis for clinical practice, but considerable need remains for development of theory and methodology.

In the area of diagnosis, promising efforts have been undertaken to develop clear statements of case history characteristics and physical symptoms that can be used to identify the presence of elder abuse or neglect (Fulmer & Wetle, 1986; Hwalek & Sengstock, 1986; Neale et al., 1991). However further refinement in this area is an ongoing need. As discussed earlier, the problems of obtaining an accurate and objective history, coupled with the similarity between physiological aging and abuse symptoms, make identification of elder abuse victims a challenging responsibility for the nurse. The task of identifying and aiding such victims is also complicated by the reluctance of abuse victims to seek help. The reluctance of elderly victims to trust others also compounds the difficulty of professionals dealing with these cases. Although such resistance may be difficult for the nurse to manage, it is understandable in light of the experiences of these victims.

Therefore the key element in the provision of high-quality care to elder abuse victims is the establishment of a trusting and insightful relationship between the victim and the primary care provider. In large part, education of the public and of those providing health, social, and psychological intervention will facilitate this process (Phillips, 1983b).

Other care providers should work through this trusted professional. All components of the care must be recorded so that all professionals can follow the progress of the client and achieve continuity in care. It is hoped that the element of trust will grow as the client becomes aware of a sincere concern on the part of the nurses who provide care.

In turn, such measures will enable the client to be more open with the nurse and will lead to greater insight into the elderly individual's physical, psychological, and social situations, resulting in more appropriate measures in the client's care. It should be recognized that diagnosis and treatment of this problem requires patience, and in many cases, long-term intervention, before the victim will acknowledge his or her predicament and discuss it with a professional willing to help.

This makes it difficult for the nurse to evaluate the effectiveness of the intervention. In many instances, nurses may have to be content with the recognition that they have helped the patient to begin the process of dealing with the problem and with the realization that final resolution of the problem may not occur until many years and several other professionals have intervened. Nurses willing to accept this challenge may gain satisfaction from the knowledge that they are forerunners in the development of methods of assistance to elderly abuse victims who have heretofore been neglected by other professionals in the health care arena.

REFERENCES

Anetzberger, G. J. (1987). *The etiology of elder abuse by adult offspring*. Springfield, IL: Charles C Thomas.

Anetzberger, J. (1989). Implications of research on elder abuse perpetrators: Rethinking current social policy and programming. In R. Filinson & S. R. Ingman (Eds.), *Elder abuse: Practice and policy* (pp. 43-50). New York: Human Sciences Press.

Atchley, R. C. (1991). *Social forces and aging* (6th ed.). Belmont, CA: Wadsworth.

Back, K. W. (1976). Personal characteristics and social behavior: Theory and method. In R. H. Binstock & E. Shanas (Eds.), *Handbook of aging and the social sciences*. New York: Van Nostrand Reinhold.

Bandura, A., & Walters, W. (1974). Catharsis—A questionable mode of coping with violence. In S. Steinmetz &

M. Straus (Eds.), *Violence in the family* (pp. 303-307). New York: Harper & Row.

Berkowitz, L. (1973, July). The case for bottling up rage. *Psychology Today, 7*, pp. 24-31.

Block, M. R., & J. D. Sinnott (1979). *The battered elder syndrome: An exploratory study*. College Park, MD: Center on Aging.

Blumberg, M. (1964, Winter). When parents hit out. *Twentieth Century 173*:39-44.

Bragg, D. F., Flanary, B., Smithers, R., Ravel, D. L., Lanier, L. C., Sutton, J., Marquardt, B., Graham, S., Gregg, G., Solis, N., Prince, M., Collins, C., McCoy, P., Guimbardo, R., Elrod, J. (1977-78). *Report on Texas nursing homes*. Submitted to J. L. Hill, Attorney General. Austin, TX: Nursing Home Task Force.

Burston, G. R. (1978, November). Do your elderly parents live in fear of being battered? *Modern Geriatrics*, p. 16.

Callaghan, J. J. (1986). Guest editor's perspective. *Pride Institute Journal of Long Term Home Health Care, 5* (4), 2-3.

Calvert, R. (1974). Criminal and civil liability in husband-wife assaults. In S. Steinmetz & M. Straus (Eds.) *Violence in the family* (pp. 88-91). New York: Harper & Row.

Case, G. B., & G. Lesnoff-Caravaglia (1978). The battered child grown old. Dallas: American Gerontological Society Annual Meeting.

Conley, D. M. (1986). Developing a comprehensive approach: The key for the future. In M. W. Galbraith (Ed.), *Convergence in aging:* Vol. 3. *Elder abuse: Perspectives on an emerging crisis* (pp. 177-188). Kansas City, KS: Mid-America Congress on Aging.

Cravedi, K. G. (1986). Elder abuse: The evolution of federal and state policy reform. *Pride Institute Journal of Long Term Home Health Care, 5*(4), 4-9.

Douglass R. L., 1988. *Domestic mistreatment of the elderly—Towards prevention*. Washington, DC: American Association of Retired Persons.

Douglass, R. L., Hickey, T., & Noel, C. (1980). *A study of maltreatment of the elderly and other vulnerable adults*. Ann Arbor, MI: University of Michigan Institute of Gerontology.

Elder abuse: Reported cases increase. (1981, September 10) *Vintage*, p. 3.

Emlet, C. A. (1984). Coordinating county based services for the frail elderly: A tri-departmental approach. *Journal of Gerontological Social Work, 8*, 5-13.

Field, M. H., & Field, H. F. (1973). Marital violence and the criminal process: Neither justice nor peace. *Social Service Review, 47*, 221-240.

Fulmer, T. T. (1989). Mistreatment of elders: Assessment diagnosis, and intervention. *Nursing Clinics of North America, 24*(3), 707-716.

Fulmer, T. & Ashley, J. (1986). Neglect: What part of abuse? *Pride Institute Journal of Long Term Home Health Care, 5*(4), 18-24.

Fulmer, T., & Ashley, J. (1989). Clinical indicators of elder neglect. *Applied Nursing Research, 2*(4), 161-167.

Fulmer, T., & Cahill, V. M. (1984). Assessing elder abuse: A Study. *Journal of Gerontological Nursing, 10*(12), 16-20.

Fulmer, T., Street, S., & Carr, K. (1984). Abuse of the elderly: Screening and detection. *Journal of Emergency Nursing, 10*(3), 131-140.

Fulmer, T., & Wetle, T. (1986). Elder abuse screening and intervention. *Nurse Practitioner, 11*(5), 33-38.

Galbraith, M. W. (1986). Elder abuse: An overview. In M. W. Galbraith (Ed.), *Convergence in aging:* Vol. 3. *Elder abuse: Perspectives on an emerging crisis* (pp. 5-27). Kansas City, KS: Mid-America Congress on Aging.

Galbraith, M. W. (1989). A critical examination of the definitional, methodological, and theoretical problems of elder abuse. In R. Filinson & S. R. Ingman (Eds.), *Elder abuse: Practice and policy* (pp. 35-42). New York: Human Sciences Press.

Gelles, R. J. (1973). Child abuse as psychopathology: A sociological critique and reformulation. *American Journal of Orthopsychiatry, 43,* 611-621.

Gelles, R. J. (1974). *The violent home.* Beverly Hills: Sage.

Gelles, R. J. (1977). No place to go: The social dynamics of marital violence. In Roy (Ed.), *Battered women* (pp. 46-63). New York: Van Nostrand Reinhold.

Gelles, R. J., & Straus, M. A. (1988). *Intimate violence.* New York: Simon and Schuster.

Gesino, J. P., Smith, H. H., & Keckich, W. A. (1982). The battered woman grows old. *Clinical Gerontologist, 1*(1), 59-67.

Gil, D. (1971). Violence against children. *Journal of Marriage and the Family, 33*(4), 637-648.

Gilbert, D. (1986). The ethics of mandatory elder abuse reporting statutes. *Advances in Nursing Science, 8*(2), 51-62.

Grambs, J. D. (1989). *Women over forty* (rev. ed.). New York: Springer.

Hackbarth, D., Andreson, P., & Konestabo, B. (1989) Maltreatment of the elderly in the home: A framework for prevention and intervention. *Journal of Home Health Care Practice, 2*(1), 43-56.

Ham, R. (1981). Pitfalls in the diagnosis of abuse of the elderly. In B. B. Harris (Ed.), *Abuse and neglect of the elderly in Illinois: Incidence and characteristics, legislation and policy recommendations* (pp. B-1 to B-7). Springfield, IL: State of Illinois.

Haviland, S. & O'Brien, J. (1989). Physical abuse and neglect of the elderly: Assessment and intervention. *Orthopaedic Nursing, 8*(4), 11-19.

Hendricks, J. & Hendricks, C. D. (1981). *Aging in mass society* (4th ed). Cambridge, MA: Winthrop.

Hickey, T., & Douglass, R. L. (1981a). Mistreatment of the elderly in the domestic setting: An exploratory study. *American Journal of Public Health, 71,* 500-507.

Hickey, T., & Douglass, R. L. (1981b). Neglect and abuse of older family members: Professionals' perspectives and case experiences. *The Gerontologist, 21,* 171-176.

Himmelstein, D. U., Jones, A. A., & Woolhandler, S. (1983). Hypernatremia dehydration in nursing home patients: An indicator of neglect. *Journal of the American Geriatrics Society, XXXI,* 466-471.

Hirst, S. P., & Miller, J. (1986). The abused elderly. *Journal of Psychosocial Nursing, 24* (10), 28-34.

Holmes, T., & Rahe, R. (1967). The social readjustment rating scale. *Journal of Psychosomatic Research, 11,* 213-218.

Hwalek, M. A., & Sengstock, M. C. (1986). Assessing the probability of abuse of the elderly: Toward the development of a clinical screening instrument. *Journal of Applied Gerontology, 5,* 153-173.

Jones, J., Dougherty, J., Scheible, D., & Cunningham, W. (1988). Emergency department protocol for the diagnosis and evaluation of geriatric abuse. *Annals of Emergency Medicine, 17*(10), 1006-1015.

Justice, B., & Justice, R. (1976). *The abusing family.* New York: Human Sciences Press.

Kallen, D. J. (1984). Clinical sociology and adolescent medicine: The design of a program. *Clinical Sociology Review, 2,* 78-93.

Kempe, G. H., et al. (1966). The battered child syndrome. *Journal of the American Medical Association, 181,* 17-41.

Kimsey, L. R., Tarbox, A. R., & Bragg, D. F. (1981). Abuse of the elderly—the hidden agenda: I. The caretakers and the categories of abuse. *Journal of the American Geriatrics Society, XXIX,* 465-472.

Kinderknecht, C. H. (1986). In home social work with abused or neglected elderly: An experiential guide to assessment and treatment. *Journal of Gerontological Social Work 9,* 29-42.

Kinney, M. B., Wendt, R., & Hurst, J. (1986). Elder abuse: Techniques for effective resolution. In M. W. Galbraith (Ed.), *Convergence in aging:* Vol. 3. *Elder abuse: Perspectives on an emerging crisis* (pp. 110-124). Kansas City, KS: Mid-America Congress on Aging.

Kransnow, M., & Fleshner, E. (1979, November). *Parental abuse.* Paper presented at the Twenty-third Annual Geronotological Society Meeting, Washington, DC.

Lau, E. A. (1986). Inpatient geropsychiatry in the network of elder abuse services. In M. W. Galbraith, (Ed.), *Convergence in aging:* Vol. 3. *Elder abuse: Perspectives on an emerging crisis* (pp. 65-80). Kansas City, KS: Mid-America Congress on Aging.

Lau, E., & Kosberg, J. (1979). Abuse of the elderly by informal care providers. *Aging* (Sept./Oct.), 10-15.

Law Enforcement Assistance Administration (1977, September 4). News release. Washington, DC: U.S. Department of Justice.

Levinger, G. (1976). Sources of marital dissatisfaction among applicants for divorce. *American Journal of Orthopsychiatry, 26,* 803-807.

Liang, J., & Sengstock, M. C. (1980). *Criminal victimization of the elderly and their interaction with the criminal justice system.* Detroit, MI: Institute of Gerontology, Wayne State University.

Michigan Women's Commission (1977). *Domestic assault.* Lansing, MI: State of Michigan.

Midwest Research Institute (1977). *Crimes against the aging: Patterns and prevention.* Kansas City, MO: Midwest Research Institute.

Neale, A. V., Hwalek, M., Scott, R. O., Sengstock, M. C., & Stahl, C. (1991). Validation of the Hwalek-Sengstock Elder Abuse Screening Test. *Journal of Applied Gerontology, 10*(4), 417-429.

Neugarten, B. L., Havighurst, R. J., & Tobin, S. S. (1968). Personality and patterns of aging. In B. L. Neugarten (Ed.), *Middle age and aging.* Chicago: University of Chicago Press.

O'Malley, T. A. (1986). Abuse and neglect of the elderly: The wrong issue? *Pride Institute Journal of Long Term Home Health Care, 5*(4), 25-28.

Pagelow, M. D. (1984). *Family violence.* New York: Praeger.

Phillips, L., (1983a). Elder abuse—What is it? Who says so? *Geriatric Nursing* (May/June), 167-170.

Phillips, L. (1983b). Abuse and neglect of the frail elderly at home: An exploration of theoretical relationships. *Journal of Advanced Nursing, 8,* 379-392.

Phillips, L. R. (1988). The fit of elder abuse with the family violence paradigm, and the implications of a paradigm shift for clinical practice. *Public Health Nursing, 5*(4), 222-229.

Phillips, L., & Rempusheski, V. (1985). A decision-making model for diagnosing and intervening in elder abuse and neglect. *Nursing Research, 34,* 134-139.

Pillemer, K., & Finkelhor, D. (1988). The prevalence of elder abuse: A random sample survey. *The Gerontologist, 28*(1), 51-57.

Pollick, M. (1987) Abuse of the elderly: A review. *Holistic Nursing Practice, 1*(2), 43-53.

Quinn, M. J., & Tomita, S. K. (1986). *Elder abuse and neglect.* New York: Springer.

Renvoize, J., (1978). *Web of violence: A study of family violence.* London: Routledge and Kegan Paul.

Rinkle, V. (1989). Federal initiatives. In R. Filinson & S. R. Ingman (Eds.), *Elder abuse: Practice and policy* (pp. 129-137). New York: Human Sciences Press.

Select Committee on Aging: House of Representatives (1985). *The rights of America's institutionalized aged: Lost in confinement* (Comm. Pub. No. 99-543). Washington, DC: U.S. Government Printing Office.

Sengstock, M. C. (1991). Sex and genter implications in cases of elder abuse. *Journal of Women and Aging, 3*(2), 25-43.

Sengstock, M. C., & Barrett, S. (1981, July). Techniques of identifying abused elders. Hamburg, Germany: Twelfth International Congress of Gerontology.

Sengstock, M. C., & Barrett, S. (1982, November). Legal services for aged victims of domestic abuse: The experience of one legal aid agency. Toronto, Ontario: American Society of Criminology.

Sengstock, M. C., & Barrett, S. (1986). Elderly victims of family abuse, neglect, and maltreatment: Can legal assistance help? *Journal of Gerontological Social Work, 9*(3), 43-61.

Sengstock, M. C., Barrett, S., & Graham, R. (1984). Abused elders: Victims of villains or of circumstances? *Journal of Gerontological Social Work, 8*(1,2), 101-111.

Sengstock, M. C., Hwalek, M. (1985-86). A critical analysis of measures for the identification of physical abuse and neglect of the elderly. *Home Health Care Services Quarterly, 6*(4), 27-39.

Sengstock, M. C., & Hwalek, M. (1986a). *The Sengstock-Hwalek Comprehensive Index of Elder Abuse* (2nd ed.). Detroit: SPEC Associates.

Sengstock, M. C., & Hwalek, M. (1986b). *The Sengstock-Hwalek Comprehensive Index of Elder Abuse: Instruction manual.* Detroit: SPEC Associates.

Sengstock, M. C., & Hwalek, M. (1986c). Domestic abuse of the elderly: Which cases involve the police? *Journal of Interpersonal Violence, 1*(3), 335-349.

Sengstock, M. C., & Hwalek, M. (1987). A review and analysis of measures for the identification of elder abuse. *Journal of Gerontological Social Work, 9,* 21-36.

Sengstock, M. C., Hwalek, M., & Moshier, S. (1986). A comprehensive index for assessing abuse and neglect of the elderly. In M. W. Galbraith (Ed.), *Elder abuse: perspectives on an emerging crisis* (Vol. 3) *Convergence in aging* (pp. 41-64). Kansas City, MO: Mid-America Conference on Aging.

Sengstock, M. C., Hwalek, M., & Petrone, S. (1989). Services for aged abuse victims: Service types and related factors. *Journal of Elder Abuse and Neglect, 1*(4), 37-56.

Sengstock, M. C., Hwalek, M., & Stahl, C. (1991). Developing new models of service delivery to aged abuse victims: Does it matter? *Clinical Sociology Review, 9,* 142-161.

Sengstock, M. C., & Liang, J. (1982). *Identifying and characterizing elder abuse.* Detroit, MI: Wayne State University Institute of Gerontology.

Sengstock, M. C., & Liang, J. (1983). Domestic abuse of the aged: Assessing some dimensions of the problem. In *Interdisciplinary topics in gerontology* (Vol. 17). *Social Gerontology.* Basel, Switzerland and New York: S. Karger.

Sengstock, M. C., McFarland, M. R., & Hwalek, M. (1990). Identification of elder abuse in institutional settings: Required changes in existing protocols. *Journal of elder abuse and neglect, 2*(½), 31-50.

Spinetta, J., & Rigler, D. (1972). The child abusing parent: A psychological review. *Psychological Bulletin, 77,* 293-304.

Steinmetz, S. (1981, January/February), Elder abuse. *Aging,* pp. 6-10.

Steinmetz, S. K. (1978, July/August). Battered parents. *Society,* pp. 54-55.

Steinmetz, S. K., & Straus, M. A. (1974). General introduction: Social myth and social system in the study of intra family violence. In S. K. Steinmetz & M. A. Straus (Eds.), *Violence in the family* (pp. 3-25). New York: Harper & Row.

Steuer, J., & Austin, E. (1980, August). Family abuse of the elderly. *Journal of the American Geriatrics Society,* pp. 372-376.

Straus, M. A., Gelles, R. J. & Steinmetz, S. K. (1980). *Behind closed doors*. New York: Anchor Books.

Strow, C., & MacKreth, R. (1977). Family group meetings—Strengthening partnership. *Journal of Gerontological Nursing, 3*(1), 31-35.

Sundeen, R., & Mathieu, J. (1976). The fear of crime and its consequences among the elderly in three urban communities. *The Gerontologist, 16* (3), 211-219.

Thobaben, M. (1989). State elder/adult abuse and protection laws. In R. Filinson & S. R. Ingman (Eds.), *Elder abuse: Practice and policy* (pp. 138-152). New York: Human Sciences Press.

Thobaben, M. & Anderson, L. (1985). Reporting elder abuse: It's the law. *American Journal of Nursing, 85,* 371-374.

Traxler, A. (1986). Elder abuse laws: A survey of state statutes. In M. W. Galbraith (Ed.), *Convergence in aging: Vol. 3 Elder abuse: Perspectives on an emerging crisis* (pp. 139-167). Kansas City, KS: Mid-America Congress on Aging.

Truninger, E. (1971). Marital violence: The legal solutions. *Hastings Law Journal, 23:* 259-276.

U.S. Department of Justice (1977). *Criminal victimization in the United States, 1974.* Washington, DC: National Criminal Justice Information and Statistics Service.

Verma, S., & Haviland, S. (1988). Ethical issues related to institutionalization. In J. G. O'Brien (Ed.), *Ethical and legal issues in care of the elderly* (pp. 44-56). East Lansing, MI: Department of Family Practice, Michigan State University.

Wolf, R. S., Halas, K. T. Green, L. B. & McNiff, M. L. (1985-86). A model for the integration of community-based health and social services. *Home Health Care Services Quarterly, 6,* 41-57.

Wolf, R. S., Strugnell, C. P. & Godkin, M. A. (1982). *Preliminary findings from three model projects on elderly abuse.* Worcester, MA: University of Massachusetts Medical Center, Center on Aging.

Wolf, R. S., Godkin, M. A., & Pillemer, K. A. (1984). *Final report from three model projects.* Worcester, MA: University of Massachusetts Medical Center, Center on Aging.

Wolf, R. S., & Pillemer, K. A. (1984). *Working with abused elders: Assessment, advocacy, and intervention.* Worcester, MA: University of Massachusetts Medical Center, Center on Aging.

Wolfgang, M. (1958). *Patterns in criminal homicide.* New York: Wiley.

Wolfgang, M., & Ferracuti, F. (1967). *The subculture of violence.* London: Tavistock.

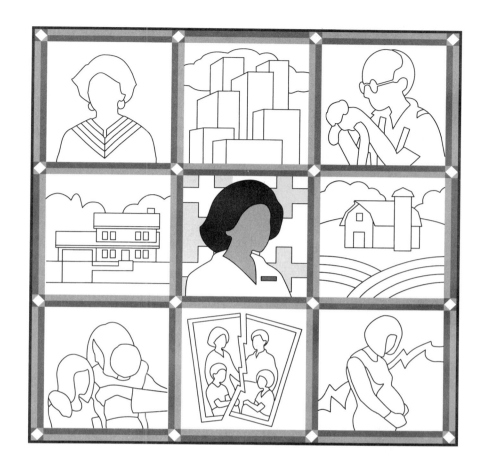

Nursing Care

CHAPTER

8

Nursing Care of Abused Children

Janice Humphreys *and* Ann Marie Ramsey

i was in pain
when i was hit by a train
i was in the hospital for a while
and it made me smile
that i was still alive
i felt dead
when i hit my head
but i was still happy that i'm going to live
to twenty five

Eric Willock, age 12*

Nursing care of abused and neglected children requires current, theory-based knowledge and individualized application. The nurse may become aware of child abuse and neglect at almost any point in practice with families. The maltreated child may be obvious or may be seen with less apparent indications of abuse and neglect. Nursing care of families is based on prevention and therefore does not require evidence of a "problem" for the nurse to intervene. Assessment for potential and actual child abuse and neglect is therefore an integral part of the nursing care of every child and parent. This chapter assists in the application of the theory and research presented in previous chapters to nursing practice.

A nursing process format is used, and a sample nursing process is also included.

Early theories of child abuse and neglect tended to suggest that only one or a few factors contributed to the occurrence of child maltreatment. More recent theoretical developments recognize the importance of multiple factors. (See Chapter 2 for a discussion of theories of child abuse and neglect.) The need for a multidisciplinary approach to interventions with abusive and neglectful families is generally recognized. Although some discussion of the benefits and difficulties of multidisciplinary interventions is presented, the primary purpose of this chapter is to discuss the nurse's role with abused and neglected children and their families. Child abuse and neglect is a complex, serious health problem requiring the best efforts of professionals from a variety of disciplines. The role of the nurse is addressed in this chapter.

---

*Reprinted from *Every Twelve Seconds,* compiled by Susan Venters (Hillsboro, Oregon: Shelter, 1981) by permission of the author.

SELF-AWARENESS

Care of abusive or potentially abusive families begins with the nurses' examination of their own feelings. Several studies have reported that certain factors influence clinicians' responses to child abuse and neglect. Kalichman, Craig, and Follingstad (1990) found differences in the responsibility attributed to the abuser, nonabusive parent, and victim based on clinician gender. Howe, Herzberger, and Tennen (1988) also found gender differences in clinicians' responses to child abuse vignettes. Consistent with previous research reports (Herzberger & Tennen, 1985; Snyder & Newberger, 1986), Howe et al. also found that clinicians' personal experience with abuse influenced perceptions and decisions to report abuse to child protective services. A nonjudgmental, helping approach to any client requires awareness and resolution of personal feelings that interfere with providing the highest quality professional nursing care.

Scharer (1979) describes two reactions that can occur when the nurse encounters abuse and neglect. "The first is a horror that a parent could injure his innocent child; as a result the helper (nurse) responds to the parent in an angry, punitive fashion. . . . The second is one of denial" (p. 15). Denial by the nurse that abuse and neglect have occurred may result from the nurse's disbelief that the parent could be responsible. Either response, anger or denial, is not helpful, can impair the safety of the child, and can limit the effectiveness of nursing care.

In a separate article Scharer (1978) identifies a third and equally damaging response to child abuse and neglect—rescue fantasy. "Rescue fantasy usually means a form of behavior observed when the nurse or any other helping person appears to feel that she can save or in some way rescue a person for whom she is caring" (p. 1483). Rescue fantasies can prevent the nurse from seeing the real needs of the family. An example of a nurse experiencing a rescue fantasy is the staff nurse caring for a neglected infant now gaining weight, who is pleasant but will not use any of the parent's suggestions regarding child care. Because the child has been neglected, the nurse assumes that only she and the rest of the health care system know what is best for the child. These feelings thus prevent the nurse from using every therapeutic interaction with the neglectful family. A discussion of how to resolve personal and professional feelings about child abuse and neglect and the implications for nursing education can be found in Chapter 15.

Nurses must examine the basis for their practice. Do they believe that people who abuse and neglect children are sick? Do parents maltreat their children because they learned to use violence from their parents? Do parents neglect their children because they are overwhelmed by the multitude of simultaneous demands placed on them and the lack of sufficient knowledge or resources to meet those demands? The answers are found by first obtaining knowledge of theories of child maltreatment and second by examining values and feelings in response. Such an examination of feelings is difficult. As discussed in Chapter 2, part of the reason that no single definition of child abuse and neglect can be identified may reflect the fear of many that the broader the definition, the closer child maltreatment comes to generally accepted child-rearing practices. Does every adult have the potential to abuse or neglect a child? Concerned professionals may deny that every adult is capable of harming a child. Yet if the nurse is interested in prevention, it is sensible to acknowledge the possibility that every adult has the potential to be a perpetrator and every child, a victim of child abuse and neglect. That does not imply that every parent *will* harm his or her child. Rather, nurses are encouraged to approach their practice prepared to assess the possibility of child abuse and neglect as they would nutritional status, immunization history, or any other aspect of child health. As with many other socially unacceptable facts, no adult will acknowledge the maltreatment of a child unless he or she is given an open opportunity to discuss it. No professional nurse will give an adult the opportunity to ask for assistance in child-rearing if she does not suspect that every parent has the potential for problems. No child maltreatment can be found by the nurse who never suspects it.

ASSESSMENT

Nursing care begins with assessment. Before any action can be taken, data are collected systematically.

Assessment for potential or actual child abuse requires the taking of a history and physical examination. The techniques of the two components of assessment can be approached using a variety of methods. This text does not teach the beginning nurse basic questions to ask or how to palpate a lesion. Rather, this chapter attempts to identify areas of particular significance in the history and physical examination for child abuse and neglect. For ease of presentation, a particular history-taking and physical examination format will be followed. However, any thorough approach to assessment could be used. Nurses are encouraged to develop the approach that works best for them, to develop expertise using the approach, and to assess every child and family in a systematic fashion. Expertise in history taking and physical examination are essential components to every nursing practice situation.

History

Every nurse out of necessity develops a particular method and style of data collection. The location of nursing practice also requires the nurse to adapt the extent and method of assessment. The nurse working in a well-child clinic practices under different circumstances than the nurse in an emergency room. However, each is exposed to child maltreatment and should routinely include assessment in this area.

Gathering historical data about child abuse and neglect can be stressful for both the nurse and the parent. However, the nurse, by providing a conducive environment and by using therapeutic communication techniques, can achieve maximum results.

It is essential that a nonjudgmental approach be maintained at all times. The role of the nurse does not require a judgment of the "rightness" or "wrongness" of certain client behaviors. Law enforcement and legal professionals accept responsibility for determining whether a crime has been committed. The nurse is also not in a position to punish or discipline parents who maltreat their children. If the nurse expects to assist abusive and neglectful parents to "come to their senses" by expressing her own anger or threats to remove their

children, this response is actually only reinforcing to the parents that the use of aggression is appropriate to aid learning. The nurse is using a subtle form of "beating some sense into them." Certainly aggression and the less obvious coercion are not the therapeutic approaches of choice to families who already experience an excess of violence in their homes. It should be remembered that mothers of abused children may well be victims of violence themselves (McKibben, De Vos, & Newberger, 1989).

Newberger and Bourne (1978) identify that health professionals face multiple dilemmas in working with abusive parents. Social policies vary from those supportive of family autonomy to those recommending coercive intervention. Professional responses to child abuse are also dichotomized: compassion ("support") versus control ("punishment"). The various combinations of possible action responses are illustrated in Table 8-1.

Working with child abuse and neglect requires a skilled clinician who can establish a trusting, honest relationship with people who are most likely afraid to trust any professional. The nurse can provide the abusive and neglectful parent with an environment of support and concern. The nurse must approach the parent with compassion and questions that give the client the opportunity to voice his or her concerns and ask for help. The nurse's role is not to "cure" the child abuse and neglect. Rather, it is to assist the family to provide a safe and nurturant environment that promotes life, health, and well-being for all its members.

From the moment of initial contact with the client and family, the nurse should communicate in an open and honest manner. The first meeting begins with the nurse's introduction and a clear statement of purpose. The setting for the interview with the abusive and neglectful parent should ideally be quiet and private. In facilities without quiet, private locations the nurse can work toward making the administration aware of the need for such accommodations. A sample presentation would be: "Hello, Mrs. C. I'm J. H. I'm a pediatric clinical nurse specialist. What that means is that I'll be talking with you and asking you some questions about your daughter Sally's health, previous to today. I'll

TABLE 8-1
Dilemmas of Social Policy and Professional Response

RESPONSE	FAMILY AUTONOMY	versus	COERCIVE INTERVENTION
Compassion ("support")	1. Voluntary child development services		1. Case reporting of family crisis and mandated family intervention
	2. Guaranteed family supports (e.g., income, housing, health services)		2. Court-ordered delivery of services
versus			
Control ("punishment")	1. "Laissez-faire." No assured services or supports		1. Court action to separate child from family
	2. Retributive response to family crisis		2. Criminal prosecution of parents

Reprinted with permission from E. H. Newberger and R. Bourne (1978). The medicalization and legalization of child abuse. *American Journal of Orthopsychiatry, 48,* 593–607.

also be doing a physical examination of Sally." The specific description of the nurse's purpose helps to allay some of the parent's fears and also sets the framework for the nurse-client encounter. The nurse next sits so that her eyes are at the same level with those of the parent. The nurse neither wishes to tower over the parent nor be dominated. The seating arrangement is such that no desk or other inhibitive object comes between the nurse and the client. The nonverbal message to the parent is "I'm interested in what you have to say and would like to help you to help yourself."

The nurse continues to be supportive and compassionate throughout the questioning. Detailed interviewing about sensitive subjects, potential or actual child abuse and neglect, can be very difficult for the parent. If the parent is too threatened by the approach of the nurse, he or she is unlikely to be completely open and honest. The nurse in turn gives the parent every opportunity to share concerns or problems with child-rearing while remaining cognizant of professional responsibilities.

The nurse begins the health history of a child who is known or suspected of being abused as any other history-taking session. There are two reasons for this. First, the nurse can follow a familiar sequence of questioning, rather than a new or differ-

ent format, and thereby increase the attention to parent responses. Second, history taking always begins with parental concerns and progresses from the general family history (nonthreatening) to specific child history (more threatening). The nurse is able to demonstrate sincere concern for the parent before asking about parent-child interactions and problems.

Eliciting parental concerns is a particularly important aspect of history taking. The parent's concerns are likely the reason the child was brought to the health facility. Although initially parental concerns may seem to have little to do with suspected abuse or neglect (e.g., vague rash, sleeplessness, weaning), they may in fact address the greatest concern to both the nurse and the parent (e.g., parental stress and fears of loss of control). By giving the parent's concerns or problems primary importance, the nurse demonstrates that she is interested in and values the parent's opinion. Primary attention to the parent's concern may also be a time-saving device; facilitating movement of the history to the area of greatest importance. The initial inquiry can be as simple as "Is there anything in particular that you are concerned about or that I should pay particular attention to?" If no area is identified, the nurse will want to follow up with "If you think of anything as we go along, please do not hesitate to bring it to my attention."

As the nurse and parent progress through the history, the nurse avoids being accusatory or confrontive. Clinical experience has revealed that giving parents an opportunity to voice areas of need or weakness can be far more productive than any accusation. The following excerpt from an actual interview demonstrates this point:

Nurse: Who helps you care for the children?
Client: Nobody.
Nurse: You mean you have to be the parent all the time? That's pretty hard work.
Client: It sure is. Sometimes I just can't stand it. And that B., he just really seems to know how to aggravate me.
Nurse: Tell me about that.

Other questions that help to elicit the information of concern are "How do you discipline your children?" or "When was the last time you spanked him?"

The power of listening can never be underestimated. The nurse can make great progress in data gathering and establishing trust with the parent by just listening. Abusive and neglectful parents are often isolated physically and socially from other adults. The opportunity to voice their worries and fears to a compassionate listener can actually be therapeutic for the parent. Because of the complex nature of child maltreatment, long-term interventions are almost always necessary. A firmly-established, trusting relationship between nurse and parent is essential for achievement of client goals. Listening to the parent from the initial encounter is critical to the development of parent trust in the nurse.

It is also desirable to interview the parent with the child present at times and absent at others. The interaction between the parent and the child can be particularly informative. During an extensive history-taking session almost every child becomes wearied and bored. The parent's method of handling the child and the child's behavior can tell the nurse a great deal about factors that may be contributing to abuse and neglect in the home.

Interactions among parent, child, and nurse during a stressful situation can provide an excellent opportunity to assist parents in using alternative child-rearing behaviors. For example, the nurse may wish to address uncontrolled behavior to the child: "I know it's scary to come to the clinic." Another approach directed toward the parent might be: "Many children feel nervous the first time they come here, because they don't know what's going to happen. You don't need to do that to him (hit him, yell at him, hold him down). Let's let him calm down with this book."

Table 8-2 provides a simple but thorough listing of historical findings that can indicate potential or actual child abuse and neglect. The table has been structured so that the "at-risk responses" listed in the right-hand column do not all necessarily indicate that abuse or neglect of a child has taken place. The "at-risk responses" include obvious evidence of abuse and neglect (child in foster home or other institutional placement for abuse/neglect) and less obvious indicators of potential child abuse and neglect (poverty, single parent, chronically ill child). The body of knowledge about child abuse and neglect is developing. Early unicausal theories have been rejected in favor of multicausal theories, yet further study is needed to determine all the factors that contribute to the development of child abuse and neglect or mediate their effects. The "at-risk responses" identified in Table 8-2 have been suggested as potential or actual indicators of child abuse and neglect. These responses are intended as clues that require interpretation and clinical judgment.

A brief clarification of terms is necessary. The medical diagnosis "failure to thrive" is often automatically perceived as a euphemism for child neglect. A child admitted to a hospital pediatric unit is often treated by health professionals as a "poor little victim" and the parent as "obviously unfit." The reality is that "failure to thrive" is very much like "fever of undetermined origin," a broad medical diagnosis that provides the child with a hospital bed and time to find out what is really wrong. Certainly there are neglected children who have occasionally been labeled as "failure to thrive." For this reason the medical diagnosis has been included among the

TABLE 8-2
Child History—Indicators of Potential or Actual Child Abuse and Neglect

AREA OF ASSESSMENT	AT-RISK RESPONSES
Primary concern/reason for visit	Historical data that do not fit with physical findings
	Vague complaints about child
	Inappropriate delay in bringing child to health facility
	Reluctance on the part of the parent to give information
	Inappropriate prenatal reaction to nurse's concern (overreacts or underreacts)
	Hyperactivity
Family health history	
Parents	Grew up in a violent home (abused as child, observed mother or siblings abused)
	Low self-esteem
	Violence between adults
	Little knowledge of child development and care
	Substance abuse
	Adolescent birth of child
Siblings	History of abuse and/or neglect of siblings
	Large family
	History of sudden infant death
	Several young, dependent children in family
Other family members	Other history of violence or violent death
Household	Violence and aggression used to resolve conflicts and solve problems
	Poverty
	Single parent
	Very young parent (early teens)
	No friends, neighbors, or other support systems available
	Problems between parents, especially over children
	Other stressors
	a. Unemployment
	b. Illness in the family
	History of child foster home or other institutional placement for abuse/neglect
Child health history	
Prenatal	Unwanted pregnancy
	Difficult or complicated pregnancy
	Early adolescent parent
	Wanted a baby so that "I would have someone to love"
	Little or no prenatal care
Birth	Cesarean section
	Prematurity
	Low birth weight
	Birth defect
	Immediate separation of parents and child
	Child not of preferred sex or appearance
Neonatal	Separation of parents and child
	Complications or identification of health problem

TABLE 8-2 *Continued*
Child History—Indications of Potential or Actual Child Abuse and Neglect

AREA OF ASSESSMENT	AT-RISK RESPONSES
Nutrition (if necessary include 24-hour dietary recall)	History of feeding problems (frequent change of formula, colic, difficult to feed) Inappropriate food, drink, or drugs Dietary intake that does not fit with physical findings Inadequate or excessive food or fluid intake Obesity, anorexia and/or bulimia
Personal/social	Negative description of child (different, troublesome, difficult) Parent has unrealistic expectations of child Multiple school absences Difficulty in school Depression History of phobias, running away from home, or delinquent acts Poor peer relationships or no peer relations Sexual problems in child (excessive or public masturbation, age-inappropriate sexual play, promiscuity) History of pregnancy Substance abuse
Discipline	Use of physical punishment, especially in an infant or adolescent Use of an object to administer physical punishment Excessive, inappropriate, inconsistent physical punishment History of parent "losing control" and/or "hitting too hard"
Sleep	"Doesn't sleep," "Awake all night" Consistent history of inadequate sleep for age
Elimination	Inappropriate, excessive home treatment of constipation Enuresis Violent or excessively severe toilet training
Growth and development	History of excessive autostimulation "Hyperactivity" Learning disability Developmental delays Excessive aggression or passivity
Illness	Disability requiring special treatment from parents History of multiple, unexplained illnesses History of menstrual disorders
Operations/hospitalization	Operations or illness that required extended hospitalization Operations for rupture of internal organs (spleen, liver) Parent refusal to have child hospitalized Significant delay in seeking hospitalization History of suicide attempt History of overdoses even in young children History of multiple, unexplained operations and/or hospitalizations
Diagnostic tests	Evaluation for failure to thrive or other problem that would explain injuries and/or lack of weight gain History of multiple evaluations and/or diagnostic tests for unexplained illnesses Severe anemia Elevated lead level

TABLE 8–2 *Continued*
Child History-Indicators of Potential or Actual Child Abuse and Neglect

AREA OF ASSESSMENT	AT-RISK RESPONSES
Diagnostic tests	Parent refusal for further diagnostic studies
	Parent insistence on further, unwarranted diagnostic studies
Accidents	Repeated
	History of preceding events does not support actual injuries
Safety	No age-appropriate safety precautions
	History of poisoning
Immunizations	None or only a few
Health care utilization	Parent "shops" for hospital care
	No consistent provider
	Significant delay in seeking health care for serious problems
Review of body systems	Changes in previously reported data
	Pertinent data not previously reported

"at-risk responses" in Table 8-2. It is also true, however, that almost every chronic illness of childhood can present itself as a failure to thrive. Parents whose child is admitted to a hospital with the possibility of finding out their child has a chronic, possibly terminal, illness are in need of expert care, not merely tolerance. Therefore, the medical diagnosis of "failure to thrive" requires the nurse to skillfully use the tools of assessment and evaluation to ensure the proper care plan.

Physical Examination

It is particularly important to consider historical data in light of physical examination findings (see Table 8-3). The information acquired from the history may cause the nurse little or no alarm, yet when contrasted with data from physical examination, may reveal quite another picture. The parent may give a history of a restless, irritable, difficult-to-feed infant. On observing the parent feed the child, the nurse observes a crying infant who immediately quiets when fed, sucks hungrily, and quickly falls to sleep after feeding. Or, a parent may report that the child was left momentarily unattended in a bath tub while the parent answered the telephone. The parent states that on returning he

found the child had accidentally turned on the hot water. Physical examination reveals second- and third-degree burns of the four distal extremities only. Some clinicians advocate that variance between historical and physical findings must be considered child abuse until proved otherwise (Smith & Kunjukrishnan, 1985). It is therefore not merely the history or physical findings in isolation that are important. It is the combination of the two sources of data and the *discrepancies* that exist between them.

The general appearance of a child is also important. The child's appearance includes not only the manner of dress, but also the behavior of the child during the assessment phase. The nurse who assesses the child can compare the affect, development, and growth of each individual against the generally accepted norms.

Every contact with parents and their children is an opportunity for the nurse to assess and intervene. The child-abusing and neglecting parent may be particularly observant of the nurse's behavior because he or she is often anxious and desperate for help. The nurse's manner of interaction between both parent and child demonstrates alternative behaviors to each. A physical examination need not be a socially acceptable means of frightening, controlling, and hurting children. Instead the nurse can

TABLE 8-3
Physical Examination of the Child—Indicators of Potential or Actual Child Abuse and Neglect

AREA OF ASSESSMENT	AT-RISK FINDINGS
General appearance	Marked passivity or watchfulness
	Fearful, anxious, hyperactive
	Malnourished-looking; constant hunger in an infant
	Poor hygiene
	Inappropriate dress for weather conditions
	Excessive detachment by parent
	Physical handicap
Vital statistics	
Height, weight, and head circumference	Failure to gain height and/or weight as expected compared with growth charts
	Less than 3rd percentile rank
	Drop off in previously identified growth trends first in height, then weight, and finally head circumference
Skin	Excessive or unexplainable bruises, welts, or scars (hypopigmented or hyperpigmented), possibly in various stages of healing
	Bruises shaped like implements (electric cord, belt buckles, bite marks)
	Cigarette or dip burns
	Wasting of subcutaneous tissue
	Infected or untreated wound
	(Skin lesion recording may most accurately be done on a diagram of the body)
Head	Patchy baldness on scalp
	Subdural hematoma
Eyes	Evidence of trauma and/or resultant visual impairment
Ears	
Nose	
Mouth	Bruising, lacerations
	Gross dental caries
	Venereal infection
Neck	
Chest	
Abdomen	Intra-abdominal injuries
	Abdominal distention
	Pregnancy
Genitourinary	Urinary tract infection
	Vaginitis
	Venereal infection
	Bruising, bleeding
	Severe diaper rash
Rectal	Poor sphincter muscle tone
	Bruising, bleeding
	Venereal infection
Peripheral vascular	
Musculo-skeletal	Skull of facial fractures
	Soft tissue swelling
	Fractured femur
	Green-stick or spiral fractures
	Limited motion of an extremity
	Multiple fractures in various stages of healing
Neurological (includes Denver Developmental Screening Test)	Developmental retardation
	Limited motion of an extremity

establish trust, identify strengths, and still conduct a thorough assessment.

It is essential that the nurse document her practice in all nursing situations. This is especially true in cases of suspected or actual child abuse and neglect. The nurse should carefully and specifically record an assessment. The use of clients' own words should be noted within quotation marks. Physical findings should be objectively recorded. Documentation of skin injuries can be noted on figure diagrams identical to those used to note burns. Some clinicians advocate the use of photographs to further document the location, nature, and extent of injuries (Smith & Kunjukrishnan, 1985).

NURSING DIAGNOSIS

The last step in the process of assessment is the development of appropriate nursing diagnoses. Potential or actual child abuse and neglect can result in a variety of nursing diagnoses. The needs of the individual child and family are used as a basis for nursing diagnosis development. Therefore there is no single nursing diagnosis for children who have the potential for or have actually experienced abuse or neglect. A sample nursing process (Table 8-4) with nursing diagnoses has been included at the end of this chapter to aid in understanding assessment.

PLANNING

The planning stage of professional nursing care requires the development of goals and nursing actions. In the case of child abuse and neglect, goals are realistic, multidimensional, and both long term and short term. Nursing intervention with child abuse and neglect is based on the three levels of prevention. The plan in the case of child abuse and neglect must of necessity be prioritized. The safety of the child must always be the first concern of the nurse. However, the development of interventions requires caution that responses to child abuse and neglect are not attempts to control.

Goals

Goals are client oriented and whenever possible developed with the client. When mutually agreed on goals are developed, "noncompliance" becomes much less of a problem. Mutually agreed on goals can even be growth producing for the abusive and neglectful parent. By working with the parent to identify realistic goals in an area of mutual concern—child welfare—the nurse is actually helping the parent to improve his or her problem-solving capabilities. Furthermore, the nurse again demonstrates to the parent that his or her opinions and participation are important—that the parent has value. Attention to and reinforcement for parent strengths contribute to increasing the parent's self-esteem and self-care capabilities.

However, conflict can arise when the abusive and neglectful parent does not identify the same problems as the nurse. To the parent, strict corporal punishment may be absolutely essential to the development of a healthy child. The parent may not perceive violent child-rearing practices as a problem that requires set goals aimed at their elimination. The nurse may be tempted to impose her own goals on the parent. Certainly in those cases where the safety of the child is questioned, the parent's wishes cannot always be strictly followed. However, in the majority of abuse and neglect cases, the safety of the child can be assured and the parent's perception of problems generally can be followed. The nurse who sets goals exclusive of the parent will likely experience frustration and disappointment when the goals are not achieved. This does not mean that problems identified by the nurse but not the parent should be forgotten. The nurse should instead realize that the problem now becomes helping the parent to identify the nurse's original area of concern. Until both parent and nurse identify the same problem areas, no goals can be developed or action taken to achieve them.

Child abuse and neglect is such a complex problem that all the appropriate goals would be impossible to list. Goals are identified in reference to the appropriate nursing diagnosis. For example, the nursing diagnosis "Alteration in parenting related to inappropriate discipline" might appropriately be associated with the goal "Parent will demonstrate age-appropriate discipline with one week." However, in another family the goal might instead be "Within one week the parent will verbalize the developmental characteristics of a 6-month-old child." The sample nursing process (Table 8-4) provides additional examples.

NURSING INTERVENTION

Nursing interventions with child abuse and neglect cover a broad spectrum. The nurse is concerned about the hospitalized infant who is severely neglected. However, the nurse would be remiss if she failed to be equally concerned about the societal problems that contributed to the infant's condition. Schein (1972) states "The new values call for the professional to be an advocate, to set out to improve society, not merely to service it, to become more socially conscious, to be more an initiator than a responder" (p. 3). The nursing literature on child abuse and neglect tends to reflect nurses as "responders"; the majority of the publications describes nursing interventions in the case of overt abuse and/or neglect. Nurses work in the community, but with few exceptions have not written about their responsibility and activities in the wider advocacy against child maltreatment (Davis & Johnson, 1978). The following discussion attempts to highlight some of the societal problems contributing to child maltreatment that require nursing intervention.

Primary Prevention

Primary prevention of child abuse and neglect includes all interventions that prevent maltreatment of children. Also included under primary prevention are child health promotion activities with both well and "at-risk" populations. The type of nursing intervention at this level varies with the location and nature of practice.

Caldwell, Bogat, and Davidson (1988) present an extensive analysis of the child abuse potential and prevention literature. They argue that although some advocate the development of services solely for "high-risk" populations, there are serious limitations to this strategy. "Even if we work for ever-increasing sophistication and accuracy in the assessment of child maltreatment risk, limitations inherent in the task (i.e., problems in methodological adequacy, definitional ambiguity, and the mathematics of predicting low base rate phenomena, and potential costs) seriously hinder the ultimate utility of these efforts" (p. 620). They conclude that primary preventive services to general populations without regard to their risk is the best approach to reducing child abuse and neglect. Families can be assisted without stigma, and healthy nonabusive interactions between parents and children can be enhanced for all.

Prenatal

The prenatal period is an optimal time for professional nursing intervention aimed at the prevention of child abuse and neglect. Nurses who practice in primary care clinics, in the community, and in the case of the pregnant adolescent, in school-based clinics, have a great opportunity to impact the health of the soon-to-be-born child.

The nursing process begins with the assessment phase. Many studies identify factors that place parents and children at risk for maltreatment. It is imperative that the professional nurse be cognizant of these risk factors. These "risk factors" can be subcategorized into parental characteristics/personality factors, and parent behavioral factors.

The prenatal assessment should include the mother and father's current family situation and family background to provide insight into behavioral and personality factors. Parental age is important; literature reports suggest that parenthood before age 20 is a risk factor for maltreatment (Milner & Chilamkurti, 1991). Marital status is also important—single parenthood is also associated with a higher incidence of child maltreatment (Milner & Chilamkurti, 1991). If the expectant mother is unmarried, her relationship with the father of the child should be explored. Jason and Andereck (1983) and Showers, Apolo, Thomas, and Beavers (1985) identified that the boyfriend is at risk for committing fatal child abuse. The mother-to-be should be encouraged to discuss her boyfriend's feelings regarding the impending arrival. A better approach is to encourage the expectant mother to have the father accompany her to her prenatal visits or to arrange for a community health nurse to visit the home and assess the couple. As discussed in Chapter 2, stress is believed to play a major role in the incidence of child maltreatment. Hence prenatal assessment should evaluate family stressors. Such factors as poverty, unemployment, poor personal health, marital discord, number of other children in the home, and family health problems all produce stress in the family.

It is important for the nurse to assess for parenting experience in the prospective parent(s). If the client is already a parent, the nurse has an opportunity to assess current parenting methods. The best assessment method uses open-ended questions, such as, "How do you let your children know what is appropriate behavior and what is not?" and "How do you discipline your children?" Themes that include "my child should know right from wrong without being told" and use of violence, such as smacking, swatting, spanking, and whipping, are "red flags" that should alert the professional nurse to the strong risk for child maltreatment. For first-time parents-to-be, these questions can be phrased in terms of how their parents let them know right from wrong and how their parents disciplined them. The literature has extensively explored and supported a relationship between a childhood history of maltreatment and the potential to maltreat as an adult (Cappell & Heiner, 1990; Steele, 1987). The literature has also supported the theory that maltreating parents have high or unrealistic expectations of their children (Kravitz, & Driscoll, 1983; Steele & Pollock, 1974; Twentyman & Plotkin, 1982).

Parental behavior can be assessed by the professional nurse using both subjective and objective data collected in an ongoing manner during the prenatal period. Perhaps one of the greatest risk factors for child maltreatment is battering of the mother. It is estimated that approximately 30% of children born into such a circumstance will be abused themselves (Kaufman & Zigler, 1987; Widom, 1989). In addition, the literature suggests that even if these children are not physically abused, they can suffer from poor interactional skills, poor social competence, and learning (Gage, 1990). Battering during pregnancy has also been associated with premature delivery and low birth weight (Bullock & McFarlane, 1989). Subjective data in this area include asking the client if her partner has ever been violent with her. This method of questioning has a varying degree of reliability, however, because the woman may deny such violent behavior. Objective data should include assessment of the woman's interaction with the health care provider during the interview, inconsistencies in injury explanations, and frequent visits to the emergency room.

Another aspect of parental behavior that has received considerable attention in both the media and the scholarly literature is that of substance abuse during pregnancy. The sequelae of substance abuse during pregnancy include premature labor, low birth weight, congenital anomalies, and complications associated with infant withdrawal. Numerous studies have linked prenatal drug abuse with future child maltreatment (Chasnoff, 1988; Densen-Gerber 1978). This area is particularly difficult to assess for several reasons. First, the type of person who abuses drugs is unlikely to value preventive health care and hence is unlikely to seek prenatal care. Second, those women who do enter the health care system while abusing drugs during pregnancy would most likely be reluctant to admit such behavior. Recently there has been controversy over whether to file criminal fetus maltreatment charges against drug-abusing pregnant women. Proponents argue that society has a responsibility to promote healthy pregnancy (Krieger, 1988) and that appropriate interventions to accomplish this include reporting mothers to child protective services and detaining these women in hospitals or other facilities. Opponents counter with the argument that such threats would alienate women from seeking prenatal care, only to have the drug abuse continue. They also note that there are insufficient rehabilitation facilities to provide services to drug-addicted women; hence prosecution of drug-addicted women is another situation of "blaming the victim" (Landwirth, 1987; Paulson, 1983). Interventions to address these prenatal risk factors include enrollment of prospective parents in prenatal and parenting classes in the community, referral to individual counseling through community mental health boards, and referral to rehabilitation facilities for substance-abusing women. Barth, Hacking, and Ash (1988) report that enrollment in a specialized program called the Child Parent Enrichment program where at-risk mothers were visited in their homes by paraprofessional women from their community resulted in a lower incidence of child maltreatment than the control group enrolled in traditional community-based programs. The professional nurse is encouraged to contact local health departments, major universities, and child protection and child prevention agencies to determine if such services are available in her community. Finally, when referring substance-abusing women to rehabilitation, the professional nurse should carefully assess the program to ensure that it meets the needs of the pregnant woman. Does the program offer on-site prenatal care; does the program offer a component on parenting and care of children; is there on-site day-care for siblings; and finally, does the program offer ongoing support services, such as assistance in securing housing after the residential program ends, referral to local food programs, and contact with the local department of social services for enrollment into Aid to Dependent Children (ADC) programs or job training/placement services.

Hospital

The hospital environment can be used to assess perinatal risk factors for child maltreatment. For mothers who have not had contact with the health care system before delivery, the hospital must then be used to assess prenatal risk factors as well. The hospital-based nurse collects both objective and subjective data from the family. There are short-term interventions that the hospital nurse can accomplish and long-term interventions that can be accomplished by referral to community health nurses. Perinatal factors can be subdivided into parental factors and infant factors.

Parental factors that may indicate an infant is at risk for child maltreatment include a mother unpre-

pared for childbirth, a difficult delivery (i.e., long labor, much pain), lack of a support person during delivery, few visitors or support persons in the postnatal period, a mother who verbalizes she has no clothing, food, or a crib for the newborn, and the mother who demonstrates disinterest in her newborn (Heindl, Krall, Salus, & Broadhurst, 1979). Finally, one research study has suggested that the baby's name may have some predictive value in early identification of families at risk for abuse. This study identified naming practices, such as not naming the baby once it is born, allowing nonparental people to name the child, or naming the child after an aversive person or stimulus, may provide insight as to parental readiness and acknowledgment of the parental role (Crittenden & Morrison, 1988).

Infant characteristics that have been associated with maltreatment include low birth weight and the treatment sequelae (placement in neonatal intensive care unit (NICU), separation from mother, irritability, poor feeding, slow weight gain); fussy, colicky infants; and infants with congenital anomalies or developmental delays. Other factors related to the infant include parental disappointment with the infant's sex, parental repulsion by normal infant behavior, such as crying, stooling, spitting up. Studies have found that children with chronic health problems in the first year of life have a greater chance of encountering maltreatment than their healthier peers (Sherrod, O'Connor, Vietze, & Altemeier, 1984).

The hospital nurse can intervene in several ways. In the case of the infant born healthy, the nurse can help provide time when the mother and/or father can spend an uninterrupted period of time with the newborn. Klaus and Kennell (1976) report that "there is a sensitive period in the first minutes and hours of life during which it is necessary that the mother and father have close contact with their neonate for later development to be optimal"(p. 14). They recommend that the parents spend 30 to 45 minutes with their nude newborn, the child's body temperature maintained by an overhead heating panel, with as few interruptions as possible. They further recommend that instillation of eyedrops be delayed until the parents have had the opportunity for extended contact with their newborn during the first hour of life.

The hospital-based nurse can further facilitate the parent-child bond by encouraging parents to participate in the care of their children as soon as they are ready. Maintaining newborns in a nursery separate from postpartum mothers may inhibit the parents' ability to develop a healthy relationship with their children. The rooming-in of the newborn with its mother during hospitalization has been shown to correlate with fewer subsequent cases of parenting inadequacy and therefore is encouraged. The nurse can further use the daily, extended contact among mother, father, and newborn to praise and reassure the parents. Criticism of parental behavior can be replaced with identification of strengths where they exist.

In addition to the traditional class on bathing the baby, the nurse on a postpartum unit can provide anticipatory guidance to parents in terms of what they can expect when they go home. Topics to be covered include infant crying, feeding patterns and developmental milestones. The nurse should emphasize that parenting is hard work and that it is okay to ask for help. Parents can be encouraged to identify and call on others who can help them adjust to the changes and stress they experience.

Nursing intervention may be even more important in the case of the birth of a handicapped or a premature infant. These infants are frequently whisked away from parents to initiate life-sustaining measures. Such parents are unable to experience the desired early contact with their children. In addition, they are grieving a loss of the anticipated perfect child and must adjust to their "imperfect" baby. Nursing interventions include providing emotional support to the family of the infant, encouraging parents to have contact whenever possible with the child, and educating parents in the care of their child. Parents are encouraged to be as involved as possible in the daily child care. Many NICUs now routinely encourage active parent participation. Nurses can advocate such policies in hospitals where they do not already exist.

The handicapped child or the child who is hospitalized for long periods, particularly during infancy, is a special concern to the nurse who practices on a pediatric unit. In a study of 51 abused children, Stern (1973) observed that "one-third of these children had either been seriously ill in the newborn period or had a persistent congenital defect" (p. 119). The separation of the parent and child or the existence of some anomaly is associated with child maltreatment. It may be simplistic to think that prematurity or birth defect alone predisposes a child to abuse or neglect. Chronic health problems, particularly in offspring, are a source of stress. In addition, financial strain, absence from work, and the need to identify alternative sources of other child care may occur. Primary prevention of child abuse and neglect in the case of the premature or handicapped child includes attention to more than just the child. Professional nurses include among their interventions contact with community social agencies, child care services, community health nurse visits, and parent groups whenever appropriate.

Community

Professional nurses who can intervene in terms of primary prevention include community health nurses, public health nurses, school nurses, and clinic nurses. Each of these roles is in a position to assess families for risk factors *before* maltreatment occurs and to refer them to appropriate resources.

The community health nurse (CHN) functions in providing skilled nursing care to the child with an identified health problem. As discussed earlier, children with chronic health problems are at significantly higher risk for abuse. The CHN providing skilled care to such a population can use frequent home visits to assess family functioning and to provide anticipatory guidance to parents. The frequent family contact in the home environment allows the CHN to assess the family in a natural setting. Generally, behavior in the home is free from influences associated with the hospital (i.e., acute illness, foreign environment). In addition, the CHN maintains contact with the family over time, which allows for assessment of parental behavior changes toward the child. Parental behaviors that should be considered "red flags"—behaviors that may signal a potential for maltreatment—include the child who is dirty or unkempt visit after visit, and parents who continuously refer to their child negatively. A major component of the CHN visit is a history and physical assessment. Factors that may indicate a potential for maltreatment include the child who is not gaining weight appropriate for age, the child who the parent reports is very fussy, inconsolable and/or irritable, and parents who do not follow up with the pediatrician or obtain immunizations for the child. The CHN should also assess support systems, those people the mother can rely on in times of need. The parent who is isolated and reports poor or nonexistent support systems is also at risk for maltreatment.

Another component of the CHN visit is teaching. Although a majority of teaching is directed toward the disease process, routine teaching should include anticipatory guidance in the area of growth and development, nutrition, and preventive health care. Finally, the CHN should be familiar with community support services and refer families when risk factors are identified.

The public health nurse's scope of practice tends to be broader than the CHN. The public health nurse (PHN) is funded through a county or city health department. The goal of public health nursing is promotion of health through prevention. The PHN makes home visits to clients referred from a variety of sources including schools, clinics, child protection agencies, hospitals, and home health agencies after skilled care is no longer needed. Because the goal of public health nursing is health promotion through prevention, the PHN is in an optimal position to prevent maltreatment. Several demonstration programs funded and operated through public health departments have shown great promise in the role of prevention. The most noteworthy programs are the maternal-child support programs that provide home visitation by professionals or paraprofessionals to pregnant and new mothers. Examples include the Child Parent Enrichment program (Barth et al. 1988) and several demonstration projects sponsored by the National Center on Child Abuse and Neglect (Gray, 1982).

Both the CHN and the PHN are in an excellent position to connect parents to appropriate resources in the community to meet their needs. Parents of children with special health care needs who are experiencing the stressors of isolation, financial burdens, and feeling overwhelmed can be referred to community-based support programs. For parent-to-parent support, parents can be referred to local support groups. The groups may be diagnosis based (i.e., seizure disorder support group), or they may be response based (i.e., parents of children with special health care needs). If the nurse is unfamiliar with locating such groups, she may contact the local hospital pediatric ward or the regional children's hospital. The clinical nurse specialist in the area of interest should be able to provide contacts for such groups. Another source of information is the local United Way, because they provide funding to many community-based groups. For families that need financial help, the nurse should contact the local health department to determine whether the state offers a program of services to crippled children (in some states this has been changed to services to children with special health care needs). Although the program may vary from state to state, the majority offer a low-cost or no-cost insurance program, family assessment, case management, ombudsman services, and, in some states, a parent support network.

Preventive services is a program sponsored by the state department of social services aimed at assisting families encountering a multitude of stressors. This program is a voluntary help program directed at prevention of maltreatment through coordination of appropriate community-based services. Anyone can make a referral to preventive services; the family can even "refer" themselves. When a referral has been accepted, the family is assigned a case worker. The case worker visits the home to make a family/environmental assessment. The prevention worker then puts the family in contact with appropriate agencies geared toward meeting the family's needs. Prevention can assist families in meeting a variety of needs, from helping them secure adequate housing and furniture to providing daycare and job training. Because the program is voluntary, families must be motivated to work with the agency to accomplish their goals. Preventive services continues to work with a family until all the goals are met, even if the process takes a year or longer.

Nurses who practice within the schools can intervene with adolescents who are just entering the child-bearing years. Nursing interventions include sex education programs that allow adolescents to be knowledgeable about sexuality and contraception. The decision of when and if to have children can be made more intelligently if adolescents and young adults are well informed about the prevention of pregnancy. Child development courses that expose the adolescent to the realities of being a parent can also assist the potential parent's decision making. If the adolescent becomes a parent, she or he is more likely to understand the child's behavior after exposure to information about child growth and development.

The pregnant adolescent presents another opportunity for primary prevention of child abuse and neglect. The school or clinic nurse can intervene with the pregnant adolescent by presenting available options. If the adolescent chooses to keep and raise the child, the nurse can work closely with the mother-to-be. The primary care nurse working with the pregnant adolescent should refer the client to available community-based maternal-child support programs.

It is important that the nurse approach the pregnant adolescent with the same respect given to any other client. The pregnant adolescent does not need recriminations from the nurse. The nurse who seeks to punish or lecture the adolescent on past behaviors ceases to be therapeutic. When the adolescent father is also involved in prenatal planning, the same nonjudgmental, supportive approach is appropriate. Group programs for pregnant mothers that allow them to complete their education by assisting with child care, parent education, and peer contacts are useful.

Clinic-based nurses who provide primary care to children and their parents routinely include anticipatory guidance as part of their health promotion teaching. Parents can be prepared for the various behaviors and changes in their children as they grow and develop. For example, the negativism of a 2-year-old may not be as aggravating to parents if they have been forewarned and understand that it is normal for that stage of development. In addition, parents need to be prepared to be angry and to want to hit their child. The nurse can problem solve with the parents to identify alternative methods of dealing with their frustration and anger, and to learn effective, nonviolent methods of discipline.

The nursing roles discussed in this section also involve the identification of family strengths and resources. Parents should routinely be praised for evidence of good child care. Even if there are 99 problems with child care identified by the nurse, the parent can be praised for the one aspect of positive parenting. The routine inclusion of praise to the parent as part of well-child care cannot be overemphasized. Parents rarely hear what they did *right* from health care providers. It is important that evidence of skillful parenting be acknowledged and rewarded. Praise from the nurse can be easily included during the history or physical examination. For example, "You've really done an excellent job at seeing that your child has a nutritious diet." Or, "Her skin is so beautiful. I can see that she's really getting the kind of care she needs." Parents are usually pleased and surprised to have their hard work noticed. By praising good parenting, the nurse increases the likelihood of its continuing, helps the parent to see his or her strengths, and increases parent self-esteem. Parents should also be encouraged to spend some time away from the child; they can be supported and reassured that time for themselves is not selfish. One approach acknowledges that "you can't be the parent all the time."

An excellent way to give both parents and preschool children time apart is to enroll the child in Head Start or another stimulating preschool program. Clinical experience has revealed that Head Start is a blessing to many parents and a delight to the children. Head Start has also been shown to assist children in their personal development, that is, increased self-esteem, advanced reading, arithmetic, and language achievement scores at all grade levels, even 15 years after Head Start experience. In a long-term follow-up of individuals at 19 to 22 years of age, those who had attended Head Start had a higher high school completion rate, a greater likelihood of attending college, less tendency to use welfare, a higher rate of employment, and lower arrest rates than those who had attended no preschool (Weikart, 1980). Programs like Head Start were developed to help break the cycle of poverty. Considering the major contribution that poverty makes to family violence, the nurse who is truly a client advocate will work for the continuation of programs that intervene to assist the poor.

Social interventions

Several authors and reports (Child Welfare League of America, 1989) have recommended changes in social policy and services that could significantly enhance the lives of children and their families. Vondra and Toth (1989) conclude that interventions that fail to address the multiple problems confronting families are unlikely to provide the full range of services necessary to help them recover and gain control of their lives. In 1971 Gil clearly identified several changes that must occur if maltreatment of children is to be eliminated in the United States. Gil's suggestions are still examples of the most basic and potentially the most pervasive form of primary prevention. The nurse who is more than just a "responder" can be actively intervening at the social policy level.

Briefly, Gil (1971) recommends that efforts be made to change the cultural sanction for the use of physical force, in all areas, against children. He says that "changing this aspect of the prevailing child rearing philosophy, and developing clear-cut cultural prohibitions and legal sanctions against such use of physical force, are likely to produce over time the strongest possible reduction of the incidence and prevalence of physical abuse of children" (p. 646). Gil does not suggest that children be treated with such permissiveness that they are never punished. He recommends that constructive, educational, nonviolent discipline be used. As he points out, ". . . rarely, if ever, is corporal punishment administered for the benefit of an attacked child, for usually it serves the immediate needs of the attacking adult who is seeking relief from his uncontrollable anger and stress" (p. 647).

The other major intervention suggested by Gil is the active pursuit of the elimination of poverty and racism. Social inequalities that prevent individuals of every race from experiencing the same opportunities result in the overrepresentation of minorities in the lowest socioeconomic strata. In addition, current social policies allow for levels of poverty that were heretofore unacceptable. Racial discrimination and poverty contribute in a complex fashion to child maltreatment. The nurse cannot expect to eliminate the maltreatment of children by family education or support alone. The culture and social environment in which the harming of children occurs and is at times condoned requires nursing intervention.

Social support and social interaction repeatedly have been identified as significant factors in child maltreatment. Although in a literature review Seagull (1987) concludes that there is little evidence that social support plays a significant role in the cause of child abuse, she suggests that support can be found for a relationship between child neglect and lack of social support. Others (Hamilton, 1989; Hoffman-Plotkin & Twentyman, 1984) have identified the social isolation that is frequently associated with child neglect. Cowen and Work (1988) propose that availability of support in early childhood and continuing support in later childhood serve to strengthen the development of resilience in children as they experience life adversity. Social interventions that support families and enhance their interactions with members in their communities serve as primary prevention for child maltreatment. "It is not the quantity but the quality of social support that is vital and its timing" (Hamilton, 1989, p. 32). Community-based (municipal, church, volunteer, etc.) and/or employer-supported child care assists families by providing child services and family resources. If families need additional services, existing relationships can support families through life events. Some authors argue that home visitors reduce both felt and actual isolation and should be supported (Cohn, 1981).

Child care that provides services to children even when they experience minor illnesses can be invaluable. Even a minor childhood illness can seriously affect families who rely on all adult members for employment income and benefits. Clearly nurses can be involved in establishing and, if necessary, initiating community- and/or employer-supported child care services. Minor childhood illness and care services can reasonably be developed in association with health care institutions and other providers. As direct client providers, nurses are an obvious choice in such programs. Given the finding in at least one study (Sherrod, et al., 1984) that maltreated infants tend to be ill more often than other infants, nursing involvement with minor illness and care services can provide an additional opportunity for early diagnosis and treatment of child abuse and neglect.

Finally, Gil recommends that comprehensive programming be undertaken in every community to reduce abuse and neglect of children. Included in each community program should be:

1. Comprehensive family planning programs, including repeal of all legislation concerning medical abortions . . .
2. Family life and education counseling programs for adolescents and adults in preparation for, and after marriage . . .
3. A comprehensive, high-quality, neighborhood-based, national health service, financed through general tax revenue, and geared not only to the treatment of acute and chronic illness, but also the promotion and maintenance of maximum feasible physical and mental health for everyone . . .
4. A range of high-quality, neighborhood-based social services geared to the reduction of environmental stresses on family life and especially on mothers who carry major responsibility for the child-rearing function . . .
5. . . . a system of social services and child care facilities geared to assisting families and children that cannot live together because of severe relationship and/or reality problems (Gil, 1971, p. 647).

Nurses can include Gil's or similar recommendations as part of primary prevention of child abuse and neglect at the community level. The framework for the existence of child abuse and neglect lies in the larger community sphere. Its impact is seen in the family.

In 1982 Michigan income tax forms had a new option for taxpayers: a box that permitted persons receiving a refund to check off to allot two dollars (or four dollars for a joint return) for child abuse prevention. Funds collected from the check-off were placed in the Children's Trust Fund within the Michigan Department of Treasury. Half of the money collected each year is invested, and half is spent for local child abuse prevention programs. Funds are distributed by a citizen's board, appointed by the governor, for local child abuse councils and local prevention services through hospitals, churches, schools, and other community organizations.

Every year since its implementation the Children's Trust Fund has received increased funds from tax check-off (Children's Trust fund, 1988/89-1989/90). As of the fifth funding cycle, 133 child abuse and neglect prevention grants had been awarded. However, in reviewing the percentage of tax returns eligible to contribute toward the fund, only 6% to 7% actually do so. Even after a legislative appropriation for increasing public awareness of the fund of $500,000, fewer than 6% of all eligible state tax returns contributed. Although they are important, programs like the Michigan's Children Trust Fund are only one step toward enhancing societal interventions with families.

Secondary Prevention

At the moment a child experiences harm at the hands of parents or some other responsible adult, professional nursing interventions are termed "secondary prevention." The goals of secondary prevention are early diagnosis and intervention to prevent recurrence. At the time of secondary prevention, injury has already been inflicted on the child. Nursing interventions are aimed at limiting the impact of child abuse and neglect.

Secondary prevention of child abuse and neglect must focus on interventions at several points in the family system. Clearly the health and safety of the children must be a first priority. Within families, however, interventions must be directed at the individual needs of members, interactions among members, and the larger family environment. Each family must be individually assessed and a specific program of care established. Nurses will be required to contribute their expertise to a multidisciplinary effort on behalf of the maltreating family. Within this general framework the nature of nursing practice with abusive and neglectful families varies depending on the nurse's role and practice setting.

Hospital

The most important type of secondary prevention of child abuse and neglect is the early identification of the maltreated child. In the case of the nurse who practices in an acute care setting, abused and neglected children may or may not be medically diagnosed at her first contact. Some forms of child abuse and neglect are not readily obvious (see Tables 8-2 and 8-3 for a complete listing of pertinent assessment findings). Some children are admitted directly to pediatric or intensive care units with the diagnosis of child abuse and/or neglect. Other children with reported "accidental" injuries seen in emergency rooms are more correctly identified as abused and neglected. Nursing interventions, although still secondary prevention, are focused on limiting the consequences of the maltreatment and preventing recurrence.

The less obviously maltreated child is the one who is encountered by the nurse in the hospital and medically diagnosed as other than abused or neglected. The child with a fractured femur who "fell out of bed" certainly needs health care to aid in the healing process. However, reduction of the fracture alone is profoundly inadequate treatment.

The first step in early identification of child abuse and neglect is a thorough nursing assessment. Other professional nursing interventions may involve consultation with other health professionals. Diagnostic tests to definitely determine child abuse and neglect usually require a physician's order. The nurse, with extended, intensive contact with hospitalized children and their parents, coupled with thorough assessment and theoretically based knowledge, often has the greatest insight into family health needs. The nurse should accurately record an assessment and alert other professionals involved in the care of the child and family.

Child abuse and neglect should be handled via collaboration by a group of health professionals. Ideally, a child abuse and neglect team exists in every hospital. The team is composed of interested representatives from several different professions—nursing, social work, medicine, etc. The child abuse and neglect team meets on a regular basis and as needed to review suspected cases, develop plans of care, and educate other members of the hospital community. Child abuse and neglect teams can be invaluable resources and aids to the early detection and treatment of child maltreatment. An important nursing intervention is the development of multidisciplinary child abuse and neglect teams in hospitals where they do not already exist.

Multidisciplinary efforts in the case of child abuse and neglect are extremely important. Cupoli and Newberger (1977) note that neither health nor social interventions alone will allay the impact of child maltreatment. However, interdisciplinary management of child abuse can be difficult. In an article showing the physician's perspective on interdisciplinary management of child abuse, Newberger (1976) identifies several factors that prevent professionals from various disciplines from working most effectively. Professionals from one discipline are often ignorant of the conceptual basis for practice of another discipline. Thus communication among members of different disciplines is often poor and compounded by institutional isolation. Confusion sometimes exists among professionals of various disciplines regarding assumption of management responsibilities. Some professionals display a chauvinistic attitude toward other disciplines and/or generally distrust or lack confidence in colleagues in different fields. Newberger suggests that, in general, all professionals suffer from too much work, a sense of hopelessness, punitive attitudes and public policies, and cultural isolation from clients. The result is often multiple professionals functioning independently in a fashion that can hurt, not help, violent and neglectful families. For the benefit of the family, the nurse can therefore ensure that a coordinated approach to child abuse and neglect among professionals is used. The nurse is in a prime position to coordinate such multidisciplinary functioning. At the minimum, nurses can be systematic and thorough in their assessments and assertive in their interventions if the best interests of the maltreated child and his or her family are to be served.

Schmitt and Mauro (1989) describe an outpatient approach to the medical treatment of children diagnosed with nonorganic failure to thrive. Nursing involvement in such an approach is obvious. They categorize types of nonorganic failure to thrive as follows: accidental, neglectful, or deliberate. Accidental failure to thrive is the result of errors in formula preparation, diet selection, or feeding technique. A mother who switches from concentrated formula to ready-to-feed and still continues to dilute the formula is an example of a mother who accidentally contributes to the failure to thrive of her child. Deliberate failure to thrive is the direct result of the intentional undernourishing of a child. Schmitt and Mauro suggest that this type of failure to thrive is rare, and that such children usually require placement in foster care. Neglectful failure to thrive occurs because the parent is overwhelmed or psychologically distressed.

> In neglectful cases, the parent caretaker does not spend enough time with the baby and neglects feeding. This neglect may occur because the parent is busy with external problems, perhaps overwhelmed with work or overburdened by more children than she can handle. In other cases, the parent is preoccupied with psychological stresses, for example depression, very poor self-esteem, marital strife, or even psychosis (p. 239).

Schmitt and Mauro (1989) recommend that the care of children and families experiencing any type of failure to thrive begin with a detailed history with particular attention to nutrition. A detailed 24-hour recall of the child's diet provides essential information. Every effort must be made to avoid leading the parent as he or she recounts the process of feeding preparation. Schmitt and Mauro conclude that in families with good mother-child interaction, with normal child development, and when there are no deprivational behaviors or inflicted injuries that management of the failure to thrive can be maintained on a monthly outpatient basis. "If the infant is over 12 months of age, the parents have a support system, or the parents have sought medical care for some previous sickness or immunizations, an outpatient approach is even safer" (pp. 243–244). The authors recommend a multidisciplinary outpatient management of mild neglectful failure to thrive according to the following steps: clearly written dietary and stimulation instructions, twice weekly visits by the public health nurse, and referral to child protective services. Even with the prospect of successful outpatient management, the providers cannot forget that every case of even suspected child abuse and neglect must be reported.

Community

Lutzker and Newman (1986) define child abuse and neglect as a community health problem and suggest a community-based treatment approach. Hence community health nurses and public health nurses play an integral role in intervention at the secondary prevention level, namely case finding and treatment.

Risk factors were discussed in the section on primary prevention. Once the nurse identifies the family at risk, the assessment must be carried one step further and the nurse must assess if child maltreatment is occurring. Assessment data that lead the nurse to strongly suspect abuse include a child who is wary of physical contact with adults and who may even shrink away from such contact; the child who winces or flinches when an adult hand is raised; the child who responds to the nurse's questions with one-word answers and who often glances toward the parent or caregiver before answering as if to seek approval; and the child who demonstrates extremes of behavior ranging from overt aggression to profound withdrawal (Heindl et al., 1979). When behavioral cues suggest abuse, a physical examination must follow. Physical assessment data suggestive of abuse include bruises or welts in unusual places and in various states of healing. It is unlikely that a child would incur numerous bruises on the expanse of the back from a fall. A fall would be expected to injure a bony prominence. Abuse injuries are often to the trunk area of the body, since this area is easy to cover to prevent discovery of the injury. Other signs include unexplained burns, fractures, cuts, and dislocations. When questioned regarding injuries, parents often appear nervous and have a "hard time remembering" what happened. Frequently the parent blames the child for being "clumsy" and may even state that the child did not inform him or her about the injury when it occurred. The caregiver should also be asked why the child was not brought for medical treatment after the injury.

Assessment data for neglect are distinctly different than those for abuse. Behavioral indicators that are "red flags" for neglect include the child who is truant from school frequently and when he or she does attend school, he or she often arrives late and leaves early. School nurses are in key positions to identify and follow up on such behaviors. Physical indicators of neglect include the child who demonstrates poor physical growth and fails to meet appropriate developmental milestones. The infant who is not stimulated and left in the crib all day may have a bald spot in the back of the head. Neglected children often are dirty and their clothes may be old, dirty, or inappropriate for environmental conditions. The children often do not receive proper medical care in terms of both preventive health care (well-child visits/immunizations) and treatment of health problems (injuries or colds).

Once child maltreatment has been identified, the professional nurse's next intervention is to report the fact to the appropriate child protective agency. There are mandatory child abuse and neglect reporting laws in every state that hold the nurse legally responsible to report all cases (see Chapter 13 for detailed discussion). Often the quickest way to report is a referral to the local Child Protective Services Agency (CPSA) followed by the written report shortly thereafter. It is important to have definite, objective data to support the claim when reporting child maltreatment. Physical findings are important, as are environmental findings, school attendance records, and verbatim parental accounts. Reports of findings such as "the mother constantly yells at the child and he seems afraid" will probably not meet CPSA standards for maltreatment. Reporting of child abuse can be made anonymously; however, CPSA may appreciate knowing who reports the abuse because this helps determine the credibility of the report. Once the nurse has given the in-

take person the data, it is the responsibility of the CPSA to assign the case and begin action. Many states have a mandatory time frame in which the CPSA must take action. In addition, many states also have a time frame within which the written report must be sent to the CPSA. The state's child protection law contains the state's guidelines in these areas.

The CPSA worker makes a home visit to the family and informs them of the referral. Ideally, the parent should be informed that the referral is being made; however, realistically most families react with anger and hostility to such accusations. The professional nurse must consider the impact of such a revelation on the therapeutic relationship with the family. It is important that the nurse not mistakenly assume that abusive and neglectful parents do not want help, and that they are content in their maltreatment of their child. It is possible that some parents do not wish to change their behavior, yet clinical experience more often reveals anxious, frightened people who do not want to lose custody of their children but who fear what harm they may do in the future. Once the CPSA worker has met with the family, the nurse can assist the family to use the variety of services available from the protective service agency. Parents often suffer under the misconception that the sole function of protective service agencies is to remove children from their families. Child protective agencies often offer a wide range of services from crisis telephone lines to emergency respite child care services.

The primary focus of secondary prevention is to assure safety of the child victim. In some cases the child will be placed in temporary foster care until the parent has completed treatment, in other cases the family will be closely monitored by CPSA while the family is in treatment. This intervention is very important; Cohn and Daro (1987) report, after an analysis of the research findings on child abuse and neglect treatment programs, that approximately one third of parents in treatment programs continue to maltreat their child(ren) during the course of therapy. The CHN of PHN may also be following such families and should be attune to the possibility of continued maltreatment despite treatment interventions.

Secondary prevention treatment program are focused on the family as a unit, rather than on select individuals. Scharer (1979) describes the role of the professional nurse when intervening with abusive and neglectful families. She describes this role in terms of six subroles: mother surrogate, managerial, technical, teacher, nurse-psychotherapist, and socializing agent. Essentially, nursing interventions are focused on gaining trust, role modeling, teaching problem solving and limit setting, attending to the parent, and facilitating the development of extrafamilial resources. Carter, Reid, and Reh (1975) see the role of the professional nurse as service coordinator. Intervention techniques used by the nurse included relationship building, modeling of appropriate methods of childcare, psychological support to the mother, collaboration with mother in planning health care, and coordination of other agency services. Modeling and reinforcement of desirable behaviors were also used. In suggested interventions with abusive and neglectful families, derived from both studies, nurses are called on to use the full range of their skills.

In the few instances in which child abuse and neglect is committed by a mentally ill parent, intensive treatment by the appropriate professional should be aimed at alleviating the illness. However, since 95% of the adults who abuse and neglect children are not psychotic, psychiatric treatment is not a frequently used treatment option (Justice & Justice, 1976).

Treatment modalities and interventions are custom tailored to meet the family's needs. When intervening with maltreating families, the nurse must use assessment data to set long- and short-term goals. Short-term goals must be directed to alleviate immediate stressors, since abusive and neglectful parents most often experience tremendous stress combined with inappropriate methods of child-rearing. Quick action by the professional nurse to alleviate some of the family stress can not only prevent recurrence of child abuse and neglect but also demonstrate to the family the nurse's commitment and ability to "deliver." The power of definitive interventions like emergency housing, supplemental food, and short-term child care should never be underestimated. Horowitz and Wintermute (1978) describe an emergency fund established in New Jersey precisely for the purpose of providing direct services to child abusive and neglectful families that were not covered by any other resource. One result of the pilot study was the realization that small, immediate stress-reducing interventions could successfully eliminate the need for more extensive agency action later.

More long-term stress-reducing interventions call for the nurse to involve the family in available community social and economic assistance programs. Even limited social and economic assistance may be enough to reduce the strain on the family and allow them to attend to alternative methods of coping and child-rearing. Ideally, the level of poverty of families would not merely be decreased in the case of poor, abusive, and neglectful families, but the cause of their poverty would be addressed as well. For example, if a father is laid off from his job as a manual laborer, he would be provided with assistance in retraining, thereby increasing his ability to get a satisfactory job, to raise his status of living, and to allow his family to be self-sufficient. Although the financially independent, nonpoor families may still commit child abuse and neglect, the chances are significantly less.

The ultimate long-term goal for abusive families is to achieve a change in behavior. Many modalities exist to accomplish this. One approach is education of parents, commonly referred to as "parenting classes." Classes are usually structured around a learning theory or approach. Four common theories used in structuring parenting classes include (1) supportive discussion that is an unstructured, parent-driven approach, (2) developmental approach that focuses on teaching parents child development with the hope that this will provide insight into the child's behavior and act as a framework for discipline, (3) a client-centered approach focused on improving the communication pattern between parent and child, and (4) a social-learning theory approach that teaches the principles of social-learning theory as a basis for parenting (Gaudin & Kurtz, 1985). The effectiveness of parenting classes, particularly of individual approaches, is difficult to assess because different outcome measures were used to determine "success." The most frequently used outcome measure was the absence of recurrent abuse. This has inherent faults because abuse may still occur but has not been reported. Hence, the effectiveness of parenting classes at this time is at best inconclusive.

Another intervention modality is the parent support group. Such groups exist to provide social support and a format for discussion and friendship for maltreating parents. Parents Anonymous is an example of such a group. Parents Anonymous is based on the theoretical approach to child abuse, which states that abuse results from (1) unresolved conflict from the parent's childhood, (2) current unmet parental needs, and (3) stressful events that are presently occurring. The group then focuses on parental factors that contribute to the occurrence of such situations. These factors include social isolation, low self-esteem, impulsiveness, passivity, negative attitude toward the child, inadequate knowledge of child development, inadequate problem-solving skills, inability to cope with stress, and inappropriate child-management techniques.

Hunka, O'Toole, and O'Toole (1985) empirically evaluated the effectiveness of a Midwest Parents Anonymous group by use of interviews and a Likert questionnaire to assess the 18 subjects' progress in the aforementioned factors. Overall, the majority of the parents reported positive change in each one of the factors. Self-esteem was reported to be the most problematic area for the subjects and also demonstrated the greatest degree of improvement after treatment. Hence it appears that this particular program was effective for these participants. It should be noted that the longer the subjects attended the sessions and the more frequently the subjects attended, the greater the differences in pretreatment and posttreatment scores. (Hunka et al., 1985).

Another treatment option is a combination of the two approaches, that is, parenting classes that also function as support groups. Soditus and Mock (1988) discuss one such program developed and implemented by public health nurses in Sacramento. The goals of the 8-week program were to increase parents' skills as nurturers, to facilitate positive parent-child interactions, and to encourage parents to see their children as individuals. Although the classes were structured, parents were encouraged to participate and share. Soditus and Mock reported that participation in the classes increased the parents' self-esteem, shown by more relaxed posture by participants over time, more smiling, and increased interaction between parents. No other empirical measures of program effectiveness were reported and there was no follow-up of families after completion of the program to assess for any recurrent abusive behavior.

The federal government has funded four major studies aimed at evaluating and determining the effectiveness of interventions aimed at treating child abuse and neglect (Cohn et al., 1981). The overall results of this evaluation concluded that lay services (such as Parents Anonymous) were found to be most effective within a treatment program that included parenting classes and individual therapy. In addition, the findings identified an optimal length of treatment to be between 7 and 18 months. Clients involved in treatment less than 6 months or longer than 19 months scored lower on success indicators than the optimal treatment time group. Success rates, however, for all the demonstration projects evaluated were disappointing—only fair to poor. Physical abuse continued to occur during the course of treatment in 30% to 47% of the cases evaluated. The authors conclude that overall current treatment efforts are not very effective.

Kempe and Kempe (1978) estimated that 20% of maltreating families experience no change in behavior, regardless of intervention; 40% of parents experience a long-term behavior change; and 40% cease to physically maltreat their children but continue to emotionally and mentally maltreat. The findings of the government studies suggest the percentages for continued maltreatment to be much higher than Kempe and Kempe estimated. Kempe and Kempe use these findings to advocate that more dollars be invested in primary prevention because secondary prevention does not appear to be effective.

Social interventions

The complex nature of child abuse and neglect and the need for multidisciplinary involvement has been presented. The nurse concerned about the status and treatment of children is likely alarmed at dramatic cutbacks of social services to children and their families. The nature of child abuse and neglect requires the involvement of many disciplines, and yet the exact agencies that are needed the most by families with the fewest resources are the agencies that experience the most severe funding cuts. The individuals who preach the sanctity of the American family are often the advocates of the elimination of the few services that might help a family stay nonviolent and together. The American Bar Association's Juvenile Justice Standards Project (1977) has taken one step further by citing the low prevailing quality of protective child welfare services in the United States and therefore recommending a sharp *restriction* of access to those services. A technique suggested for decreasing the number of referred cases of child abuse and neglect is the change of mandatory reporting to discretionary reporting. Social policies and beliefs that promote such a backward movement of child welfare services are of great concern and a focus of intervention for nursing.

Over the past 30 years the problem of child abuse and neglect has become more familiar to both the professional and general public. Of the cases of child abuse and neglect reported to child protective services in 1988, 26% came from sources other than institutions and community agencies (National Center on Child Abuse and Neglect, 1988). Approximately 68% of the reports were from professionals (education, health care, law enforcement, social agency). Hospitals and public health agencies accounted for 10%. Unfortunately, as many cases and possibly even more went unreported.

Friedrich (1977) reports that after a 2-week media campaign in Houston, Texas, aimed at educating the public and professionals about their role in child abuse, a significant increase in reported cases of child abuse occurred. The greatest apparent effect of the campaign was on the professionals, and the increase in reports came under the category of the "less severe" type of abuse (soft tissue abuse, abuse with neglect). "Possibly the campaign had the effect of increasing potential reporters' awareness of the many types of abuse rather than just the severe

types like burns, fractures, and gunshot" (pp. 161-162). As suggested in previous chapters (see Chapter 2), many cases of child abuse and neglect go unreported. Nurses thus have a responsibility to see that media campaigns like the one described by Friedrich take place in their community. Until abusive families are identified and given assistance, the child-victim will likely continue to suffer.

The increasing literature reports on resilience in children offer hope to professionals and families alike. The work of Cowen and Work (1988) has already been cited for its important insight in the role of support in the development of resilience in children as they experience life adversity. Mrazek and Mrazek (1987) conclude that there are generic life circumstances and abuse-specific protective factors that can help children to be less vulnerable to the debilitating effects of abuse and neglect. Generic life circumstances that can support children include: good health, educational, and social welfare services. According to Mrazek and Mrazek (1987), these factors can foster resilience in children regardless of the stressors. Abuse-specific protective factors include quick and full acknowledgment of an offender regarding abuse, and timeliness and permanence of legal actions affecting the child's custody. Although these factors alone cannot ensure that detrimental effects on children are minimized, they are recognized as significant factors that should be considered in the development of any plan of care for abused and neglected children.

Tertiary Prevention

Ideally, child abuse and neglect is never allowed to progress to this stage of intervention; however, as social resources are eliminated, more children are likely to be identified for the first time at this late stage. Tertiary prevention is the level of intervention required when the damage of child abuse and neglect is done and the disability is irreversible. The goal of tertiary prevention is rehabilitation to the maximum level of functioning possible within the limitations of the disability.

Tertiary prevention is also necessary when, after thorough assessment and interdisciplinary consultation, it becomes clear that the abusive and neglectful family cannot safely function together. Of necessity the child is removed from the home, either voluntarily or by court action. At the time of the removal, the child is placed in an alternative living arrangement, usually a foster home. In certain areas where emergency custody programs exist through the courts, the nurses in such facilities will find themselves in an excellent position to provide services from crisis intervention to health promotion.

The Child Welfare League of America has developed *Standards for Service for Abused or Neglected Children and their Families* (1989). These standards were developed by a multidisciplinary committee that sought to address both the generic components of child welfare practice as well as specific information on children and families experiencing abuse and neglect. These standards provide guidelines for multidisciplinary practice with maltreated children and their families. The role of child protective services and the legal system are discussed in detail. In addition, these standards describe multidisciplinary practice with abusive families and community responsibilities directed toward the protection of children. Standards as the ideals or goals for practice with abused and neglected children and their families provide important guidelines for the nurse who seeks to restore these individuals to their highest level of functioning. The Child Welfare League of America, in the case of abuse and neglected children and others, provides important information on meeting human responses to serious child health concerns.

Separation of children from their families is often necessary to ensure the safety of children, but it does not solve the family's problems. If prior separation from children is thought at least partly responsible for the lack of positive parent-child relationship, subsequent separations can only be expected to exacerbate the problem (Watters, Parry, Caplan, & Bates, 1986).

Foster home placement for an abused and neglected child is often identified as a "temporary" action designed to provide care to the child when the family cannot. However, in Massachusetts, Derdeyn (1977) reports that in a cross-sectional study, 60% of the children in foster care had been in foster care for 4 to 8 years. Interestingly, one of the factors impeding return of children to their families, cited by the Jenkins and Norman (1975) study of children in foster care in New York City, was the extreme poverty of their mothers.

Derdeyn also discusses that foster home placement often is not temporary, and that many children live in multiple homes during their placement. Adoption is often an impossibility. Even if a family wished to adopt a child, the biological parents usually refuse to give up custody. It appears that foster children, in the eyes of the court, have even fewer rights than children in general. Derdeyn recommends permanent foster placement for children who cannot be returned home or placed by adoption.

Generally, institutions—foster homes, group homes, or large child welfare institutions—are unacceptable and do not benefit the abused and neglected children in them (Bush 1980). The 370 children surveyed by Bush lived in a variety of settings at the time of the study. The majority of children living in institutions "felt less comfortable, loved, looked after, trusted, cared about, and wanted than children in any other form of surrogate care (foster home) or than children who had been returned to their original families. In general, institutions were reported to be run on the basis that the children in them had 'problems' and were in need of treatment" (p. 249). Another frequent comment of the children interviewed by Bush was that environment and activities were organized primarily to facilitate the running of the institution.

When the abused and neglected child is in poor physical condition as the result of parent maltreatment, the nurse can use interventions based on healing and restorative principles. For example, the malnourished infant requires nursing interventions that alleviate the child's alteration in nutrition. The burned child experiences the same alterations in skin integrity as any other burn victim. In addition to physical needs, the abused and neglected child is likely to have difficulties relating to adults, to be limited in communication, and to otherwise be developmentally delayed.

The appropriate nursing interventions directed at the psychological, social, and developmental needs of the abused and neglected child at the level of tertiary prevention are rehabilitative. The harm inflicted on the child is irreversible, and nursing care must seek to limit the extent of the disability as much as possible.

As always, the nurse first addresses the safety of the child. As discussed previously, often when the child's safety can be secured, the living environment is hardly desirable. The child experiences an unsafe, unhealthy childhood in the home of his biological parents only to be moved, "for his own good," to a safe but still questionably healthy alternative home. It is doubtful that an abused and neglected child would learn to be a successful parent in either setting.

The most important intervention for the abused and neglected child is the securing of a positive, loving home. If the home of the biological parents cannot be made safe, then the nurse should support the other professionals involved in the welfare of the child in foster home placement. Ideally, the biological parents' home should be made safe and the child returned as soon as possible.

The plan of care with the abusive and neglectful parents should include interventions that reduce stress on the parent and increase parent self-esteem, problem-solving skills, and knowledge of child development. Family counseling and therapy are most likely necessary to terminate the maladaptive family members' interactions. See Chapter 10 for a detailed discussion of overall family nursing care.

While in foster care the abused and neglected child needs ongoing nursing intervention. Indeed, it is possible that the nurse is the only consistent person in the life of the child in the transition from abusive and neglectful home to foster home. The nurse seeks to ensure that the foster home provides the child with an environment that is supportive, understanding, consistent, and nonviolent. Often the move to a foster home involves relocation to another part of town. Nursing intervention can ensure that schooling and health care services con-tinue in the new location where past services ended. A child need not restart his or her immunizations just because no one kept track of the shot records.

Nursing intervention aimed at helping an abused and neglected child overcome past trauma may include psychological therapy, special education, or both for the emotionally disturbed. The child who does not require special assistance in school still needs the support of his or her school nurse who receives a referral on the child from his or her public health nurse.

The preschool child can also be involved in an educational program appropriate to his or her needs. Many abused and neglected children have received either no developmental stimulation or the wrong kind. As soon as possible, they need to experience developmentally appropriate, positive stimulation.

Many severely abused and neglected children experience permanent physical disabilities as a result of their maltreatment. These children are entitled to many of the same state, federal, and charitable health and financial benefits available to other disabled children. The nurse can see that the abused and neglected child uses all available services as soon as possible in an effort to reduce the impact of physical disability.

In a qualitative study Korbin (1989) proposes a framework for understanding the most severe form of child abuse and neglect, fatal maltreatment. Korbin's study was limited to mothers. She concluded that although extreme in outcome, fatal maltreatment was not a homogeneous entity. She further noted that although the specifics of each case varied, each was characterized by a *recurrent* pattern of abuse culminating in fatality. Korbin's progression of events leading to child fatality is briefly discussed below.

The women in Korbin's study reported life histories rampant with adverse conditions and risk factors. These include past and/or concurrent family violence, difficulties (real and/or perceived) in child management, and financial stressors. Korbin reported that within a pattern of recurrent abuse, the women gave signals to others that problems existed. "Like suicide victims, abusive parents may give signs or clues that they consciously or unconsciously hope will be interpreted as pleas for help and alert others to the problems that they are experiencing. Such signals may be provided to professionals and public service agencies or to individuals such as kin, neighbors or friends in their personal networks" (p. 484). Especially noteworthy was Korbin's finding that the presence of visible injuries was a significant point in the evolution toward child fatality. When the mothers were faced with visible evidence of their maltreatment, they were often shocked into seeking help or telling others of their behavior. For the women in Korbin's study, however, these warnings and pleas for help went unrecognized and therefore untreated. "This was a pivotal stage in the progression towards the fatality. The women could exit the cycle into intervention (that might or might not be successful), or they could engage in denial that contributed to a continuing pattern of abuse and culminated in the fatality" (p. 486). At this point the mothers entered a cycle of denial and continuing abuse. The lack of response by others who knew of the abuse contributed to the mothers' denial of the seriousness of their actions. Two of the women in Korbin's study had been reported to child protective services and either the deceased child or another had been removed from the home. Fontana and Alfaro (1987) found that a previous court-ordered placement was among the few factors that differentiated fatal from nonfatal abuse. Korbin concluded that regardless of the reason for removing the child, the reuniting period may be particularly dangerous for the child. Korbin's research supports the need for early identification and intervention with families at-risk or experiencing child abuse and neglect. Her findings further suggest that removal of the child from the home ensures the safety of the child often only in the short term.

It would seem that leaving an abused and neglected child in an unsafe home is unacceptable. However, placing a child in a foster home, group home, or state institution is also no solution. The energies of the nurse, in the case of child abuse and neglect, are best directed toward an earlier level of prevention, ideally primary. Social policies in the United States must become intolerable to the nurse until children are given the same rights and opportunities as granted by the Constitution to adults.

It should also be noted that all three levels of prevention of child abuse and neglect may be necessary in the nursing interventions with an individual family. For example, the professional nurse may become familiar with a family when intervening to safely return an abused child to his or her home from foster care (tertiary prevention), when securing supplemental food program benefits for underfed siblings (secondary prevention), and when providing health promotion to parents of a healthy newborn (primary prevention). The demands on the nurse are great and require skillful, creative nursing care.

EVALUATION

The final step of the nursing process is evaluation. At this point the professional nurse reviews the changes that have occurred based on the identified goals. Again, the nurse must be realistic in her evaluation of child abuse and neglect. She can also praise even small evidences of progress. Praise to a parent who is having difficulty in child-rearing can be a new experience and a strong reinforcer.

SAMPLE NURSING PROCESS

A sample nursing process in a case of child abuse and neglect has been included in this chapter to demonstrate how each of the four steps can be applied to a hypothetical case. A brief description of the case has been recorded. An in-depth assessment composed of both historical and physical findings would naturally have preceded its development. The total assessment is not completely reported. In addition, each child and family are unique and require individualized plans of care. The sample nursing process (Table 8-4) is included as a starting point for professional nursing practice.

TABLE 8-4
Sample Nursing Process

Brief background

Kent is a 15-month-old white boy admitted to the general pediatric unit of the hospital with a medical diagnosis of child abuse and neglect. Kent lives with his 22-year old mother and two siblings. The family's sole source of income is Aid to Dependent Children. Kent's mother describes him as a "difficult" child who willfully disobeys her and refuses to be toilet trained. She reports that he holds his bowel movements "just to make me angry." In addition, Kent's mother reports that he "won't eat" and drinks only KoolAid in his bottle. Kent's mother is the primary caretaker who knows no one in the neighborhood and moved to the area to be with Kent's father, who has since deserted the family.

The nurse's physical examination of Kent includes, but is not limited to the following:

General appearance	Thin, 15-month-old white boy who appears to watch all activities in the room, but remains quiet and passive through all procedures including subsequent blood drawing.
Vital statistics	Height and weight below 3rd percentile.
Skin	Multiple discrete, circumscribed 1 cm in diameter second-degree burns in various stages of resolution about the distal arms and legs. Scant purulent drainage noted at lesions. Generalized decreased subcutaneous tissue.
Neurological	Abnormal score on DDST (Failed language and personal/social).

Three of the nursing diagnoses are identified in order of priority

Family-focused nursing diagnosis

I. Altered family process: potential for subsequent violence (child) related to lack of parent support systems, inadequate financial resources, mother's knowledge deficit regarding growth and development, and ineffective parent behavior

CLIENT GOALS	NURSING INTERVENTION	EVALUATION
I. Family will not experience additional violence as evidenced by:	I. The nurse will:	Because the nursing process is still in the development phase, no evaluation is possible. When appropriate, evaluation should be ongoing and based on the achievement of identified family goals measured against the stated criteria.
A. Short term (before discharge) 1. No additional child injuries during hospitalization	A. 1.a. Provide continuous, but discrete supervision of mother-child interaction 1.b. Provide mother with age-appropriate child safety precautions for hospitalization	

TABLE 8-4 *Continued*
Sample Nursing Process

CLIENT GOALS	NURSING INTERVENTION	EVALUATION
2. Demonstration of nurturant behavior by parent toward child	2.a. Role model nurturant child care behaviors for mother, especially during bath, play, and feeding	
	2.b. Encourage mother to actively participate in daily child care	
	2.c. Praise mother's attempts at nurturant behaviors expecting closer approximations of goal qd	
3. Mother's voicing of factors contributing to past episodes of violence toward child	3.a. Spend at least 20 min qd encouraging mother to talk about herself	
	3.b. Use therapeutic communication techniques to elicit factors contributing to violence toward child	
	3.c. Use therapeutic communication to increase mother's awareness of factors contributing to violence against child	
4. Mother's identification of alternative methods of expressing anger	4.a. Use therapeutic communication and problem-solving techniques to assist mother in identification of nonviolent expressions of anger	
5. Mother's identification of key aspects of child behavior and development during the toddler stage	5.a. Provide mother with information about child development	
	5.b. Demonstrate to mother how information about child development can be used in daily life (discipline, play, feeding, toileting)	

TABLE 8-4 *Continued*
Sample Nursing Process

CLIENT GOALS	NURSING INTERVENTION	EVALUATION
6. Mother's agreement to participate with child protective and other agencies	6.a. Provide mother with information about child protective and other agencies 6.b. Contact appropriate agencies and establish client contact before discharge 6.c. Reassure mother that all agencies are concerned with child safety and helping her to care for her child	
B. Long term (6 mo postdischarge) 1. No additional child injuries during hospitalization	B.1.a. Referral to public health nursing for continued, intermittent monitoring of child, home, and family	Long-term evaluation will be carried out by the public health nurse following the family and will be ongoing and based on the achievement of identified family goals as measured against the stated criteria.
	1.b. Public health nurse will have contact with mother and child before discharge 1.c. Public health nurse will secure and coordinate child protective and other agency services to family	
2. Improved DDST age-appropriate score	2.a. Public health nurse will enroll child in an educational preschool program 2.b. School will educate, encourage, and support mother in parenting skills 2.c. Public health nurse or school will administer DDST 6 mo postdischarge	
3. Demonstration of consistent nurturant parent behaviors	3.a. See I.B.1.a. 3.b. Public health nurse will continue activities described in I.A.2.a. and c.	

TABLE 8-4 *Continued*
Sample Nursing Process

CLIENT GOALS	NURSING INTERVENTION	EVALUATION
4. Documented demonstration of mother using nonviolent methods of dealing with anger	4.a. See I.B.1.a. and c.	
5. Demonstration by mother of age-appropriate techniques of child discipline	5.a. See I.B.1.a.	
	5.b. See I.B.4.a.	
	5.c. Public health nurse will praise all attempts by mother to use nonviolent discipline	
6. Documented active participation with other agencies	6.a. See I.B.1.a. and c.	
7. Documented use (as appropriate) of alternative child care services	7.a. See I.B.1.a., 2.b.	
	7.b. Public health nurse will provide information to mother regarding daycare centers and emergency child care services	
	7.c. Public health nurse will use problem-solving techniques to assist mother in identifying friends and/or relatives who might assist or exchange child care	
8. Mother's participation in social or other organizations (church, school, etc.) that increase circle of acquaintances	8.a. Public health nurse will assess mother for areas of social, educational, recreational, religious, or community interest	
	8.b. Public health nurse will provide information about appropriate organizations in community and arrange for personal contact as desired	
	8.c. Public health nurse will praise all evidence of mother decreasing her social isolation	

TABLE 8-4 *Continued*
Sample Nursing Process

CLIENT GOALS	NURSING INTERVENTION	EVALUATION

Child-focused nursing diagnosis

II. Impairment of skin integrity related to partial-thickness burns and poor hygiene

CLIENT GOALS	NURSING INTERVENTION	EVALUATION
II. Client will experience improved skin integrity during hospitalization(2 wk) as evidenced by:	II. The nurse will:	Because the nursing process is still in the development phase, no evaluation is possible. When appropriate, evaluation should be ongoing and based on the achievement of identified client goals measured against the stated criteria.
A. Healing of skin lesions	A.1. Note size, shape, location, and condition of lesions	
1. No additional child injuries during hospitalization	A.2. Exact diagram of lesions will be recorded and included in initial nursing assessment	
	A.3. Skin lesions will be cleaned and gently debrided after 15 min of soaking during AM bath	
	A.4. Lesions will then be left open to air	
	A.5. Progress of lesions will be monitored	
	A.6. Provide adequate diet (see Nursing Diagnosis #3)	
B. Decreased signs of infection (redness, tenderness, swelling)	B.1. Monitor vital signs	
	B.2. Monitor skin lesions for increased redness, tenderness, and swelling	
	B.3. Monitor laboratory data (i.e., CBC)	
	B.4. Keep client's fingernails clean and short	
	B.5. Inform mother of all signs of improvement	
C. No new skin lesions	C.1. Monitor client's skin qd	
	C.2. Provide supervision of mother-child interaction	
D. Evidence of good personal hygiene	D.1. Serve as role model to mother	
	D.2. Provide information to mother	
	D.3. Praise mother's efforts to assist in attainment of goal and identify strengths	

TABLE 8-4 *Continued*
Sample Nursing Process

CLIENT GOALS	NURSING INTERVENTION	EVALUATION

Child-focused nursing diagnosis

III. Alteration in nutrition: less than body requirements, probably related to parent knowledge deficit and inadequate finanical resources

III. Client will experience adequate nutrition during hospitalization (2 wk) as evidenced by:	III. The nurse will:	Because the nursing process is still in the development phase, no evaluation is possible. When appropriate, evaluation should be ongoing and based on the achievement of identified client goals measured against the stated criteria.
A. No loss in weight	A.1. Provide client with age-appropriate diet qd: Protein 1.8 (g/kg) Energy 100 (kcal/kg) Fat>30%,<50% Carbohydrate 50 to 100g	
	A.2. Record all food and fluid intake	
	A.3. Provide a varied selection of food (color, taste, texture)	
	A.4. Prepare food so that it is mild and of comfortable temperature	
	A.5. Provide three nutritious finger-food snacks (10:00 AM, 3:00 PM, 7:30 PM)	
	A.7. Encourage mother's involvement in feeding a. Serve as role model to mother b. Provide information to mother c. Praise mother's efforts to assist in attainment of goal and identify strengths	
	A.8. Weigh qd	
B. Good skin turgor and moist mucous membranes	B.1. Provide client with adequate fluid intake qd: (120 to 125 ml/kg)	
	B.2. Record all fluid intake	
	B.3. Offer 4 oz of fluid (vary type) every waking hour	

TABLE 8-4 *Continued*
Sample Nursing Process

CLIENT GOALS	NURSING INTERVENTION	EVALUATION
	B.4. Encourage drinking from cup a. Assist as necessary b. Praise mother and child efforts B.5. Measure urine specific gravity each shift	
C. Laboratory findings that show no worsening of physical condition	C.1. Monitor laboratory tests and alter diet as necessary	
D. Mother's identification of key aspects of nutrition, child behavior, and development during the toddler stage and appropriate available resources	D.1. Inform mother about nutrition, growth, and development D.2. Arrange consultation with nutritionist D.3. Inform mother regarding available supplemental food programs D.4. Recommend parent-child educational daycare center to mother D.5. Contact social service agency to arrange for enrollment before discharge	

SUMMARY

Nursing care of the abused and neglected child is approached from a family framework and based on the limited available nursing research. The use of the nursing process in practice with abusive and neglectful families involves four steps—assessment, goals, planning, and evaluation. Assessment for child abuse and neglect can be included in the practice of every nurse who provides care to children and their families. Particular attention should be paid in assessment to certain warning signs that can indicate potential or actual abuse. Although three levels of prevention of child abuse and neglect are discussed, nursing practice should be directed toward primary prevention since *no* level of maltreatment of children can be acceptable to the nurse whose philosophy is to promote the life, health, and well-being of her clients.

REFERENCES

American Bar Association. Juvenile Justice Standards Project (1977). *Standards relating to abuse and neglect.* Cambridge: Harper & Row.

Barth, R. P., Hacking, S., & Ash, J. R. (1988). Preventing child abuse: An experimental evaluation of the child-parent enrichment project. *Journal of Primary Prevention, 8,* 201-217.

Browne, K., & Saqi, S. (1988). Mother-infant interaction and attachment in physically abusing families. *Journal of Reproductive and Infant Psychology, 6,* 163-182.

Bullock, L. F., & McFarlane, J. (1989, September). The birth-weight/battering connection. *American Journal of Nursing, 89,* 1153-1155.

Bush, M. (1980). Institutions for dependent and neglected children: Therapeutic option of choice or last resort? *American Journal of Orthopsychiatry, 50,* 239-55.

Caldwell, R. A., Bogat, G. A., & Davidson, W. S. (1988). The assessment of child abuse potential and the prevention of child abuse and neglect: A policy analysis. *American Journal of Community Psychology, 16,* 609-624.

Cappell, C., & Heiner, R. B. (1990). The intergenerational transmission of family aggression. *Journal of Family Violence, 5,* 135-152.

Carter, B. D., Reed, R., & Reh, C. J. (1975). Mental health nursing intervention with child abusing and neglectful mothers. *Journal of Psychiatric Nursing and Mental Health Services, 13,* 132-140.

Cersonsky, J. (1988). Cocaine abusers as mothers. *Pediatrics, 82,* 136.

Chasnoff, I. J. (1988). Cocaine abusers as mothers. *Pediatrics, 82,* 136-137.

Child Welfare League of America. (1989). *Standards for service for abused or neglected children and their families.* Washington, DC: Child Welfare League of America.

Children's Trust Fund. (1988/89-1989/90). *State plan for years 1988/89 and 1989/90.* Lansing, MI: Children's Trust Fund.

Cohn, A. H. (1981). *An approach to preventing child abuse.* Chicago: National Committee for Prevention of Child Abuse.

Cohn, A. H., & Daro, D. (1987). Is treatment too late: What ten years of evaluative research tells us. *Child Abuse and Neglect, 11,* 433-442.

Cowen, E. L., & Work, W. C. (1988). Resilient children, psychological wellness, and primary prevention. *American Journal of Community Psychology, 16,* 591-607.

Crittenden, P. M., & Morrison, A. K. (1988). An early parental indicator of potential maltreatment. *Pediatric Nursing, 14,* 415-417.

Cupoli, J. M., & Newberger, E. H. (1977). Optimism or pessimism for the victim of child abuse? *Pediatrics, 59,* 1356-1360.

Davis, N. L., & Johnson, G. H. (1978). A way of caring: Nurses initiate community action to prevent child abuse. *AORN Journal, 27,* 631-35.

Densen-Gerber, J. (1978). *Child abuse and neglect as related to parental drug abuse and other antisocial behavior.* New York: Odyssey.

Derdeyn, A. P. (1977). A case for permanent foster placement of dependent, neglected, and abused children. *American Journal of Orthopsychiatry, 47,* 604-614.

Fontana, V., & Alfaro, J. (1987). *High risk factors associated with child maltreatment fatalities.* New York: Mayor's Task Force on Child Abuse and Neglect.

Friedrich, W. N. (1977). Evaluation of media campaign's effect on reporting patterns of child abuse. *Perceptual and Motor Skills, 45,* 161-62.

Gage, R. B. (1990). Consequences of children's exposure to spouse abuse. *Pediatric Nursing, 16,* 258-260.

Gaudin, J. M., & Kurtz, D. P. (1985). Parenting skills training for child abusers. *Journal of Group Psychotherapy, Psychodrama and Sociometry, 38,* 35-54.

Gil, D. G. (1971). Violence against children. *Journal of Marriage and the Family, 32,* 637-48.

Gough, D., & Taylor, J. (1988). Child abuse prevention: Studies of ante-natal and post-natal services. *Journal of Reproductive and Infant Psychology, 6,* 217-228.

Gray, E. B. (1982). Perinatal support programs: A strategy for primary prevention of child abuse. *Journal of Primary Prevention, 2,* 138-152.

Hamilton, L. R. (1989). Variables associated with child maltreatment and implications for prevention and treatment. *Early Child Development and Care, 42,* 31-36.

Heindl, C., Krall, C. A., Salus, M. K., & Broadhurst, D. D. (1979). *The nurse's role in the prevention and treatment of child abuse and neglect* (DHEW No. 79-30202). Washington, DC: U.S. Department of Health, Education and Welfare.

Herzberger, S. D., & Tennen, H. (1988). Snips and snails and puppy dog tails: Gender of agent, recipient, and observer as determinants of perceptions of discipline. *Sex Roles, 12,* 853-865.

Hoffman-Plotkin, D., & Twentyman, C. T. (1984). A multimodal assessment of behavioral and cognitive deficits in abused and neglected preschoolers. *Child Development, 55,* 794-802.

Horowitz, B., & Wintermute, W. (1978). Use of an emergency fund in protective services casework. *Child Welfare, 57,* 432-437.

Howe, A. C., Herzberger, S., & Tennen, H. (1988). The influence of personal history of abuse and gender on clinicians' judgments of child abuse. *Journal of Family Violence, 3,* 105-119.

Hunka, C. D., O'Toole, A. W., & O'Toole, R. (1985). Self-help therapy in parents anonymous. *Journal of Psychosocial Nursing, 23,* 24-31.

Jason, J., & Andereck, N. D. (1983). Fatal child abuse in Georgia: The epidemiology of severe physical child abuse. *Child Abuse and Neglect, 7,* 1-9.

Jenkins, S., & Norman, M. (1975). *Beyond placement: Mothers view foster care.* New York: Columbia University Press.

Justice, B., & Justice, R. (1976). *The abusing family.* New York: Human Sciences Press.

Kalichman, S. C., Craig, M. E., & Follingstad, D. R. (1990). Professionals' adherence to mandatory child abuse reporting laws: Effects of responsibility attribution, confidence ratings, and situational factors. *Child Abuse and Neglect, 14,* 69-77.

Kaufman, J., & Zigler, E. (1987). Do abused children become abusive parents? *American Journal of Orthopsychiatry, 57,* 186-192.

Kempe, R. S., & Kempe, C. H. (1978). *Child abuse.* Cambridge: Harvard University Press.

Klaus, M. H., & Kennell, J. H. (Eds.). (1976). Maternal-infant bonding. In *Maternal-infant bonding* (p. 10-21). St. Louis: Mosby-Year Book.

Korbin, J. E. (1989). Fatal maltreatment by mothers: A proposed framework. *Child Abuse and Neglect, 13,* 481-489.

Krieger, L. M. (1988, July 2). Mothers accountable for fetuses health. *San Francisco Examiner,* p. 1.

Landwirth, J. (1987). Fetal abuse and neglect: An emerging controversy. *Pediatrics, 79,* 508-514.

Levinthal, J. M. (1988). Can child maltreatment be predicted during the perinatal period: Evidence from longitudinal cohort studies. *Journal of Reproductive and Infant Psychology, 6,* 139-161.

Lutzker, J. R., & Newman, M. R. (1986). Child abuse and neglect: Community problem, community solutions. *Education and Treatment of Children, 9,* 344-354.

McKibben, L., De Vos, E., & Newberger, E. H. (1989). Victimization of mothers of abused chidren: A controlled study. *Pediatrics, 84,* 531-535.

Milner, J. S., & Chilamkurti, C. (1991). Physical child abuse perpetrator characteristics. *Journal of Interpersonal Violence, 6,* 345-366.

Mrazek, P. J., & Mrazek, D. P. (1987). Resilience in child maltreatment victims: A conceptual exploration. *Child Abuse and Neglect, 11,* 357-366.

National Center on Child Abuse & Neglect (1988). *Study of National Incidence and Prevalence of Child Abuse and Neglect: 1988.* (Contract No. 105-85-1702). Washington, DC: U.S. Department of Health and Human Services.

Newberger, E. H. (1976, April). A physician's perspective on the interdisciplinary management of child abuse. *Psychiatric Opinion, 2,* 13-18.

Newberger, E. H., & Bourne, R. (1978). The medicalization and legalization of child abuse. *American Journal of Orthopsychiatry, 48,* 593-607.

Oates, R. K., Davis, A. A., Ryan, M. G., & Stewart, L. F. (1979). Risk factors associated with child abuse. *Child Abuse and Neglect, 3,* 547-553.

O'Connor, S., Vietze, P. M., Sherrad, K. B., Sandler, H. M., & Altermeier, W. A. (1980). Reduced incidence of parenting inadequacy following rooming-in. *Pediatrics, 66,* 176-82.

Paulson, M. J., Afifi, A. A., Thomason, M. L., & Chaleff, A. (1974). The MMPI: A descriptive measure of psychopathology in abusive parents. *Journal of Clinical Psychology, 30,* 387-390.

Pelton, L. H. (1978). Child abuse and neglect: The myth of classlessness. *American Journal of Orthopsychiatry, 48,* 608-617.

Scharer, K. (1979). Nursing therapy with abusive and neglectful families. *Journal of Psychiatric Nursing and Mental Health Services, 17,* 12-21.

Scharer, K. (1978). Rescue fantasies: Professional impediments in working with abused families. *American Journal of Nursing, 78.*

Schein, E. H. (1972). *Professional education. Some new directions.* New York: McGraw-Hill.

Schmitt, B. D., & Mauro, R. D., (1989). Nonorganic failure to thrive: An outpatient approach. *Child Abuse and Neglect, 13,* 235-248.

Seagull, E. A. (1987). Social support and child maltreatment: A review of the evidence. *Child Abuse and Neglect, 11,* 41-52.

Sherrod, K. B., O'Connor, S., Vietze, P. M., & Altemeier, W. A. (1984). Child health and maltreatment. *Child Development, 55,* 1174-1183.

Showers, J., Apolo, J., Thomas, J., & Beavers, S. (1985). Fatal child abuse: A two decade review. *Pediatric Emergency Care, 1,* 66-70.

Smith, S. M., & Kunjukrishnan, R. (1985). Child abuse: Perspectives on treatment and research. *Psychiatric Clinics of North America, 8,* 665-683.

Snyder, J. C., & Newberger, E. H. (1986). Consensus and difference among hospital professionals in evaluating child maltreatment. *Violence and Victims, 1,* 125-139.

Soditus, C., & Mock, D. (1988). Interrupting the cycle of child abuse. *MCN, 13,* 196-199.

Starr, R. H. (1988). Pre- and perinatal risk and physical abuse. *Journal of Reproductive and Infant Psychology, 6,* 125-138.

Steele, B. F. (1987). Psychodynamic factors in child abuse. In R. E. Helfer & C. H. Kempe (Eds.), *The battered child* (4th ed., pp. 81-114). Chicago: University of Chicago Press.

Steele, B. F. & Pollock, C. B. (1974). A psychiatric study of parents who abuse infants and small children. In R. E. Helfer & C. H. Kempe (Eds.), *The battered child* (2nd ed., pp. 92-139). Chicago: University of Chicago Press.

Stern, L. (1973). Prematurity as a factor in child abuse. *Hospital Practice, 8,* 1-19.

Twentyman, C. T., & Plotkin, R. C. (1982). Unrealistic expectations of parents who maltreat their children: An educational deficit pertaining to child development. *Journal of Clinical Psychology, 38,* 497-503.

Vondra, J. I., & Toth, S. L. (1989). Ecological perspectives on child maltreatment: Research and intervention. *Early Child Development and Care, 42,* 11-29.

Watters, J., Parry, R., Caplan, P. J., & Bates, R. (1986). A comparison of child abuse and child neglect. *Canadian Journal of Behavioural Science, 18,* 449-459.

Weikart, D. P. (1980). *Research report.* Ypsilanti, MI: High/Scope Education Research Foundation.

Widom, C. S. (1989). Does violence beget violence? A critical examination of the literature. *Psychological Bulletin, 106,* 3-28.

CHAPTER

9

Nursing Care of Abused Women

Jacquelyn Campbell, Laura Smith McKenna, Sara Torres,
Daniel Sheridan, *and* Karen Landenburger

scared frightened and
all alone
cant go back to my home
left with only the clothes
on my back
wondering if I'll make it
on the right track
all i have is my daughter and me
made it to the shelter
we are free
now all i have to do is make
a life for katie and me
you gave me hope, courage
and most of all love
and so now i can spread my wings
take off again and go on

N.L.*

I am writing a poem
and it is one of thanks
to the women who've come seeking shelter
to those who have given me strength
its easy to share all your laughter
its harder to share your own tears so
thank you my sisters, my neighbors
for helping me deal with my fears
its you who have given me courage
to face my own life as it is
and its you who have taken the 1st step
so your children can grow up and live
there are some who can't work in a shelter
and your right it's not all peaches and cream
But its worth all the petty displeasures
just to watch someone learning to dream
(we grow from each other's growing)

Kathy Clair*

T his chapter focuses on the planning of nursing care with and for battered women in a variety of health care settings. Professional nursing care of battered women is based on theoretical foundations (see Chapter 4) and is individualized to the needs and goals of battered women dealing with various types and levels of abuse. In any health care setting, routine assessment for battering of all women seeking care, especially in situations identified as high risk for the occurrence of battering, must be a priority for nursing. Nursing interventions are needed

at all three levels of prevention. An awareness of the scope of the problem, combined with a knowledge base that directs nursing assessment and interventions, is basic to nurses' developing and retaining sensitivity to the significance of cues of abuse presented by clients. Research on nurse identification and intervention in cases of domestic violence suggests that the nurse's responsibilities begin before the initial client interaction.

ESTABLISHING THE NURSE-CLIENT RELATIONSHIP

Although nurses already have the necessary skills to plan the care of clients in a variety of clinical

---

*Both poems reprinted from *Every Twelve Seconds*, compiled by Susan Venters (Hillsboro, Oregon: Shelter, 1981) by permission of the authors.

settings, experience and research demonstrate that nursing interventions with women victims of domestic violence are consistently inadequate. King and Ryan (1989) state that the identification of such clients in health care settings is impeded by nurses' adherence to societal myths about domestic violence, and that inappropriate interventions result from nurses' misperceptions of the cues presented by battered women. Lack of basic content about abuse of women in educational programs was reported by the majority (90%) of the nurses in this study, who consistently deferred direct questioning that might lead to the woman's disclosure of the violence. Barriers to effective intervention also involved the nurse's fears of the client's response and fears of inability to respond to the client's needs.

Nurses must examine their beliefs and values related to violence against women and create learning situations that allow them to explore the dynamics of and alternate solutions to the problem of violence against women in intimate relationships. Desensitization to women's stories, exploration of one's own exposure to violence in the family, and information about community resources available to female victims of violence are necessary components of the knowledge base that will lead to appropriate interventions with such clients. Limandri (1987) describes several responses that facilitate battered women seeking help from health care providers, along with responses that inhibit help seeking. She also recognizes the importance of the effect of the client's situation on the nurse.

For example, there is frustration inherent when the nurse suspects abuse, sees the woman only once, and battering is denied. Such frustration may be easily transmitted into anger at the abused woman. It is helpful for the nurse to know that denial is a normal response to battering and an important step in grieving the losses experienced by the woman abused in an intimate relationship. The nurse should allow the abused woman this defense until she is able to confront the situation. However, for some nurses, allowing denial means condoning it, and nurses fear they will be responsible for the woman remaining in the abusive situation. As with all responses to bat-

---

Principles of Empowerment

Mutuality and reciprocity
Sharing information
Giving choices
Brainstorming solutions
Making sense of it

---

tered women, nurses are better prepared to intervene more effectively if they have thoroughly examined their own attitudes about wife abuse and anticipated their possible responses to such clients. They must carefully sort their own reactions to the myths about battering and examine their general responses to victims of violence. It is helpful to imagine a scenario in which the nurse is the victim of abuse at the hands of an intimate partner who is deeply loved, as impossible as that may seem, and place that scene at a time when her or his own self-esteem was at its lowest ebb. Once nurses realize that abuse could have happened or could happen to them in the future, they can better empathize with the woman, accept her reactions, and anticipate their own responses. Clinical discussion groups and role-plays with other nurses also help develop the sensitivity and provide the support necessary to continue working with this high-risk population.

The general model of nursing care in this chapter is an empowerment model derived from several nursing frameworks (e.g., Orem, 1991; Parse, 1987) and the grass-roots battered woman's movement. The general principles of empowerment are outlined in the following box. They are referred to throughout the chapter. The chapter also is based on the premise that the nurse needs to be sensitive to the cultural background of the abused woman.

WORKING WITH BATTERED WOMEN FROM DIFFERENT CULTURES

Quality nursing care with battered women must be culturally sensitive. The nurse must be aware of cultural issues important to the battered woman that may affect her response to treatment. Unless culture is considered, interventions with battered women will fail (Torres, 1987).

Culture refers to the cumulative deposit of knowledge, experience, meanings, beliefs, values, attitudes, religion, concepts of self, concepts of the universe, self-to-universe relationships, and time concepts acquired by a large group of people in the course of generations through individual and group strivings. Culture manifests itself both in patterns of language and thought and forms of activity and behavior.

Culture is important because it is central to how a battered woman organizes her experience. For instance, Torres (1991) found that although there were more similarities than differences between the two groups, Anglo-American battered women perceived more types of behavior as abusive and exhibited a less tolerant attitude toward abuse than did a group of Mexican-American abused women. Thus culture shapes how a battered woman views violence and the degree of hopefulness or pessimism she has toward recovery. Culture is vital to how she seeks assistance (help-seeking behavior), what she understands as the causes of psychological difficulties, and the unique, subjective experience of being a battered woman. Certain cultural beliefs, values, and practices are likely to increase the number of stressors to which the battered woman is exposed. Culture also determines the battered woman's attitudes about sharing troublesome emotional problems with nurses, attitudes toward her emotional pain, expectations of the treatment, and what she believes is the best method of addressing the difficulties presented by the abuse.

Most cultural behaviors make sense within the culture even if they do not make sense outside the culture. The nurse must view the woman's behavior from inside the culture, taking into account the following: the woman's family structure, gender roles, marriage patterns, sexual behavior, contraceptive patterns, pregnancy and childbirth practices, child-rearing practices, diet, dress, personal hygiene, housing arrangements, sanitation arrangements, religion, migrant status, occupation(s), use of chemical comforters, leisure pursuits, self-treatment strategies, and lay therapies.

The degree of assimilation and socioeconomic class are also important factors. The degree of acculturation or assimilation into the dominant culture must always be considered with battered women who are identified as ethnic minorities. The degree of acculturation determines the degree to which the woman has assumed the values and customs of the dominant culture. However, it is important to remember that even the most acculturated middle-class person has a tendency to revert to his or her cultural past in organizing coping strategies after a stressful event. There are instruments that measure the degree of acculturation. However, in the clinical area, the nurse can assess acculturation by determining:

1. Command of English
2. Language spoken at home and language preference with friends, television, and radio programs
3. Educational attainment and socioeconomic status
4. Religion and degree of religious faith
5. Stresses of migration and length of time in the United States
6. Community of residence and opportunities for linking with fellow countrymen/women

The nurse can determine this information through regular contacts with battered women by asking specific questions in this area in a culturally sensitive manner. It is important to realize that the stresses of migration can make women more vulnerable to abuse and limit their social networks and resources for coping with the abuse.

It is essential that nurses prepare for cross-cultural work. First, it is important for the nurse to explore her own attitudes to minimize biases. What are her racial, cultural, and class prejudices? Does she tend to be culture blind, a "bleeding heart" liberal, or culturally liberated? The nurse's attitude is critical. It is important to respect the cultural traditions of the individual woman and not assume that complete acculturation is the most healthy state. Cultural insensitivity or inappropriate treatment procedures can result in the inadvertent retraumatization of clients. In this regard, Silver (1986) has used the term *sanctuary trauma* to characterize the revictimization that may occur when a trauma survivor perceives that persons or environments (e.g., treatment settings) anticipated to be helpful and protective are instead experienced as being unresponsive and nonsupportive.

An important issue nurses encounter when working with battered women from a different culture or ethnic group is that of "difference"—the battered woman feels different from the nurse, and as a result she feels that the nurse is not able to help or understand her. The nurse must work to overcome this feeling. The nurse must become familiar with the woman's culture. She can read about the culture, become a participant in that culture, and talk to informants and experts from that culture. However, familiarity with the woman's culture is not enough. Nurses must develop skills for cross-cultural care.

Two essential skills the nurse needs to overcome the client's feeling of "difference" are developing "credibility" and being *perceived* as "giving." It is important that the culturally different woman views the nurse as credible. There are two types of credibility: acquired and ascribed. *Acquired* credibility is gained by status (position) and education. *Ascribed* credibility is gained not only by being empathic and having knowledge but also by communicating an awareness of the woman's world view. Thus the woman ascribes to the nurse the ability to help her. Giving is important because the culturally different battered woman must feel that she is benefiting from the helping relationship with the nurse. Giving can occur in many forms, for instance, teaching stress reduction or assisting with obtaining or negotiating social services.

There are several strategies that the nurse can use to increase communication effectiveness when working with a battered woman who has difficulty with English. The nurse can learn some words of greeting and basic sentences in the woman's language. This makes the woman feel that the nurse cares and respects her culture enough to try communicating in her own language. Speaking slowly and clearly in English, without using slang, idioms, or difficult medical terminology, and allowing time for the woman to respond aids communication. Women whose first language is not English go through a process that includes hearing in English,

translating mentally to the native tongue, thinking of a response in the native language, then translating mentally, and finally responding in English.

A three-way relationship is required when an interpreter is used. To build rapport between the interpreter and woman, it is helpful to introduce the two. It is important to have the interpreter translate exactly what the woman says; the nurse should look directly at the woman, not the interpreter, when she speaks, watching her facial expressions and body language. It is better to use a trained interpreter than a family member, because the woman may be embarrassed to discuss some issues in front of family members.

Considering a woman's culture in nursing intervention is a difficult task. If possible nurses should be supervised by experts when they begin to work with battered women from other cultural groups. Ideally, the expert would be a woman from the cultural group who is familiar with both the minority and dominant culture to assist the nurse in translating cultural behaviors into nursing care. The expert should also be sensitive to the issues battered women face.

ASSESSMENT

The nurse's initial approach to the battered woman is important in establishing a nurse-client relationship that allows the woman to disclose her abusive situation. Nurses may encounter battered women in any health care setting. However, nurses are more likely to encounter abused women in the following health care settings where clients are known to be at high risk for battering: emergency trauma units, perinatal and women's health care settings, community health settings, primary care settings, occupational health settings, and inpatient and outpatient mental health settings. In addition to assessing women for abuse if there are overt injuries or signs of conflict in the marital or cohabiting relationship, routine questions related to violence in intimate relationships should be asked of any woman who indicates a close relationship with a man. Lichtenstein (1981) recommends asking, "Have you ever been physically hurt by anyone?" while inquiring about past trauma or injuries (p. 244) or dealing with

ABUSE ASSESSMENT SCREEN

1. Have you ever been emotionally or physically abused by your partner or someone important to you?

YES ☐

NO ☐

2. Within the last year, have you been hit, slapped, kicked or otherwise physically hurt by someone?

YES ☐

NO ☐

If YES, by whom _____

Number of times _____

Mark the area of injury on body map.

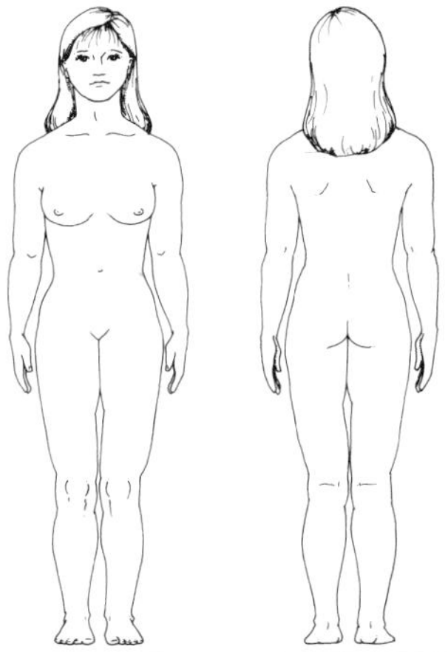

3. Within the last year, has anyone forced you to have sexual activities?

If YES, who _____

Number of times _____

4. Are you afraid of your partner or anyone you listed above?

YES ☐

NO ☐

Figure 9-1

Abuse Assessment Screen. Adapted from the Nursing Research Consortium on Violence and Abuse, 1991.

physical aggression as part of the psychosocial history when inquiring about methods of conflict resolution. Tilden and Shepherd (1987) suggest the question be framed to normalize the event: "Many families have difficulty expressing anger. What is that like in your family?" (p. 30). Another way to frame the assessment within the context of inquiring about the person's most important relationship is to ask "How do you and your partner (husband) resolve disagreements?" and to listen for indications that one partner is invested in power and control or for mention of frequent fighting. If fighting is mentioned, the nurse can ask, "Does the fighting

ever get physical?" The question about solving disagreements can be followed by "What happens when he (or she) gets really angry?" "Does it ever involve pushing or shoving?" Pushing or shoving is the least violent of aggressive conflict resolution methods and often is the start of abuse. It is also the easiest for a survivor to acknowledge. If a woman admits to pushing and shoving or more violent tactics, then a more thorough assessment of the nature of the violence can begin. It is important that the nurse develop a personal repertoire of abuse-related questions that are comfortable, natural, and culturally sensitive for both the nurse and the setting.

The Nursing Research Consortium on Violence and Abuse (Parker & McFarlane, 1991) developed a four-question assessment tool that directly asks about the characteristics of abuse in a relationship and can be incorporated into the nurse-client interview or a written history (see Figure 9-1). These questions can be prefaced or followed by giving the client information about the incidence of battering in the United States, acknowledging the sensitivity of the issue and the woman's possible emotional response, and assuring the client of the routine nature of assessment of abuse in intimate relationships given the epidemic proportions of the event in this country. Indication of the nurse's familiarity and the widespread nature of the problem is usually helpful in reassuring abused women that they are not alone in this predicament.

Although battered women rarely report abuse to primary health care providers without being asked, they describe a desire to tell of the abuse (Blair, 1986; Finkelhor, Gelles, Hotaling, & Straus, 1983). Asking the question facilitates the battered woman's self-disclosure. When the woman is not abused, asking the question as a routine part of nursing assessment educates her about the incidence and nature of the problem and can be an important nursing intervention at the primary prevention level. Routine assessment for battering must be conducted in a nonjudgmental manner, in private, and with assurances of confidentiality. Battered women frequently feel shame over being abused and are appropriately frightened of the abuser's response if he discovers the violence has been discussed. In addition, battered women often have had previous experience with the health care system that has engendered mistrust. Therefore it is important that the nurse be aware of her own values in relation to violence against women in intimate relationships and be careful of her own nonverbal cues and proxemics (use of space) in interactions with victims of violence.

Although it is often difficult to interact with clients privately in an active trauma unit, in the event of physical trauma to a female client, regardless of the plausibility of the explanation or solicitousness of the spouse, nursing assessment for possible abuse is a priority. Research not only documents the failure of health care workers to identify battered

women in primary care settings (Kurz, 1987; McLeer & Anwar, 1989; Stark, Flitcraft, & Frazier, 1979) but also the necessity to rule out battering as the cause of trauma to a female patient, especially if she is pregnant (Helton, 1986; Parker & McFarlane, 1991). Since abuse is the primary cause of trauma to women in the United States, protocols must be established to keep any accompanying male in the waiting room until abuse is ruled out in emergency settings.

In studies of women coming to hospital emergency rooms and other health care settings, the majority of abused women are never clearly identified as such in the medical record (Goldberg & Tomlanovich, 1984; McLeer & Anwar, 1989; Stark et al., 1979; Warshaw, 1989). In nursing research Drake (1982) and Goldberg and Tomlanovich (1984) found that the majority of abused women were not asked specifically if they had been abused when they sought health care. Drake (1982), Kurz (1987), and Brendtro and Bowker (1989) all found that health care to abused women is generally impersonal and insensitive to their needs, with minimal to no support given by health care providers. One of Drake's (1982) subjects said "I just wish somebody would of come right out and asked me. I always hope they'll do that." (p. 45). Nurses must find a secluded place and do just that—*ask*.

The community health nurse also finds privacy at a premium. The battered woman is usually reluctant to discuss the problem in front of her children, and the abusive spouse frequently finds a reason to be present when any helping professional is in the home. Suggesting a short walk with the wife, using the reason that the weather is fine or the nurse is restless, may be an effective way to create privacy. A battered woman may sometimes resist to the idea of home visitation; she has usually been warned to keep strangers out of the house. Meeting her at other locations, such as a restaurant, a social service agency, or a child care center, may be a useful strategy to create privacy for interaction around the abuse.

When privacy has been obtained and a nonauthoritarian atmosphere created, sensitivity and directness are mandatory. However, although direct questions allow the client to disclose information about the abuse to the nurse, the nurse cannot expect the abused woman to always respond as directly. Battered women frequently use denial as a means of coping with the violence and may minimize its occurrence at first. In this situation, it is important to document the indicators of abuse, as well as the assessment process so that subsequent nurses and health care providers can add current information to data gathered later.

If a woman takes advantage of this opportunity to discuss the abuse with a concerned professional, it should be remembered that the woman has **chosen** that professional for her disclosure. Therefore it is unethical to only make a referral to some other member of the health care team (e.g., social work) without assessing the situation further and discussing the woman's options for intervention with her. This is true even in a hectic emergency situation. A systematic nursing assessment of the abusive situation can act as intervention, increasing the battered woman's awareness of the seriousness of the violence and of changes in abusive behavior over time. A nonthreatening confrontation with information about a pattern of increasing severity and frequency helps the woman define the situation, often influences her decision making, and can facilitate help-seeking behavior. The abused woman who admits to being hit may minimize the seriousness of the problem. This often takes the form of blaming herself for the incidents, blaming her husband's alcohol use, asserting that the violence is permanently over, attributing its occurrence to a period of family stress, or using other forms of rationalization or intellectualization. It is useful to view minimization as partial denial, an appropriate reaction to a devastating situation, and a necessary part of the grieving process. Sensitive exploration of the history of abuse allows the nurse to gather data while helping the woman define the characteristics of the abusive situation and assists her in making decisions. As Goldberg and Carey (1982) suggest, "assessment of the battered woman can be viewed as intervention, and made an integral part of the therapeutic plan" (p. 66). This is especially important when the battered woman may not be seen again. As indicated, the thorough assessment of any woman in an inti-

mate relationship with a man routinely includes questions about a history of violence. Findings in the history and physical examination that should alert the professional nurse to the possibility of wife abuse are presented in Tables 9-1 and 9-2. No single at-risk finding in the tables necessarily indicates abuse, but several such findings warrant at least an at-risk nursing diagnosis. As with all assessments, the nurse must be systematic in collecting data, and all assessment data must be validated with the client. When violence or abuse is acknowledged by the client or strongly suggested by the nurse's assessment data, several areas of assessment specific to battered women must be carefully explored.

History

When violence has been indicated, the most effective means of obtaining the history of abuse is to use a communication model that allows the woman to talk about the problem from her perspective (Kinlein, 1977), "not interrupted," and "given time for full scope, emphasis and even repetition" (p. 58). This can be initiated with a request to "tell me about the hitting," or another open-ended statement. If the woman asks where to begin, telling her "anywhere you would like" works well. If the information about abuse has come up in the middle of a systematic history, the nurse can indicate an interest in pursuing the topic further with the woman. The woman is given the choice of talking about it then or returning to the issue at the end of the more formal history.

The nurse's role during the narration is to listen empathetically, and if following the Kinlein (1977) model completely, to record every word that is said. This approach emphasizes the importance the nurse is imparting to the woman's words and provides a useful record for future reference. Verbatim recording skills develop with practice, but regardless of whether the record is kept verbatim, specific documentation of the client's description of her situation is extremely important. It is particularly important to state *who* and *when* the woman says hit her. The nurse or the medical record may be needed in court to document the abuse, and both the abused

TABLE 9-1
Indicators of Potential or Actual Wife Abuse from History

AREA OF ASSESSMENT	AT-RISK RESPONSES*
Primary concern/reason for visit	Unwarranted delay between time of injury and seeking treatment
	Inappropriate spouse reactions (lack of concern, overconcern, threatening demeanor, reluctance to leave wife, etc.)
	Vague information about cause of injury or problem; discrepancy between physical findings and verbal description of cause; obviously incongruous cause of injury given
	Minimizing serious injury
	Seeking emergency room treatment for vague stress-related symptoms and minor injuries
	Suicide attempt; history of previous attempts
Family health history	
Family of origin	Traditional values about women's role taught
	Spouse abuse or child abuse (may not be significant for wife but should be noted)
Children	Children abused
	Physical punishment used routinely and severely with children
	Children are hostile toward or fearful of father
	Father perceives children as an additional burden
	Father demands unquestioning obedience from children
Partner	Alcohol or drug abuse
	Holds machismo values
	Experience with violence outside of home, including violence against women in previous relationships
	Low self-esteem; lack of power in workplace or other arenas outside of home
	Uses force or coercion in sexual activities
	Unemployment or underemployment
	Extreme jealousy of female friendships, work, and children, as well as other men; jealousy frequently unfounded
	Stressors such as death in family, moving, change of jobs, trouble at work
	Abused as a child or witnessed father abusing mother
Household	Poverty
	Conflicts solved by aggression or violence
	Isolated from neighbors, relatives; few friends; lack of support systems
Past health history	Fractures and trauma injuries
	Depression, anxiety symptoms, substance abuse
	Injuries while pregnant
	Spontaneous abortions
	Psychophysiological complaints
	Previous suicide attempts
Nutrition	Evidence of overeating or anorexia as reactions to stress
	Sudden changes in weight
Personal/social	Low self-esteem; evaluates self poorly in relation to others and ideal self, has trouble listing strengths, makes negative comments about self frequently, doubts own abilities

TABLE 9-1 *Continued*
Indicators of Potential or Actual Wife Abuse from History

AREA OF ASSESSMENT	AT-RISK RESPONSES
Personal/social	Expresses feelings of being trapped, powerlessness, that the situation is hopeless, that it is futile to make future plans
	Chronic fatigue, apathy
	Feels responsible for spouse's behavior
	Holds traditional values about the home, a wife's prescribed role, the husband's prerogatives, strong commitment to marriage
	External locus of control orientation, feels no control over situation, believes fate or other forces determine events
	Major decisions in household made by spouse, indicates far less power than he has in relationship, activities controlled by spouse, money controlled by spouse
	Few support systems, few supportive friends, little outside home activity, outside relationships have been discouraged by spouse or curtailed by self to deal with violent situation
	Physical aggression in courtship
Sleep	Sleep disturbances, insomnia, sleeping more than 10 to 12 hours per day
Elimination	Chronic constipation, diarrhea, or elimination disturbances related to stress
Illness	Frequent psychophysiological illnesses
	Treatment for mental illness
	Use of tranquilizers and/or mood elevators and/or antidepressants
Operations/hospitalizations	Hospitalizations for trauma injuries
	Suicide attempts
	Hospitalization for depression
	Refusals of hospitalization when suggested by physician
Personal safety	Handgun(s) in home
	History of frequent accidents
	Does not take safety precautions
Health care utilization	No regular provider
	Indicates mistrust of health care system
Review of systems	Headaches, undiagnosed gastrointestinal symptoms, palpitations, other possible psychophysiological complaints
	Sexual difficulties, feels husband is "rough" in sexual activities, lack of sexual desire, pain with intercourse
	Joint pain and/or other areas of tenderness, especially at the extremities
	Chronic pain
	Pelvic inflammatory disease

*At-risk responses are derived from clinical experience and review of the literature.

woman and the nurse must be able to evaluate the history for patterns. The purpose of the record and limited confidentiality must be explained to the woman. Her greatest fear may be that the record will somehow be available to her spouse. Once she knows the record is available only with her consent, the presence and availability of the record is a powerful resource in any future legal actions. The woman is more likely to need such records for custody actions than for criminal prosecution.

After the narration, the nurse may need to clarify certain aspects of the story. Kinlein (1977) suggests

TABLE 9-2

Indicators of Wife Abuse from Physical Examination

AREA OF ASSESSMENT	AT-RISK FINDINGS
General appearance	Increased anxiety in presence of spouse
	Watching spouse for approval of answers to questions
	Signs of fatigue
	Inappropriate or anxious nonverbal behavior
	Nonverbal communication suggesting shame about body
	Flinches when touched
	Poor grooming, inappropriate attire
Vital statistics	Overweight or underweight
	Hypertension
Skin	Bruises, welts, edema, or scars, especially on breasts, upper arms, abdomen, chest, face, and genitalia
	Burns
Head	Subdural hematoma
	Clumps of hair missing
Eyes	Swelling
	Subconjunctival hemorrhage
Genital/urinary	Edema, bruises, tenderness, external bleeding
Rectal	Bruising, bleeding, edema, irritation
Musculoskeletal	Fractures, especially of facial bones, spiral fractures of radius or ulna, ribs
	Shoulder dislocation
	Limited motion of an extremity
	Old fractures in various stages of healing
Abdomen	Abdominal injuries in pregnant women
	Intra-abdominal injury
Neurological	Hyperactive reflex responses
	Ear or eye problems secondary to injury
	Areas of numbness from old injuries
	Tremors
Mental status examination	Anxiety, fear
	Depression
	Suicidal ideation
	Low self-esteem
	Memory loss
	Difficulty concentrating

only clarifying what has been previously said, not opening new areas of concern. This is probably the most useful approach if the nurse will see the woman again or is sure that her total health needs will be addressed elsewhere. However, certain aspects of the situation should be explored in order for the woman herself to make a complete assessment. If follow-up is assured, these areas may be assessed in subsequent sessions, but they should not be forgotten.

Although the woman's feelings about the abuse need to be expressed, she may need to intellectual-

ize or disassociate herself from her feelings to describe the situation. If she is not able to respond to
sensitive questioning, it can be assumed that this
process is necessary, at least temporarily. However,
an abused woman may not describe her feelings
because she assumes that her emotions are somehow unacceptable. She may fear the intensity of her
feelings or find her fantasies of retaliation unacceptable. The 46 battered women in Star's (1978) study
were significantly less able to express anger than the
control group of 12 not physically but emotionally
abused women. Whatever the feelings, the abused
woman needs reassurance that it is normal for her
to have strong and frequent, socially undesirable
emotions. It is often helpful for the nurse to describe
the whole gamut of feelings that the abused woman
describes, from feeling angry, trapped, despairing,
and hopeless to feeling great love for the abuser and
confidence that violence will not recur. The nurse
should also stress that conflicting emotions may be
felt simultaneously and that the woman may frequently vacillate between them. Although the
woman may not "own" her emotions at the time of
assessment, should she later become aware of these
reactions, it may be helpful for her to recognize their
normalcy and acceptability.

Part of the process of initially minimizing the
abuse is to avoid labeling the violence as *abuse* or
battering. The majority of women who are physically
or sexually assaulted, or both, even many times
within the past year, do not label themselves as
abused or battered women. In recent research Campbell (1991) found that such women may label their
situation as emotional abuse but consider abused or
battered women to be pathetic victims rather than
the strong women they actually are. However, recognition that their situation is in fact abuse seems to
be a turning point for these women. They reported
that this recognition was accompanied by blaming
themselves less for the violence, being more sure
that their partner was the one who needed to
change, and becoming less invested in the relationship (or in love). In that research, many women said
it was helpful to them for the nurse to point out that
experts would label their situation as abuse or battering. Therefore it may be therapeutic to point this

out to women, but without forcing this label on
them, and to continue using terminology that the
woman prefers.

Assessment of danger

Another important aspect of history is a description
of the pattern of abuse in the relationship, and assessment of the risk of homicide. Violence that escalates over time or, following Walker's (1979a; 1984)
cycle of violence pattern, increases in severity, must
be described carefully. The Danger Assessment
(Campbell, 1986) is a nurse-developed instrument
useful in assisting the nurse and the battered
woman to determine together the risk of homicide
that exists in her particular situation (see Figure
9-2). This 15-item instrument asks the woman to
respond with yes-no answers to questions identifying the risk factors associated with the incidence of
homicide in violent relationships; it takes approximately 10 minutes to complete. The instrument has
been used in several research studies and has acceptable reliability and construct validity, but it has
not been sufficiently tested to yield a cutoff score or
concrete prediction (Campbell, 1992). The instrument can be copied and used either clinically or in
research, but users are asked to correspond thereafter with the author so that it can be developed
further.

Initially, the nurse asks the woman to record all
episodes of violence during the past year on a calendar and then to assess whether the abuse has
become more frequent or more violent over time
(items 1 and 2). Women can easily recall the approx-
imate timing of abusive incidents (exact dates are
not important) by anchoring them to holidays and
other important events. This recording often helps
the woman look at the pattern of abuse realistically
if she has minimized its occurrence and is thus another instance of assessment as intervention.

After completion of the calendar, the nurse informs the client that several risk factors for homicide
in violent intimate relationships have been identified and invites her to see how many factors apply
to her situation. Escalation of violence is identified
as a serious risk factor for homicide in battering relationships, as is access to or the presence of a gun

---

DANGER ASSESSMENT

Several risk factors have been associated with homicides (murder) of both batterers and battered women in research that has been conducted after the killings have taken place. We cannot predict what will happen in your case, but we would like for you to be aware of the danger of homicide in situations of severe battering and for you to see how many of the risk factors apply to your situation. (The "he" in the questions refers to your husband, partner, ex-husband, ex-partner, or whoever is currently physically hurting you).

___ 1. Has the physical violence increased in frequency over the past year?
___ 2. Has the physical violence increased in severity over the past year and/or has a weapon or threat with weapon been used?
___ 3. Does he ever try to choke you?
___ 4. Is there a gun in the house?
___ 5. Has he ever forced you into sex when you did not wish to do so?
___ 6. Does he use drugs? By drugs I mean "uppers" or amphetamines, speed, angel dust, cocaine, "crack", street drugs, heroin, or mixtures.
___ 7. Does he threaten to kill you and/or do you believe he is capable of killing you?
___ 8. Is he drunk every day or almost every day? (In terms of quantity of alcohol.)
___ 9. Does he control most or all of your daily activities? For instance, does he tell you who you can be friends with, how much money you can take with you shopping, or when you can take the car? (If he tries, but you do not let him, check here ___)
___ 10. Have you ever been beaten by him while you were pregnant? (If never pregnant by him, check here ___)
___ 11. Is he violently and constantly jealous of you? (For instance, does he say, "If I can't have you, no one can.")
___ 12. Have you ever threatened or tried to commit suicide?
___ 13. Has he ever threatened or tried to commit suicide?
___ 14. Is he violent towards the children?
___ 15. Is he violent outside of the home?

___   TOTAL YES ANSWERS

THANK YOU. PLEASE TALK TO YOUR NURSE, ADVOCATE, OR COUNSELOR ABOUT WHAT THE DANGER ASSESSMENT MEANS IN TERMS OF YOUR SITUATION.

Figure 9-2

Danger Assessment. (From J. Campbell. Copyright © 1985, 1988.)

in the home. Threats of using a weapon or homicide often begin as abuse escalates and often precede lethal violence. Substance abuse by the batterer (alcohol and certain drugs), sexual abuse, threats of lethal violence, and the use of violence outside the home are additional risk factors assessed in the tool. Research indicates that abusers who killed their partners or who were killed by their partners were more likely to have threatened their partners with lethal violence and to be violent outside their homes (Browne, 1987). Control of the woman's daily activities, battering during pregnancy, extreme jealousy, abuse of children, and threats or attempts of suicide are additional factors the woman should consider while using the information generated by this tool for future decision making.

When the woman completes the Danger Assessment, she is encouraged to assess the degree of danger herself. If the woman and nurse validate the abuser's potential for committing lethal violence, the nurse is obliged to inform the woman that changing her own behavior within the relationship has been found to be basically ineffective in avoiding further incidence of abuse. She may be able to do things like disarm or discard a weapon, ask police to impound any guns, or ask neighbors to call the police if they hear sounds of physical assault. Information about other alternatives also can be discussed, with particular attention on a plan for providing physical safety for the woman and her children. Because the woman may be most at risk for homicide when she actually leaves or lets the abuser know that she is leaving permanently, a plan for physical safety is necessary whenever the woman talks to the nurse about leaving. If the abuse involves the children and the woman is unable to take action to provide for their physical safety, the nurse may need to call child protective services, the police, or both. There is usually sufficient evidence of physical injury, old if not current, in such situations to warrant such actions. Immediate removal of the children and the woman to a shelter is another possibility.

After homicide risk has been assessed, and if immediate danger is not present, the pattern of abuse can be examined to identify the events that trigger the abusive incidents. It is important during this part of the assessment to avoid blaming the woman. The focus of this assessment is on the stressors that occur within the relationship to help the woman understand the mechanisms that are operating. It may also be useful to determine the amount of violence that occurred in the batterer's family of origin to help the woman connect his childhood learning with his present abusive behavior and thereby understand how deeply his behavior may be rooted in previous experience.

Social support

Patterns of psychological abuse and controlling behavior, including jealousy and enforced isolation, should be explored with the woman. It is important to see the pattern of abuse as part of the total relationship and useful for women to identify possible sources of feelings of entrapment, low self-esteem, and depression. Systematic assessment of personal networks and support systems are important to evaluate, especially when an abused woman describes isolation from family, friends, or both.

Findings related to personal networks of battered women indicate that the majority of battered women are not socially isolated, have the quantity of members in their personal networks similar to other women, and see them as frequently (McKenna, 1985). However, although the size of the network of an abused woman may be similar to that of another woman, the amount of support available to her is much less, and loss of network members is much greater. The following box lists several questions to explore with a battered woman to help her assess the support she may or may not have available to her through her personal network.

When a health care provider assesses social isolation in an abused woman, it is important to assess the reason for the loss of network members. Some batterers purposely isolate women from their social contacts, and like the degree of violence, the enforced isolation begins subtly and increases over time. However, this is only one of the possible patterns. At least as often, the woman isolates herself from network members in a strategic effort to protect herself from any actual or potentially nonsupportive response from the network member. For example, the concerned family member who

---

Personal Support Systems Assessment

Ask the woman to make a list of the names of people in her life who are important to her.
For each person, ask the woman:

1. Does (s)he know about the abuse in your relationship with your partner?
2. If *yes,* can this person be called on to help you in any way as you deal with this situation? If *no,* could this person be called on to help you in any way if (s)he knew about the abuse?
3. If *yes,* indicate the type of support this person could be called on to provide (e.g., childcare, transportation, financial assistance, emotional support, safe shelter).
4. Are there any other people in your life who could be called on to help you deal with this situation?

Adapted from McKenna, 1985.

encourages the abused woman to leave her situation when she has not yet decided to deal with the violence by leaving is experienced as stressful rather than supportive. Minimizing contact with nonsupportive family members may be useful to the abused woman in maintaining her mental health. Assessment of this important aspect of social support can assist the woman to maintain adequate supportive relationships while she avoids the nonsupportive responses that increase her level of stress.

The woman's dependency on the marriage is also important to assess, both in light of the amount of loss she can expect to confront and in terms of her potential ability to leave. Kalmuss and Straus (1982) identified two distinct areas of dependency on marriage: (1) objective dependence, or conditions that tie the woman to marriage in terms of economic survival (e.g., young children or few financial resources), and (2) subjective dependence, the degree of her emotional investment. Using data from the first nationally representative survey of 2,143 couples, Kalmuss and Strauss found that subjective dependence significantly correlated by multivariate analysis with less severe physical aggression, whereas objective dependence was strongly related to abuse. Mahon (1981) also found an "internalized . . . total commitment to marriage" present in her extremely small sample (N = 11) of battered women in long-term relationships (p. 153). Strong indications of both objective and subjective dependence on the marriage and heavy commitment to it would predict intense grieving reaction in the woman and less ability to contemplate leaving the relationship without interventions.

The woman's perceptions about her children are also an important part of the history. Children of abused women are also frequently abused, probably more often and more seriously by the male partner but also by the woman (Stark & Flitcraft, 1985). Indications of child abuse must be reported as they would in any other situation. The woman is also frequently and justifiably concerned about the effect of the violence on the children, and the facts about intergenerational transmission of violence need to be shared. Conversely, she may describe her children as the reason that she stays in the relationship,

and this needs to be carefully considered with her. She may be able to outline, with the help of the nurse, the pros and cons of the relationship in terms of the children, which can be helpful in her assessment of the ramifications of the abuse.

Sexual abuse

The area of sexual abuse needs to be explored with the woman. Research indicates that sexual abuse occurs in at least 40% to 45% of battered women, but it is a topic that will seldom be initiated by the woman (Campbell, 1989b). An introduction about the frequency of the dilemma can be useful in approaching the topic of sexual abuse. The question "Does your partner (husband) ever force you into sex that you do not wish to participate in?" avoids language that the woman may not identify with and yet will explore experiences that would be labeled sexual abuse or marital rape. It is not important that the woman labels being forced into sex or sexual activities as abuse (unless she wants to bring criminal charges against her partner), but she needs to disclose either emotional or physical distress from the sexual relationship. In one study, women who were sexually and physically abused had significantly lower levels of self-esteem than those who were physically abused only (Campbell, 1989b).

Thus the history part of the nursing assessment with an abused woman includes all the routine areas of questioning, but also incorporates some areas specific to battering. (See Table 9-1 for indications of potential or actual wife abuse.) In the first narration the woman may include at least some of the areas spontaneously, but if she does not, the nurse must decide which additional areas to explore in light of-time restrictions, possibilities of continued contact, and priorities suggested by the woman's verbal and nonverbal cues. The areas postponed in terms of history should be noted for further follow-up or passed on as topics to be covered in subsequent assessment by the professional to whom the woman is referred.

Physical symptoms from abuse

It is important to realize that many physical conditions may have direct links to physical abuse or be indirect sequelae related to the stress of physical and emotional trauma and fear. Wife abuse is a significant risk factor for medical diagnoses of pelvic inflammatory disease, nonulcer dyspepsia, irritable bowel syndrome, and chronic pain (e.g., head, back, abdominal) (Drossman et al., 1990; Goldberg & Tomlanovich, 1984; Schei, 1991). Although abused women have been found to be more frequently and severely distressed by physical symptoms of stress (Campbell, 1989a), the physical symptoms may be the result of physical damage from old injury as well as related to stress. For instance, a woman "slammed" against kitchen cupboards approximately once a month can suffer back and/or neurological damage from both impact and whiplash-type injury. This kind of serious injury can be caused by the "pushing and shoving" that so often occurs in intimate relationships but sounds like a relatively mild instance of abusive tactics. Much is known about the neurological damage incurred by boxers, but an abused woman is more likely to be referred for counseling than for a neurological workup if she complains about frequent headaches. Marital rape has been associated with such physical problems as vaginal and anal tearing, hemorrhoids, pain with intercourse, and infections that may result in pelvic inflammatory disease (Campbell & Alford, 1989). These kinds of physical symptoms from injuries have been listed in Table 9-2.

Physical Examination

The physical examination of the battered or suspected abused woman should be conducted as any other physical assessment of an adult female. In addition to the standard protocol used for all clients, careful attention must be directed to any signs of injury, past and present, with exact measurement of even the most insignificant-looking bruise. Use of a body map (see Abuse Assessment Screen, Figure 9-1) to record the site of injuries and/or photographs are valuable means of documentation. Since most injuries to the battered woman are to the face, chest, breasts, and abdomen, special attention should be paid to these areas (Stark et al., 1979). A thorough

neurological examination may be indicated, as may be x-ray films for old as well as current fractures (Campbell & Sheridan, 1989). When conducting the physical examination, the nurse should remember that many conditions may be related to old injuries from abuse, and the nurse should ask specifically about the background of each such finding. For instance, hearing loss in one ear may be related to an untreated rupture of the tympanic membrane from a blow to the ear. The incidence of accompanying sexual abuse would also indicate careful examination of the genitalia and a pelvic examination for physical signs of such. Extreme gentleness is important in light of the body image damage that has been done.

The general appearance of the woman should include observations about her behavior as well as physical appearance. Nonverbal behavior that indicates a sense of shame about her body is fairly common in battered women and understandable in terms of body image insult. Other affective behaviors can give clues as to how the woman deals with feelings.

Mental Status Examination

During mental status examination signs of depression, high anxiety, low self-esteem, and posttraumatic stress disorder (PTSD) (see the box on p. 280) should be carefully noted. Especially when clients seem to overreact to apparently minor physical or emotional complaints, the nurse should remember that abused women tend to respond with greater than average anxiety to threats to their current well-being (Trimpey, 1989). This is understandable given the reality of threat and physical danger in their situation.

Several studies have described higher levels of depression in abused women when compared with samples of women where the incidence of abuse is unknown (Bergman, Larsson, Brismar & Klang, 1987; Kerouac, Taggart, Lescop, & Fortin, 1986; McKenna, 1985). When Campbell (1989a) compared abused women with other women having serious problems in an intimate relationship with a man, she found approximately equal mean levels of depression, suggesting that the level of depression was related to grief and stress about the relationship ending rather than being hit per se. However, the abused women were more likely to be seriously depressed. Depression is a common response to situational stress, especially when resources are inadequate or when multiple losses lead to prolonged grieving (Carpenito, 1992). Although not all persons who commit suicide are clinically depressed, thorough assessment of suicide potential is also important. Because battered women are more likely to attempt suicide than nonbattered women, suicidal intent must be considered as a real possibility (Bergman et al., 1987; Carmen, Rieker & Mills, 1984).

Assessment of self-esteem is also an important part of the mental status examination. Nurses may assess self-esteem by asking the woman to list her strengths and weaknesses, by asking her to evaluate herself in comparison to her friends, or by inquiring about how near she believes she is to the person she would like to be. Another clue to self-esteem is if the woman blames herself for the abuse. Although the minority (20%) of women blamed themselves for their problems in the relationship in Campbell's (1989a) sample of battered women, those who did were more likely to be severely depressed and have low self-esteem. In light of the prevalence of low self-esteem in battered women, a more objective measure like the Culture-Free Self-Esteem Inventories (CFSEI) for Adults (Battle, 1981) may be used. When the setting does not allow for use of standardized tests to measure the response of the client, the woman's response to the structured interview questions should be carefully noted. When the setting does allow for use of a standardized instrument, it is strongly recommended that the tool be used as an integral part of the nurse's interview rather than self-administered before the interview. This suggestion is based on research that indicates self-disclosure of highly sensitive information may be increased when the client interacts with a nurse who engenders a sense of trust and who responds in an accepting, nonjudgmental manner (McFarlane, Christoffel, Bateman, Miller, & Bullock, 1991).

NURSING DIAGNOSIS

The diagnostic aspect of assessment is best begun by sharing with the abused woman her strengths as the nurse sees them. This is extremely important in terms of the potential low self-esteem and the generally prevailing attitude of battered women that they will be condemned for their behavior—if not in terms of inciting the beatings in some way, at least for not ending the relationship. Abused women are frequently extremely creative in finding ways to deal with a violent spouse and in bringing up their children with a minimum of damage. They need recognition and support for those efforts. At this point it is also helpful to explain how normal her reactions (such as depression) and behavior are in light of the impact of being beaten in a marriage. It is important for the nurse to remember how much blame and fault-finding the woman usually receives from the batterer and to enthusiastically praise the woman in terms of her specific strengths. Clinical experience has shown that it is useful to record these strengths and show the woman that they are part of the record and therefore considered as important as any problems she may have.

The next part of the diagnostic process is to ask the woman to list any concerns she has and what priority she places on them. To the nurse's surprise, the woman may focus on a problem that seems peripheral to abuse. This may be part of a testing process for the woman and/or may be what seems central to her existence at that moment. These feelings must be respected in deciding the course of nursing interventions. When the woman has listed the areas that she believes need attention, the nurse can add others, asking if the woman agrees that they also need inclusion. At this point the nurse may need to explain the holistic nature of nursing; some women may think that the nurse is primarily interested in physical injury.

Another important aspect of the nurse's contribution to the diagnostic process is to help the woman determine any patterns of stress-related symptoms. Battered women frequently report problems such as headaches, gastrointestinal symptoms, and heart palpitations. In one study abused women were significantly more likely to have more frequent

TABLE 9-3
Nursing Diagnoses to Consider with Abused Women*

NURSING DIAGNOSIS	DEFINITION
1. Ineffective individual coping related to response to identifiable situational stressors	Useful when the woman is unable to manage long-term situational stressors (relocation, inadequate finances, lack of support system, poor self-esteem)
2. Impaired adjustment related to response to multiple losses and inadequate support	Useful for period immediately following acute battering when woman experiences extended disbelief, shock, or anger and is unable to orient her thinking to the future
3. Grieving related to actual or perceived loss related to wife abuse	Useful when the woman anticipates or is actually aware of losses (status, relationship, person, etc.) related to the abuse; when the grief is unresolved or prolonged, consider dysfunctional grieving as subsequent diagnosis
4. Posttrauma response related to wife abuse	Useful when the type of violence experienced stimulates a sustained emotional response that interferes with interpersonal relationships and precipitates self-destructive behavior (suicide attempts, substance abuse); often seen in women who have a history of victimization (sexual assault, child abuse, etc.)
5. Decisional conflict related to wife abuse and conflict with personal values or beliefs	Useful in situations where the woman finds herself unable to decide about a course of action because of the losses involved or where the decisions she perceives as necessary conflict with her values or the values of her support system
6. Anxiety related to ongoing threat of wife abuse	Wife abuse threatens a woman's self-concept and interferes with her sense of security, roles, and values; fear may be a more useful diagnosis when the violence or threats of violence pose a direct threat to the woman's physical safety

*Not inclusive of all diagnoses that might be used with abused women.

and more severe symptoms of stress than non-abused women (Campbell, 1989a). The woman may not see these complaints as related to the almost constant stress experienced and may need help in connecting their occurrence to patterns of beating. The emphasis should be on the normalcy of these symptoms in her situation, although the possibility of further medical diagnosis and intervention should also be discussed. As mentioned, the nurse should also remember that these symptoms may be related to old injuries or a decreased immune re-sponse that can also be the result of stress but necessitates medical intervention.

Nursing diagnosis in the case of battered women may cover a range of concerns. A list of applicable nursing diagnoses (Table 9-3) and a sample nursing process have been included in this chapter (see Table 9-6). Although other nursing diagnoses may be appropriate to specific abused women, the diagnoses listed will assist with many women attempting to deal with violence in intimate relationships.

PLANNING

The planning stage of the nursing process requires working with the battered woman to develop goals and interventions that seem appropriate to her. Short-term goals should be fairly simple and concrete. Achievement of these first goals has immeasurable value in showing the woman that some of her problems can be solved, that she is capable of achieving solutions even in her restricted situation, and that working for long-term goals is also feasible. The battered woman may seem passive in the goal-setting phase, because of her feelings of being trapped, her mistrust of helping professionals, and/or the protective mechanism of not looking toward the future, trying to deal only with each day as it comes. The nurse must recognize such behavior as normal and help the woman to formulate her own goals. This may be considered as partially an intervention; it is helping the woman develop problem-solving techniques.

Long-term goals may be more difficult for the abused woman to develop. The nurse must be careful not to prematurely impose a goal of leaving the abuser during this process. The majority of abused women do, in fact, eventually leave the violent relationship or manage to make the violence end (Campbell, in press; Okun, 1986). Leaving the abuser and/or otherwise dealing with the violence is best considered a process. The woman may leave and return several times before leaving permanently. In one study the average number of times women left and returned before making a final break was 5.2 times (Okun). This process of leaving and returning is best conceptualized as a **healthy** testing of the partner's promises to reform, testing her children's ability to cope without their father, and testing her own economic and personal resources. The first few times she leaves, the woman may fully intend to return; she is making a point that the abuse needs to end, not the relationship. Later in the process of leaving she may try the notion of leaving for good, and she is more likely to use a shelter than go to family or friends. The battered woman may take months or years to reach the point of leaving permanently, and she may never reach it. She may, however, inquire whether the nurse believes this should be a goal, because she is often used to this advice. The nurses may need to explore their own thinking on the subject. If the woman is not yet ready to contemplate the future, long-term goals may be set later in the course of the relationship.

The process of planning is mutual, with the final decisions left to the woman. Support and suggested alternatives can be offered by the nurse. It is difficult for nurses to imagine the battering situation, especially if unemployment, several young children, and a dearth of support systems accompany the problem. Clinical experience has shown that abused women have often thought of anything that traditional nursing has to suggest. The women themselves, with encouragement to think as widely and fancifully as they can, usually discover the germs of effective solutions that can be refined, explored, and expanded with the nurse. Such a process can often be enjoyable for both the woman and the nurse. There is nothing more useful for raising self-esteem for the woman than determining her own solutions and being praised effusively for them.

NURSING INTERVENTION

Professional nursing interventions for the problem of wife abuse are based on the three levels of prevention. Identifying and caring for the individual battered woman is insufficient; nurses must seek the societal causes and work to eliminate their influence.

Primary Prevention

Primary prevention involves (1) interventions at the societal level, (2) identification of women at risk to become abused, and (3) implementation of nursing care, both with those women at risk and with their potential abusers. Because wife abuse originates in sexism and the patriarchal social structure, prevention must start at this point. As Lichenstein (1981) asserts, "To prevent abuse, social attitudes toward women must be changed. Dependence of women must be eliminated. This means economic, social, and psychological dependency" (p. 249).

Health promotion: interventions at the societal level

Political activism is a mandatory role for nurses in changing the social structure so that women are no longer so dependent. Each individual nurse cannot be expected to take on every political cause that has impact on these issues. However, each nurse can make one such issue something that she becomes truly involved in, and then at least vote and write to elected officials about the rest. Support for legislation directed toward gender equality is an obvious starting point, and the issue of equal compensation for work of comparable worth is an area of immense implication for the profession of nursing as well as for the economic dependence of all women. The lack of affordable, responsible child care for working mothers also remains a significant block to economic independence for women. Private industry and government need constant prodding to make daycare a reality for every woman who needs it. The lack of viable job training for women without advanced education or technical skills is an ongoing problem. Nurses can join with other women in advocating change in these areas and can thereby realize the enormous strength of women working together that is necessary in challenging deeply embedded values and structures.

To eliminate sexism, the child-rearing patterns of our culture must be radically altered. Problems with male identification leading to macho attitudes can be assuaged by full participation of fathers in all aspects of parenting. Boys can be encouraged toward this kind of behavior in parenting classes in high school, and prenatal classes are also important in this regard. Fathers involved in labor and delivery may be more likely to be involved in child-rearing later. Nurses can also participate in public education to promote male participation in child-rearing; the proliferation of cable television health programs presents excellent opportunities.

The sexism, male dominance, and violence portrayed on television and in children's books must be protested frequently and vehemently. On an adult level, pornography, especially that depicting violence against women, must be curtailed. Laboratory and field studies (Donnerstein, 1980; Malamuth & Check, 1981) suggest that viewing erotic films depicting women as victims of violence increases men's aggression and acceptance of interpersonal violence against women. Erotica and pornography can be differentiated by mutuality and reciprocity in the sexual acts portrayed in the former, whereas the latter depicts the humiliation and domination of women, if not actual violence (Sandelowski, 1980; Steinem, 1978). With these differentiations in mind, individuals can argue effectively against pornography without tangling with the issues of freedom of speech and open attitudes toward sex. Feminists advocate women banding together against pornography, demonstrating against movies depicting violent sex, confronting men who buy pornographic materials, and educating the public as to the dangers of such media (MacKinnon, 1981).

The adult male in today's society often feels threatened. The feminist movement has challenged his traditional prerogatives, and economic malaise is eroding his chances to attain power and prestige in the work environment. He receives mixed messages in the media and from women as to whether strength and macho characteristics, or gentleness and advocating sexual equality, are preferable. Activities for health promotion for men should include supporting men's groups for discussion of the evolving male role and for helping men to get in touch with their feelings and learn to express them without aggression. Nursing advocacy is also needed to create better school systems, less discrimination, job training, and job opportunities for young men in our society. Facing a future without viable opportunities to be productive or support a family, young men, especially those of minority ethnic groups and from poverty backgrounds, often believe their only way of finding status is through a tough reputation that often includes controlling their female partners. Nursing assessment of individual men, including boys and adolescents, should include a discussion of these issues and how the man deals with them. This is as important as assessing for physical problems.

Women also need help in overcoming psychological dependence on men. This need has been addressed well in women's support groups as an outgrowth of the women's movement. However, these groups remain predominantly organized and used by middle-class women. Poorer women generally do not perceive themselves as having the leisure time, the child care, or the transportation to take advantage of such groups and are not sure of their welcome. They are often overwhelmed by the problems of everyday living. However, discussions of women's roles and gaining support from each other can be part of groups organized around more "practical" aims, groups that can be held in poor neighborhoods with child care provided. Waiting rooms of hospital and public health clinics can be used to engage men and women in meaningful conversations on all kinds of issues. Professionals often complain that people do not take advantage of educational programs and discussion groups offered, and yet they allow the people they are trying to reach to sit for hours in a variety of waiting rooms or stand in endless lines to initiate contact with social and health services. The target groups are there; a more creative way than videotapes is needed to fill this time. Women who are clients of the mental health system need such discussions regardless of their presenting symptoms. All women's roles are changing, and all women are dealing with this at some level. The women may not ask for "feminist therapy," but mental health nurses should lead the struggle to ensure that therapy for women does not further cripple them with reinforcement of traditional psychiatric myths about female dependency. Problems in self-esteem and susceptibility to depression are natural outgrowths of growing up female in a sexist society.

School nurses and community health nurses are in a good position to deal with these issues with adolescent girls. The high prevalence of dating violence should be discussed with these young women. Jealousy can be discussed and redefined as an issue of ownership rather than love. Adolescent mothers can be approached singly or in groups by maternal-child health nurses for discussion of issues related to dating, sexuality, and women's roles. These young women are at high risk of becoming caught in poverty and external crippling of potentials. Dependence on a man can seem attractive as a

way to escape, and such young women need help in growth of the self before they can make wise decisions about intimate relationships with men.

Interventions with women at risk

There are no consistent factors that have been identified as placing an individual woman at risk to be abused (Hotaling & Sugarman, 1986, 1990). However, women who are intimately involved with men displaying macho characteristics are at risk, especially those who are unemployed, lack power at work, are in highly stressful situations from other causes, abuse alcohol, or were themselves exposed to a violent home as a child. (Other characteristics indicating risk are in Tables 9-1 and 9-2). There is also recent evidence that abuse is more frequent in couples cohabiting, separated, or divorced than in those currently married (Hotaling & Sugarman, 1990). This underscores the need to assess all women for abuse, not just those who are married.

A woman at risk who has not actually been beaten may respond affirmatively to questions like, "Has your spouse ever threatened to hit you?" or "Have you ever been afraid that he would hit you?" It is useful to suggest a women's group for these women and to inform them that increased family stress may begin a cycle of battering; they need to know how to obtain crisis intervention in such a situation. It is also helpful to encourage women to plan a scenario of what they would do if they actually were beaten. This rehearsal usually lends support if beating occurs and does not frighten the woman unnecessarily as might be imagined; she has usually thought of the possibility previously, but without support, has not thought it through completely.

Women at risk frequently subscribe to the myth that they can somehow save a man with problems—problems with alcohol or drugs or a violent temper or a rotten childhood—that enough love and patience from her will cure him. Women need to understand that they cannot be held responsible for a spouse's behavior and that such problems require professional intervention, not just a partner's support. Convincing the man to accept help is, of course, a difficult issue. The man who exhibits a macho male identity finds it almost impossible to admit a need for help. The individual woman is the best judge of conditions under which the man may be willing to seek help, and the nurse can help her to accomplish these conditions. An authoritarian message that help is necessary from a male physician can sometimes be useful in persuading the man. If the female partner thinks this would be helpful, it can be arranged by the nurse.

Other attitudes frequently displayed by the woman at risk for abuse are that all men are unreasonably jealous, at least occasionally resort to violence, and need to be dominant. Gentleness in male behavior may be woefully absent in her experience and community. A middle-class nurse from a different culture may be considered a useless source of information on male behavior in her world. Another nurse or health team member from a similar background may be more persuasive. Even more useful is a group of women who are her peers, some of whom have encountered or successfully demanded different standards of behavior. Such experiences can be difficult to arrange, but the results are worthwhile.

Assertiveness training is also helpful for both women who are at risk for battering and abused women themselves. Assertiveness classes have been more prevalent for middle-class women than those who are poor. Creativity is needed in making such classes available for the traditionally underserved: at lunch hours in workplaces like factories, office buildings, hospitals, and shopping centers where women are frequently employed; at neighborhood centers; or at Head Start classrooms when the children are occupied. Special care must be taken to be sure that poor women feel invited, that small groups of friends are encouraged to come, and that the relevance to their situation is emphasized.

Primary prevention can also take the forms of fighting poverty at the societal level or helping the individual man or woman at risk to find a job. It may also include promoting nonviolence in our culture and in individual families. Preventing wife abuse is certainly an almost overwhelming task, but fortunately others are involved. Nurses must band together with women and concerned men every-

where. Many groups of professionals can also be included—social workers, psychologists, concerned physicians, feminist lawyers, and some police. Coalitions of nurses with individuals from these groups can be formed. Nurses are welcome on boards of agencies and groups involved with wife abuse and can help set policy in this kind of position. The opportunities for nurses to significantly make an impact on the quest to prevent the battering of women, both in terms of health promotion and identification and intervention for those at risk, are extensive and varied. Nurses *can* make a difference.

Secondary Prevention

Secondary prevention of wife abuse involves diligent efforts at early case finding and interventions with women in the beginning stages of wife abuse. Drake (1982), basing her conclusions on Walker's (1979a) cycle of violence theory, suggests that the ideal time for nurses to intervene is between the end of phase two (the acute battering incident) and the beginning of phase three, when the husband may be contrite and reestablish the bonds between the couple. At this point the woman is most likely to seek medical or nursing care for her injuries and come to the attention of nurses. The woman may be in crisis at this point and especially open to help, regardless of the setting to which she presents herself.

Case finding

The emergency room nurse is important in case finding. An estimated 18% to 25% of all women seen in emergency rooms are victims of wife abuse (Goldberg & Tomlanovich, 1984; Stark et al., 1979). Wife battering is the leading cause of trauma to women in the United States (McLeer & Anwar, 1989). With that fact in mind, wife abuse should be ruled out before other causes are investigated. Therefore any male partner coming to an emergency room with an injured woman should be kept in the waiting room as a matter of policy until abuse is ruled out (Campbell & Sheridan, 1989). Questions about abuse should be direct, such as: "Who hit you?" or "Who did that to you?" This approach minimizes the chances of the woman making up a story and conveys that the nurse is knowledgeable about abuse.

It is appropriate that the professional nurse takes responsibility for determining battering since the nurse is more likely to be female and therefore less threatening, and because abuse, with all its psychological and social ramifications, is more logically within the wider scope of nursing than medicine (Warshaw, 1989). There may be a social work department that can help the woman also, but nurses should not make the referral until and unless the woman chooses to talk to a social worker. The woman may come to the emergency room with fairly minor injuries in an attempt to seek help for the primary problem. It is tempting to treat such clients quickly with a lecture about the misuse of emergency rooms. A high index of suspicion for abuse in nurses will prevent these women from going away not truly served.

Since the most frequent area of injury is the face, it is easy for both the woman and the emergency staff to focus on this kind of obvious trauma and not conduct a complete physical examination. A superficial but bloody face wound may hurt more than the more serious head injury or internal injuries (Campbell & Sheridan, 1989). Given the high incidence of sexual abuse, a pelvic examination may be conducted if the woman so indicates.

If the injuries are serious enough to warrant hospitalization, this should be considered as beneficial in terms of protecting the woman temporarily and allowing her to really think, removed from the batterer and the stresses of home. The emergency room nurse can alert the inpatient staff of the possibility of abuse if it has not been confirmed, so that the woman's nurses can discuss the issue with her. Another alternative is to keep the woman in the emergency department for a few hours until the nurse has time to sit and talk with her.

An abused woman may also present herself to mental health facilities with a variety of psychiatric symptoms in an effort to reach out for assistance. In clinical experience with battered women, they have often recounted how the psychiatric staff tended to "dope me up" as a primary intervention, which generally lessened their pain, but also interfered

with their resolve to take effective action. As soon as their symptoms subsided, they were usually released without any interventions to solve the underlying problems. This general course of events did not seem to alter whether they told of the abuse. Battering must be assumed to be a possible cause of or related to depression, anxiety, substance abuse, and marital problems in the mental health arena, and it should receive specific inquiry and intervention. Researchers have begun to document the prevalence of abused women in both inpatient and outpatient mental health facilities.

The widespread incidence of battering during pregnancy suggests another important arena where wife abuse can be identified, often in early stages, and attended to by nursing. Prenatal clinics, private obstetrical offices, childbirth education classes, and inpatient postpartum floors are all places where nurses can be alert for wife battering (see Chapter 7).

In community health nursing, nurses are in clients' homes and deal with families on a regular basis. In such settings, wife abuse may easily be revealed if the professional nurse is alert to the possibility and gently asks the right questions. As previously mentioned, many battered women seem anxious to tell if asked empathetically in a safe and private situation. One area of community health nursing where nurses may have contact with women in early battering situations is in birth control clinics. A nursing study in a Planned Parenthood clinic demonstrated that 8.2% of 793 women responded that they were abused on the four abuse assessment screening questions shown in Figure 9-1 (Bullock, McFarlane, Bateman & Miller, 1989). The actual prevalence was undoubtedly higher because nurses actually interviewing women about abuse will discover more. This type of clinic is also an excellent setting in which to identify young women who are in relationships that are beginning to be characterized by excessive control by the man and by violence. Descriptions of the spouse making all the decisions about birth control or "forcing" the woman in any manner are indications that abuse may be present. Follow-up appointments for the woman are therefore important even if not mandatory in terms of the chosen birth control method.

Occupational health is another important case-finding setting. Abuse is frequently known by co-workers and friends of the woman in the workplace before it comes to the attention of professionals. A vigorous campaign of distributing information about wife abuse in the workplace, coupled with suggestions to approach the occupational health nurse if abuse is known, can be useful in early identification. The woman may also be absent recurrently and show evidence of facial bruises, perhaps covered with heavy makeup. She may be defensive about questions regarding her absenteeism and indicate powerlessness in the relationship by saying she is not able to spend her salary according to her own desires, to work overtime, or to rearrange her schedule because of his objections. The workplace is an excellent setting to provide nursing care to a battered woman because of her separation from the spouse.

Primary care settings and physician's offices are other health arenas where abuse, especially abuse in middle-class homes, can be detected (King & Ryan, 1989). Battered women may often seek medical attention because of stress-related symptoms, chronic pain, or both. Inclusion of questions about abuse in nursing assessment or careful review of physician's findings can be used to identify the battered woman.

Regardless of the setting in which abuse is identified, documentation is crucial. The record should clearly state who (by name) the woman says has injured her. This can be put in quotes after the phrase, patient states . . ., so there is no question of the nurse making a judgment about the perpetrator. In this way abuse can be established for future court action, even if the woman states she has no intention of leaving or taking legal steps at the time of the nursing assessment. The court actions for which the records are most often needed are child custody suits, since the abuser often tries to obtain custody of the children if she leaves him. The woman may also decide later that she wants to press charges or may need the records in a court action against her for assault or homicide. The records should also contain a complete description of any visible signs of injury, old as well as new. These injuries should

be recorded on a body map with the description, date of injury, and photographed if possible. The nurse can discuss the record with the woman and how she can obtain it if she ever needs it. This gives her an important possible tactic to use and is therefore an empowerment strategy.

A Theoretical Framework for Intervention

To understand the abused woman, it is helpful to study her behavior in the context of the midrange nursing theory developed by Landenburger (1989) that also has elements of similarity with a grieving framework (Bowlby, 1980; Flynn & Whitcomb, 1981; Silverman, 1981; Weinfourt, 1979; Werner-Beland, 1980). Her reaction can thus be seen as normal process in a situation of multiple and severe losses. In Western patriarchal society a successful marriage is often seen as the single most important achievement for women. This picture is starting to change, but any battered woman is still dealing with a significant loss, that of the idealized version of marriage. The woman is typically thought to be responsible for the success of the marriage, and to acknowledge that it is in shambles entails considerable loss of self-esteem. Support for this interpretation was found by Campbell (1989a), who found abused women and other women with serious problems in their primary relationships to have similar, but significantly lower than the instrument norms, scores on self-esteem and depression. For the abused woman, body image loss because of the physical injuries and sexual abuse incurred is also a part of the picture (Campbell, 1989b). The abused woman has lost a great deal of trust in her mate and in the world as a safe place, and she has also lost her illusions that the man is basically good for her and an appropriate object of her love and affection. When she contemplates leaving the man, she must face the potential losses of status in marriage, financial security or some semblance thereof, a father for her children, her home, and various support systems. The tendency of many abused wives to stay married to their husbands, return to them after leaving, drop assault charges against them, and/or idealize them even after leaving has baffled and exasperated the scholars in the field and those working with battered women. This behavior can be perhaps best understood as a normal process of commitment to a relationship and then reaction to the multiple losses as the woman becomes aware of them.

Such reframing from a picture of victimization and pathology to one of normalcy and recognizing strengths has also been labeled a survivor framework (Gondolf, 1988a; Hoff, 1988). The advantages of using such a framework are that it views the response patterns as essentially healthy and as a process to be worked through and supported by nursing care. Being perceived as survivors rather than victims is also an approach that most battered women prefer themselves.

Binding

Landenburger's (1989) midrange theory of the process of entrapment in and recovery from an abusive relationship was derived from a grounded theory study of abused women and has support from several independent research projects. Her research indicates that a woman passes progressively through a process including four phases: binding, enduring, disengaging, and recovering. As with grieving, the process takes considerable time and the behaviors vary in their appearance, sequence, intensity, and length of time required to experience them. The first phase of binding incorporates the initial development of the relationship and the beginnings of abuse within the relationship. As in any intimate relationship, the woman is trying to create a loving, long-term partnership. She has made a commitment to try to make this relationship work, and she works very hard at that, despite warning signals that begin to develop. She chooses to interpret the signs of ownership or jealousy that are almost always present as symbols of the love and attention she needs rather than as troublesome. She concentrates on the positive aspects and overlooks or passes over the negative.

Similarly, all the authors who have traced the grief response have identified an initial period of shock and denial that follows significant loss. When the abuse first begins, the woman experiences a tremendous sense of loss of the idealized relationship she has worked to achieve. Other research has also found that the battered woman may deny or minimize the importance of the initial battering in a variety of ways (Ferraro & Johnson, 1983). At first, the abuse is typically only a small part of the relationship (Landenburger, 1989). The woman may explain the occasional push or shove as a temporary aberration in an essentially loving relationship, or she may blame the stress that the man is currently undergoing or her own behavior. She may admit the violence but blame it on alcohol or a temporary loss of control in her spouse. His typical blaming such factors that minimize his responsibility supports her denial. However, once a man has used violence with his wife, a psychological barrier seems to have been broken, and a pattern of abuse is started. The initial shock and denial of the woman, a perfectly normal response, may be perceived by the man as a form of acquiescence, a sign that the man's goals have been achieved, or both. Through no fault of hers, this may serve to reinforce his abusive behavior.

As the violence recurs, the impact and meaning become apparent. She begins to question what is happening as her attempts to make things right are obviously futile (Landenburger, 1989). For the woman, this is a transitional period into the next phase. Many strong feelings may be experienced by the woman. However, the intermittent pattern of some abuser's beatings may allow the woman to return to denial during quiescent periods. The feeling that first surfaces is sometimes anger, and the woman may try to fight back, either verbally or physically. This is a strategy that many abused women try at various points during the relationship; therefore her acts of aggressiveness should be interpreted in that light (Campbell, in press). If the woman finds that fighting back only worsens the violence directed against her, she will stop fighting back and therefore have to suppress her anger. In a traditional psychological interpretation, it can be predicted that the anger may be dealt with by turning it inward, by displacement onto others, by projection, or by developing somatic symptoms.

Enduring

In Landenburger's (1989) second phase, enduring, the woman sees herself as putting up with the abuse. Feeling responsible is an important aspect of this phase. The related concept of guilt is another strong feeling associated with loss and grief, and it has been noted in much of the literature that battered women frequently blame themselves for the abuse, at least at first. Their guilt is reinforced by the psychological abuse and blame dealt out by the spouse. However, in a sample of 97 battered women from the community, only 20% blamed themselves for the abuse (Campbell, 1989a). Frieze (1979) found that another sample of abused women blamed themselves for the abuse less as time went on, signifying a lessening of the guilt as the battering continued. As Landenburger found, many women who do not blame themselves for the abuse feel responsible in another way; they feel responsible for helping their partner.

Bargaining is a mechanism identified in a grieving framework, and a similar mechanism labeled placating was described by the women in Landenburger's sample. The battered woman frequently makes a pact, either overtly or covertly, with her husband that she will correct whatever behavior he sees as a problem in return for an absence of violence. She also bargains with him about returning to him or staying with him only if he changes his behavior or seeks treatment for the violence or substance abuse. This can be a very effective strategy for entering abusive men into treatment. Gondolf (1988b) found that the strongest predictor of women in shelters returning to their partner was that he was in counseling. However, as Gondolf (1988b) points out, "Unfortunately batterers often use counseling as a form of manipulation . . ., dropping out as soon as the threat of separation is over" (p. 286).

The feelings of helplessness, despair, and loss of control so often identified by abused women and clinically seen as depression, are a normal part of grieving. The period of enduring is extremely painful as the woman struggles with her feelings of responsibility to the relationship and trying to determine why she is being abused. Women in both Landenburger's (1989) and Ulrich's (1991) samples describe a loss or shrinking of self as the abuse continues and escalates. The battered woman doubts her ability to cope without the man and may feel totally worthless. She cannot be expected to make the difficult decisions and plans necessary for leaving when she is in this stage. Instead, she tries to hide the abuse and finds it difficult to disclose to anyone. This should also be interpreted as a normal desire to avoid the stigma associated with abuse and to protect her partner. Even to herself, she usually does not label what is happening to her as abuse or battering (Campbell, 1991).

Disengaging

Acceptance of the loss, along with realistic plans for change, either within the relationship or outside of it, comes slowly for most women. The degree of loss, in terms of time and energy invested in the relationship, perceived ability to cope without it, and the love felt for the spouse, may prolong the time needed to opt for change. Some women may never actually work through the grieving process. For some women, the process may resemble the chronic grieving that individuals with permanent disabilities and chronic illnesses frequently display (Werner-Beland, 1980).

However, most women next enter a stage of disengaging (Landenburger, 1989). They begin to identify with other women in similar situations through media accounts of abuse, friends or family members, or in community or shelter support groups. All are therefore important adjuncts to other kinds of intervention, and the media should be encouraged to continue informed news coverage of abuse and abuse-related entertainment programs. After seeing such media, the abused woman for the first time may label what is happening as abuse, and herself as an abused or battered woman. Women in Campbell's (1991) longitudinal study stated that this labeling process was accompanied by a significant change in how they thought about the relationship and what they did. They recounted shifts in blame from themselves to him, feeling like he was the one who had to change, not her, and deciding that the relationship would have to end.

In a nursing study of 51 women who had left abusers, Ulrich (1991) found that the two most frequent categories of reasons for leaving were safety and personal growth. The safety category included fearing for their own, others', or their children's physical safety, or their children's emotional safety. The personal growth category included sudden changes in awareness, having reached a personal limit or being concerned for their own potential.

Women in the disengaging phase begin to actively seek help to end the relationship (Landenburger, 1989). Gondolf (1990) noted that women in his large sample of women in shelters more actively sought help as the abuse increased in severity and frequency. Bowker (1983) also noted that women's help-seeking switched from family and friends to more formal systems as time elapsed, and the more formal systems were found to be more helpful.

During disengagement, anger often reemerges and may become rage, and the woman may fantasize about killing her partner (Landenburger, 1989). Her partner senses that she is close to a breaking point, and he often escalates his threats and violence to keep her in the relationship. These situations are extremely volatile, and serious injury or homicide of either partner may occur. This is the most dangerous part of the process but also the stage where the woman's self starts to reemerge.

Recovering

Progress is seldom direct and without vacillation between stages. The recovering phase includes the initial adjustment to leaving the relationship and may encompass a temporary return to him. It takes considerable work, effort, pain, and assistance from others for a woman to survive on her own (Landenburger, 1989). Part of the recovering phase is a struggle for survival, in terms of the necessities of life, dealing with her children's losses, and justifying her leaving to her partner, children, and critical others. Idealization of the spouse may be seen during this period, which is also characteristic of grieving. This mechanism is often difficult for professionals working with the abused woman to understand, and it may lead her to return to the spouse, especially if she is having problems with survival and depression. When viewed as a normal part of a process to be worked through, it is more acceptable.

The response is also compounded by the fact that the man is not dead even if the woman has left him, and constantly reappears in her life when she is psychologically vulnerable.

Part of this aspect of the recovery process is a search for meaning in the experience and her behavior, which includes determining why she stayed so long. Successfully working through the multiple losses and searching for meaning may well depend on the support given to the abused woman through the process. Nursing can be instrumental in providing that support.

Secondary Prevention Nursing Interventions

Interventions at the secondary prevention level are based on an assessment of where the abused woman is in her entrapment and recovery process. The early denial and minimization must neither be disparaged nor encouraged. The battered woman needs to know the facts about wife abuse, primarily that it generally tends to escalate. During early abuse she frequently wants to know if it is possible for the violent spouse to change. This is possible, but the woman should be aware that he must want to change and be willing to undergo treatment of some kind. She needs to direct her efforts toward that end, rather than try to change her behavior to please him more and thus avoid abuse. A useful approach is to concentrate on assisting the woman to be as healthy as possible despite the batterings. This usually seems logical to both the abused woman and the nurse, and it avoids such pitfalls as encouraging the woman to be more submissive. Areas of concern, such as low self-esteem and lack of assertiveness, can be approached in a variety of ways. Individual counseling aimed at raising self-esteem and teaching assertiveness skills can be useful, as can group and class situations. Once the abused woman feels better about herself she may be able to set firm limits at home, but without these strengths, suggestions of such may be premature.

Efforts to improve the health of the victim of early abuse can also focus on stress-related symptoms she may be experiencing. Relaxation training, exercise programs, role-playing, coping skills development, and teaching the woman to be more in touch with her physiological self may all be helpful to her. It should also be remembered that battered women may be kept socially isolated by the spouse or may find their support systems detrimental rather than helpful. The nurse can discuss the importance of the woman having positive support systems and problem solve with her to try to find and develop new supportive networks or maintain existing ones. Alleviating some of the external stressors in the relationship, such as lack of child care or difficulties in finding financial resources, may be addressed through referral to social work or other community resources. The woman may need help in finding a job, which could be instrumental in improving her self-esteem and decreasing her economic dependence on the spouse. Many batterers find their spouses' employment threatening, but alleviation of some of the financial burdens may seem attractive enough to overcome their objections.

A woman in the early stages of battering frequently seeks some way of maintaining the relationship. Marriage or couple counseling may be dangerous to the women. If she discloses the abuse in the sessions, she may be beaten for it; if she does not disclose, this crucial issue will not be addressed by the therapist. However, *if* violence has only recently begun in the relationship, couple counseling is desired by *both* partners, and the woman has considered the possible danger, it may be a potential recourse. The nurse can be instrumental in making sure the counseling is provided by someone knowledgeable about abuse, a clinician who is not interested in only keeping the couple together to the detriment of the wife. Rather than traditional marital therapy, models have been developed based on behavioral and social-learning theories (Watts & Courtois, 1981). The man is encouraged to take responsibility for the violence, using confrontation if necessary, and to learn new ways of dealing with anger. The couple is encouraged to expand their definitions of sex role behavior and taught better methods of communication. Stopping the violence completely becomes the primary goal, and if this cannot be done by rebuilding the relationship, the couple is helped with dissolution. Nurses can con-

duct this kind of marital counseling themselves with proper background and training, or they can learn where such counseling is provided and work with the woman separately.

As well as providing interventions for individual abused women, the nurse should be concerned with institutional measures at the secondary prevention level. It is not enough that the individual nurse include questions about battering in her own practice; protocols should be officially established in all the settings mentioned so that all health professionals assess for abuse. The battered woman's movement, several concerned physicians, and the Nursing Network on Violence Against Women have been encouraging hospitals to have both protocols and training to systematically assess and intervene with these women. A nursing research effort by Tilden and Shepherd (1987) found a significant increase in emergency nurses' documentation of battering (from only 9.2% of abused women documented as such to 22%) after staff training and implementation of a protocol. In response to the work of the advocacy groups, in 1992 the Joint Commission on the Accreditation of Healthcare Organizations (JCAHO) adopted guidelines for written policies and procedures on family violence and sexual assault throughout the life cycle (Table 9-4). The 1992 guidelines include spouse and partner abuse as well as requiring member health care organizations to maintain appropriate family violence referral lists, perform thorough documentation, and provide family violence intervention education to key personnel. Nurses also need to support training about abuse for the police, legal professionals, social workers, physicians, and clergy, as well as for nurses. Workshops for professionals and interested key people and public education on abuse are needed and can be conducted by nurses.

Tertiary Prevention

Tertiary prevention is aimed at helping the severely abused wife to recover. The severely battered woman has been victimized by physical and psychological abuse for a significant amount of time and usually has experienced considerable physical

TABLE 9-4

Joint Commission on Accreditation of Healthcare Organization (JCAHO) Guidelines for Written Policies and Procedures

Adult and Child Victims of Alleged or Suspected Abuse or Neglect Emergency Department/Service and Ambulatory Care Services

JCAHO STANDARDS	GUIDELINES
ES.5.1.10.1 HO.3.2.15	Criteria needed to identify possible abuse victims

ES.5.2.10.1.1
HO.3.2.15.1.1
	Types of abuse to be addressed:
	    Physical assault
	    Rape or sexual molestation
	    Domestic abuse of elders, spouses, partners, and children

ES.5.1.2.10.2
HO.3.2.15.2
	Procedures for patient evaluation:
	    Patient consent
	    Examination and treatment
	    Hospital's role in collection, retention, and safeguarding of specimens,
	        photographs, and other evidence
	    Notification/release of information to proper authorities

ES.5.1.2.10.3 HO.3.2.15.3	Referral list of private and community-based family violence agencies available through the hospital

ES.5.1.2.10.4
HO.3.2.15.4
	Medical record documentation to include examinations, treatment, referrals
	    to other care providers and community-based agencies, and required
	    notification of authorities

ES.5.1.2.10.5 HO.3.2.15.5	Requires appropriate staff to be trained in the identification and procedures needed to work with abuse survivors

From The Joint Commission Accreditation Manual for Hospitals, 1992 edition, Chicago.

and psychological damage. However, she has usually also developed strong resolve as a result of her ordeal and has many insights into her own nature and that of her husband. Tertiary prevention interventions are often performed in wife abuse shelters or in mental health settings. The woman is usually experiencing many of the strong emotions associated with grieving and often can be helped at this point to achieve necessary acceptance of the losses and final resolution.

Harassment in abusive relationships

One of the difficulties in recovering from an abusive relationship is the harassment to which the abuser all too often subjects the woman, especially while she is trying to leave the relationship. The women in Campbell's (1991) longitudinal study described the harassment as lasting anywhere from a month to several years, with an average of 1 year after they left the abuser. This behavior may make it more difficult for her to leave permanently.

To date, no research focuses directly on harassment of battered women, and none of the research instruments designed to measure various aspects of abuse contain items addressing harassment. However, this behavior has been described extensively in much of the literature on abuse (e.g., Walker, 1979a). Sheridan (1992) has created a Harassment in Abusive Relationships: A Self-Report Scale (HARASS) instrument. Based on extensive interviews with battered women survivors and family violence clinical experts, a list of harassing male behaviors has been identified that are applicable to many battering situations (Table 9-5). The instru-

TABLE 9-5
Harassment in Abusive Relationships: A Self-Report Scale (HARASS) Selected Descriptions

The Behavior		How Often Does It Occur
		0 = Never
		1 = Rarely
		2 = Occasionally
		3 = Frequently
		4 = Very frequently

MY PARTNER

MY FORMER PARTNER   (Circle One)

		0	1	2	3	4
1.	Scares me with a weapon	0	1	2	3	4
2.	Threatens to harm our pet	0	1	2	3	4
3.	Threatens to harm the kids if I leave him	0	1	2	3	4
4.	Tries to get me fired from my job	0	1	2	3	4
5.	Destroys my property	0	1	2	3	4
6.	Threatens to kill himself if I leave him	0	1	2	3	4
7.	Calls me on the phone and hangs up	0	1	2	3	4
8.	Follows me	0	1	2	3	4
9.	Threatens to take the kids if I leave him	0	1	2	3	4
10.	Frightens my family	0	1	2	3	4
11.	Leaves notes on my car	0	1	2	3	4
12.	Threatens to kill me if I leave or stay away from him	0	1	2	3	4
13.	Shows up without warning	0	1	2	3	4
14.	Makes me feel like he can again force me into sex	0	1	2	3	4
15.	Sits in his car outside my home	0	1	2	3	4
16.	Frightens my friends	0	1	2	3	4
17.	Agrees to pay certain bills, then doesn't pay them	0	1	2	3	4
18.	Reports me to the authorities for taking drugs when I don't	0	1	2	3	4
19.	Leaves threatening messages on the telephone answering machine	0	1	2	3	4
20.	Refuses to grant me a divorce	0	1	2	3	4

© 1992, Daniel J. Sheridan. Reprinted with permission. Requests to use this instrument must be sent in writing to Daniel J. Sheridan, MS, RN, Family Violence Consultant, Trauma Program—UHN 66, Oregon Health Sciences University, 3181 SW Sam Jackson Park Road, Portland, OR 97201.

ment can be used clinically as an assessment tool and as a stimulant for discussion in battered women's support groups. In addition, research is being conducted to further explore the psychometric properties of the instrument and its correlation with battered women being able to remain out of an abusive relationship.

Nursing roles in shelters

Shelters for abused women have been established in most major cities in the United States and have been invaluable to battered women as a haven of physical safety for them and their children and as a setting for effective interventions of many types. Most shelters provide individual and group counseling; help with bureaucratic institutions, such as the police, legal representation, social services, child care, and children's programming; and aid the woman in making future plans, such as employment counseling and liaisons with housing authorities. Best of all is the support and knowledge that they are not alone that is gained by the women from each other in the shelter setting.

Unfortunately, many shelters are in desperate financial straits. Funding traditionally has been unstable, and most of the original government and private grants used for initial start-up have expired. Money for battered women's programs has become a low priority in the present political climate; these programs have become the victims of the same backlash against feminism seen in many arenas over the past decade. Nurses are desperately needed at the policy-making level, on governing boards of shelters, on boards of social service funding agencies, and at the state planning level to advocate for the establishment of more shelters where they are needed and to ensure that existing shelters remain open.

Shelters are usually run with a combination of professional and volunteer staff, drawing from social workers, psychologists, occupational therapists, and child care professionals as paid staff. In addition, many formerly abused women, feminists, nurses, lawyers, and others have been involved in the planning, operations, and volunteer services of shelters. Professional education programs, including nursing programs, have found shelters to be an excellent clinical experience for students.

Health services are usually recognized as a necessary part of shelters, and they are obtained in a variety of ways. It would be ideal to have a professional nurse as part of the paid staff of all shelters, and nurses involved in their planning can advocate for this. When this is not feasible, community health nurses can be contracted for on a part-time basis, or arrangements can be made to refer women and children to nurse clinicians. However, in-house nursing care is preferable considering the dangers involved whenever the woman leaves the shelter, the transportation difficulties, and the traditional mistrust of the health care system held by the poor

and undeserved in general, and the battered woman specifically. Nurses can fill the gap by volunteering at shelters and performing a variety of roles while there. Shelter staff may need some demonstration of the expanded autonomous roles of professional nursing; at first they may envision the responsibilities of nurses as only that of monitoring blood pressure, teaching health classes, establishing first aid procedures, or giving advice about the endemic children's diarrhea problems that come with change of diet and new environment. These roles may be important, but there is much more that nurses can do in wife abuse shelters.

The group sessions conducted in most shelters can be successfully led by nurses. Several nursing experts have described models for groups for battered wives based on their experiences in a shelter (Campbell, 1986b; Henderson, 1989; Janosik & Phipps, 1982). They suggest that the major goal be crisis intervention, allowing the women to initiate the topics and find their own solutions, finding meaning in the abuse experience, and offering and receiving peer support. The women come and go from the group because of their varying lengths of stay in the shelter, necessitating constant readjustment to differing stages of progress and different faces. The women may also be in a variety of phases of the entrapment and recovery process. Janosik and Phipps (1982) see this as an advantage in terms of older group members providing role models for the newer.

Nurses can also lead groups dealing with parenting issues or general health concerns that may include sexual abuse. Clinical experience in shelters suggests that it is generally beneficial to allow the women to decide what areas to explore with the nurse, rather than using a set agenda. Topics may range from race relations among shelter staff and residents and among residents themselves to breast self-examination. Group sessions can be fun or serious depending on clients' needs. Flexibility and openness are important when the nurse acts as group leader.

Women in shelters can also be seen individually for a variety of health needs. A shelter is a wonderful place to practice a range of nursing skills, from physical assessment to one-to-one counseling. Campbell and Humphreys (1987) and Hollencamp and Attala (1986) have described nursing care in shelters in detail.

The woman's length of stay in the shelter is variable, and the relationship with the nurse may be a single contact or may be of a fairly long-term nature. It is important to have a good community resource network established with actual names and some knowledge of other nurses to whom women can be referred for follow-up. Once a battered woman has had beneficial contact with a nurse, she is usually enthusiastic about her long-term health care being handled by a nurse unless she has an acute problem needing medical diagnosis. Nursing often provides an excellent avenue through which she can meet her health care needs; battered women frequently express their pleasure with the woman-to-woman contact and the holistic possibilities of nursing care.

Tertiary-level individual interventions ideally start with building on the woman's strengths found in the nursing assessment. It takes a great deal of courage to go to a shelter. One of the most poignant images from our clinical experience in shelters is the sight of the battered woman arriving, usually with several children in tow, at a completely strange place, with all of her hastily gathered belongings in a black plastic garbage bag. How many of us would be willing to leave our homes, with few if any financial or material resources, when we have been the victims of wrongdoing, and place our future as human beings in the hands of complete strangers? It is imperative to continually praise the abused woman for that act of courage alone.

Other strengths shown by the woman's appearance at the shelter include the mere fact of physical survival, the successful and often carefully planned escape, and the caring for the children shown by leaving. These need to be recognized as strengths and pointed out to the woman. Additional individual strengths found in assessment are important to stress to help combat the woman's feelings of being trapped and helpless. These also serve as a base for further developing problem-solving strategies. The woman may feel she has exhausted all her resources in just getting to the shelter and may need to be reminded that if she was able to do that, she can do just about anything with a little help and a little time. The first few days at the shelter may need to be just that—some time to rest and recoup and gather her resources, in safety finally. The newly arrived shelter resident should not be expected to do much future planning until she has had a chance just to be relieved. However, it is important that her injuries be carefully documented for future legal proceedings. Because the nurse is often not present on her arrival, staff can be instructed how to measure and describe the physical problems. Photography of injuries is usually desirable. There also may be need for immediate medical intervention, and the nurse can be helpful in setting up protocols within the shelter and making contacts with the nearest emergency room.

Care for the physical injuries to battered women can require much ingenuity on the part of shelter staff and nurse consultants. Examples of women with injuries from clinical experience include a woman with a broken jaw that had been wired internally and set with a metal brace, a woman bleeding internally who had not been thoroughly examined in the emergency room, and a 4-day postpartum mother who had been raped by her husband as soon as she got home from the hospital. The latter woman required hospitalization for hemorrhage, and she left her newborn baby and two siblings at the shelter. It is extremely helpful if the shelter has a nurse to call in such situations for consultation.

Other serious health problems include medication for chronic diseases that has been left behind, dangerously high blood pressure necessitating transportation by ambulance, and severe asthma in a child. Chronic conditions are often exacerbated by the stress of the situation, and communicable diseases are common in communal living situations. The nurse can devise a short health history form for the woman and her children that can be completed on arrival so that shelter staff members are alerted to health problems needing immediate attention. Women are also at high risk for AIDS because of unknown sexual infidelity of their partner or drug abuse, and because part of a relationship of control of the woman may include the man's refusal to use a condom.

Individual nursing assessment can determine other physical health problems for which the woman seeks help for herself, her children, or both. It has been found helpful to announce a specific day and time that the nurse will be at the shelter to see any women who wish to seek care. Staff members can also make referrals for such problems as substance abuse or observable poor nutritional status. Communication with staff about health problems is important, and the regular shelter records of the women can be used to enter short nursing entries for assessment and interventions. With professional nursing care, the women have often found the shelter a good place to begin working on health problems that have been bothering them, which may or may not be directly connected with abuse.

The woman experiencing severe abuse and in a shelter is usually starting to experience the strong emotions of the grieving process. She may need help in combating depression, dealing with her anger, or both. Perhaps the most helpful intervention is letting the woman know how normal these feelings are in her situation and helping her recognize and accept the ambivalence she often feels about the abuser and her relationship to him. The woman can be helped to recognize her many losses and to grieve for them. Tears can be useful and healing, and the battered woman must not be hurried into decision-making activities until she has had a chance to mourn. Just as a grieving widow needs to talk about the deceased, the abused woman must be allowed to express herself fully about the man, including the good points and happy memories. Other residents and staff may not encourage this as much as they might; the shelter atmosphere sometimes appears to be very much against all men, and this is natural. However, the individual woman may even need to idealize her man before she moves on, and the nurse can provide and encourage this opportunity.

The woman's anger also needs expression. The shelter, with its close living quarters, many responsibilities, and strong feeling tones, can sometimes be an explosive place. Children are noisy; people don't always attend to chores; privacy is elusive.

Anger that has built up over the duration of an abusive relationship without any safe means of expression for fear of further beatings can be released over a minor incident between residents, against staff, or against confused and restless children. The battered woman may feel resentful if she perceives that she is being judged by staff and other residents for the way she has and is handling the abuse, or for the way she mothers her children. The legal system and social services system she has to deal with to build a future life can also be frustrating. All these factors can underlie and trigger angry outbursts. These outbursts are best handled as they occur, and the women involved are helped to see where the anger comes from and encouraged to express it verbally and assertively. This approach is helpful in both dealing with the situation at hand and in teaching the woman how to deal with anger constructively.

The guilt that the abused woman may feel is also best dealt with by encouragement of expression first. As angry as it may make the nurse to hear the woman blame herself or worry about her spouse, this is a necessary part of grieving and recovery and cutting her off is not helpful. Again, assurance that this is normal is the beginning of intervention. Then the woman can be helped to review events with an emphasis on the batterer's behavior, which helps her realize that usually what she said and did made no real difference in the final outcome. She also needs help in recognizing that no one can take responsibility for another's actions. She may need time to think through events again with this fact in mind, and although unable initially to progress beyond some measure of guilt, she eventually may report a successful resolution of the situation.

The nurse's role in shelters can thus be seen as multifaceted. The nurse works as part of the shelter staff team, and the nature of her interventions is based on the needs of the staff and the residents. There is room for several nurses to work at once at one shelter, either working in a rotating sequence or performing a more specialized role. Nursing roles may evolve over time, as staff and residents recognize what kinds of services are available. There is a definite need for nursing in all shelters, and nurses are urged to become involved.

Interventions in mental health settings

The nurse may also give tertiary-level interventions for abused women at both inpatient and outpatient mental health institutions. The middle-class battered woman may be more likely to seek help in these settings or in a private psychiatrist's or psychologist's office than in a shelter. The abused woman frequently presents with symptoms of depression, including suicidal intent, anxiety, or may be referred for marital difficulties. Revealing the abuse and labeling it as such is the first task. The second is to assess the woman's danger, either from herself in terms of suicide or from the batterer, and to do crisis intervention if necessary on that basis. The third step is to assess for posttraumatic stress disorder.

Posttraumatic stress disorder (PTSD). *Posttraumatic stress disorder* is a useful perspective in determining the seriousness of and treatment for the psychological effects of severe abuse. PTSD is a cluster of symptoms that arises from exposure to severely traumatic event(s). The stressor is generally outside the range of usual human experiences. Any environmental stimulus perceived as dangerous, whether it produces physical injury or not, can be sufficiently traumatic to precipitate a posttraumatic stress disorder. The disorder has been noted in survivors of induced human trauma, such as war, assault, rape, incest, and wife abuse; and to natural catastrophes, such as fires, hurricanes, and earthquakes. Human-induced trauma is generally more difficult to recover from. The symptoms of PTSD according to the DSM III-R are listed in the box (American Psychiatric Association, 1987).

The experience of a significant, recognizable stressor or trauma is followed by recurrent subjective reexperiencing of the trauma. It is important to realize that the reexperiencing can be of feelings associated with the trauma rather than actual "flashbacks." For instance, one battered woman told of seeing a friend of her abusive husband in a shopping mall about 6 months after she left him and being overwhelmed with a terrible fear that she did not understand. There is also a general numbing of responsiveness, and cognitive or somatic symptoms of irritability, anxiety, aggressiveness, and depres-

---

Posttraumatic Stress Disorder (DSM III-R)

1. Existence of a recognizable stressor
2. Reexperiencing of the trauma as evidenced by at least one of the following:
   Intrusive recollections of the event
   Recurring dreams, nightmares
   Sudden acting or feeling as if the trauma were recurring, stimulated by an emotional or environmental event
3. Psychological numbing as evidenced by:
   Diminished interest in activities
   Feelings of estrangement
   Constricted affect
4. At least two of the following symptoms that were not present before the trauma:
   Exaggerated startle reflex, anxiety
   Sleep disturbance
   Survival guilt
   Impaired concentration or memory
   Avoidance of activities that are reminders of the trauma
   Intensification of symptoms by exposure to events that symbolize or resemble the traumatic event
   Irritability, hypersensitivity

---

sion may follow. As well as recurring dreams and nightmares, sleep disturbances such as insomnia often occur. Psychic numbing, or emotional anesthesia in relation to other people and to previously enjoyed activities is also common. Alcohol and other substances may be used in an attempt to maintain control and soothe emotions.

Onset of PTSD varies among individuals and can be from a few hours or days to months or years after the stressor. Acute PTSD has an onset within 6 months of the traumatic event, and symptoms last for less than 6 months. Chronic PTSD, or the delayed stress response, is characterized by an onset of symptoms at least 6 months after the traumatic event or symptoms last for at least 6 months. This type of PTSD is seen especially in Vietnam veterans, but it also has been reported in survivors of catastrophe and human-induced trauma. Symptoms are similar to those in the box on the previous page but they are more severe.

Victimization takes its toll, especially when it continues over an extended period of time, as with battered women. When individuals experience chronic victimization by someone close to them, the impact is intensified and complicated by the profound betrayal of trust. There are many factors that are important in the readjustment to a traumatic event such as wife abuse. The frequency, intensity, duration, and nature of the abuse affect the severity and duration of symptoms. PTSD stressors have been classified into two categories—bereavement and personal injury—with different kinds of symptomatology. Battered women experience both. Therefore they can be expected to experience sadness over loss and discomfort over discovered personal vulnerability (bereavement), as well as fear of repetition of the event and feelings of responsibility (personal injury). Having taken an active role during the trauma itself and immediately after has been linked to a better adjustment, but often abused women have been forced into a passive role in the situation. Lack of helpful support systems and socioeconomic problems have also been linked with slower and more difficult posttrauma readjustment. Finally, instead of the trauma being a single occurrence or time limited (tour of duty), abused women have continued exposure to the trauma over long periods of time. Thus battered women may be suffering from serious PTSD, which obviously needs to be recognized.

PTSD is definitely responsive to treatment. The major focus in PTSD is education to normalize the reactions and provide information about PTSD in terms of its patterns and occurrence. This explanation of the syndrome can assist women in their quest to make sense of their response to the abuse. Treatment in a group modality such as formalized support groups with mental health professionals as group leaders is the treatment of choice. Sometimes antidepressants are prescribed to control intrusive thoughts and depression.

Other mental health-related interventions. Women with less serious symptoms can be treated in other kinds of groups. Consciousness-raising groups have been found to help women increase self-esteem, increase their sense of control, and significantly decrease depression. Weitz (1982) defines such groups as regular meetings in which women discuss and search for similarities among their personal experiences. Groups then use this knowledge of commonalities to develop an understanding of power relations between the sexes and of the role structures and socialization processes that maintain these power relations. Such groups can be appropriately organized and led by nurses and held in mental health settings. Battered women can be referred to this kind of group consisting of women from various situations.

Individual therapy with abused women in mental health settings deals with many of the issues discussed as individual interventions with women in shelters. Walker (1979b) advocates "feminist psychotherapy" for battered women, carefully explaining that she does not suggest a therapist who tries to make feminists out of women who hold traditional values in regard to sex roles, but ideally a woman therapist who "believes in the strength of being a woman" (p. 75). Walker further describes therapy that helps the woman explore her own psychological self in relationship to the battering and helps her separate those issues from the ones that result from sexist society and her spouse's background and therefore are not her fault.

Concomitant interventions for the abuser are necessary at the tertiary level. Both partners need to understand that the violence will escalate in severity and frequency if he does not receive treatment specifically for battering. If he refuses such intervention, and the confirmed abuser often will, the woman must be helped to understand that strategies designed to end the violence while remaining in the relationship are not likely to succeed. Abused women have no real control over their batterer's violent behavior. The nurse and abused woman should explore other options for her, and she should have a plan for escaping or otherwise staying safe if the situation becomes dangerous.

Interventions for violent men

It is ironic and aggravating that the abused woman must flee her home or be labeled as sick and receive treatment, while the batterer stays home and is seldom identified as needing interventions. Most abusers do not fit current definitions of mental illness, yet their behavior clearly must be changed.

Batterers may come to the attention of the mental health system through alcoholic treatment programs, and specific questions about abuse should be included in the histories of such men. Their wives should also be asked about physical violence in the relationship, because the man frequently denies such occurrences or treats them lightly. It cannot be assumed that resolving alcohol problems will also solve the problems of violence in the relationship; specific interventions for abuse need to be implemented also.

There are now specific programs for abusive men in most localities, certainly a needed development. Some communities are experimenting with mandated counseling for batterers through the law enforcement system. Group treatment seems to be the avenue of choice, based on the Men's Aid program model started in England (Melville, 1978). Telephone counseling and drop-in services have also been a part of Men's Aid. Confrontation is used to get the abusers to admit their responsibility, and ways of dealing with anger besides hitting are taught. The men are also encouraged to get in touch with their other feelings and learn how to express them, and also to deal with changing sex roles and the difficulties in being a man today. To be effective, such groups must deal with attitudes as well as behavior. Research evaluation of batterer treatment groups has been mixed, and many of the research designs have been flawed. From the evidence accumulated to date, it appears that court-mandated participation is most successful; otherwise, most men drop out of treatment (Dutton, 1988). Male therapists or co-therapists, male and female, are generally used in leading such groups, to provide a role model and to better be able to challenge these men.

The nurse as advocate

Where such programs for abusive men do not yet exist, the nurse can be instrumental in the community in advocating for their establishment. Once begun, nurses need to encourage this as a useful intervention for battering and to advocate with the police, lawyers, judges, and probation officers to make use of them, as a mandatory alternative to jail or legal proceedings, if necessary. Establishment of these programs should work in conjunction with the formation of shelters for abused wives in all communities.

Advocacy also includes working at the local and state level to make it easier for abused women to find housing if they want to leave the abuser. Liaisons can be formed with shelters and other programs for battered women and urban housing programs. In many cases, vacant houses can be rehabilitated to provide a home for two abused women and their children. The women can receive support from each other, build on a friendship started in a shelter or group, and pool their resources to make a home. The housing situation for battered women can also be helped by advocacy with public housing authorities. When they understand the desperate need and the funding rules that limit the women's stay in shelters, they are often helpful in cutting "red tape" for battered women.

Advocacy can also take the form of working with the police and the legal profession, as outlined in Chapters 12 and 14. In addition, the nurse should discuss battering and what battered women and their children need in all her professional and social contacts. Shelters always need donations of time, money, supplies, clothing, and food. When talking about abuse, nurses frequently are told of personal battering by acquaintances and fellow professionals. As battering becomes more of a public issue, individual women feel more comfortable in talking about their own abuse. Advocacy for battered women and demonstration of knowledge on the subject of abuse become a novel means of case finding and an opportunity for intervention.

EVALUATION

Evaluation of nursing care for abused women is based on achievement of goals set by the individual woman or group. When the goals are truly formulated by the women themselves, the nurse can avoid the trap of being dissatisfied with interventions that do not necessarily result in the woman leaving the relationship, even when the nurse has decided that this course of action would be best. The goals set for nursing care may be limited, depending on the amount of intervention possible in the particular setting. Achievement of the goals, however modest, can still be a powerful statement of possibilities to the battered wife. Praise for her progress, however small, can be an important reinforcer for the woman to seek further help and to have confidence in her own ability to address the underlying problems.

When working with battered women, the nurse needs to become accustomed to measuring gains in small steps and to deal with the women in a variety of stages of resolution of this significant health problem. The nurse can begin to recognize that for every abused woman who is still in denial of the seriousness of abuse, there is another woman who is close to rebuilding a healthy life for herself. It is easy for professionals to become discouraged when working with battered women; similar feelings are expressed by nurses who work with clients with chronic health problems. These feelings can be dealt with by sharing with others who work with abuse and by taking pride in evaluation of what has been achieved when working with the abuse victim. Shelter staffs also often need help with such feelings. Nurses can help by pointing out that women who return to the abusive relationship may still have gained a great deal of support and insight by staying in the shelter, feel less alone in dealing with the problem, know where they can go if they are in danger, and be farther along in their grieving process than when they first arrived.

During evaluation the nurse may also need to deal with her own feelings of anger against the batterer, especially if the woman has not experienced them during the period of nursing intervention.

This is a frequent dilemma of professionals dealing with abused women. If the nurse works in a shelter situation or with other professionals cognizant of wife abuse, it is appropriate for the nurse to delay her feelings of anger and discuss them later with her colleagues. Even if she does not have a good professional support system, it is important that the nurse not let her own anger show when she is with a woman not feeling anger. However, the feelings must be dealt with constructively, or the nurse will find anger against specific batterers becoming generalized to many men, and this will interfere with effective nursing practice. Even in shelters, the nurse and staff must be careful to deal with their understandably strong feelings about situations in private or the women will suspect that staff "talks about us" behind their backs. Working with abuse victims engenders many strong feelings, and the nurses and other professionals involved need to form their own support systems carefully so that they will not become incapacitated by the feelings or become "burned out." Evaluation includes the nurse's careful reevaluation of her own feelings and how they affect her nursing care.

Evaluation of nursing care with the battered woman includes making plans for the future. It is important for the woman who stays in the relationship to have a variety of choices of helpful services that she can rely on if she decides to seek further assistance. The nurse must make sure that the individuals to whom she refers the woman are knowledgeable about abuse and immediately can put the woman at ease.

SAMPLE NURSING PROCESS

A sample nursing process has been included to show how each of the four steps might be applied to a hypothetical case of wife abuse (Table 9-6). This is not intended to be applicable to all cases of battered women; instead, it is provided as an illustration of some of the aspects of wife abuse that might be included in nursing care and as a means of suggesting the wording of possible nursing diagnoses. Only a brief description of the case is presented. An

TABLE 9-6
Sample Nursing Process

Brief background

Anne is a 27-year-old black woman, married to John who is 28. They have two children, 5 and 7 years old. Anne works as a sales clerk; John has been unemployed for 2 years. Anne was seen in the emergency room of the local hospital 1 week ago following miscarriage in the second month of pregnancy. She also had multiple bruises, two fractured ribs, and disclosed to the emergency room that she had been beaten by her husband just before the miscarriage. Referral was made to the local Public Health Department, nursing division, for abuse and follow-up care of her injuries.

The community health nurse's initial assessment of Anne includes but is not limited to the following:

Significant history	History of abuse over last 6 years. Says husband is extremely jealous about her work relationships with other men and imagines that she is having affairs.
	Abuse has escalated over time in frequency and severity. Husband beats her with fists and "shoves her around" at least once a month at current time. He has never used a weapon. Anne believes that being hit "now and then" is to be expected in marriage. She does not attempt to retaliate because the few times she has, she has been beaten more severely. She reports severe headaches at least once a week. Reports extreme soreness in rib area and generalized fatigue because of "not sleeping well." States wanted baby but does not feel she can talk about it.
General appearance	Energetic, neatly dressed young woman, average height and weight. Speaks quickly with many gestures; smiles when discussing miscarriage and violence.
Skin	5-cm oval-shaped contusion on left arm just above elbow, tender to touch.
Musculoskeletal	Fracture of 9th and 10th right ribs diagnosed by x-ray examination.
Neurological	Alert, oriented to time, place, person. Uses humor describing situation. No display of sadness when discussing loss of baby. Unable to list personal strengths.

Nursing diagnoses (Carpenito, 1992) that could be used in this situation include:

1. Dysfunctional grieving related to loss of baby and wife abuse as evidenced by prolonged denial and inability to discuss feelings.
2. Pain related to fractured ribs as evidenced by client's report of extreme soreness and difficulty sleeping.
3. Anxiety related to ongoing threat of physical violence (wife abuse) as evidenced by headache, excessive rate of speech, and insomnia.
4. Self-esteem disturbance related to wife abuse as evidenced by inability to identify strengths.
5. High risk for injury related to history of wife abuse.

TABLE 9-6 *Continued*
Sample Nursing Process

NURSING DX	CLIENT GOALS	NURSING INTERVENTION
I. Dysfunctional grieving related to loss of baby and wife abuse as evidenced by prolonged denial and inability to discuss feelings.	Short term Client will acknowledge the loss of the baby within 2 visits and express sorrow related to loss. Long term Client will acknowledge losses related to wife abuse and identify related losses.	1. Discuss with client what pregnancy meant to her when she indicates readiness. 2. Encourage client to contact her sister whom she has identified as supportive. Form helping relationship with client. 1. Discuss with client losses described by others in wife abuse situations. 2. Encourage client to explore expectations of marriage and possible losses related to violence from spouse.
II. Pain related to fractured ribs as evidenced by client's report of extreme soreness and difficulty sleeping.	Short term Client will report decreased pain in ribs within 1 wk and less difficulty sleeping.	1. Plan with client for brief periods of rest throughout day. 2. Tape ribs for support and show client how to do herself. 3. Heat to area when resting to promote healing (hot showers/baths, heating pad/hot water bottle).
III. Anxiety related to ongoing threat of physical violence (wife abuse) as evidenced by headache, excessive rate of speech, and insomnia.	Short term Client will experience a decrease in anxiety-related symptoms within 4 wk, specifically: Decreased incidence of headaches Reporting 7 hr of sleep per night Reporting feeling less tension and decreased rate of speech Long term Client will identify triggers to anxiety and institute stress management strategies.	1. Help client identify anxiety-producing situations and identify symptoms related to anxiety. 2. Discuss current coping strategies with client and help her identify those that are effective. 3. Teach client relaxation exercises to use before sleep and during rest periods daily. 4. Help client plan a regular exercise regimen. 5. Discuss sleep patterns with client and encourage sleep-enhancing mechanisms that she has used in the past.
IV. Self-esteem disturbance related to wife abuse as evidenced by inability to identify strengths.	Short term Client will begin to increase self-awareness/self-exploration by the end of 3 wk as evidenced by: Comparing her own situation with situation of other women experiencing wife abuse Identifying personal strengths used in dealing with her difficult situation	1. Encourage increased social interaction such as joining a woman's group. 2. Discuss incidence of wife abuse and relationship to woman's role in society. 3. Identify strengths observed and discuss these with client.

TABLE 9-6 *Continued*
Sample Nursing Process

NURSING DX	CLIENT GOALS	NURSING INTERVENTION
		4. Praise efforts at problem solving.
		5. Explore feelings and behaviors with her.
		6. Help client identify what she can control and what she cannot.
		7. Provide self as a role model in self-exploration.
	Long term	1. Continue to explore client's attitudes, feelings, and values with her.
	Client will increase self-esteem by the end of 6 mo as evidenced by:	
	Client being able to list at least 10 significant personal strengths	2. Help her to identify long-term goals and plans.
	Client being able to identify long-term goals and confidently express realistic plans to achieve them	
V. High risk for injury related to history of wife abuse.	Client will realistically assess own danger and plan for safety by the end of 4 wk, specifically:	1. Share facts about wife abuse with client.
	State realistically the pattern of abuse in the relationship	2. Help client identify incidence and patterns of abuse using a calendar and body map.
	Identify husband's patterns of abusive behavior	3. Discuss behavior of children in wife abuse homes in general and assist her to compare with behavior of her children.
	Identify effects of violence on children	4. Discuss characteristics of abusive men with her and relate to husband's behavior.
	Establish plan for physical safety in case of future abuse	5. Identify community and personal resources for physical safety (e.g., a wife abuse shelter or home of a supportive friend or relative).
		6. Discuss legal alternatives with her (restraining orders, crime of wife abuse).

Evaluation of nursing interventions is based on achievement of goals as perceived by client and nurse and takes place at intervals identified.

in-depth assessment, including a complete history and physical assessment, would be indicated in most actual situations. Evaluations of nursing interventions are based on achievement of goals as perceived by client and as indicated by criteria met.

SUMMARY

Nursing care of abused women is based on thorough assessment, identification of strengths and areas needing nursing intervention, goal setting and planning with the client, performing nursing interventions and working with other professionals in providing services, and evaluating outcomes. Primary prevention includes interventions with women at risk to be battered as well as assertive actions at the societal level directed toward eliminating sex role patterns that allow and encourage violence against women. Secondary prevention necessitates active case finding. A direct, knowledgeable, and empathic approach to women suspected of being abused is important. Nursing interventions at the secondary prevention level are aimed at eliminating abuse before the patterns become entrenched. These interventions are performed in a variety of settings and follow the theoretical framework of accepting the woman at her current level of progress through the process of entrapment and recovery from an abusive relationship (Landenburger, 1989). This has many characteristics of a grieving process, a reaction to multiple losses. Tertiary-level interventions may find the nurse providing care in shelters or in community or inpatient mental health settings. Nursing care at secondary and tertiary levels also includes advocacy for better services for battered women, their children, and batterers. Empirical validation of these interventions is needed to document their impact and build practice theory.

REFERENCES

American Psychiatric Association. (1987). *Diagnostic and statistical manual III-R*. Washington, DC: American Psychiatric Association.

Battle, J. (1981). Culture-free SEI self-esteem inventories for children and adults. Seattle, WA: Special Publications.

Bergman, B., Larsson, G., Brismar, B., & Klang, M. (1987). Psychiatric morbidity and personality characteristics of battered women. *Acta Psychiatrica Scandinavica, 76*, 678-683.

Blair, K. A. (1986). The battered woman: Is she a silent victim? *Nurse Practitioner, 11*, 38-47.

Bowker, L. H. (1983). Beating wife-beating. Lexington, MA: Lexington Books.

Bowlby, J. (1980). *Attachment and loss: Vol. 3, Loss*. New York: Basic Books.

Brendtro, M., & Bowker, H. L. (1989). Battered women: How can nurses help. *Issues in Mental Health Nursing, 10*, 169-180.

Browne, A. (1987). *When battered women kill*. New York: Free Press.

Bullock, L., McFarlane, J., Bateman, L. H., & Miller, V. (1989). The prevalence and characteristics of battered women in a primary care setting. *Nurse Practitioner, 14*(6), 47-55.

Campbell, J. C. (in press). Prediction of homicide in and by battered women. In J. Campbell (Ed.), *Prediction of future dangerousness in cases of child abuse, wife abuse and sexual assault*. Newbury Park: Sage.

Campbell, J. C. (1986). A support group for battered women. *Advances in Nursing Science, 8*(2), 13-20.

Campbell, J. C. (1989a). A test of two explanatory models of women's responses to battering. *Nursing Research, 38*(1), 18-24.

Campbell, J. C. (1989b). Women's responses to sexual abuse in intimate relationships. *Women's Health Care International, 10*, 335-346.

Campbell, J. C. (1991, May). *Qualitative analysis of women's responses to battering over time*. Paper presented at the third National Nursing Network on Violence Against Women Conference, Detroit, MI.

Campbell, J. C., & Alford, P. (1989). The dark side of marital rape on women's health. *American Journal of Nursing, 89*, 946-949.

Campbell, J. C., & Humphreys, J. (1987). Providing health care in shelters. *Response, 10*(11), 20-23.

Campbell, J. C., & Sheridan, D. J. (1989). Emergency nursing interventions with battered women. *Journal of Emergency Nursing, 15*(1), 12-17.

Carmen, E., Rieker, P. P., & Mills, T. (1984). Victims of violence and psychiatric illness. *American Journal of Psychiatry, 141*(3), 378-383.

Carpenito, L. J. (1992). *Nursing diagnosis application to clinical practice*. Philadelphia: J. B. Lippincott.

Donnerstein, E. (1980). Aggressive erotica and violence against women. *Journal of Personality and Social Psychology, 39*, 269-277.

Drake, V. K. (1982). Battered women: A health care problem in disguise. *Image, 14*, 40-47.

Drossman, D. A., Leserman, J., Nachman, G., Li, Z., Gluck, H., Toomey, T. C., & Mitchell, C. M. (1990). Sexual and physical abuse in women with functional or organic gastrointestinal disorders. *Annals of Internal Medicine, 113*(11), 828-833.

Dutton, D. G. (1988). *The domestic assault of women.* Newton, MA: Allyn & Bacon.

Ferraro, K. J., & Johnson, J. M. (1983). How women experience battering: The process of victimization. *Social Problems, 30,* 325-339.

Figley, C. R. (1985). *Trauma and its wake: The study and treatment of post-traumatic stress disorder.* New York: Bruner/Mazel.

Finkelhor, D., Gelles, R. J., Hotaling, G. T., & Strauss, M. A. (Eds). (1983). *The dark side of families.* Beverly Hills: Sage.

Flynn, J. B., & Whitcomb, J. C. (1981). Unresolved grief in battered women. *Journal of Emergency Nursing, 7*(6), 250-254.

Frieze, I. R. (1979). Perceptions of battered wives. In D. Bar-Tal, J. S. Carroll, & I. R. Frieze (Eds.), *New approaches to social problems* (pp. 79-108). San Francisco: Jossey-Bass.

Galanti, G. A. (1991). *Caring for patients from different cultures.* Philadelphia: University of Pennsylvania Press.

Goldberg, W., & Carey, A. (1982). Domestic violence victims in the emergency setting. *Topics in Emergency Medicine, 3,* 65-75.

Goldberg, W. G., & Tomlanovich, M. C. (1984). Domestic violence victims in the emergency department. *Journal of the American Medical Association, 251,* 3259-3264.

Gondolf, E. (1988a). *Battered women as survivors.* Lexington, MA: DC Heath.

Gondolf, E. W. (1988b). The effect of batterer counseling on shelter outcome. *Journal of Interpersonal Violence, 3*(3), 275-289.

Gondolf, E. W. (1990). *Battered women as survivors.* Holmes Beach, FL: Learning Publications.

Helton, A. S. (1986). Battering during pregnancy. *American Journal of Nursing, 86*(8), 910-913.

Henderson, A. D. (1989). Use of social support in a transition house for abused women. *Health Care for Women International, 10,* 61-73.

Hoff, L. A. (1988). Collaborative feminist research and the myth of objectivity. In K. Yllo & M. Bograd (Eds.), *Feminist perspectives on wife abuse* (pp. 269-281, Chapter 13). Bevery Hills: Sage.

Hollencamp, M., & Attala, J. (1986). Meeting health needs in a crisis shelter: A challenge to nurses in the community. *Journal of Community Health Nursing, 39*(40), 201-209.

Hotaling, G. T., & Sugarman, D. B. (1986). An analysis of risk markers in husband to wife violence: The current state of knowledge. *Violence and Victims, 1*(2), 101-124.

Hotaling, G. T., & Sugarman, D. B. (1990). A risk marker analysis of assaulted wives. *Journal of Family Violence, 5*(1), 1-14.

Janosik, E. H., & Phipps, L. B. (1982). *Life cycle group work in nursing.* Monterey, CA: Wadsworth Health Sciences Division.

Joint Commission on the Accreditation of Healthcare Organizations (1992). *AMH accreditation manual for hospitals.* Terrace, IL: JCAHO.

Kalmuss, D. S., & Straus, M. A. (1982). Wife's marital dependency and wife abuse. *Journal of Marriage and the Family, 44*(2), 277-286.

Kerouac, S., Taggart, M., Lescop, J., & Fortin, M. (1986). Dimensions of health in violent families. *Health Care for Women International, 7,* 413-426.

King, M. C., & Ryan, J. (1989). Abused women: Dispelling myths and encouraging intervention. *Nurse Practitioner, 14,* 47-58.

Kinlein, M. L. (1977). *Independent nursing practice with clients.* Philadelphia: Lippincott.

Kurz, D. (1987). Emergency department responses to battered women: Resistance to medicalization. *Social Problems, 34,* 501-513.

Landenburger, K. (1989). A process of entrapment in and recovery from an abusive relationship. *Issues in Mental Health Nursing, 10,* 209-227.

Lichtenstein, V. R. (1981). The battered woman: Guidelines for effective nursing intervention. *Issues in Mental Health Nursing, 3,* 237-250.

Limandri, B. J. (1987). The therapeutic relationship with abused women. *Journal of Psychosocial Nursing, 25,* 9-16.

MacKinnon, C. A. (1981). Feminism, Marxism, method, and the state: An agenda for theory. In M. Z. Rosaldo, B. C. Gelpi, & O. K. Nannerl (Eds.), *Feminist theory: A critique of ideology* (pp. 1-30). Chicago: University of Chicago Press.

Mahon, L. (1981). Common characteristics of abused women. *Issues in Mental Health Nursing, 3,* 137-157.

Malamuth, N. M., & Check, J. V. P. (1981). The effects of mass media exposure on acceptance of violence against women: A field experiment. *Journal of Research in Personality, (15),* 436-446.

McFarlane, J., Christoffel, K., Bateman, L., Miller, V., & Bullock, L. (1991). Assessing for abuse: Self-report versus nurse interview. *Public Health Nursing, 8,* 245-250.

McKenna, L. S. (1985). Social support systems of battered women: Influence on psychological adaptation. *Dissertations Abstracts International, 47*(5A), 1895.

McLeer, S. V., & Anwar, R. (1989). A study of battered women presenting in an emergency department. *American Journal of Public Health, 79*(1), 65-66.

Melville, J. (1978). A note on men's aid. In J. P. Martin (Ed.), *Violence and the family* (pp. 311-13). Chichester: John Wiley & Sons.

Okun, L. E. (1986). *Woman abuse: Facts replacing myths.* Albany, NY: SUNY Press.

Orem, D. (1991). *Nursing: Concepts of practice* (4th ed.). St. Louis: Mosby-Year Book.

Parker, B., & McFarlane, J. (1991). Identifying and helping battered pregnant women. *Maternal Child Nursing, 16,* 161-164.

Parse, R. R. (1987). *Nursing science, major paradigms, theories, and critiques.* Philadelphia: W. B. Saunders.

Parson, E. R. (1985). Ethnicity and traumatic stress: The intersecting point in psychotherapy. In C. R. Figley (Ed.), *Trauma and its wake: The study and treatment of posttraumatic stress disorder* (pp. 314-337). New York: Bruner-/Mazel.

Sandelowski, M. (1980). *Women, health, and choice.* Englewood Cliffs, NJ: Prentice Hall.

Schei, B. (1991). *Trapped in painful love.* Trondheim, Norway: TAPIR.

Sheridan, D. J. (1992). HARASS: Harassment in abusive relationships instruments. Unpublished paper.

Silver, S. M. (1986). An inpatient program for posttraumatic stress disorder: Context as treatment. In Figley, C. R. (1985). *Trauma and its wake: Traumatic stress, theory, research, and intervention* (pp. 213-231). New York: Bruner-/Mazel.

Silverman, P. R. (1981). *Helping women cope with grief.* Beverly Hills: Sage.

Star, B. (1978). Comparing battered and non-battered women. *Victimology: An International Journal, 3*(1-2), 32-44.

Stark, E., & Flitcraft, A. (1985). Woman-battering, child abuse and social heredity: What is the relationship? In N. Johnson (Ed.), *Marital violence.* London: Routledge & Kegan Paul.

Stark, E., Flitcraft, A., & Frazier, W. (1979). Medicine and patriarchal violence: The social construction of a "private" event. *International Journal of Health Services, 9*(3), 461-493.

Steinem, G. (1978, November). Erotica and pornography: A clear and present difference. *MS,* 53-54, 75-78.

Sue, D. W., & Sue, D. (1990). *Counseling the culturally different: Theory and practice.* New York: John Wiley & Sons.

Tilden, V. P., & Shepherd, P. (1987). Increasing the rate of identification of battered women in an emergency department: Use of a nursing protocol. *Research in Nursing & Health, 10,* 209-215.

Torres, S. (1987). Hispanic-American battered women: Why consider cultural differences? *Response, 10*(3), 20-21.

Torres, S. (1991). A comparison of wife abuse between two cultures: Perceptions, attitudes, nature, and extent. *Issues in Mental Health Nursing, 12*(1), 113-131.

Trimpey, M. L. (1989). Self-esteem and anxiety: Key issues in an abused women's support group. *Issues in Mental Health Nursing, (10),* 297-308.

Ulrich, Y. C. (1991). Women's reasons for leaving abusive spouses. *Health Care for Women International, 12*(4), 465-473.

Walker, L. E. (1979a). *The battered woman.* New York: Harper & Row.

Walker, L. (1979b). How battering happens and how to stop it. In D. Moore (Ed.), *Battered Women* (pp. 59-78). Beverly Hills: Sage.

Walker, L. E. (1984). *The battered woman syndrome.* New York: Springer.

Warshaw, C. (1989). Limitations of the medical model in the care of battered women. *Gender & Society, 3*(4), 506-517.

Watts, D. L., & Courtois, C. A. (1981). Trends in the treatment of men who commit violence against women. *Personnel and Guidance Journal, 60,* 245-249.

Weinfourt, R. (1979). Battered women: The grieving process. *Journal of Psychiatric Nursing and Mental Health Services, 17*(4), 40-47.

Weitz, R. (1982). Feminist consciousness raising, self-concept, and depression. *Sex Roles, 8,* 235-37.

Werner-Beland, J. (1980). *Grief responses to long-term illness.* Reston, VA: Reston.

C H A P T E R

10 Nursing Care of Families Using Violence

Doris Campbell *and* Jacquelyn Campbell

"Breaking away"
I have to escape from beneath this dark cloud
cold, ominous easy to hide in
Need to let sunshine into my life
I'll be blinded by the sudden burst of light
Like a child taking first steps
Falling down sometimes
Get up and try again
Raising my children not to hide beneath the cloud
Laughing and free, we'll grow together
getting our strength
from warmth
of the light

Linda Strawder*

A violent family is in pain. Without understanding the underlying dynamics or necessarily labeling the violent behavior as a problem, violent family members are hurting each other emotionally and physically. Even those members who are not victims or perpetrators are learning that violence is acceptable and are highly at risk to use violence themselves, either in the family or outside it. They are also hurt by the destructive family dynamics. Their homes are academies in which the children learn to become violent adults. Nurses see such families in hospitals, clinics, homes, and mental health settings. Effective nursing care can be crucial in preventing further violence and in helping these families to end the pain they are causing each other.

A violent family is considered to be one in which at least one family member is using physical or sexual force against another, resulting in physical and emotional destructive injury or both. The issue of when physical discipline of children becomes destructive is important, but is discussed in Chapter 2. In most cases there is also intent to injure on the part of the violent family member, although this is frequently difficult to determine. Thus a violent family can be one in which there is child abuse, wife abuse, abuse of elderly members, severe physical aggression between siblings, violence by adolescents against parents, or any combination thereof. A family in which there is incest is also considered to be violent, because even if physical force is not actually used, it is implied, and destructive injury is a consequence.

The nursing care section of this book begins with this chapter describing the nursing care of violent or

---

*Reprinted from *Every Twelve Seconds*, compiled by Susan Venters (Hillsboro, Oregon: Shelter, 1981) by permission of the author.

290

potentially violent families in which the family as a whole is considered the focus of intervention. The suggested interventions are based on the theoretical frameworks of violence and kinds of family abuse described in previous sections. This chapter also suggests nursing measures for decreasing violence in society generally, which will have the effect of decreasing the legitimacy of violence within families. Specific nursing interventions for victims of elder abuse, child abuse, and abuse of female partners are described in Chapters 7, 8, and 9.

Four areas of theoretical background are important in setting the stage for nursing care of violent families. It is necessary to understand:

1. Family theoretical perspectives and approaches
2. Why the family seems especially prone to use violence as a conflict resolution strategy
3. The evidence suggesting the intergenerational transmission of violence
4. The connections between wife abuse and child abuse

FAMILY THEORY AND FAMILY THERAPY PERSPECTIVES

A theoretical framework is useful in guiding clinical efforts in any area of nursing. Theories from nursing, family social sciences, and family therapy may all be useful in assessing problems, defining goals, and planning appropriate interventions with families experiencing violence. Relevant discussions of nursing theories and family nursing process are found in Oermann (1991), Fitzpatrick (1982), and Friedman (1992). Jones (1980) provides a comparative analysis of the major conceptualizations of family therapy, and Luepnitz (1988) gives a critical analysis of various family therapy approaches from a feminist perspective. Empirical studies based on many of these theories and models provide important information on their utility for guiding the involvement of professionals with violent families. With more research, it is likely that the formulation of more effective family intervention and prevention strategies will become possible.

The following frameworks from the family social sciences and family therapy are examples of prominent family theoretical perspectives.

Systems Approach

Based on a systems theory framework, the family is viewed as an open social system with boundaries, self-regulatory mechanisms, interacting and superordinate systems and subcomponents. The family system is comprised of a set of interacting subsystems that are logically related (e.g., a spouse subsystem, a parent-child subsystem, a sibling subsystem). Important assumptions of a systems perspective are (1) a change in one member of the system ultimately results in changes in the entire system, (2) the system is greater than the sum of its parts, and (3) the system is capable of self-regulation and can adapt and change (Friedman, 1992).

A nurse whose practice is guided by a systems perspective assesses the individual members of the family as well as the family as a whole. Intervention strategies should be directed toward the family as an interacting system as well as toward the larger systems with which the family must relate.

Structural-Functional Approach

This perspective also views the family as a social system, but with more of an outcome orientation than a process orientation. The structural-functional approach is grounded in Gestalt psychology, which emphasizes that one must view the whole and its parts and explore the interrelationships between them. The general assumptions of the structural-functional perspective are that the family is (1) a social system with functional requirements, (2) that it is a small group possessing certain generic features common to all small groups, and (3) that as a social system, the family accomplishes functions that serve the individual in addition to the society (Friedman, 1992).

The concept of structure refers to how the family is organized, the manner in which units are arranged, and how these units relate to each other.

Important dimensions of family structure include role structure, value systems, communication processes and power structure. These elements are intimately interrelated and interacting. Family structure is ultimately evaluated by how well the family is able to fulfill its functions—the goals important to its members and society.

Family functions are defined as outcomes or consequences of the family structure (e.g., what the family does). Examples of family functions to be assessed from this theoretical perspective are the family's affective function, its socialization and social placement function, reproduction function, economic function, and health care function. Relationships between the family and other social systems (e.g., the health care system) are also examined (Friedman, 1992; Oermann, 1991).

The nurse whose practice is grounded in structural-functional theory finds it a useful framework for examining the family as a holistic unit and to assess how the family interacts with other institutions. This approach is compatible with general systems theory and interfaces well with a developmental perspective of the family.

Developmental Approach

Theories of family development attempt to account for changes in the family over time based on the idea that families are long-lived groups with a natural history or life cycle. Family development theory describes family life over time by dividing the family life cycle into a series of discrete stages. The most widely used formulation of family developmental stages is the eight-stage family life cycle devised by Duvall and Hill (1948).

Family developmental theory is based on common, normative stages or general features of family life (such as changes in the family when new members are added or subtracted, changes in the developmental stages of the oldest child, child-rearing, and discipline practices). Family developmental theory does not address situational or nonnormative stressors, and this is its major weakness. The assumption of homogeneity of families and stability within each stage presents a middle-class bias that

fails to consider the diversity in American families. Despite these limitations, family developmental theory does increase understanding of families at different points in their life cycles and generates "typical" descriptions of family life during the various stages (Friedman, 1992; Oermann, 1991).

The nurse can use a developmental perspective to guide the assessment of the family's developmental stage and its performance of the tasks appropriate to that stage. The nurse can then develop guidelines for analyzing family growth and health promotion needs and should be able to better provide the support needed for smooth progression from one stage to another.

Interactional Approach

The interactional approach focuses on how family members relate to one another. Family dynamics or family processes are the core of the framework. Processes that are considered important to investigate include roles, status relations, communication patterns, decision-making patterns, and socialization. The interactional perspective does not examine the family within its external environment, nor how the external social system interfaces with the family. The interactional approach is therefore limited by the fact that the family is viewed as self-contained (Friedman, 1992; Oermann, 1991). However, it is a valid approach to use when exploring the meaning or perception various acts or symbols have for people in the process of interaction.

Family Ecological Perspective

The family ecological perspective incorporates the family environment into any examination of the family. It is sometimes referred to as the *ecosystem approach* because it explores relationships between a changing environment and a changing family. The major concepts of the theory are (1) the environed unit (family), (2) the environment, and (3) the patterning of interactions and transactions between them (Oermann, 1991). The family ecomap can be used to perform an ecological assessment of the family.

The family ecologic framework proposed by Bronfenbrenner (1979) is an example of a systems approach in which the family is pictured as part of three nested structures: the microsystem, mesosystem, and macrosystem. The individual family members are nested within the immediate setting that includes the family (the microsystem). The microsystem is situated within and affected by a mesosystem, which includes not only the individual family members but also the immediate larger social environment. The mesosystem is nested within a macrosystem, an even larger environment and social setting that includes a community's ideology, values, and social institutions (Friedman, 1992).

The family ecosystem approach is the conceptual approach that forms the basis for the Roberts and Feetham (1982) Feetham Family Functioning Survey (FFFS). The FFFS measures relationships among the family and broader social units such as (1) school and work, (2) the family and subsystems within the family, and (3) the family and individuals within the family.

Family Paradigm Theory

Family paradigm theory assumes that the family's basic beliefs guide its interpretation of and responses to a variety of social situations. This model of the family, developed by Reiss (1981), explains variations in families that are based on their shared beliefs about the social world and their family's place within it.

Four family paradigms that are based on distinct approaches used by families to problem solve are (1) consensus-sensitive (closed) families, (2) achievement-sensitive (random) families, (3) environment-sensitive (open) families, and (4) distance-sensitive (synchronous) families. Reiss (1981) and a team of researchers have presented some evidence in support of the major concepts of this theory.

Family rituals are mechanisms used by families to stabilize identity, clarify roles, delineate boundaries, and thus conserve the family's paradigm or world view. Examples of family rituals are family traditions, family celebrations, and patterned family interactions (Campbell, 1991). Ritual use in families can be explored to provide clues to difficulties families face in maintaining the family's paradigm, its shared identity, during challenging periods of change or conflict (Campbell, 1991).

The nurse can use ritual assessment to evaluate the extent to which the family has had to give up certain rituals and routines because of a severe clinical problem such as family violence. The nurse can also help the family to consider ways to adapt cherished rituals or develop new and meaningful ones.

Family Stress Perspective

The family stress model (*ABCX*) was conceptualized by Hill (1949) to describe variations in how families coped with stress. Hill postulated that *A* (the stressor event) interacting with *B* (the family's crisis meeting resources) interacting with *C* (the definition the family makes of the event) produces *X* (the crisis). In this model, Hill defined a stressor as a situation for which the family has had little or no prior preparation. A crisis is defined as any sharp or decisive change from which old patterns are inadequate (McCubbin & Patterson, 1982).

Hill's original conceptualization has been expanded by McCubbin and Patterson (1982), who added postcrisis variables to the model in an effort to describe the additional life stressors and changes that may influence the family's ability to achieve adaptation. The model is referred to as the Double ABCX model of family stress and coping. In this framework, the *aA* factor represents family demands or pileup, which include event-related stressors and family hardships, as well as prior strains that continue to affect family life. The double B (*bB*) factor refers to the family's existing resources as well as resources strengthened or developed in response to the demands of the crisis. The double C (*c C*) factor is the meaning the family gives to the total crisis situation that includes the stressor believed to have caused the crisis as well as stressors and strains that have accumulated since the onset of the event. The Double X (*xX*) factor refers to the outcome of family efforts or family adaptation (Oermann, 1991). A more recent version of the Double ABCX Model is the T-Double ABCX Model of Family Adjustment and Adaptation proposed by McCubbin and McCubbin (1987). This variation adds the T-factor, which addresses those family types and strengths and capabilities that explain why some families are better suited than others to adjust and adapt to changes. Four family types identified by McCubbin and McCubbin (1987) are (1) regenerative, (2) resilient, (3) rhythmic, and (4) ritualistic. The typologies are based on dimensions of family strength, such as family hardiness, family coherence, family bonding, family flexibility, family time and routines, valuing of that time, family celebrations, and family traditions (Oermann, 1991).

Family stress models have relevance for nursing because they provide a framework for assessment and intervention with the family in a variety of areas. For example, the aA factor can guide the nurse to view family violence in terms of the stressors and hardships it has placed on the family. The cC factor can guide the nurse to try to understand the meaning the family gives to the violence and to the total crisis situation surrounding it.

Feminist Perspectives

Feminist theory focuses on women and attempts to understand patterning of the human experience from a paradigm that incorporates assumptions and beliefs about the origins and consequences of gendered social organization, as well as strategic directions and actions for social change. Issues of gender, inequality, power and privilege, patriarchy, and the subordination of women can all be examined from a feminist perspective. Luepnitz (1988), Goldner (1988), and Yllö and Bogard (1988) have critiqued the strengths and limitations of family systems theories in guiding the understanding of generation and gender issues. They argue that current family theories and the therapies based on them are inadequate explanatory and treatment models and describe how feminist theory can foster knowledge and understanding of both generational and gender issues. Research based on perspectives from feminist theory is needed to help answer such questions

as why the family takes the form it does at the present time. Could families be differently constituted? Feminist theory could also provide a framework for studying the social genesis of such problems as wife battering, incest, and other problems that occur frequently among women but have been largely neglected by family therapists (Luepnitz, 1988; Yllö and Bogard (1988). This approach guides nurses to be aware of the gender-related power imbalances within families that maintain many forms of family violence.

In summary, theoretical models describing multifactorial and multilevel contributions to the development and maintenance of family violence increase understanding of family violence in the context in which it takes place. Collectively, the various family theories and family therapy approaches can provide perspectives for understanding the individual, family, societal, cultural, and contextual factors that contribute to family violence. Increased understandings in these areas can lead to more effective intervention with families experiencing violence.

There is no unifying family theory that ties together the various types of family violence under one conceptual umbrella, and it is unlikely that such a model can be constructed, given the qualitatively unique developmental and life-span issues associated with violence directed toward children, adults, and the elderly (Ammerman & Hersen, 1991). Since numerous factors mediate the extent, severity, and impact of family violence, the level of intervention required for treatment (primary, secondary, tertiary) varies.

The essence of family-centered nursing involves understanding the dynamics of the family and all the forces, both internal and external, that affect it. Nursing may be required to gain insights into concepts from a variety of highly complex theoretical and intervention models to deliver effective nursing care to families experiencing violence.

THE FAMILY AS A VIOLENCE-PRODUCING INSTITUTION

The national survey by Straus (1983) and his associates showed that 33% of 2,143 conjugal pairs used some form of physical aggression toward a spouse during 1975, and 72% of 1,146 couples with children in the home used some form of violence toward them (Dibble & Straus, 1980). The 1985 national survey by these same researchers indicated that 16% (one of six American couples) experienced an incident involving a physical assault during 1985 and that 110 of every 1,000 children were assaulted by a parent in a way regarded as "abuse" (Straus & Gelles, 1988). In addition, there is growing evidence that elderly family members are abused.

Although there appears to be substantial reductions in the rates of child abuse and wifebeating between the 1975 and 1985 resurvey, it is obvious that the rates of intrafamily violence remain extremely high. These kinds of data explode the myth that the American family is a nonviolent institution. Gelles and Straus have suggested several factors that they believe contribute to the family in general using violence (Gelles & Straus, 1979; Straus & Gelles, 1990).

The first characteristic of families is that there is a great deal of "time at risk" for violence between family members. They spend many hours of every day interacting with each other, time which has the potential of becoming violent. Closely related is the idea that the wide range of family activities and interests affords many possible areas of conflict.

The intensity of involvement in families is another potentiating factor. What may be a minor irritation in a relationship with a friend or co-worker may be seriously upsetting between family members. The activities of family members may also impinge on each other's privacy, usage of family equipment, and ability to engage in activities of their own. The many different ages and the difference in sex among family members is also a conflict-generating factor (Gelles & Straus, 1979; Straus & Gelles, 1990).

In addition, there is the concept that family members have the right to try to influence the behavior and values of each other, which sets the stage for disagreements. Children have no choice about belonging to this particular group of people; thus solving problems by leaving the group is usually impossible for them. Major life stressors, inherent in the development of the family, also contribute

to the possibilities of physical aggression, yet the nuclear family of today is frequently isolated from the support systems of relatives. Finally, the American culture sanctions a certain amount of violence within families both overtly, as in approval of physical punishment for children, and covertly, as in the widespread tolerance, even if not approval of hitting wives by men (Gelles & Straus, 1979; Straus & Gelles, 1990).

The cumulative effect of these characteristics of families is that the family can become a very stressful, conflict-producing arena where people spend much time together. The family is expected to "absorb emotional tension from external situations as well as internally generated family stresses" (Steinmetz, 1977, p. 108). Adults also may have been taught in their childhood that violence is an acceptable way to solve problems and therefore be more apt to use physical aggression in response to stresses experienced in normal family life.

THE INTERGENERATIONAL TRANSMISSION OF VIOLENCE

Social-learning theory (see Chapter 1) provides the background for understanding the evidence that there is an intergenerational transmission of violence within families. When children are hit by their parents, even as a disciplinary measure, the child learns a powerful message. First, the parents are demonstrating that violence is an acceptable way to deal with conflict, and second, that love and violence are intertwined. As Gelles explains, "The child learns that those who love him or her the most are also those who hit and have the right to hit" (Gelles & Straus, 1979, p. 554).

In a study of 57 demographically varied families, Steinmetz (1977) found that families primarily used one of three methods of conflict resolution: discussion, verbal aggression (screaming, yelling, threatening), or physical aggression. The form to which the husband and wife were primarily exposed in their families of orientation was most likely to be used in their family of procreation. This was true of husband-wife conflicts, parent-child disagreements, and sibling to sibling problems (Hotaling, Straus, & Lincoln; 1990; Steinmetz, 1977).

The national survey by Straus, Gelles, and Steinmetz (1980) also indicated that "the people who had been hit as teen-agers tended to be the most violent to their own husbands or wives and to their own children" (p. 116). They also found that the siblings who had experienced the most violence at the hands of their parents were most likely to be severely physically aggressive toward each other. Children also hit parents in violent families. Of the children Straus et al. studied, 18% had hit one of their parents during the survey year. Not surprisingly, these children had also been frequently and often severely the victims of parental violence. Finally, the survey showed that, "When a child grows up in a home where parents use lots of physical punishment and also hit each other, the chances of becoming a violent husband, wife, or parent are the greatest of all" (Straus, Gelles, & Steinmetz, 1980, p. 119).

More recent critiques of the research suggest a lack of convincing empirical support for the intergenerational transmission of violence in the family as the major or sole cause of family violences (Straus et al., 1980). Bolton and Bolton (1987) concluded that the presence of childhood victimization does not mandate adult perpetration. Nor does the absence of childhood victimization insulate against possible family violence perpetration, especially if the learning of social skills or controls against violence were inadequate during the childhood experience.

THE CONNECTIONS BETWEEN WIFE ABUSE AND CHILD ABUSE

The data summarized in the previous section suggest that families who are abusive toward each other at the spousal level or toward children would be prone to be involved in the other form of abuse also. The information available is not conclusive in this regard. Most studies have surveyed samples of abused wives or child abusers for evidence of the other kind of abuse so that a generalizable picture is difficult to obtain. However, the same national survey cited earlier found that couples who did not use physical aggression toward each other at all were

the least likely to be abusive toward their children. Conversely, "28% of the children of these high violence couples had been abused during the year" (Coleman, 1980; Gayfard, 1979; Renvoize, 1978; Rounsaville & Weissman, 1977-78).

The studies of samples of abused women and children have also emphasized the interrelationship between spouse and child abuse. Estimates vary regarding the amount of overlap, but most research indicates a higher rate of child abuse for violent couples and a higher rate of wife abuse in parents documented as child abusers than in the normal population (Steinmetz, 1977; Stark & Flitcraft, 1984). This evidence seems logical in terms of the idea that certain families tend to be violent in all of their attempts of resolution of serious conflicts.

The factors associated with the family as a violence-prone institution—the intergenerational transmission of violence and the connections between wife abuse and child abuse—suggest that there are families that are violent or prone to being violent that need interventions as a total unit. Nursing interventions with these families are based on the nursing process and begin with assessment of the family. Nursing care should take place within the context of the family's social and cultural background; therefore family assessments should incorporate important elements of the family's social and cultural world.

CULTURALLY SENSITIVE CARE

Culturally sensitive family nursing care is based on understanding and respect for the diversity of backgrounds and perspectives found in American families today. The United States is definitely a multicultural society with many ethnic and cultural groups represented.

Cultural groups in multicultural societies tend to vary according to power hierarchies forming dominant groups and minority groups. Dominant groups are generally defined by the control they have over resources (material and nonmaterial), whereas minority groups are accorded a status based on a relative lack of power (Hess, Markson, & Stein, 1989). The lack of power of minority groups corresponds with the general societal constraints placed on such groups (e.g., lack of opportunity for upward mobility, grossly inadequate provisions for education and health care) that may severely limit the resources available to minority group families, leaving large numbers poor and poorly prepared for coping with the kinds of chronic stress that have been associated with extreme interpersonal violence. Such restrictions may erroneously contribute to the myth that violence is a problem of poor and minority or ethnic families. Cultural values, beliefs, ethnicity, and life histories, among others, are important factors that influence behavior and how a family and its members view themselves collectively and in relation to others. These variables, unfortunately, have not been studied extensively in research on violence. It is currently unknown to what extent they contribute to the social-structural context causing violence.

Sensitivity to one's own cultural identity can help foster an understanding of and appreciation for the influence that different sociocultural perspectives have on one's attitudes, values, beliefs, and behaviors. An especially knowledgeable, caring, and sensitive nurse is required to provide effective preventive and interventive care with families experiencing violence. The nurse should have a clear notion of the meaning of such concepts as culture, ethnicity, acculturation, accommodation, ethnocentrism, cultural relativism, cultural shock, and minority families. *Culture* is generally defined as circumscribed guides used by societies and ethnic groups to solve their problems and derive meaning from their lives. Culture denotes patterns of learned behavior and values that are transmitted from one generation to the next (Friedman, 1992). Basic texts in psychiatric mental health nursing and in family health nursing that may be helpful in further defining and differentiating these concepts include Gary and Kavanagh (1991) and Friedman (1992).

Assessment of the family's cultural orientation is critical to understanding and working efficaciously with families from cultures different from the nurse's own background. It is important to realize that discussions of how to assess and intervene with various cultural groups run the "risk of promoting stereotypes that misrepresent and oversimplify the cultures involved" (Gary & Kavanagh, 1991, p. 149). Nonetheless, the nurse must be willing to try to understand the complexities and life conditions under which different groups have developed their world views and under which they function. For example, Gary and Kavanagh (1991) suggest that a black in Harlem, a Mexican migrant in Texas, a Native American in Arizona, and a white nurse in Minneapolis would each have perspectives on the world shaped by the life experiences and conditions under which they have lived.

Friedman (1992) recommends that the following areas guide a general assessment of the cultural orientation of a family:

1. Ethnic/racial identity
2. Languages spoken
3. Place of birth
4. Geographical mobility
5. Family's religion
6. Ethnic group affiliation
7. Neighborhood affiliation
8. Dietary habits, dress
9. Household appearance
10. Use of folk systems
11. Acceptance by community

Cultural assessment questions that cover these basic areas should be integrated throughout the entire family assessment. The results will provide the nurse with comprehensive data about cultural influences related to how the family is organized (role, power, values, and communication patterns), child-rearing practices, affective responses, health care practices and beliefs, and coping strategies (Friedman, 1992). This information is invaluable in developing an effective data base from which to plan care for the family experiencing family violence.

ASSESSMENT

Before the nurse can make an effective assessment of violence in a family, she must first examine her own feelings about the subject and be committed to the idea that violence is an important health problem and within the scope of nursing. Violence is not an easy area to explore with families, and it is usually easier to just avoid it. Strong feelings of anger and despair may be aroused in family members, and of justifiable fear in the nurse. Before she begins routinely to explore violence in family nursing care, it is useful for the nurse to attend workshops on the issue and/or arrange for group discussions with her colleagues. In such settings, role-playing can be used to help nurses anticipate dealing with confrontations within families. Once a family member has been identified as violent or potentially violent, that information affects the nurse's interactions with him or her. Nurses need to be able to share their fear with peers and explore ways of handling it through discussion.

The incidence of physical injury and death from violence outside and especially within the home indicates the seriousness of the problem. Nurses are probably in people's homes more than any other professionals. If nursing care of families does not include assessing for and intervening with violence, it will probably not be identified as a problem until someone has been seriously injured or killed. Rather than waiting for that to occur and letting the police, courts, or social worker intervene at that point, with demonstrably poor results, nursing can work for early identification and prevention as with any other serious health problem. After examining her feelings and working to gain knowledge and expertise, the nurse is in a prime position to make a significant impact in the prevention of morbidity and mortality from violence.

The other aspect of feeling exploration to be noted is the idea that family conflict resolution is a private, family matter. These feelings can also be discussed in workshops or nursing conferences in the agency involved. The families may also share this view and perceive their privacy as being invaded by questions in this area. If the nurse handles her questions in this realm as a routine area of assessment with a matter-of-fact demeanor, the inquiry will seem more comfortable. If the family questions the need for such exploration, the nurse can share the facts about the prevalence of abuse and injuries from violence. This is valuable not only in making the family feel more at ease, but also in

educating the public about the problem of violence. The first few times the nurse includes a detailed assessment about violence may be uncomfortable for her, but just as nursing has learned to include sexual functioning assessment without discomfort, violence in the family can also be learned to be handled easily with practice.

An important area to consider in any family assessment is family strengths. The healthy areas of family functioning need to be explored with the family, both to see the total picture and to identify areas that can be built on in nursing interventions. A model of family well-being can be used as a framework for identification of family strengths (Meister, 1984). Using this framework, the nurse assesses for areas of family functioning, both past and present, where needs of individual members are met by the family and the family has adequate physical and affective resources. An inventory of social supports both within and outside the family can be developed. Such an inventory can be used to identify those who are providing direct aid, emotional support, and/or affirmation to members or the total family unit. Relationships that can be strengthened and utilized further tend to become evident. Healthy coping mechanisms used to deal with normative life changes and developmental issues are identified. Areas where the family feels a sense of accomplishment and problems considered effectively solved need as thorough an exploration as areas of difficulty. Family actions that foster appropriate help-seeking and utilization behavior can be identified as actions to be encouraged for future referrals. As a general indication of family well-being, each individual member can be asked about their personal sense of their own life as a whole and their perception of their family. Family functions that have enhanced individual and total unit perceptions of well-being in the past are identified as important family mechanisms to be encouraged by nursing care.

Assessment of a total family is usually done in primary health care settings, in community nursing, and in mental health settings when an entire family has been referred. Whenever a family history is being taken, it is important that patterns of family conflict resolution be explored. Questions about this area of concern should also be included in the social/personal section of the history of individuals. Physical assessment of family members includes watching for signs of trauma. Observation of intra-familial interactions are also important in family assessment. The history, physical examination, and nursing observations, conducted with an awareness of the possibility of violence in the family, reveal potential and actual problems the family is having with violence.

History

There are several areas of the history of families that can indicate that the family may have or is prone to have problems with violence. These areas, along with at-risk findings, have been outlined in Table 10-1. In addition, as part of the data collection, the nurse should use direct questions about physical aggression. Questions about methods of disciplining children, including physical punishment, are usually routinely asked in the nursing history of families, but in the past direct inquiry about other

TABLE 10-1

Indicators of Potential or Actual Violence in a Family from Nursing History

AREA OF ASSESSMENT	AT-RISK RESPONSES
Information from genogram	Severe physical punishment or husband-wife violence in parental families of origin
	Violent death or serious injury from violence in genogram
	Family members in parental families of origin using violence outside the home
	Wife abuse in husband's previous marital relationship
Family structure	Single-parent home
	Dependent grandparent in home
	Blended family (involving stepparents and/or step-children)
Family resources	Unemployment; poverty
	Inadequate housing
	Elderly member with controlled resources
	Financial problems
	Total control of monetary resources by male head of household
	Perception of inadequate "fit" of family resources to family demands
Family roles	Rigid traditional sex roles
	Individual or family dissatisfaction with roles family expects individuals to fulfill
	Roles incompatible
	Roles rigid, unchangeable
Family boundaries	Boundaries rigid; mistrust of all outsiders
Family communication patterns	Family communications nonnurturing; destructive to some members
	Communications ambiguous
	Lack of communication among family members
Family conflict resolution patterns	Extensive use of verbal aggression; many threats of violence
	Evidence of physical aggression used in husband-wife, parent-child, sibling-sibling or parent-grandparent conflict resolution
Family power distribution	Autocratic decision making by father
	Children have no power
	Grandparent in home who is powerless
	Frequent power struggles

TABLE 10-1   *Continued*
Indicators of Potential or Actual Violence in a Family from Nursing History

AREA OF ASSESSMENT	AT-RISK RESPONSES
Family values	Violence considered acceptable or valued
	Great incongruence of values among family members or between family and society
	Differing values among family members considered intolerable
Emotional climate	High tension in home
	Lack of visible affection
	Scapegoating
	High anxiety in family member(s)
	Lack of support between family members
	Frequent disparagement between family members
Division of labor	Rigid division of labor according to sex
	Members highly dissatisfied with division of labor
Support systems	Family isolation
	Family inhibitions to helpseeking
	Children not forming close, supportive peer relationships (especially same-sex peer relationships)
	Lack of support systems considered useful for direct aid, emotional support, and/or affirmation
	Relatives are highly critical; tension among extended family
	Sudden withdrawal by adolescent from social activity and peers
	Violence in extended family
Developmental stages	More than one family member facing difficult developmental crisis
	Lack of knowledge in parents of what to expect at various developmental stages in children, selves, and grandparents
Stressors	At-risk scores on stress scale
	Lack of successful coping mechanisms to deal with stress in the past
	Situational crises
	Stress-related physical symptoms in family members
Socialization of children	Physical punishment used
	Only one parent disciplines children
	Lack of nurturance of children
	Children displaying aggressive behavior, at home or outside of home
	Juvenile delinquency or sexual promiscuity in children
Health history	Frequent trauma injuries to family members
	Adolescent suicide attempts
	Serious illness in a family member
	History of treatment for mental illness or vaginal trauma
	History of venereal disease or genital trauma in children
	Drug or alcohol abuse
	Substance abuse in adolescents

forms of violence has often been neglected. The nurse needs to ask whether there is ever hitting between any family members.

Nursing judgment is required in assessing how many of the at-risk findings constitute a real problem with physical aggression in the family. Physical punishment of children is usually considered normal with little follow-up questioning. On initial assessment the nurse needs to inquire more about such child-rearing practices, how often physical punishment is used, whether or not such implements as belts are ever used, whether the form of such punishment is spanking or slapping or hitting with fists. After a relationship with the family is established, this area can be readdressed and the nurse can discuss the implications of even the mildest forms of physical punishment.

Another area that is infrequently explored fully is sibling fighting. Keeping in mind the Steinmetz (1977) findings that sibling conflict resolution mirrors adult and parent-child methods in both form and severity, the full picture of sibling fights and how they are handled needs to be carefully assessed. Children often learn how to handle anger in their relationships with brothers and sisters and how the parents guide such interactions. When brothers and sisters are allowed to use unrestricted physical aggression against each other, they also learn that violence is endorsed as a way to solve problems. The potential for severity in such conflicts is also frequently overlooked. Extrapolating from their findings in the large national survey of family violence, Straus et al. (1980) estimate that "2.3 million children in the United States have at some time used a knife or gun on a brother or sister" (p. 117). Siblings using physical aggression against each other can no longer be considered necessarily normal, nor can this be considered an area not needing intervention. Guns in the home are more than 40 times more likely to kill a family member (by accident, homicide, or suicide) than kill an intruder (Kellerman & Reay, 1986). Therefore the nurse should assess for the presence of a handgun in the home and strongly advocate for gun-free households.

Sexual abuse within the family is difficult to assess and may only be revealed after intense in-volvement with the family. It is important that nurses be aware of the possibility of incest and try to elicit information about its occurrence when there are indications that it may be a possibility. Taking an individual history on each family member before, during, or after conducting the physical examination in private may be an avenue to use for uncovering sexual abuse. Victims of incest are usually able to disclose the activity to helping professionals when directly asked about it (Burgess & Holmstrom, 1979). Changes in the behavior of the child or indications of vaginal irritation and/or trauma are important suggestions that incestuous activities have occurred. It is also important to assess the relationship, by observation and history, of female children to adult males who are in and around the home frequently. It must be remembered that sexual abuse is frequently carried out by uncles, cousins, and close family friends as well as by fathers and stepfathers. The mother of the child may have uneasy feelings or suspicions of the incest, and as the relationship with the nurse develops, she may ask oblique questions concerning "normal" sexual activity or make general references to problems in the sexual relationship between herself and her spouse. It is important that these questions be followed up, and if there is any indication of possible sexual abuse, direct queries should be made about it. For a young child the question might be "Has anyone ever touched your private parts or other parts of your body with their private parts or hands or body in a way that hurt you or made you feel bad?" The nurse should substitute the term the child uses for vagina or penis for private parts. For an adolescent, the question could be "Has anyone ever forced or pressured you into sexual activities you did not wish to participate in?"

The incestuous family is often very closed and isolates itself from helping professionals if possible. An aura of secrecy in the general family feeling tone and a closed attitude toward the nurse's questions during the history-taking phase may alert her to the possibility of incest. It is important to keep the lines of communication open with these families and delay closing the case until further assessment can be made. It may take a long time before trust can be engendered in these families, and the nurse must be patient. Another way to obtain the needed information is to elicit the help of another adult who the child trusts; often a teacher or school nurse can be helpful in this regard. The nurse can share her uneasiness about the possibility of sexual abuse in the family and ask the other professional to approach the child if she herself has not yet formed a trusting relationship with the child. If the suspicions of incest are strong, protective services must be informed as with any other case of child abuse. There is no such thing as consensual sex between an adult family member and a child. As Herman (1981) states,

> Because a child is powerless in relation to an adult, she is not free to refuse a sexual advance. Therefore, any sexual relationship between the two must necessarily take on some of the coercive characteristics of a rape, even if, as is usually the case, the adult uses positive enticements rather than force to establish the relationship (p. 27).

Assessment Tools

The genogram or kinship diagram is an important tool of family assessment. The genogram can fruitfully include questions on violence as well as other health problems. This must be asked about specifically or it will not be revealed. Remembering the intergenerational transmission of violence, the genogram should include inquiries about wife and child abuse, violent injury and death, histories of incarceration for violent crime, and family members' use of violence in interpersonal relationships outside the home. Cultural sensitivity and an awareness of differential treatment by the law according to race and class is necessary when assessing this information, however. Questions that start with asking about people ever having been hit and followed up with asking about how often the hitting occurred and how severe it was are more useful than using the word *abuse*. Many people do not recognize a history of significant violence as abuse when it has happened to them or a family member.

Nursing assessment of families may include more formal assessment tools that tap areas of con-

cern, especially for determining potential for violence. The Feetham Family Functioning Survey (FFFS) has been shown to be a reliable and concurrently valid nursing measure that can quickly indicate perceptions of dissatisfaction with family functioning (Roberts & Feetham, 1982). The instrument is designed to be self-administered and can be completed in 10 minutes. When scores on this instrument indicate perception of problems in family functioning, it provides a useful starting point for discussion about the areas indicated as problematic (for example, the FFFS indicator, "Disagreement with Spouse"), which includes questions about possible violence. Other family assessment tools are available and have been reviewed for their appropriateness and usefulness (Spear & Sachs, 1985).

Physical Assessment

In addition to physical examination of individual family members, an important part of the objective portion of assessment is observations of family interactions. Physical examination of at-risk findings for abuse of individuals can be found in Tables 8-3 and 9-2 in the chapters on nursing care of abused children and abused wives. Table 10-2 instead focuses on important areas of observation that the nurse must make to assess the possibility of violence in the family. Objective observation of family members interacting with each other is vital in highlighting discrepancies between what actually happens and what has been described. Home visits with as many family members present as possible are invaluable in this regard. Community health nursing home visits often take place when only the mother and preschool children and/or a grandparent are at home, and the nurse may miss important elements. Creativity is needed to ensure a total assessment of the family, and interventions for family problems with violence are almost impossible if the nurse only has a relationship with the mother. The nurse should attempt to have fairly lengthy visits of initial assessment. Children may be able to maintain their "best behavior" for a short time, but a longer visit often allows interactions to become

TABLE 10-2

Indicators of Potential or Actual Violence in a Family from Nursing Observation

AREA OF ASSESSMENT	AT-RISK OBSERVATIONS
General considerations	Observations differ significantly from information gathered on history
Family resources	Family members inadequately clothed and groomed
	One family member inadequately clothed and/or groomed, but the rest are not
	Household totally disorganized and family members indicate displeasure with the lack of organization
Family roles	One parent looks at the other to hold major interaction with children
	One parent answers all questions
	One parent looks to other for approval before answering questions
Family communication patterns	Members continually interrupt each other
	Members answer questions for each other; one member never talks for him or herself
	Negative nonverbal behavior in other members when one family member is speaking
	Members frequently misunderstand each other
	Members do not listen to each other
Family conflict resolution	Verbal aggression used in front of nurse
Family power distribution	Members act afraid of another member
	One person makes all decisions
	Power struggles
Emotional climate	Nonverbals unhappy, anxious, fearful
	Excessive physical distance maintained between members
	Members never touch each other
	Tense atmosphere
	Secretive atmosphere
	Voice tones sharp, nonaffectionate, disparaging

(Also include observations from Tables 8-3 and 9-2.)

more nearly what they are without a stranger in the home.

The nurse also often finds that complete assessment with relation to observations about possible violence comes over time.

As the relationship with the family develops and the members become more comfortable with the nurse, more normal interactions are conducted in her presence. The family may also reveal more about the nature of their relationships verbally as the helping relationship is formed. The nurse can return to areas of the history that she thinks the family was reticent or uncomfortable about in the working stage of the relationship. It is often useful to have shown the family that the nurse is empathetic, knowledgeable, and helpful in other more concrete or traditionally nursing areas of family concern before attempting to fully assess and intervene with potential or actual violence.

Nursing Diagnosis

Family assessment data are now synthesized into family nursing diagnoses. As with an individual, the nurse must work with the family in the identification of problems and concerns. The first priority of this final stage of assessment is a listing of family strengths as both the nurse and the family perceive them. This starts diagnosis in a positive note and identifies areas of competence that can be further developed. Even the family badly disintegrated by violence has strengths that need to be recognized by all as a basis for confidence that problems can be resolved. Problems with violence may not be the primary concern of the family at first. If the nurse's judgment does not indicate serious danger to any of the family members or suspicion of child or other dependent person abuse, which must be immediately reported, she can indicate her observations concerning potential violence but wait to work on the problem until the family is ready or has had their more immediate health problems met. It is often useful to state the concern about violence in terms of ways of solving disagreements or methods of disciplining children rather than using the words *violence* or *abuse*, which can appear judgmental and threatening to the family.

The sample nursing process at the end of the chapter (Table 10-3) indicates several possible nursing diagnoses that may be used for a family experiencing potential or actual violence. These are only hypothetical diagnoses, but they may be helpful in working or providing a base for modification according to each particular family.

PLANNING

The first step of the planning process is setting goals with the family. This can be difficult when working with an entire family, because goals for one member may not match those of another. The process is best done with the entire family and can provide a form of intervention as the family discusses what they really want in terms of conflict resolution. Frequently, members are encouraged in such a setting to express desires for the future that no one else realized they had. Parents are often surprised at how much fighting between each other assumed to be "in private" is actually known and of concern to children. Children are almost always aware of parental verbal and physical aggression toward each other, and open discussion with the nurse acting as role model and referee if necessary, is helpful, both as clarification to parents and children as to what is

happening and as a starting point of goal setting.

If it cannot be arranged for the whole family to work together with the nurse to identify goals, a family meeting can be suggested before the next session with the nurse. It is vital that every member of the family, no matter how young, has input into the planning process. A group process of learning how to conduct family discussions and family problem-solving sessions can be a new experience for a family and is an important intervention itself. Goal setting is an excellent starting point because it focuses on ideas for the future, often less conflict generating than problems in the past. It is useful for the problem identification, goal setting, and planning to be done on paper with a copy for the family. They can then work on reformulations when the nurse is not present. If the whole family cannot be persuaded to work together, at the least, space should be left on the sheets for input from absent family members.

The family must be helped to set concrete and easily achievable short-term goals as well as more idealistic long-term goals. They can be encouraged to see that the short-term goals are steps toward the long-term solutions and therefore more easily achievable but important to set and evaluate in terms of marking progress toward the future goals. Goal setting, when done correctly, can serve as an important motivator for all family members. Achievement of short-term goals is a valuable reinforcer of the effort being expended.

When the entire family has been involved with goal setting and planning interventions, there is greater likelihood of successful nursing care. The family is also better equipped to decide what is actually feasible for them than the nurse. The nurse can make suggestions, ensuring that each family member has input, and can encourage exploration of alternatives, but she must be careful not to impose solutions on the family. The inclusion of children in the planning process is a good way to obtain valuable, creative suggestions for interventions. It also helps their sense of being important to the family and models a truly democratic way of solving family problems. Family members may be uncomfortable with this mode of group interaction at first, especially if they have been accustomed to an autocratic method of family decision making. It is important that the nurse try to arrange a total family interaction time when she or he can be present for the planning process. Absent family members may sabotage the interventions if they have not had input. The nurse should also be present to guide the interaction and teach the family methods to achieve their goals if they are not used to such a process. This is the basis for continued interventions.

NURSING INTERVENTIONS

Nursing interventions with families experiencing violence can be considered at the societal and community level, as well as with individual families. Nursing care is directed toward the prevention of violence in families and the identification and treatment of families who are already involved with the problem. From incidence statistics and the aspects of family life that make violence a possibility, it is readily apparent that there is much to be accomplished. The first task is to prevent the seeds of violence from being planted in this unfortunately fertile ground, the family.

Primary Prevention

Primary prevention of violent families is a task to be undertaken by many segments of our society, including nurses. To prevent families from becoming violent, nursing must promote nonviolence in family interactions and in society in general, take specific measures to try to eliminate physical aggression from the family arena, and identify and intervene with families who are at risk to become violent.

Promotion of Nonviolence

Elimination of violence from our society is an awesome undertaking. However, there are some specific measures that nurses can advocate for on a societal level that can make a difference. The first is to decrease the amount of violence in the media. Based on social-learning theory, less violence on television, in children's books, and in movies will decrease the amount of modeling for violence that is needed for learning.

Measures have been instituted to rate movies for violence (and sex) so that young children may be prevented from seeing films that are problematic for them. These ratings are unclear guidelines for parents concerned about violence. The PG (Parental Guidance) rating is the most troublesome in terms of violence. Diligent reading of movie reviews and inquiries of other parents are needed to determine if a movie rated PG contains a great deal of violence. The raters seem to be more concerned with graphic sex than with the murder and mayhem depicted in some PG films. The context of the violence is also important. For children old enough to distinguish fantasy from reality, an obviously unrealistic movie containing violence may have less of an aggression-producing result (Sawin, 1981). When the hero of the film uses force to achieve laudable aims or violent characters are not punished for their acts, a message of the legitimacy of using violence is conveyed. Nurses need to advocate a rating system that differentiates PG films on the basis of violence.

Violence on television continues to be a problem for parents. Despite the laudable efforts of the Parent Teachers Association and American Medical Association, children's television programming continues to be violent, and evening programs, even in the so-called family hour, are filled with physical aggression. Parental supervision of children's TV viewing is only part of the solution. Whenever public outcries lose momentum, the networks seem to return to violence. Nurses need to help in maintaining pressure on the programmers to decrease the violence being shown.

Another aspect of societal advocacy that nurses can join is the fight for gun control legislation. Gun ownership has been found to correlate strongly with the roles of suicide and homicide by guns (Lester, 1988; Lunde, 1986), and strict gun control legislation has been associated with a temporary reduction in firearm assaults (Jung, 1988). Advocating for gun control is not the only answer to violence, but it is a start. It would not only prevent some arguments from becoming lethal, but also would create a climate of negative sanction toward violence.

Historically, nurses have not been involved in political advocacy. However, the American Nurses' Association and state nurses' associations are beginning to lead the profession in using their potential political power. Individual nurses can be effective by writing their legislators, but this impact can be magnified many times by working through the local and state units of the ANA. Linkages can be formed with other organizations concerned about these issues, and nurses can spearhead national campaigns that could have considerable power. There is considerable support for decreasing media violence and gun control legislation. What remains is mobilization and effective political action.

The other arena in which nurses can have considerable impact is child-rearing. Whole cultures are totally nonviolent, and their way of living can be mainly traced to the way their children are raised and the strong sanctions against aggression in their cultures. High school parenting classes and childbirth education classes are the places to start with strong messages about raising children without using physical punishment. Both laboratory studies of aggression and anthropological research on nonviolent cultures suggest that cooperation, empathy, nurturance, tenderness, sensitivity to feelings, and an abhorrence of violence need to be taught as primary values to young children of both sexes. In other words, boys need to be socialized more like girls are. Nurses can also be useful in supporting the teaching of nonaggressive problem solving to children in preschools. The use of physical punishment in schools must be abolished wherever it is found. When schools use physical aggression to discipline students, they are only teaching that our society sanctions the use of violence, and they are teaching it not only to the children being punished, but to the rest of the students in that school system as well. Wherever nurses have contact with parents—in clinics, in school nursing, in community health nursing, in inpatient and outpatient pediatric settings—the message of nonviolence can be spread.

Another important societal and community in-tervention is for nurses to advocate for and teach special classes to schoolchildren on sex and violence. Important gains can be made in the prevention and early detection of incest if children know what is inappropriate sexual contact and who they should tell if any occurs. A full discussion of incest with children, including the invariable threats to not tell and protestations of normalcy and affection by the offender, arms children with the knowledge necessary to get help immediately before serious physical and emotional damage has been done. Such discussions can best be held within the context of a general health curriculum. This kind of curriculum includes general sex education, health promotion, and emotional health content, incorporating how to deal with violence and the promotion of nonviolence values and problem-solving methods. The curriculum would be taught at every grade level, with age-appropriate teaching methodologies. Nurses can advocate for the establishment of such curricula both as school nurses and community health professionals and as concerned citizens and parents.

A final area of broad nursing intervention is the promotion of healthy attitudes toward the elderly and advocacy of programs that allow older Americans independence and useful functioning as long as possible. Nurses can be in the forefront in helping the young respect the aging process, rather than dread and fear it. Learning institutions and social service agencies need to take advantage of the potential participation of older adults. Programs that provide home health care or daycare to the elderly must be advocated. It is unrealistic to expect that all dependent elderly can be totally cared for in their children's homes. Nurses are ideal to begin and administer such programs. Promotion of third-party payments for nurse-administered daycare centers is also needed.

Families at Risk

The identification of families at risk to become violent includes both performing assessment in one's own professional practice and advocating for its inclusion by other health professionals. Any family that uses physical punishment or any form of physical aggression can be considered at risk to become violent, because violence tends to escalate under stress. Families under a great deal of stress, from poverty, unemployment, recent divorce or death in the family, severe illness in a family member, developmental crises in family members, remarriage, and changes in location or job can be considered to be at risk also. This is especially true if their methods of conflict resolution are problematic to any of the family members. In addition, families in which communications are unclear or discordant or at a very low level can be identified as at risk to become violent. An absence of emotional nurturance or psychological abuse can also be considered as at-risk indicators. A final category of families at risk for violence are those with a dependent elderly person in the home, especially if there is a history of verbal or physical aggression or both in the family, or the elderly family member is adding considerable financial or emotional stress to the home (see Chapter 7). An overall framework to identify families at risk is to evaluate the "fit" of family resources to demand (see Chapter 3).

Interventions with such families consist primarily of helping them to develop democratic ways of solving problems in the family. Steinmetz's (1977) study showed that the more democratic the family was in terms of power relationships and conflict resolution, the less likely members were to use physical aggression. She also found that the most effective outcomes of conflict, in family members' perceptions, were those that were treated as a shared problem that could be solved with mutual benefits. Destructive resolutions were those that became adversary contests, power struggles between family members. Nurses need to help families evolve more constructive ways to deal with the inevitable disagreements that characterize family life. It is useful to meet with the entire family and help members work through a relatively minor conflict that has developed among them; one that is not rife with deep emotions or a long-standing history of arguments is best. Once the family has seen how

this kind of disagreement can be solved without creating a power struggle or aggressive argument, they can start to practice the same methods with more difficult problems.

Effective means of disciplining children, without the use of physical punishment, need to be discussed and modeled by the nurse. This idea may seem foreign to the parents, and careful elementary groundwork is necessary before any suggested alternatives will be considered. It is frequently useful to explore with the parents how they themselves were punished as children and how they perceived hitting by their parents. The perceptions of the physical aggression can also be explored with the children. If the nurse can show how effective her use of positive reinforcement can be with the family's children, this is a powerful teaching method. Getting the parents to at least try other methods of correction and carefully evaluating their results is also useful. Children who are becoming aggressive themselves, both within and outside the home, are a good example for the nurse to associate with the use of physical punishment in the home. This is a troublesome area of intervention, and the development of a firm, trusting relationship is necessary before parents will listen to the nurse on the subject of discipline.

Another aspect of intervention is to help the family develop and more fully use various support systems. Today's nuclear family has become more isolated from relatives, the church, and neighbors. It is more likely to move frequently than families of the past. Community agencies and groups may be able to take the place of some of the more traditional support systems, but the family may need help in finding groups that are suitable and of interest to them. They also may want someone to attend such a group with them for the first time. The nurse may be that person, or she may be able to suggest another family in the area who could go also.

Other interventions with families at risk may include helping to alleviate some of the stressors the family is facing. The nurse may be able to work with social services in helping family members to obtain jobs, further education, or work training. Anticipatory guidance for developmental crises, such as adolescence, birth of the first child, and retirement, can be helpful for families. Part of the intervention is to help the family assess how much stress they are experiencing and the normalcy of tension in the home in particularly stressful times. How the family members can help each other with stress, including helping to arrange for times and places of privacy for the individuals, can be useful.

Problems with family communications, a lack of nurturance of family members, or both can best be addressed through sessions conducted with the whole family to improve communications. The professional nurse can easily conduct such family intervention with the extensive background in therapeutic communications that is provided in most nursing education. The principles are the same; the family is helped to see blocks that the members are presently using in communication with each other, and members are taught to use active listening and therapeutic techniques of exploration of feelings. The most widely used block in family interactions is giving advice, and modeling of shared problem solving can be done by the nurse to provide an alternative. Family members can be taught to present clear, unambiguous messages. They need to be helped to respond to each other in ways that are nurturing and self-worth enhancing rather than destructive. Almost all families at risk can benefit from at least a few sessions of this kind of family intervention.

A final possible intervention is referral to agencies directed toward the prevention of child abuse or referral to other agencies offering classes in parenting or other such services. Some of these programs offer respite care of children for families under a great deal of stress, and a variety of groups for parents to help them deal with stress. These kinds of alternatives are useful as an adjunct to nursing care. Daycare programs for the elderly or home health agencies that offer help with household management as well as health care for dependent elderly persons can offer the same kind of assistance to families hard-pressed to deal with an ill grandparent or one who has more needs to be filled than the family can provide on a daily basis without inordinant stress.

Secondary Prevention

Secondary prevention interventions include identification of families that are beginning to use violence beyond the physical punishment of children. Such families may be referred because of possibilities of abuse or because a child is becoming violent in school. Nurses may identify incestuous families secondary to the diagnosis of venereal disease in young children. This may be considered a definite sign of sexual abuse, and almost definitely incest, because the child would have been more likely to have told of the sexual contact unless it was with a relative or close family friend. Adolescent female runaways are also frequently incest victims; one estimate is that 70% of the children who run away from home are sexually abused (Dunwoody, 1982). Male and female runaways may also be fleeing other forms of violence in the home. Adolescents in trouble with the criminal justice system often reflect the violence in their families, and sexually promiscuous teenage girls are frequently the victims of incest and other forms of violence. When a child (or adolescent) is identified as a problem because of aggression toward his or her parents, it must be remembered that the child may be retaliating for abuse received, or he or she may be intervening to protect the mother from wife abuse. These families begin to use violence toward each other in a variety of ways and must be intervened with as quickly as possible to prevent further physical and emotional damage.

Immediate intervention may frequently take the form of crisis intervention. If a particularly violent episode resulting in serious physical injury has occurred, or a son or daughter has run away or been arrested, or incest has just been discovered, the family may be in a situation for which they have no previously learned coping mechanisms. In such a state, the family is extremely open to assistance offered by the nurse, but may not be able to participate as fully in mutual assessment and planning as has been suggested previously because of high anxiety. The nurse may need to make a quick assessment, based primarily on the crisis situation, and offer concrete assistance that will decrease the anxiety.

Crisis intervention also includes helping the family members define the situation for each of them in terms of their feelings about it and their intellectual understanding of what has happened. The nurse may be able to clarify for family members exactly what is likely to happen next, because much of the anxiety generated in a crisis is fear of the unknown. Supportive networks need to be established, for instance relatives, friends, or clergy called, so that the family will have continued support and people to whom to express feelings after the nurse has gone. It is important that family members themselves indicate who they perceive as supportive; the sources may not be traditional (refer to Chapter 3).

The healthy coping mechanisms that the nurse observes should be encouraged and family members helped to understand that strong feelings are normal in the situation and may not always be handled nicely. The family may experience much denial in the crisis situation, especially at first, while they gather their resources. They may deny the seriousness of the situation or blame it on irrelevant external factors. The denial must be allowed (although not encouraged) and insight supported as it begins to appear. Family members are often adept at helping each other begin to see the ramifications of the crisis situation and should be encouraged to interact as much as possible.

The entire family is affected by violence and thus needs to be considered the focus of intervention. Younger children may misunderstand or be frightened by what has happened, and the first impulse of parents is often to send them away to a friend or relative. This may be useful for infants and toddlers, and the nurse can help to arrange it, but older children are better served if they are allowed to stay and participate in discussion. The nurse can make sure that the children understand what is happening, reassure them that they are not to blame in some way, and determine whether they themselves would rather stay or go.

The final part of crisis intervention is to ensure that the family will be followed up by concerned professionals. This may actually be done by the primary nurse, depending on her or his professional role, or by another nurse or professional to whom the family is referred. During the 4 to 6 weeks immediately following the crisis-precipitating event, the family is particularly open to learning new coping mechanisms and working on eliminating the violence from the home. It is imperative that this time of crisis be used to full advantage in terms of promotion of growth. This may be the only time when violent family members are willing to accept help, and referral must be swift and appropriate. This may be the most important nursing intervention of the crisis period, and the nurse must be sure that the referral to agency or person is acceptable to the family and they will be seen immediately.

Nursing intervention at the secondary prevention level frequently involves working with protective services. If the violence is directed toward children, either physically or sexually, a report to protective services is mandatory. They can also be helpful in working with the families by providing counseling and a variety of social services. The same is true of adult branches of protective services that operate in most cities. Although not as strongly mandated by law, reporting of elderly or spouse abuse to adult protective services may be appropriate, especially if the family is resistive to other interventions. An investigation by the agency will ensue that impresses on the family the seriousness of the problem and may prompt their seeking help through protective services or other agencies. The nurse may have the advantage of being able to work with the family through and after adult or child protective service investigation. Even when there is not enough evidence to warrant abuse or assault charges, the nurse can continue to work with the family in preventing further violence. Nurses need to be aware, in advance of referral, exactly how protective services operate in the particular community in which they practice. They need to be able to explain to families precisely what will ensue and how much time will be involved. It is helpful if the nurse is on personal terms with the professionals at the local protective services so that coordination and continuity efforts are successful and the nurse is informed of current agent protocol and policy.

Other agencies may be used as referrals by the nurse. Community mental health clinics and private psychiatrists, psychologists, and social workers knowledgeable about violence in families may be helpful. Nurse-to-nurse referrals are often preferable, when the identifying nurse's professional role does not include the kind of long-term home visitation or therapy sessions required by such families. Psychiatric mental health clinical nurse specialists, nurse family therapists, and family nurse practitioners are often available as consultants in community health agencies or as part of community mental health centers or primary care clinics. Nurses practicing in other settings need to contact these nurse specialists and make sure they are knowledgeable about violence. Then linkages can be formed so that the nurse-to-nurse referrals are conducted with a minimum of red tape and waiting for the families.

The identifying nurse may continue to work with the family in resolving some of their other health concerns and in reinforcing and supporting the therapy being conducted by other professionals. It is beyond the scope of this book to teach the basics of family therapy with a seriously dysfunctional family (Whall, 1982). However, some descriptions of aspects of family therapy specific to families experiencing violence are described.

Family therapy with violent families requires the nurse to have a firm, personal support system of colleagues with whom she can discuss the progression of therapy. Violent families, including those who are incestuous, engender strong feelings in the nurse and can be extremely draining. In addition, the intrafamily dynamics are powerful and the nurse can easily become caught up in them. The Minuchen (1974) model of "joining" the family can be helpful in gaining a true appreciation for the values of the family and engendering trust, but enmeshment with a severely violent family can cloud judgment if careful self-awareness is not maintained. Frequent discussions with a supervisor or colleague can help the nurse remain objective. It also must be kept in mind that these families have usually taken several years to reach such a destructive stage, and the roots of the violence may have preceded the present situation by several generations. Therefore progress in eliminating the violence requires much time and hard work on the part of all participants.

A behavioral family therapy model is frequently suggested for working with violent families (Watts & Courtis, 1981). This is helpful in assisting the family with understanding how violent interaction patterns are learned, and in keeping the interactions focused on the present situation, thereby escaping a pattern of blaming individual members for past parts in the violence. At the same time, it is imperative for individual members to take responsibility for their own violent behavior. Regardless of the model of family therapy used, it may be necessary for the nurse to use considerable confrontation in making sure that this occurs. The therapy then focuses on the extinction of violent behavior on the part of all family members by establishing enforceable, definite, and undesirable consequences for further violence, coupled with reinforcement of nonviolent behaviors and the teaching of new ways to deal with stress and arguments. Contracts with the nurse and among family members may be helpful in specifically delineating the consequences of physically aggressive behavior. The family members must monitor each other's behavior between therapy sessions, and it is imperative that everyone understand exactly what will happen. It is not sufficient that the violent relationship of primary concern (such as wife abuse) is the subject of behavior elimination or reinforcing; all the physical aggression in the household must be stopped and new methods of dealing with anger instituted.

In addition to using behavioral techniques, it is important that the communication patterns between family members be analyzed and improved. Family members should also have a chance to express their feelings and learn how to accept both positive and negative feelings from their kin. The power distribution among family members also should be analyzed and equalized in most violent families. All these types of intervention are difficult and demanding.

If possible, especially if the family is large and includes several adolescents, a co-therapist arrangement is ideal. There is so much happening in a violent family that two therapists are more likely to be able to detect all the underlying dynamics. They can also support each other in confrontation and prevent triangulation attempts that frequently occur with just one therapist in a violent family. If the therapists are male and female, it is helpful because many of the family problems may stem from sex role difficulties.

Homework assignments are a useful intervention with violent family therapy. This allows work to be continued on problems between sessions, which is valuable in light of the difficulty of the problems being addressed. Assignments can be in the form of monitoring conflicts and how they were resolved and assessing the resolution. Members of the family can also be assigned to spend specific periods of time with other members with whom communication has been strained. Activities designed to enhance communication and which both members have decided would be fun can be decided for these periods. Family activities with all members can also be assigned with input from the members as to what would be enjoyable. Violent families are often in such conflict that they have forgotten how to have fun together. It is valuable if the nurse can accompany the family on at least one outing. This helps to cement the therapeutic relationship and allows the nurse to observe the family away from home or office.

Secondary prevention measures may also include working with the criminal justice system. The nurse may be called on to testify in court and/or to create liaisons between the enforcement agencies or lawyers and the family and other professionals involved. She may also help by being a supportive, knowledgeable person for the family in the courtroom and during the court proceedings. All of these activities necessitate a working knowledge of the law (as it applies to family violence) and of the criminal justice system. Background information on these subjects can be found in Chapters 13 and 14. In addition, the nurse needs to advocate for the education and sensitization of judges, district attorneys, police, and defense lawyers to the issues surrounding family violence and the plight of the victims. With such background, the court experience can be therapeutic and of practical assistance for the family, rather than a traumatizing experience (Dunwoody, 1982).

Secondary prevention of violence in families can thus be seen as a potential area for nursing to make considerable impact. Identification of families using

violence in conflict resolution may take place in many nursing settings, including inpatient areas, where this is routinely assessed. Nurses in community health settings, mental health agencies, and primary care facilities may be in prime positions to provide effective interventions, case coordination, and important referrals. Nurse specialists in family therapy and family functioning may continue the interventions in the form of family therapy and long-term case management and follow-up.

Tertiary Prevention

Tertiary level nursing interventions for violence are usually carried out with families who have broken up because of violence. This may include working with parents who have had a child or children placed in foster homes because of abuse; families who have a member incarcerated because of sexual, elderly, wife, sibling, or child assault or intrafamilial homicide; and families who have gone through a divorce or have a child who has run away permanently because of violence. Some significant emotional and perhaps physical damage has been done, and the nurse is mainly concerned with helping the family return to as healthy functioning as possible and to grieve for their losses.

Part of intervention on the tertiary level is to work with the children. They need to have the emotional effects of the violence assessed and handled and to be involved with learning different ways to cope with anger to counteract the learning of violent means that has already occurred. More detailed means of working with the children are outlined specifically in Chapter 8.

The adolescents of violent families may act out their disturbances in school, by running away, and by engaging in sexual or delinquent activities. Coordination efforts are needed with the professionals working directly with these teenagers as a result of their behavior. Nurses can play a significant role in runaway programs for adolescents. It would be helpful for a nurse to be part of the paid staff of such agencies, where teenagers who have run away from home are frequently housed temporarily. These adolescents may have a variety of health problems, including sexual abuse, other sexual concerns, drug abuse, and alcohol misuse, that can effectively be managed by a nurse. Group sessions on health matters are a useful mode of intervention with these young people. If a full-time or part-time nurse cannot be hired for the program, community health nurses or volunteer nurses can involve themselves with such agencies on the planning level as well as in direct services.

All the family members need concerned, empathetic family sessions with the nurse concerning the effects of the violence on them. The family needs to grieve for the lost family member and the loss of the family as a total unit. The nurse can support family members through their stages of mourning and encourage expression of feelings about the events. The family should also examine the impact of violence on their lives and work to eliminate any remaining physical aggression between members. Identification of serious psychological or physical aftereffects is also needed, and appropriate referrals should be made where indicated. Another type of tertiary intervention is provided for the mother and other siblings of abused children in hospitals. This is a good opportunity for intervention while supervising the mother's hospital visits to help her devise a safety plan that will keep her and her children together and free from violence.

EVALUATION

The evaluation of nursing care of violent families is based on achievement of the goals set with the family during the planning stage of intervention. Evaluation is an ongoing process that begins with the short-term goals with revisions of the plans and long-term goals as needed. As part of evaluation, it is also important to reassess the family periodically. It is important to conduct evaluation with the entire family so that praise can be given for progress achieved and so that no family member feels judged in his or her absence. Ongoing evaluation also includes frequent contacts with other professionals and agencies involved to maintain continuity.

Self-evaluation is also done by the nurse on the basis of the goals. When working with violent or po-

tentially violent families, it is important that the nurse continually study herself and reevaluate her perceptions and feelings. The problems may be more extensive than was originally assessed. The full extent of the violence often does not become evident until the nurse has worked with the family for some time. Long-term interventions with such families can become draining, and the nurse may decide that her or his effectiveness as primary therapist or case manager has eroded over time. In such cases it is best to discuss these feelings with the family as well as with a supervisor. If the nurse transfers the family to another professional without a full airing of the dilemma with the family, they may feel abandoned or fear that their case is hopeless.

Final evaluation is the time when the family is encouraged to make realistic plans for the future. If nursing intervention is ending before the problems with violence have been completely resolved, the family needs referrals of people who can be contacted for future interventions. These contacts can also be made if the family experiences a period of particular stress when the physical aggression is apt to exacerbate. If the family can anticipate problems and seek help early, another round of violent interaction may be prevented.

SAMPLE NURSING PROCESS

A sample nursing process for a hypothetical case has been included (Table 10-3). This illustration of nursing care is intended to show how nursing care can be provided to victims of family violence. The sample is not meant to be all-inclusive of possible nursing diagnoses or interventions for the problems of violence, but illustrates what might be used in a hypothetical case. The background given is brief, and the history and observations only indicate findings related to the violence. In actual nursing care, a much more detailed and holistic history and physical assessment would be conducted.

SUMMARY

Nursing care of violent or potentially violent families is based on theoretical framework that because

TABLE 10-3
Sample Nursing Process

Brief background

   The Smith family is a white middle-class family consisting of the mother, Dora; her second husband, Bill; Patty, a 14-year-old daughter from Dora's first marriage; and Billy, a 10-year-old son of this marriage. Dora's mother, Eileen, also lives with the family and is incapacitated by chronic arthritis. Patty has approached the school nurse with a "twisted" arm that also has several elongated bruises around the wrist. Patty admits to the school nurse that her stepfather has twisted her arm. On direct questioning, Patty indicates that the incident occurred when her stepfather approached her sexually and he grabbed and twisted her arm after she refused his advances. The school nurse obtains permission from Patty and her mother to make a home visit. The stepfather is not present when she arrives, but Patty, Dora, Eileen, and Billy are there.

   The nurse's observations and history of the family include, but are not limited to the following:

Significant history	Dora states that she and Bill have a satisfactory sexual life. Bill is under a great deal of stress because of a new boss and being "behind" with the bills, and he is extremely irritable toward Dora and she does not feel as "close" to him as she would like. Bill makes all of the decisions in the family and believes in "taking a belt to the kids" when they don't behave. She expresses horror at the news that Bill has tried to have a sexual relationship with Patty. Eileen is totally quiet during the interview and Dora talks for her, even when a question is directly asked of Eileen. Dora says that Eileen is becoming very difficult to care for as her arthritis worsens. Billy has been in trouble in school because of frequent fights with other children and cursing at teachers. Dora expresses a high degree of commitment to "making this marriage work."
Significant observations	Nonverbals are highly anxious and Eileen looks afraid of Dora. Patty sits very close to Dora and they occasionally touch. Affectionate tones of voice and glances are used between them. Both Eileen and Billy sit apart from the other two. Billy has a sullen expression and answers questions abruptly and without elaboration. Dora's tone of voice is disparaging when she talks about Eileen.

Three of the family nursing diagnoses identified are listed in order of priority:

  I. Potential for violence (incest) related to spousal marital problems, family stress, inadequate family and individual (father) coping mechanisms, unequal power relationships, and dysfunctional communication patterns.
 II. Potential for violence (elderly) related to family stress, dysfunctional communication patterns, chronic illness in grandmother, increased role responsibilities (mother), and inadequate family and individual (mother) coping mechanisms.
III. Aggressive behavior patterns (father and son) related to corporal punishment, observations of aggressive behavior, family stress, and destructive conflict resolution patterns.

TABLE 10-3 *Continued*
Sample Nursing Process

FAMILY GOALS	NURSING INTERVENTION
I. Potential for subsequent violence (incest) Overall No further sexual advances toward Patty as evidenced by: 1. Patty reporting no further advances 2. Protective service investigation showing no further advances 3. Patty's fear of stepfather diminishing	The nurse will: Report incident to protective services after discussion of such with family on first home visit. Initiate and maintain contact with protective services to coordinate care. Refer family for family therapy with a family nurse practitioner working in a community mental health center. Initiate and maintain contact with family nurse practitioner to reinforce and support therapy. See Patty regularly in school to discuss the progress being made in the family, monitor events in the home according to her perceptions, and help her express feelings about what is happening and has happened. Make regular home visits when all family members are present to obtain the perceptions of other family members and to make continued assessments. Build on observed strength of closeness between Patty and Dora by encouraging mother-daughter interactions.
Long term Increased satisfaction with marital relationship at the end of 3 mo as evidenced by: 1. Signs of decreased tension in the home 2. Dora reporting feeling "closer" to husband	Form therapeutic relationship with family: Discuss fully the marital relationship with mother and father. Help parents see the relationship of the stress in home with their relationship. Build on mother's commitment to marriage as a motivator to improve relationship. Support expression of feelings to nurse and of partners to each other. Help partners develop more effective coping mechanisms to deal with stress and to help each other cope. Suggest regular times for partners to be together alone, including weekends away. Help to arrange for babysitting and suggest Patty learn to care for grandmother at times. Teach family how to listen effectively to each other and communicate with respect for the other person. Teach parents how to encourage feeling expression to each other as a coping mechanism for dealing with stress and as a relationship-enhancing strategy.

TABLE 10-3 *Continued*
Sample Nursing Process

FAMILY GOALS	NURSING INTERVENTION
II. Potential for subsequent violence (elderly) Short term Increased family sharing of responsibilities of physical care of grandmother at the end of 2 wk as evidenced by: 1. Mother feeling less tied down 2. Signs of decreased anxiety in grandmother 3. Less disparaging communication patterns toward grandmother by mother 4. Other family members taking care of grandmother's needs when possible	The nurse will: Refer grandmother to physician for complete medical workup and suggestions of arthritis treatment. Encourage contact of mother's siblings for help in caring for grandmother on selected weekends. Help family work out a schedule of care for grandmother that all can participate in. Point out the communication patterns that mother has been using in relationship to grandmother and teach more effective communication skills. Help grandmother express feelings about situation. Help grandmother and mother really communicate with each other by role modeling and pointing out blocks as they occur. Praise mother's care of grandmother and encourage other family members to express appreciation for it.
Long term Demonstration of improved individual and family coping mechanisms at the end of 3 mo as evidenced by: 1. Mother feeling less tension 2. Family showing less conflict in communications 3. Family holding regular discussions to solve problems	The nurse will: Support coping mechanisms being developed in family therapy. Encourage family to problem-solve with health concerns together during regular home visits; praise their efforts. Teach supportive communication techniques. Help mother develop individual coping mechanisms, such as relaxation techniques, spending time with friends while other family members take care of grandmother, and expressing feelings openly.
III. Aggressive behavior problems Short term Recognition within family of the connections between aggressive behavior in son and aggressive behavior in father at the end of 2 wk as evidenced by: 1. A decision by father to refrain from physical punishment 2. Reports from family therapist of constructive conflict resolution 3. Reports from Patty of same	The nurse will: Discuss the intergenerational transmission of violence with family. Identify with father how he learned violence in family of origin. Encourage and praise efforts made. Suggest family members keeping a log of conflicts, how they were solved, and how effective the solutions were perceived to be. Discuss these logs with the family.
Long term Less aggressive behavior in Billy at the end of 3 months as evidenced by: 1. Less nonverbal negativity in Billy 2. Fewer reports of aggressive behavior in school	The nurse will: Support interventions being given to Billy through his school; maintain coordination with professionals there and provide communication between Billy's school and family. Encourage father to spend at least half hour every day in some kind of one-to-one activity. Encourage feeling expression between Billy and father. Praise Billy for nonaggressive behavior and efforts to change. Encourage family to use a great deal of praise with Billy also.

Evaluation is based on achievement of goals as perceived by family and as indicated by criteria met.

of the nature of family interaction, violence can easily develop, that physically aggressive interaction modes are transmitted through family socialization from one generation to the next, and that families who are found to be abusive in one form may also be abusive in another. Thus nursing care based on the total family unit is frequently indicated. The nature of the suggested nursing practice is necessarily based on clinical experience and family nursing principles because of the paucity of nursing research specific to family violence. Assessment of families for possible violence includes direct questioning about forms of conflict resolution. Other indications that the family may be at risk for or actually experiencing violence were summarized in Tables 10-1 and 10-2. The assessment for violence ends with nursing diagnoses being formulated with the family, a process that should include identification of family strengths. On the basis of the problems listed, the family works together with the nurse to formulate short-term and long-term goals and interventions. This process of planning together can be a form of intervention itself.

Interventions are based on the three levels of prevention and include interventions of societal and community advocacy for nonviolence as well as measures taken with individual families. The nurse is in an excellent position to work with the entire family, as well as to be a liaison between the family and other professionals and agencies. Nursing care is finally evaluated with the family on the basis of the goals set. The nursing care of violent families is both challenging and rewarding and has the potential for being an arena where nurses can make a significant impact on decreasing the violent nature of American society.

REFERENCES

Ammerman, R. T., & Hersen, M. (1991). Family violence: A clinical overview. In R. T. Ammerman & M. Hersen (Eds.), *Case studies in family violence* (pp. 3–12). New York: Plenum.

Bolton, F. G., & Bolton, S. R. (1987). Critical issues in the violent family's social environment. In F. G. Bolton & S. R. Bolton (Eds.), *Working with violent families: A guide for clinical and legal practitioners* (pp. 81-85). Newbury Park: Sage.

Bronfenbrenner, U. (1979). *The ecology of human development: Experiments by nature and design.* Cambridge, MA: Harvard University Press.

Burgess, A. W., & Holmstrom, L. L. (1979). *Rape: Crisis and recovery.* Bowie, MD: Robert J. Brady.

Campbell, D. W. (1991). Family paradigm theory and family rituals: Implications for child and family health. *The Nurse Practitioner: The American Journal of Primary Health Care, 16,* 22, 25, 26, 31.

Coleman, K. (1980). Conjugal violence: What thirty-three men report. *Journal of Marriage and Family Therapy, 6,* 210.

Dibble, U., & Straus, M. (1980). Some social structure determinants of inconsistency between attitudes and behavior: The case of family violence. *Journal of Marriage and the Family, 42,* 73.

The duel over gun control. (1981, March 23). *Time,* p. 33.

Dunwoody, E. (1982). Sexual abuse of children: A serious, widespread problem. *Response, 5,* 1-2, 13-14.

Duvall, E. M., & Hill, R. (1948). Report of the committee of the dynamics of family interaction. Washington, DC: National Conference on Family Life.

Fitzpatrick, J., Whall, A., Johnston, R., & Floyd, J. (1982). *Nursing models and their psychiatric mental health applications.* Bowie, MD: Robert J. Brady.

Friedman, M. M. (1992). *Family nursing: Theory and assessment* (2nd ed.). Norwalk, CT: Appleton-Century Crofts.

Gary, F., & Kavanagh, C. K. (1991). *Psychiatric-mental health nursing.* Philadelphia: J. B. Lippincott.

Gayfard, J. J. (1979). The aetiology of repeated serious physical assaults by husbands on wives. *Medicine, Science, and The Law, 19,* 23.

Gelles, R. J., & Straus, M. A. (1979). Determinants of violence in the family. In W. Burr, R. Hill, F. I. Nye, & I. Reiss, (Eds.), *Contemporary theories about the family* (Vol. 1) (pp. 549-577). New York: The Free Press.

Goldner, V. (1988). Generation and gender: Normative and covert hierarchies. *Family Process, 27,* 17-31.

Herman, J. (1981). *Father-daughter incest* (p. 27). Cambridge: Harvard University Press.

Hess, B. B., Markson, E. W., & Stein, P. J. (1989). *Sociology.* (3rd ed.). New York: Macmillan.

Hill, R. (1949). *Families under stress.* New York: Harper & Row.

Hotaling, G. T., Straus, M., & Lincoln, A. (1990). Intrafamily violence and crime and violence outside the family. In M. Straus & R. Gelles (Eds.), *Physical violence in the American family.* New Brunswick, NJ: Transaction.

Jones, S. L. (1980). *Family therapy: A comparison of approaches.* Bowie, MD: Robert J. Brady.

Jung, R. & Jason, L. (1988). Firearms, violence, and the effects of gun control legislation. *American Journal of Community Psychology, 16*(4), 515-524.

Kellerman, A. L., & Reay, D. T. (1986). Protection or peril? An analysis of firearm related deaths in the home. *New England Journal of Medicine, 314,* 1557-1560.

Lester, D. (1988). Gun control ownership and suicide prevention. *Suicide and Life-threatening Behavior, 18*(2), 176-180.

Luepnitz, D. A. (1988). *The family interpreted: Feminist theory in clinical practice.* New York: Basic Books.

Lunde, D. (1986) *Murder and madness: Suggestions for homicide prevention.* Second Annual Symposium in Psychiatry and Law. *American Journal of Forensic Psychiatry, 7*(2), 40-47.

McCubbin, M. A., & McCubbin, H. I. (1987). Family stress theory and assessment: The T-Double ABCX model of family adjustment and adaptation. In H. I. McCubbin & A. L. Thompson (Eds.), *Family assessment inventories for research and practice* (pp. 14-32). Madison, WI: University of Wisconsin.

McCubbin, M. A., & Patterson, J. M. (1982). Family adaptation to crises. In H. I. McCubbin, A. E. Cauble, & J. M. Patterson (Eds.), *Family stress, coping and social support* (pp. 26-47). Springfield, IL: Charles C. Thomas.

Meister, S. B. (1984). Family well-being. In J. Campbell & J. Humphreys (Eds.), *Nursing care of victims of family violence* (pp. 54-73). Reston, VA: Reston.

Minuchin, S. (1974). *Families and family therapy.* Cambridge: Harvard University Press.

Oermann, M. H. (1991). *Professional nursing practice: A conceptual approach.* New York: J. B. Lippincott.

Reiss, D. (1981). *The family's construction of reality.* Cambridge, MA: Harvard University Press.

Renvoize, J. (1978). *Web of violence.* London: Routledge & Kegan Paul.

Roberts, C. S., & Feetham, S. L. (1982). Assessing family functioning across three areas of relationships. *Nursing Research, 31*(4), 231-235.

Rounsaville, B. J., & Weissman, M. A. (1977-78). Battered women: A medical problem requiring detection. *International Journal of Psychiatry in Medicine, 8,* 191-202.

Sawin, D. (1981). The fantasy-reality distinction in televised violence: Modifying influences on children's aggression. *Journal of Research in Personality, 15,* 329.

Spear, J., & Sachs, B. (1985). Selecting the appropriate family assessment tool. *Pediatric Nursing, 11,* 349-355.

Stark, E., & Flitcraft, A. (1984). Woman-battering, child abuse and social heredity: What is the relationship? In N. Johnson (Ed.), *Marital violence.* London: Routledge & Kegan Paul.

Steinmetz, S. (1977). *Cycle of violence.* New York: Praeger.

Straus, M. A. (1983). Ordinary violence, child abuse and wife beating: What do they have in common? In D. Finkelhor, R. J. Gelles, G. T. Hotaling, & M. A. Straus (Eds.), *The dark side of families: Current family violence research* (pp. 213-234). Beverly Hills, CA: Sage.

Straus, M. A., & Gelles, R. A. (1990). *Physical violence in American families.* New Brunswick, NJ: Transaction.

Straus, M. A., & Gelles, R. J. (1988). The prevalence of family violence. In G. Hotaling, D. Finkelhor, J. Kirkpatrick, & M. Straus, (Eds.), *Family abuse and its consequences* (pp. 14-52). Newbury Park, CA: Sage.

Straus, M. A., Gelles, R. J., & Steinmetz, S. K. (1980). *Behind closed doors.* Garden City, NY: Doubleday.

Watts, D., & Courtis, C. (1981). Trends in the treatment of men who commit violence against women. *Personnel and Guidance Journal, 60,* 246.

Whall, A. A. (1982). Family systems theory: Relationship to nursing conceptual models. In J. Fitzpatrick et al. (Eds.), *Nursing models and their psychiatric mental health applications* (pp. 69-94). Bowie, MD: Robert J. Brady.

Yllö, K., & Bogard, M. (1988). *Feminist perspectives on wife abuse.* Newbury Park, CA: Sage.

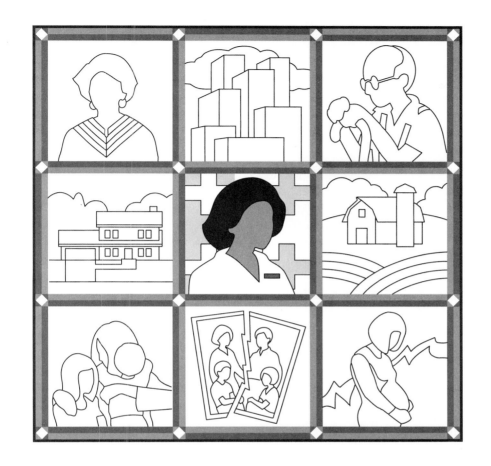

Nursing and the
Justice System

The Nurse and the Police
Dealing with abused children

Isaiah McKinnon *and* David G. Blocker

Reports of child abuse and neglect continue to increase every year. In 1986 more than 1.5 million children nationwide were reported as abused and neglected, a 74% increase since 1980. The spectrum of serious child abuse appears to be changing. Today children are more likely to have severe injuries resulting from sudden, impulsive acts of violence. Substance abuse, depression, isolation, and a history of abuse in the parents' own childhood have all been linked to child maltreatment (Kessler & Hyden, 1991).

The role of law enforcement in cases of child abuse and neglect begins with a report or suspicion of child maltreatment and ends with the securing of safety for the child.

The goal of preventing child abuse and/or neglect at every level is common to both law enforcement and nursing. This chapter describes the role and responsibilities of law enforcement personnel in cases of suspected or actual child maltreatment. In addition, the interface with nursing is discussed to increase the sensitivity of both disciplines, law enforcement and nursing, to each other and facilitate a cooperative effort in the prevention of child maltreatment. No single agency or professional discipline can work in isolation to prevent and treat the problem. Only through concerned community effort can real changes occur.

Generally, society believes that law enforcement officers' emotional responses to crimes become hardened because of the nature of their work. However, a problem such as child abuse or neglect raises the wrath of private citizens and the police alike. Child abuse is not exclusive to any particular geographical area, but is prevalent in many areas throughout the country. Adults who abuse and neglect children are not a homogeneous group. They vary in levels of background and education and may be found in all levels of society, as documented in the national media. Child abuse may occur as an isolated incident, or it may be chronic. Factors such as poverty, unemployment, patterns of parental discord, and difficulties in the parent-child relationship may create a climate where child abuse can occur (Kessler & Hyden, 1991). Every ethnic, professional, and social group in the United States has been affected in some way by this crime. There is no definitive list of causes explaining all physical abuse or neglect, but certain elements are seen more often than are others. One common factor is that the potential to abuse is learned behavior. Abusive parents had poor parent models and were themselves usually abused or neglected by their parents.

A second common factor is society's general acceptance of the use of violence and force in conflict resolution and the corporal punishment of children in the name of discipline (Kessler & Hyden, 1991).

A third common factor is the use of illegal drugs and the abuse of alcohol by the abuser. Adults who normally would not hurt a child may become irrational or lose inhibitions while drinking or using illegal drugs, or they may be too involved in drinking and drug use to care for a child (Bete, 1987).

The actual incidence of child abuse and neglect is difficult to ascertain, but the reports continue to increase every year. Departments of social services and protective services keep various records of the cases of child abuse and neglect in all states.

DEFINITION OF CHILD ABUSE AND NEGLECT

The term *child abuse* carries many connotations and can be defined generally as any act by parents or other persons legally responsible for the child's welfare that causes injury or places the child in danger.

To assist in identifying the instances of child abuse and neglect, law enforcement uses the following statutory definitions (Detroit Police Department Training and Information Bulletin, 1978):

Child: A person under 18 years of age.

Child abuse: Harm or threatened harm to a child's health or welfare by a person responsible for the child's health or welfare that occurs through nonaccidental physical or mental injury, sexual abuse, or maltreatment.

Child neglect: Harm to a child's health or welfare by a parent, legal guardian, or person who has custodial care of the child that occurs through negligent treatment, including the failure to provide adequate food, clothing, shelter, or medial care. (p. 1)

REPORTING CHILD ABUSE AND NEGLECT

In an effort to protect children from being abused, Michigan legislators passed the Michigan Child Protection Law in 1975. The Child Protection Law of 1975 (Public Act 238) was revised in May 1989 and mandates that certain persons (e.g., nurses, dentist, psychologists, social workers, teachers, regulated child-care providers, physicians, and law enforcement officers) make an immediate oral report of all suspected child abuse and neglect cases to the Michigan Department of Social Services. A written report must follow within 72 hours; this written form is commonly known as DSS-3200 (Michigan Child Protection Law P.A. (MCPLPA) 238, 1975). A person required to report an instance of suspected child abuse or neglect and who fails to do so is civilly liable for the damages proximately caused by that failure; if a person *knowingly* fails to do so, he or she is guilty of a misdemeanor (MCPLPA 238, 1975).

There are no fixed criteria; any person can report what he or she believes to be suspected child abuse or neglect. If there is any question, doubt should be resolved in favor of the child and the situation reported. Anyone reporting suspected child abuse or neglect in good faith will be granted immunity from civil or criminal liability under the Child Protection Law (MCPLPA 238, 1975).

PROTECTIVE SERVICES

Child welfare had its beginnings in this country at the turn of the century when, for the first time, a child was protected from abuse by court action under laws that had been passed to protect animals.

The problem of child abuse grew in national recognition. By 1965 most states had passed legislation to protect children and require reporting of possible incidents of abuse.

Michigan Act 98 (1964) and Act 71 (1966) served to meet this need. A national trend toward having a single agency responsible for protecting abused and neglected children throughout the community led to Michigan appropriations for this purpose in 1970. Wayne County, Michigan, was among the first to provide around-the-clock protective services for children.

Michigan Public Act 238 of 1975 mandated the Michigan Department of Social Services (MDSS) to be the single responsible agency for child protective services.

According to the MDSS, protective services are necessary because children have a basic right to the care, guidance, protection, and love required for normal health, growth, and development, and there is a need to protect these rights. Protective services are social agencies designed to ensure that children are protected from physical or emotional harm resulting from parental abuse, neglect, or exploitation, and to assist parents or guardians to function appropriately in providing the necessary care for their children.

LAW ENFORCEMENT INVOLVEMENT

Nationally, police have the initial responsibility for investigating circumstances involving violation of law, prevention of crime, and preservation of peace. Child abuse is a crime. It may be a social problem; it may be the product of a disordered mind; it may indicate an overall family dysfunction . . . but it is always a crime (Child Abuse Investigation and Prosecution. *Wayne County Prosecutor's Office Handbook*).

In 1975 the Detroit Police Department organized a specialized unit within the Youth Section known as the Child Abuse Unit. This unit is responsible for investigating all matters of child abuse and neglect that occur within Detroit that are reported to the Detroit Police Department, excepting sex crimes, homicides, and child pornography. These offenses are handled by other specialized units within the Detroit Police Department.

The Detroit Police Child Abuse Unit and the MDSS, Protective Services work together in investigations of child abuse and neglect. In addition to child abuse and neglect complaints, the Child Abuse Unit is responsible for reports involving adults contributing to the delinquency of minor children, which includes nonfatal, self-inflicted gunshot wounds and underage children being home alone.

THE PATROL OFFICER

Historically, the uniformed police officer has been considered the backbone of the police department. The uniformed police officer is the first line of defense in the majority of criminal acts. That fact cannot be overemphasized in the protection of battered, defenseless children. In Michigan the statutory authority to remove a child from the home is as follows:

> Any municipal police officer, sheriff or deputy sheriff or state police officer, county agent or probation officer of any court of record may, without the order, immediately take into custody any child who is found violating any law or ordinance or whose surroundings are such as to endanger his health, morals or welfare. Whenever any such officer or county agent takes a child coming within the provisions of this chapter into custody, he shall forthwith notify the parents or parent, guardian or custodian, if they can be found within the county. While awaiting the arrival of the parent or parents, guardian or custodian, no child under the age of 17 years taken into custody under the provisions of this chapter shall be held in any detention facility unless such child be completely isolated so as to prevent any verbal, visual, or physical contact with any adult prisoner. Unless the child requires immediate detention as hereinafter provided, the arresting officer shall accept the written promise of said parent or parents, guardian or custodian to bring the child to the court at a time fixed therein. Thereupon such child shall be released to the custody of said parent or parents, guardian or custodian (Michigan Compiled Laws Ann. (1975) 712A.14)

Under normal circumstances, the police must ask permission, possess a warrant or probable cause to arrest, or believe that a crime is in the process or has been committed before entering the domicile of any citizen. More importantly, officers can usually enter a home if an emergency situation arises, such as cries for help, or it there is imminent danger to a citizen, other officers, or themselves. Traditionally in Michigan, when dealing with family dispute calls, the police officer does not have the right to enter a home without consent, a warrant, or probable cause to arrest (Search and Seizure, *Spinelli v. U.S. 393*).

INVESTIGATION

The primary concern of patrol officers responding to complaints of suspected child abuse or neglect is the safety and protection of the child. It must be determined if the child has been abused, if the child is in danger at home, or if the officer must take immediate action to ensure the child's safety.

The traditional police role in child abuse cases involves the receipt of a report, an investigation, possible detainment, and prosecution.

In Detroit, reports to the police department of child abuse and neglect are initially investigated by the uniformed officers who patrol the area. Investigative techniques vary with individual officers; however, once the officer is inside the house, he or she usually quickly isolates the child and questions him or her as to the nature and origin of any injuries. Officers listen closely to the child's explanation, then carefully note the parents' version for any inconsistencies.

When a child is injured and the parents are evasive, vague, angry, or reluctant to give information regarding how the injury occurred, they may be trying to hide the real reason.

Abused children often display signs of stress. The anxiety they feel is likely to affect all aspects of their lives to some extent. The following behavioral indicators are commonly seen as symptoms of abuse and neglect: submissiveness; aggressive acting out behavior; sudden changes in appetite, moods, and personal grooming; and severe depression or suicidal feelings (Kessler & Hyden, 1991).

Once the uniformed patrol officer has assessed the situation, the Detroit Child Abuse Unit and the

MDSS must be contacted as soon as possible for further instruction. In cases of serious physical injury, patrol officers are advised to remove the injured child from the home and to seek immediate medical attention for the child. In many cases of less serious injury or neglect, patrol officers are instructed to bring the child to the office of the Detroit Child Abuse Unit for additional questioning by the child abuse investigator. Often the injured or neglected child is placed in foster care through the MDSS or released to a suitable relative pending further investigation.

Child abuse cases are often difficult to investigate because children are normally taught to obey adults. Children are totally dependent on adults who hold positions of power and authority over them. An adult's mere physical size plays an important part in the child's world and enhances the dominating presence, which causes the child not to cooperate if so instructed by the parent or adult.

In many cases the child is too young to provide a history. There are no visible signs of physical abuse, but it is apparent the child is in distress and needs medical attention. Often parents explain the injury as an accident or of unknown origin. These initial statements given to the uniformed officers are helpful to the investigator during the follow-up investigation.

Investigations by the Detroit Child Abuse Unit often include photographs of the scene and injuries to the child, collection of evidence, interviews with any and all witnesses, medical documentation from physicians and nurses, records of previous contacts or history with the MDSS, and thorough check of police records.

Detroit Child Abuse investigators also have the responsiblity of interviewing the abused or neglected child. Guidelines found in the Role of Law Enforcement in the Prevention and Treatment of Child Abuse and Neglect are useful in such instances.

At the very beginning of the interview, the interviewer must try to determine the emotional state of the child. Is fear, hatred, defiance, shock, confusion, love, jealousy, or anger apparent? Is the child ready to tell the truth, lie, or exaggerate?

The interviewers should attempt to gain the child's confidence. The interview should be conducted on a friend-to-friend basis rather than as police officer to child.

The investigator should not appear to take sides against the parents. Under no circumstances should the interviewer indicate horror, disgust, anger, or disapproval of parents, child, or the situation. Children will often become defensive if they feel outsiders are critical of their parents, even if they feel the same way.

The interview should be conducted in language the child clearly understands. Particularly in cases of sexual abuse, the officer should accept and use whatever terms of genitals and sexual acts the child uses while also asking for clarification and eliciting specific information regarding what has occurred.

Children should be permitted to tell about incidents in their own way. They should not be pressed for details they may be unwilling or unable to give. The officer should limit questions to necessary information and should use open-ended questions whenever possible. Younger children may be more at ease if the situation is discussed in terms of fantasy.

The interview should include a discussion of what will happen next and how the officer will use the information the child has given.

If the child is an adolescent and the officer feels a "person in need of supervision," petition or a similar order will be necessary, the officer should so inform the child. The officer should also inform adolescents of their Miranda rights.

INTERFACE WITH NURSING

Health care professionals—nurses, physicians, and hospital personnel—play a critical role in not only detecting but also preventing child abuse. Nurses often see injured or ill children who may have been abused or neglected.

Parents seeking medical attention for children are asked to provide a history of the child's illness or injury. When a child is taken to the hospital by police, the investigating officers will have recorded the parents' story regarding the cause of the child's injuries and relayed it to the examining health care provider, who may conclude that the injuries did in fact occur in the manner as stated (Kessler & Hyden, 1991).

An adequate history, or lack of it, is critical in identifying abuse and neglect in children. Any injury without an adequate explanation, especially in a young child, raises concerns about either nonaccidental injury or neglect.

Delay in seeking health care, especially for significant injuries, should be carefully evaluated because it indicates a high risk of abuse. Discrepancies or contradictions in the explanation of an injury or accounts that change often indicate nonaccidental trauma (Kessler & Hyden, 1991).

Child abuse investigators consult with health care providers in many cases because of the lack of obvious physical injury. The nurse's knowledge of child abuse and neglect can provide invaluable information and assistance to the investigating officer. At all times the nurse can be the advocate of a child. The nurse involved in the day-to-day care of the abused or neglected child is often able to gain the child's confidence and may dispute the history of an injury provided by the parent.

In cases of child abuse in which the child is unable to testify in a court of law because of factors such as age, serious physical injury, and mental or emotional states, the physician or nurse may be required to give testimony on behalf of the child. This testimony is based on medical documentation of the child's injuries, the physician's professional opinion, nursing notes, the nurse's personal contact with the child, and observation of parent-child interaction during hospital or clinic visits. Nurses also share information with the protective services worker involved in the case.

ARREST

Police officers rarely have enough information or evidence to make an immediate arrest in child abuse and neglect cases. In many cases the police department is not notified until a medical examination reveals inconsistent explanations for the child's injury.

Some cases of abuse and neglect are referred to the police department by protective services. These cases are referred after the worker has made contact with the family and feels that the case is criminal in nature.

In cases of child abuse involving extremely young children, often there are no eyewitnesses to the abuse. Cases must be thoroughly investigated by trained police personnel. Cases lacking an eyewitness are often developed by a set of circumstances based on the collection of other evidence.

Police departments depend on several agencies to reach the desired results in the protection of the child. Child abuse and neglect cases are often sensitive issues that have an impact on the entire family and community. Arresting the responsible parent is not always in the best interest of the child or the family.

SUMMARY

Child abuse and neglect continues to be a growing problem in the United States. Each year the number of reports and arrests increases. With each report and each arrest, the family suffers further division and possible separation.

Nurses, physicians, hospital social workers, protective services workers, and law enforcement officers all play a significant role in the detection and prevention of child abuse and neglect. If the incidence of child abuse is to be reduced in this country, people must continue to be educated about the causes and effects of abuse and neglect.

REFERENCES

Bete, C. L. (1987). *About alcohol, child abuse, and child neglect.* South Dearfield, MA: Spyrographic.

Child Abuse Investigation and Prosecution. *Wayne County Prosecutor's Office Handbook.* Wayne County, MI.

Child Protection Law, Public Act #238 of 1975, revised, State of Michigan, 5/89. Section 722.621, 722.636. Michigan Compiled Laws.

Detroit Police Training and Information Bulletin. (January, 1978). Pub. No. 78-5.

Guidelines. Role of Law Enforcement p. (1991).

Kessler, D. B., & Hyden, P. D. (1991). Physical, sexual, and emotional abuse of children. *Clinical symposia.* 43(1), 23-35.

Michigan Compiled Laws Ann. 712A.14.

Michigan Act 98 (1964).

Michigan Act 71 (1966).

National Center on Child Abuse and Neglect (1991). *The role of law enforcement in the prevention and treatment of child abuse and neglect.* Denver: National Center on Child Abuse and Neglect.

Search and Seizure. *Spinelli v. U.S. 393.* U.S. 410.89 Supreme Court 583.216 (E.D. 2d 637).

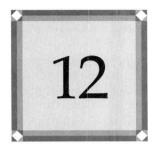

The Nurse and the Police
Dealing with Abused Women

James Bannon

O ne of the most frustrating and intransigent problems confronting the working police officer is wife abuse, or as it is known in law enforcement, domestic violence. The officer feels poorly equipped to deal with these calls for service in any meaningful way. His or her training is inadequate or nonexistent. Agency policy is unclear, nonexistent, or contrary to general policy.

As a result, the officer resents or avoids to the greatest extent possible any involvement in domestic violence cases, or alternatively, gives them short shrift. This chapter examines some of the issues that have caused police officers to adopt "hands-off" attitudes toward domestic violence.

SCOPE OF THE PROBLEM

Historically, no data have been collected on domestic violence separate from assaults. With rare excep-

tions, no effort has been made to research the issue so that reliable estimates can be made of the number of such assaults that occur. Thus "guesstimates" range from 50% to one third of all married couples are commonly thought to have some violent encounters.

To determine some notion of the size of the problem, Marie Wilt, a criminologist, and I undertook a study in Detroit, Michigan, in 1972.[1] The findings of that study, published by the Police Foundation, clearly indicated that at least 50% of all domestic assaults are never reported. In addition, it became clear that even fewer assaults are reported by the victim herself. Frequently, children, other family members, or residents in the household notify the police. Neighbors, themselves disturbed, often call as well.

Although it has proved difficult, if not impossible, to find hard data (simply because no such data are collected), it is widely believed that in many jurisdictions at least one third of all calls for police service are domestic violence calls. Of course, in larger jurisdictions with multiple crime problems, the ratio of such calls decreases dramatically. It should be understood that the reason for this decrease is entirely unrelated to the actual incidence of abuse. On the contrary, it is related to the work load of the agency and the policies of that agency designed to manage its work load.

In 1980 through 1982, the average monthly calls for police response to domestic violence cases for the city of Detroit were about 3,900 to 4,000. These figures represent all types of calls related to domestic violence. For many reasons, it is believed that this represents only a fraction of the total number of actual incidents.

One of the most notable facets of law enforcement attitudes toward domestic violence is the seeming indifference of police administration to the physical safety of its officers in responding to domestic violence calls. Federal Bureau of Investigation reports consistently indicate that about one third of all police fatalities occur during response to social conflict calls. It is also believed that most of these are domestic violence calls, although it is impossible to be precise. Similarly, a large proportion of disabling injuries (i.e., those requiring either hospitalization or release from work related to injury) are the result of attempted interventions in domestic disputes. For these reasons, it would seem that the competent police administrator would want to develop strategies for successfully dealing with these cases. Unfortunately, this has not been the case.

Although I personally indict the police for failure to adequately address the issue of abused women, in fairness, it should be noted that many police attitudes flow directly from the society of which they are a part.

It is too complex an issue to explore in this chapter, but readers are aware that historically wifebeating has been regarded in most societies as legitimate male behavior (see Chapter 4). It has been sanctioned by the courts, by the clergy, and by public opinion. There was and still remains a strong belief that the male assumes the responsibility for regulating the behavior of all in his household. Therefore it is expected that at times he may be required, in fulfilling his role, to mete out physical discipline.

It is true that in some socioeconomic groups in our society these expectations are carried out with greater public notice than in others. However, it is unreasonable to believe that there are substantial differences in attitudes about the appropriateness of the behavior. There are certainly differences in reporting by members of the upper socioeconomic strata. These differences are related to such diverse matters as living arrangements of the poor, lack of privacy, lack of alternatives for the victim and the abuser, differential concerns over public image of the affluent, and, the most important consideration of the affluent, the risk of monetary and status loss in the event of dissolution of the marriage. It should be noted that I am aware of the increasingly popular "less than married" relationships. When the term "married" is used, it defines any cohabitation that features consensual sexual access and economic interdependence. This definition would not exclude homosexual relationships. It would exclude casual sexual liaisons. I believe that the battering syndrome necessarily contains within it a requirement of dependency—social, economic, legal and emotional—that inhibits or overcomes the natural instinct to flee or vitiate the assault on one's person.

Traditional socialization of male/female children carries with it the ingredients necessary to cast the male in the dominant role and the female in the passive. However, dominance and passivity as conditioned responses are not adequate to explain violence in the relationship.

Other socialization issues as they pertain to female/male differences require examination. Most notable are the necessary male strengths of body and spirit. Men do not cry; they are physically strong, brave. They fight their own battles. They will not be cowed by another, nor will they suffer any interference with their affairs. Meanwhile, the female child is taught not only that it is okay to cry, to be sensitive, frightened, and dependent, but that it is also the most feminine thing to do. Moreover, the more feminine she is, the more she will attract her polar opposite, that is, the masculine, physical male.

Because Americans are socialized to believe that the male is acting appropriately and the female has the burden to recognize and surrender to this, it is also expected that all accommodation will be made by the woman. It is her responsibility to satisfy, pacify, and acquiesce to the demands of the male. She fails as a wife if she does not. She fails as a woman if she fails as a wife. Most often, it is her sense of failure that inhibits her from telling others of the ongoing abuse.

More definitive information on the role of the female/male socialization in the issue of spouse abuse is presented in Chapter 4. It is too complex and lengthy an issue to be discussed here. However, it is important to remember that all members of society have been exposed to the same conditioning. Although not all may be violent or victims of violence, society's thoughts on such matters are directly related to common socialization. Thus police officers have been conditioned to believe in and aspire to the "macho" man image. In fact, many have been attracted to law enforcement because of its seeming comportment with the masculine role model. The effects of this on their behavior are discussed later in this chapter.

HISTORICAL BACKGROUND*
Traditional Police Response

Although minor differences existed in police response to domestic violence calls in different parts

---

*Throughout this chapter, I have used the masculine pronoun "he" when referring to police officers. This was not a sexist convention or a design to economize on energy and space. It was done self-consciously to emphasize that until the last 10 years, policing was almost solely a male-dominated discipline. The few "policewomen" there were did not do patrol work and thus did not respond to domestic violence calls.

It is too soon to know, but perhaps neither this chapter nor this text would have been necessary if women had not been systematically excluded from patrolling our nation's cities in the past.

of the country, the result was virtually the same regardless of where the assault occurred. Changes began to occur in the late 1960s and continue today. The changes have been slow, sporadic, and reluctant. Some of the reasons are presented below.

First, it must be remembered that the police not only are a part of their own society, sharing in its beliefs and values, but also represent only one component of the criminal justice system. The other components are the prosecutorial, the courts, and corrections. Not only do these other components share social values with their society, they also have different interests and concerns than do the police on any given issue.

The police officer might desire to make an arrest and bring a charge against a man who has beaten his spouse, even if only because he is tired of repeatedly returning to the same household. Conversely, the prosecutor may not want to proceed because of his belief that the victim will not follow through, or more importantly, that it will affect his or her conviction rate. The court may also be reluctant because of concerns with an overloaded docket or the alternatives available if the spouse is convicted.

It then becomes clear to the police officer that the other components of the system simply do not want to handle these cases. The officer also realizes that his own agency does not value domestic violence arrests. Sometimes this realization is direct. The universal statement in police manuals that reads: "You should remember that domestic assaults are civil in nature and arrest should be avoided if at all possible" is the classic example.[2]

Although the statement is universally used in police procedural manuals, it is untrue. Domestic assaults are legally no different than stranger-to-stranger assaults. For whatever reasons, police administrators over the years have adopted an assumption of noncriminal behavior for the act of a man beating his wife. There is nothing in the law that permits the police executive to do this; however, the premise went unchallenged until 1975, when lawsuits were filed in Oakland, California, and in New York City.

These class action suits, settled out of court, sought to have the police treat domestic violence as a crime just like any other crime, which they legally are. As a result of these and other civil suits, police policies were changed in many (but not all) parts of the United States.

Even more pervasive and influential to an officer's judgment on such arrests, however, was the silent message that was conveyed. There simply was no recognition by the officer's superiors of the value of superior service to domestic violence victims nor of arrests for domestic assault. The latter was a function of so few of these cases resulting in prosecution and conviction of the assailant. Add to these direct messages the fact already discussed, that these cases often end in an assault, sometimes fatal, of the officer, and it is not difficult to imagine the police officer's desire to avoid all involvement.

The dilemma is obvious. The police officer is required by his dispatcher to respond to a domestic violence call, but the agency is ambivalent at best, if not actually hostile, to such calls. The officer has a policy that tells him to avoid arrest if possible. The prosecutor does not want these cases, nor does the court. The police officer has no training in how to handle such matters, and he may believe that physical resolution of conflict is the appropriate solution. His superiors will not recognize superior performance. Finally, while the officer spends an inordinate amount of time attempting to do what he knows he is not competent to do, other police work is backlogging. Worse yet, from the officer's perspective, he may be losing the opportunity to do "real" police work that is not only personally satisfying, but also obtains both public and agency acclaim. This is "the stuff that promotions are made of."

In 33 years of experience, I have never seen an award for excellence given to an officer for successful resolution of a domestic violence case, except posthumously.

Police officers have used a number of strategies to handle domestic violence calls. Some police officers confronted with the frustration of having to do something but lacking the training, the support, and the mandate, frequently fell back on their masculine role images. They would simply beat the abuser, or at least make that threat. Knowing the

effects of pain or the threat of pain on inhibiting certain behavior, many claim this was not an ineffective device.

Unfortunately, the message it delivers is that physical violence is in fact, under some circumstances, an appropriate vehicle for invoking authority. It must be remembered that the abusive male sees himself as the authority figure. The lesson he learns is not that violence is wrong but that he needs to be more circumspect so that other authority figures who also use violence are not summoned.

Some officers, without formal training, would attempt to counsel the parties, perhaps doing more harm in the long run than if they had actually beaten someone. Others—and this is the most common approach—would slough off the complaint by telling the victim to see the detectives Monday through Friday between the hours of 9 A.M. and 5 P.M. They would not take a report even though it was clear a crime had been committed. The officers knew fully that the detectives themselves had a full range of strategies to discourage the complainant's pursuit of a legal, criminal remedy.

The detective would try to dissuade the victim from prosecution, pointing out that she and the children would suffer adverse economic effects if her spouse was jailed. It was likely, however, that in the detective's entire career, he had never known an abuser who went to jail.

The detective would explain the difficulty to be encountered in sustaining the prosecution, the inconvenience of multiple court appearances, the embarrassment of public disclosure, etc. If the victim persisted, the detective might advise her to go home and think it over, to bring back medical proof of injury, or to bring her assailant in the next time she comes back.

If the victim persevered, the detective might ultimately have been compelled to submit a write-up to the prosecuting attorney, who would restart the process designed to discourage prosecution. The prosecutor's tactics might include counseling (equally untrained), intimidation, insistence on medical proof, pictures of the injury, threats of a cross-complaint, and demands for an assurance bond (a cash bond posted to guarantee prosecution). As a last resort, the prosecutor may have offered the victim a so-called peace bond, a worthless document written in appropriate legalese, which was tantamount to being a promissory note to prosecute the abuser if he assaulted the victim within the time frame stipulated in the document. Because such a subsequent assault would have constituted another crime, no such commitment was necessary.

One device used by police to avoid responding to domestic violence calls, although illegal, at least had the dubious virtue of candor. This was the call screening used in Detroit, Michigan, from about 1965 through 1973 or 1974. Call screening was deemed necessary because calls for service exceeded the department's capacity to respond to all calls. To reduce the work load, it was decided to obtain enough information from the caller to determine the exact nature of the complaint, and make a conscious decision not to send a response unit in certain cases.

In Detroit, the domestic dispute was selected as the first type of call to be screened out. The rationale for this decision was again the refusal of women to follow up on prosecution. No consideration was given to an attempt to enhance the police's willingness or capacity to prosecute, nor was any consideration given to the obvious history of the criminal justice system in discouraging prosecution.

The policy did provide that the police would be sent if a weapon was involved. The victims, on becoming aware of this exception to the no-response rule, invariably alleged a weapon. Thus the policy, it was said, was effectively vitiated.

Wilt and I took issue with this claim by raising the substantial objection that a police officer responding to an alleged assault with a weapon would react in an entirely negative fashion if there was no weapon. Often he would even threaten to arrest the caller for having made a false felony report. It is still impossible to estimate the residual effects of such a policy on a community long conditioned to rebuff when making a domestic violence complaint call. It is certain that several generations will pass before these effects disappear.

Although it is not possible to quantify the effects mentioned, it is possible to study one statistic that we believe directly reflected the abandonment of the victim—domestic homicide. We believe that the rate of such homicides rose dramatically as a direct result of the call screening policy.

Other researchers disagree with this interpretation, pointing out that all homicides had increased during the same period.[3] However, domestic homicides are frequently not categorized as such because a narrow definition of the required relationship between the assailant and the victim is used. I recommend that the required relationship be cohabitation with consensual sexual access and economic dependency.

Contemporary Developments

Although not proving the relationship between call screening and other policies designed to separate wife abuse complaints from other crimes, a rash of widely publicized trials of women accused of murdering their husbands merits attention. Such trials are not new, but the defense offered is. Women in effect are asking for an expansion of the self-defense doctrine based not on traditional legal issues, but rather on the failure of society and the legal system to protect them. Two Michigan cases are notable. The first, involving Francine Hughes, was widely publicized. The defendant was acquitted because of temporary insanity, not self-defense. However, the facts adduced at trial clearly showed a victim forced by neighbors, family, friends, and the criminal justice system to rely on her own resources to escape the unending cycle of violence. She waited until her husband was asleep, soaked him in gasoline, and lit his bed. He burned to death.[4]

The second case, that of Janet Smith, is directly related because it not only showed the same indifference of society and its system, but led to an acquittal of Mrs. Smith on the grounds of self-defense. This defense prevailed despite the fact that the threat to her, and thus the danger, was not contemporaneous with her killing of her husband. The defense focused on her accumulated experience of assault and inability to rely on the system for protection or redress.[5]

In the early 1970s, several developments occurred that began to raise domestic violence from the position of a private problem to that of a public issue. First, the feminist movement, often embodied in the National Organization for Women, recognized the plight of the battered wife as an issue of national and immediate concern. The organization adopted this issue as a primary focus for consciousness raising and action programs. At about the same time in Michigan, two female law school students, Eisenberg and Micklow, began to take an interest in the issue, desiring to focus the attention of fledgling lawyers on the matter. Their work, "Catch 22," became one of the first expositions available in writing.[6] These authors are widely credited with disseminating information both to feminist organizations and professionals in related fields.

Throughout the country, although not uniformly so, consciousness was raised and the media began to address the issue. There was confrontation between the criminal justice system and concerned women's groups. Some of this confrontation created much more unrest than enlightenment, but it finally began to stimulate an interest on the part of public officials in examining their own practices and procedures. At first, this self-examination was purely defensive. Later, some of the more sensitive administrators, prosecutors, and judges recognized and admitted the system's failures.

To their credit, police agencies were generally far more willing to critique and change than were the other components of the criminal justice system. However, there have been some false starts and unfortunate, unnecessary battles over details that have been costly in terms of cooperation; it may be beneficial to study some of them. First, there was a great deal of denial on the part of the police. This was countered by allegations that the police were frequently involved in their own violent personal relationships. Both sides were correct to a certain extent, but both lost sight of the central fact that the police have both a private and a public face. Often the police officer can and does function effectively in his public role, although privately he may engage in the same behavior he is required to police in his public role. Gambling, drinking, and traffic violations come readily to mind.

The obvious fact that agencies control police behavior through policy was lost in this debate. No policy existed, or if it did, it was contrary to the law. It was not necessary to enter the debate about private police behavior. Only if the policy was published and violated without sanction would the issue of private behavior need to be examined.

Another damaging and unnecessary debate was engaged in (and still is to some extent) over the assertions of criminal justice practitioners that their "hands-off" policy toward domestic violence was related to the failure of women to follow through on prosecution. Feminists responded strongly to this claim, pronouncing it an outright lie. Some members of the feminist movement reacted vehemently because they simply could not understand how a woman could be abused and not want to pursue all available avenues of redress.

While criminal justice personnel insisted that it was true and relied on such myths as "She must have caused it, she likes it, she loves the guy," etc., feminists insisted it was not true. In fact, it *is* true that there is much attrition in these complaints. This may in part be because of the battered women's own socialization to expect and accept male dominance and physical punishment. It may in part be related to her emotional and economic dependency or her legal confusion over her rights. Nevertheless, there is attrition in prosecution in *all* kinds of criminal prosecutions. The reasons are numerous, ranging from fear of retaliation to simple disgust over the awkwardness of the system. Yet only in the case of domestic violence victims is the failure to pursue the matter held against the victim in future complaints. Significantly, it is only in these cases that a pattern of attrition by some complainants is used to disenfranchise *all* such victims. This approach is the reason that I have described the criminal justice system's response to domestic violence victims as a systematic pattern of discrimination every bit as pervasive as that practiced in race discrimination cases.

The question becomes, how is the class of victim identified? It is clear that female victims of stranger-to-stranger violence do not experience this discrimination. Nor is the boundary fixed by the state of marriage or cohabitation since women who have long ago terminated their relationships continue to be disenfranchised.

I believe that the only common denominator among these victims was prior sexual access. Since there is nothing in the act of coitus itself to imply a surrender of autonomy on the part of the female, further reflection was needed. I concluded that consensual sexual access is widely interpreted in our society as denoting a proprietary right of the man over the woman. Although she may initially be empowered to deny the conferring of property status through access to her body, once given, she no longer exercises control over its continuation. This property notion explains abuser attitudes and behaviors—"I have a right and duty to discipline her." Since it appears to be a widely, if not universally shared notion, it also explains how the criminal justice system determines her to be less worthy of the rights extended to female victims of crime generally. It appears that once conferred, the property right can only be renounced by the man himself. He will not accept even legal dissolution orders. There are many cases of men periodically seeking out former wives and assaulting them, some after more than 25 years. Amazingly, these cases are usually treated by the criminal justice system as though the parties still cohabitated.

Despite the skirmishes and occasional battles, many police executives were willing to address the problem of their agency's neglect or outright hostility to the abused wife. It would be reassuring to report that once they had been made aware of their own culpability in contributing to the problems of conjugal violence, police executives immediately set out to correct the problem in the same way they would address a traditional crime control problem, that is, to look at and change policy, procedures, and philosophy where necessary, and to monitor compliance and address continued malfunctions in the organization. This was not the case.

Basically, no policy or operational changes were made. The problem was turned over to behavioral scientists for recommendations on how best to respond. They did not view spouse abuse as a crime, but instead saw it as a social issue calling for a crisis intervention. This intervention was not the traditional criminal intervention involving arrest and charge, but an intervention requiring police officers to act as counselors, mediators, and conciliators. It was precisely what some of them had been doing for generations without the specialized training to perform that role. The concept was one of specialized teams of highly motivated, specially trained, and selected officers who would respond to the scene and attempt to reconcile any dispute. Experiments with such a schema were carried out and reported as highly successful. The result was replication in 23 cities in the United States at a cost of $8 million.[7]

Only later did it occur to critics that the "success" of police as counselors had been predicated on the criteria of "lack of callback" (the absence of additional calls to the police). Some suggest that success may not be the only reason for lack of callback. The parties may have moved, or they may have separated, or one could be dead. I believe a more likely scenario finds the victim unwilling during any future conflicts to call for the team which, in her view, did not perform the functions she expected or felt were necessary.

In our society, police officers perform many different functions and duties, but central to our conceptualization of them when we are victims of crime is that they will arrest and charge the accused. What would be our reaction if we were victimized by a burglar, and the responding officer spent his time attempting to establish the culprits underlying desire or need to steal? Clearly the officer would not be performing the role expected of him. Should we be victimized in the future, such officers would not be called, and if they responded, they would not be welcome.

In short, a police officer therapist is a contradiction in terms. This does not mean that officers do not, in their daily routines, often and in many different contexts, function as advisors, counselors, and confidants. However, there is a substantial difference in performing these functions on an ad hoc basis and instructing police officers to routinely perform those functions.

First, there is no legal basis for officers to perform these functions. Even the naive, poorly educated abuser knows the officer's right to intervene is based solely on his right to arrest. Although such a person may not (but sometimes does) physically resist an extralegal intrusion into his home to deliver therapy, he does recognize his right to refuse to accept such an offer. In fact, this knowledge allows him to maintain an element of power and control that he would not have in an arrest situation. Unfortunately—at least in my opinion—this "police-officer-as-specialized-therapist" concept persists in parts of the country.

In 1976 the Detroit Police Department adopted new policies and procedures for its response to domestic violence calls. First was the unequivocal policy declaration that interspousal assault was no different than the same act committed by strangers. Second, if there was probable cause to believe a crime had been committed, an arrest should be made if legally permissible. Third, a report of the crime was mandatory. This report must be assigned to an investigator for follow-up and prosecution. In addition, medical documentation, pictorial evidence, and third-party witnesses were not required unless they were required in all other similar cases.

Because compliance with such major policy changes is often not complete or voluntary, a special computer program was established to permit administrators to monitor compliance. All domestic violence calls were coded in a "3900" series. Whether these were injunction violations or homicides, they were so coded. Supervisors were required to monitor compliance with the new policies and procedures. They were to censure noncompliance and acknowledge superior performance.

All public-generated complaints of poor performance were followed up with complete investiga-

tions, and punishment or corrective action was taken when appropriate. Soon voluntary compliance became the norm, and only rarely are complaints received.

Recognizing that mere policy change unaccompanied by special training designed to overcome the myths surrounding domestic violence would not be successful, Detroit police administrators determined to develop a training package. It was believed that two types of training were essential. First, a training model for recruits would be more extensive than for experienced officers. Because it would not primarily be geared to overcoming established preconceptions and experience, the recruit training would be substantially different as well as longer in duration.

Training of tenured officers would be briefer, but would also attempt to change a set of attitudes and beliefs officers had acquired over a long period of time. It could also be expected that because these attitudes had been shaped by the officers' experiences, their peers, and their agency, they would be extremely difficult to change. In fact, it was recognized that attitudinal change may not be possible. In such an event, only behaviors were thought to be susceptible to meaningful change.

It was difficult to develop the two required modules because staff members could not identify any extant programs that sought to accomplish the agency's goals. Virtually every module reviewed was designed by behaviorists whose goal was clearly to train the officer as mediator, counselor, or therapist. Because it already had been decided that this was not the desired model, such modules were rejected. Finally, Detroit's own model was created.

Although the adopted training curriculum is too long and complex to consider here, some of the principles governing its design merit discussion. First, the decision was made not to confront the officer with his presumed lack of sensitivity, concern for the victim, or discriminatory behavior. It was assumed that these were not the officer's fault, but rather that of the system of which he was a part. Furthermore, the officer was not going to be regaled with horror stories of victims; he had seen this firsthand. Perhaps he had seen incidents even more atrocious than the trainer. The woman's failure to follow through with prosecution, her tendency to return to the abusive male, or to sometimes turn on the officer and assist in his assault would all be acknowledged as true, thus removing his source of denial or excuse.

The training module focused on the procedural and legal aspects of police involvement in the domestic call. The police officer would be instructed of the very real dangers inherent in these cases and how best to cope with them: what to be alert to and safeguard against; how to approach the scene and the situation; what to say to the parties; how to elicit information sufficient to arrest or make a report. The officer would be encouraged to do these things in sequence and to depart after having achieved the various levels. Only after it became clear that an arrest was not possible or desirable would the officer be given information that would allow him to offer further assistance through referral.

Officers were given complete and comprehensive information on other services available, which ones would be appropriate, and how the client could begin to use these services. They were equipped with referral forms that were also sent to the referred agency, which was encouraged to provide feedback information to the officer on referred clients. Whenever possible, all private and public agencies offering services to abused women were asked to participate either directly or as resource persons during the actual training.

Although lectures, review of the law department policy, and orders remained an integral part of the training, role-playing was used extensively. At first, professional actors played the roles. Later the officers themselves did so. The skits were designed to examine some of the more prevailing myths as well as the dynamics of spouse abuse itself. The officer was assisted in formulating his own understanding of each of these situations.

The training was neither preachy nor righteous, but sought to direct the officer to the inevitable conclusion that there was a victim, in every sense of the word, who required his professional police atten-

tion. If she did not avail herself of his help or that to which she was referred, she was no less worthy than any other citizen victimized by a stranger.

Although it was not a part of the program, officers often concluded that not only was this victim equally entitled to police protection, but because of the extraordinary circumstance of living with the abuser, she might have an even greater need to be protected. It became clearer to the officer why the abuser needed a strong, direct, and clear message that his behavior was wrong.

An unanticipated but nonetheless welcome side effect of this officer training was the relatively large number of police officers who recognized in themselves the propensity to use violence in their own relationships. Many sought professional help. As a result, the already existent Personal Affairs Section, heretofore specializing in alcohol and substance abuse, found itself offering counseling services for officers and their spouses.

Unfortunately, Detroit's deteriorating fiscal situation forced the postponement of this training before it was completed for the entire department. In addition, because only recruit and frontline officers were initially trained and they were laid off in fiscal cutbacks to be replaced by older but untrained officers, much of the anticipated benefit remains unrealized. As the city's fiscal situation improves, the program may be completed.

Although not directly a Detroit Police Department function, a series of events in 1977 and 1978 are important to the police role in domestic violence.

The process of reviewing spouse abuse laws began with the formation of the Social Conflict Task Force. As the result of the work of the task force, proposed legislation was introduced in Michigan's House of Representatives by the Honorable Connie Binsfield of Traverse City. The proposed legislation that many had recommended sought to strengthen the hand of law enforcement and also provide for protective services for the abused spouse.

A joint legislative task force was formed that recommended legislation designed to achieve these goals. In 1978 the Michigan legislature passed these bills, and they were signed into law by Governor

William Milliken. There are two distinct pieces of legislation, but because they thoroughly complement each other, they are considered together.

The police-related issues of these laws are discussed first. Police officers are empowered to make arrests for misdemeanors not committed in their presence in spouse abuse cases. Previously, the officer was often required to leave the victim in a continuing dangerous situation, lacking the power to arrest or the ability to defuse the situation. For the first time, disobeying the terms of a spouse abuse protective order was made a criminal offense. Heretofore, such a violation was only civil contempt, and the officer could not arrest without a warrant for such violation. This law was amended in 1979 to permit extension of its protection to unmarried cohabitants, and even those married women not filing for divorce. Finally, the law required all police agencies to report spouse abuse to the Michigan State Police so that a data base could be started.

With regard to nonpolice-related issues, the legislation created a Domestic Violence Prevention and Treatment Board. This board was empowered to expend state funds to establish and continue operating domestic violence shelters to house such victims. In addition, the board was charged with the responsibility for public awareness and education programs, as well as programs designed for the prevention and treatment of domestic violence.

The board now funds 42 shelter programs and a resource library. In addition, the board conducts seminars and training programs for shelter personnel and assists in such programs for a range of professional groups, including law enforcement, legal officers, courts, and medical personnel.

I served as chairperson of the Domestic Violence Prevention and Treatment Board from 1978 to 1991. Unfortunately, the needs of battered women for shelters have severely hampered efforts in the public education, prevention, and treatment responsibilities of the board; the latter have suffered the inevitable setting of priorities inherent in the need to provide immediate protection and assistance to women most in need. These shelter programs offer an invaluable resource to police officers and other professionals who generally encounter cases of domestic violence.

INTERFACE WITH NURSING

A common thought is that the first person to have direct contact with the victim of domestic violence is the police officer. This is only partially true. The Bannon and Wilt study (1977) documented that at least 50% of all known victims of domestic violence cases required medical treatment. It should be remembered that only about 50% of all domestic violence cases are reported to the police. It is unknown what proportion of these respective ratios overlap, or how many of the 50% of cases reported to the police are the same as those seen by health care personnel.

To date, there has been no significant effort to correlate the activities and knowledge of the two disciplines. I believe that medical administrators have openly opposed or resisted medical personnel playing an active role with the police in identifying these cases, cooperating in the obtaining of evidence, and preserving it for subsequent presentation in court. It is suspected that potential legal liability for misassessment is not the whole story. Doctor-patient privilege is certainly an issue; A substantial concern for privacy issues remains. There may also be concern with the potential loss of services of staff because of documentation and evidential needs that influences these judgments. A standard emergency room walk-in patient, bearing signs of blunt force trauma or perhaps stab or cutting wounds is a good example. The patient is often accompanied by a man who is either actually (or presumed to be) the spouse. The health care professional seeing this patient is told that the injury occurred in a certain manner. The explanation is often improbable, if not impossible; however, it is recorded and no further information is sought. In fact, the interview usually continues in the presence and obviously under the influence of the person suspected of causing the injury.

Despite state statutes that either require or permit medical personnel to notify local law enforcement agencies of the injury, no such notification, in fact, usually occurs. When authorities *are* notified, the file is so incomplete that it is virtually useless for evidential purposes. It is often impossible to even determine who made the notations in the file. Moreover, when the essential information is on the official medical record, law enforcement personnel have extreme difficulty in obtaining this evidence without a court order.

Emergency room personnel should be sensitive to and trained in the dynamics of domestic violence. They should be aware of its symptoms as well as the inherent need for the client to deny its occurrence, because of embarrassment, fear, confusion, or self-doubt. There should be a firm institutional policy of notification of authorities, along with a fixing of responsibilities for such notification. There should be an established protocol to enable nursing personnel to elicit information regarding the nature of the injury and the patient's description of how the injury occurred. These documents should be separate from the medical records, and copies should be provided to the law enforcement agency, the institution, and the person reporting.

It is obvious that the hospital administration must take a leading role in establishing the policies empowering and supporting staff to perform these functions. In addition, hospitals should ensure that their assigned social worker staff is thoroughly familiar with spouse abuse. Such staff members should be directed to follow up with patients who the nursing personnel suspect are victims of domestic violence, but who may initially deny the cause of the injury. One case dramatically illustrates the value of high levels of awareness, commitment to serve, and intelligent observation of nursing personnel. A patient was admitted suffering from what was diagnosed as peritonitis due to a ruptured colon. She casually related to one of her nurses that her husband routinely abused her by rendering severe blows to the stomach, sometimes with his feet. She denied, when questioned further by the nurse, that such an assault had preceded this particular admission. However, she did admit continuing distress since the last assault some weeks previously.

The nurse recorded this information and reported it to her supervisors, who in turn notified the Michigan State Police. Officers interviewed the patient, who denied that she had been beaten or that she had even told the nurse that such was the case.

A short time later, the patient died. The police agency reopened its case and was able to locate additional witnesses who could attest to the patient's having complained to them of the assaults. In fact, other corroborating evidence was obtained. The husband was indicted and awaits trial for second-degree murder. This would not have been possible if the nurse ignored the patient's claim of prior abuse, failed to record it, or did not notify her supervisors or the police agency.

The most interesting aspect of this case is that the nurse involved and the state police detective who took a personal interest in following up the case, despite the patient's recanting of her story, had both participated in a community seminar on spouse abuse conducted by a local shelter program. Thus both had had their own awareness raised as well as their commitment increased to bring heightened awareness to their respective professional lives.

Like police officers, nursing personnel wear at least two hats—their professional serving, caring hat as a health care professional, and their citizen, member-of-the-community hat. It is within the community context that nurses can provide almost as vital a service as in the professional milieu. They are uniquely qualified as sensitive, caring professionals to convey to the community their knowledge of the magnitude and seriousness of the issue of domestic violence.

It is also true that by training and temperament, most nurses are superbly qualified to serve as volunteer staff in programs offering direct victim services. Yet, the capacity to serve is not limited to health care delivery. Generally, nurses are excellent role models for women who lack the confidence in themselves necessary to break the vicious circle of dependency, low self-esteem, and feelings of entrapment. Often it is in association with such role models that the process of empowerment begins. Nurses generally bring to their professional lives a sense of caring and concern without the need to overpower the patient or to think for her. In other words, they enable the client to do for herself, rather than attempt to do for her.

Nursing personnel can make substantial contributions when they encounter battered women, either professionally or personally. Some of the areas they can address are briefly outlined.

First, nurses should prepare themselves by learning as much as possible about the issue of domestic violence. They then are in a position to understand the concerns of the victim and the requirements for successful prosecution. Most importantly, they should be aware of all the resources available in the community to the battered woman. In addition, the nurse should be familiar with her legal rights and responsibilities in relation to domestic violence. The nurse has some protection with respect to maintaining confidentiality (see Chapter 14). However, the nurse also has an obligation to report any weapon-related injury or suspicious trauma to the police.

Nurses should be aware that prosecution is not always possible. They should have some knowledge of the legal requirements and limitations on the prosecutorial possibilities. Nothing confuses the victim more than the well-intentioned but erroneous representation that arrest and prosecution are always possible. Well-intentioned insistence that the victim must prosecute is often counterproductive since the victim who does not prosecute her abuser may feel some self-recrimination or even disloyalty if she fails to do so.

Nursing personnel should advise the battered woman that prosecution is probably available and should be pursued if the case meets the legal requirements for an indictment. Such personnel should also become familiar with the procedures in the local jurisdiction for appealing lower-level decisions that adversely affect the client's rights. Often such redress is available within the police organization itself. If not, many groups designed to act as advocates for the victim are often available in the community. These include legal aid societies and women's justice groups. Advice on the existence of such groups is always available through shelter programs, legal aid societies, and feminist groups.

Finally, nursing personnel should be familiar with the rudiments of evidence that may be required for presentation in court. As with rape victims, victims of domestic violence often have a revulsion to articles associated with the crime itself.

They may burn or discard bloody clothing, weapons, or other instruments used in the assault. It is not uncommon for the woman to shower and change clothes before seeking medical or other professional help. It has even been recorded that the victim will call the police and then clean up, almost thoroughly obliterating all evidence of the assault, before opening the door for the responding officers. This behavior is difficult to understand without appreciation of the level of embarrassment the victim feels because she is a victim.

Generally, all physical and trace evidence should be preserved. A record of witnesses should be obtained. It is important to specify to the client that a witness need not have actually *seen* the assault. They may have heard something or witnessed some part of the transaction not directly involved in the assault itself. These witnesses must be identified to the responding officers so their report reflects this information. All physical evidence including medical diagnosis, x-ray films, pictorial representation, and notes of medical observations must also be preserved and reported. Finally, and often most difficult, nursing personnel must make a commitment to testify in court regarding their actions and observations. In many cases, this may entail personal sacrifices in both time and perhaps wages.

ARREST AS A DETERRENT

This material was written by Janet E. Findlater.

Law enforcement response to domestic violence has been the subject of much scrutiny and debate during the last 20 years. It is no less so today.

In the 1970s, as part of the women's liberation movement, women began advocating for change in the perception of and response to domestic violence. They spoke and wrote about the lives of battered women and established safe home networks and shelters. They also went to their legislatures and courts seeking safety and justice for women and their children.[8]

A basic tenet of the battered women's movement is that domestic violence is criminal conduct and should be treated as such. Historically, society has regarded domestic violence as a private matter, not a public one. Criminal laws have not been enforced in these cases. Police department policies usually provided that arrest was to be avoided if at all possible in domestic violence calls; mediation or conciliation was the appropriate response.

Battered women and their advocates used a number of strategies in the 1970s and 1980s to change the "arrest only as a last resort" response of the police to domestic violence. They filed lawsuits against police departments, seeking new department policy, money damages, or both.[9] Perhaps the most publicized suit was that by Tracey Thurman in 1984 against the city of Torrington, Connecticut.[10] A jury awarded Thurman, whose repeated requests for assistance from the police had been denied, $2.3 million after she was almost killed by her husband. In the wake of the *Thurman* decision, many police departments, concerned about liability for failure to respond to domestic violence calls, adopted policies providing that domestic violence is a crime and arrest is the appropriate response.

In addition, battered women and their advocates went to the legislatures. In some states, arrest is now mandatory in domestic violence cases.[11] In many states, police may now arrest for violation of an order of protection.[12] Police arrest powers in most states have been expanded to permit arrest without a warrant for domestic misdemeanor assaults not committed in the officer's presence.[13]

Changing the police response from mediation to arrest should not occur in a vacuum. The police are only one component of the criminal justice system, and the criminal justice system is but one part of the community. Until the entire community responds consistently and appropriately by holding the assailant responsible for his criminal behavior and refusing to tolerate domestic violence, women will not be safe and justice will not be served.

The model for a coordinated community response to domestic violence is the program started in Duluth, Minnesota in 1982. The Duluth program has been replicated in communities throughout the country. In Duluth, when there is probable cause to believe a crime has been committed, the assailant is arrested and held in jail overnight. Charges are filed, and either the assailant pleads guilty or the prosecutor takes the case to trial. Generally, if it is his first offense, the assailant, on conviction, is given a 30-day suspended sentence, put on probation, and ordered to complete a 26-week batterer's education program. If he fails to attend the batterer's program, he is sent to jail to serve 30 days. If he is arrested and convicted again for domestic violence, his sentence is longer. Ellen Pence, one of the founders of the Duluth project, reports that during the 10 years the program has been in effect, no Duluth women have been killed in a domestic homicide.[14]

It is in light of the work over the past 20 years that the recent and much-publicized call for abolition of mandatory arrest laws by criminologist Lawrence Sherman must be considered.[15] In 1984 Sherman and Berk conducted a study in Minneapolis of the deterrent effect of three police interventions in domestic violence calls: arrest, mediation, and separation. They found that arrest was more likely to result in a reduction in violence than either mediation or separation.[16]

The National Institute of Justice funded six studies to replicate the Sherman and Berk Minneapolis experiment.[17] Sherman conducted one of those studies in Milwaukee and found that, at least in some cases (short-term arrest of unemployed men living in poverty ghetto areas), arrest resulted in an increase in violence.[18] Because Sherman had found in Minneapolis that arrest had a deterrent effect, his finding in Milwaukee, that in some cases it had a criminogenic effect, drew considerable attention. The significance of that finding deserves further study.[19]

Of concern to battered women and their advocates, however, was Sherman's immediate call for a reversal in policy with regard to arrest in domestic violence cases. Such a call, based on the Milwaukee study, seems premature, at best. Many questions have been raised by Sherman's findings, but his rush to conclude that mandatory arrest laws should be repealed is puzzling.

In the Milwaukee study, the deterrent effect of three police interventions was examined: warning, short-term arrest (assailant in custody 2.8 hours), and long-term arrest (assailant in custody 11.1

hours). Only the short-term arrest was found to have a criminogenic effect.

A few observations can be made. First, the finding that short-term arrest produces a criminogenic effect is simply not relevant in jurisdictions where arrest is not a short-term intervention. In Michigan, for example, state law requires that assailants be arraigned before being released or be held in custody 20 hours.[20] In the Duluth program, assailants are held in jail overnight after arrest.

In addition, Sherman's findings are not inconsistent with a call for arrest in the context of a coordinated community response to domestic violence.

In considering the arrest studies, it is important to remember that battering is learned behavior. A batterer chooses to use violence as a way to gain and maintain control over his partner. That a single arrest intervention does not change that behavior and stop the violence is not surprising. An appropriate police response to domestic violence is critical. But the message that domestic violence is a crime and it will not be tolerated cannot be delivered by the police alone. The entire criminal justice system must treat domestic violence as a crime. In addition, shelter and other support must be available to battered women and their children. It is in the context of a coordinated community response that the effectiveness of arrest should be studied.

SUMMARY

To summarize briefly, domestic violence is a serious national problem, and its costs in emotional and physical pain are astronomical. Costs in real dollars through medical payments, lost wages, and other related costs are incalculable.

The problem is not, as it has been in the past, a personal problem of the victim. The impact of domestic violence on society is so great that it becomes a clear public issue. As a public issue, it demands the efforts of all members of society to ameliorate its effects and attempt to interdict its tragic consequences.

Nursing professionals and the police share the responsibility to perform their duties so that the victim of domestic violence is not further brutalized by the system designed to protect and serve her. Nei-

ther discipline has performed its duties as well as it could. A major premise of this chapter is to specify nursing and law enforcement obligations, but more importantly to urge a joint, cooperative effort to do everything possible to redress not only past neglect but also future discrimination. Increased contact and exchange between the disciplines of law enforcement and nursing serve as avenues for mutually beneficial collaboration.

The real issue is violence generically. Violence is learned behavior, and it is learned in the home. However, it is differentially learned. That is, violence is appropriate male behavior, but inappropriate female behavior. Thus one half of our society is identified at conception as potential, if not probable, victims; the other half is identified as potential, if not probable, assailants—all without regard to who or what they are or to what they achieve or fail to achieve. Such biological determinism should be repugnant to all of us. Only through a conscious and combined effort will society be able to interdict the intergenerational transmission of violence by men against women.

REFERENCES

1. James Bannon and Marie Wilt, Domestic Violence and the Police: Studies in Detroit and Kansas City (1977).
2. Joan Zorza, *The Criminal Law of Misdemeanor Domestic Violence*, 1970–1990, 83 J. Crim. L. & Criminology 46, 48-49 (1992).
3. Lawrence Sherman, Crime and Justice: A Review of the Research Attacking Crime, in 15 Modern Policing (Michael Tonry & Norval Morris eds., 1992).
4. Faith McNulty, The Burning Bed (1980).
5. People v. Janet Smith, Otsego County Circuit Court (1978).
6. Sue E. Eisenberg & Patricia L. Micklow, *The Assaulted Wife: "Catch 22" Revisited*, 3 Women's Rts. Rptr. 138 (1977).
7. National Criminal Justice Association, The Function of the Police in Crisis Intervention and Conflict Management, A Training Guide (1974).
8. Del Martin, Battered Wives (1983); Susan Schechter, Women and Male Violence: The Visions and Struggles of the Battered Women's Movement (1982).
9. Executive Deputy Chief Bannon discussed the suits in Oakland, California and New York City earlier in this chapter.
10. 595 F. Supp. 1521 (Dist. Conn. 1984).

11. These states include, among others, Oregon, Washington, Connecticut, Wisconsin, Iowa, New Jersey and Maine. Current information on the status of mandatory arrest can be obtained from the National Center on Women and Family Law, 799 Broadway, Room 402, New York, N.Y. 10003.

12. These states include, among others, Oregon, Washington, Minnesota, Michigan, Massachusetts, New Jersey, Texas, and Wisconsin.

13. For a good discussion of these issues see Joan Zorza, *The Criminal Law of Misdemeanor Domestic Violence*, 1970–1990, 83 J. Crim. L. & Criminology 46 (1992).

14. Jan Hoffman, *When Men Hit Women*, N.Y. Times Magazine, Feb. 16, 1992, 23, 25.

15. *Arrest Can Increase Domestic Violence, Milwaukee Study Finds*, Crime Control Digest, vol. 25, n. 47, Nov. 25, 1991; *Do Arrests Increase the Rates of Repeated Domestic Violence?*, N.Y. Times, Nov. 27, 1991, at C8, col. 4.

16. Lawrence Sherman and Richard Berk, *The Minneapolis Domestic Violence Experiment*, 1 Police Found. Rep.1 (1984).

17. For reports on the arrest studies in Charlotte, North Carolina, Omaha, Nebraska, and Colorado Springs, Colorado see 83 J. Crim. L. & Criminology (1992).

18. Lawrence Sherman, *The Variable Effects of Arrest on Criminal Careers: The Milwaukee Domestic Violence Experiment*, 83 J. Crim. L. & Criminology 137 (1992); Lawrence Sherman, *From Initial Deterrence to Long-Term Escalation: Short-Custody Arrest for Poverty Ghetto Domestic Violence*, 29 Criminology 821 (1991).

19. For commentaries by Cynthia Grant Bowman, Lisa A. Frisch, Lisa G. Lerman, David B. Mitchell, Daniel D. Polsby and Joan Zorza on the arrest studies see 83 J. Crim. L. & Criminology (1992).

20. Mich. Comp. Laws Ann. Sec. 750.582a.

C H A P T E R

The Nurse and the Legal System
Dealing with Abused Children

Joyce Underwood Munro

THE LEGAL CONCEPT OF CHILD ABUSE

Every case of child abuse and neglect encountered has legal ramifications for the nurse. The nature of nursing practice is such that entry into the lives of families is personal and frequent. Child abuse as a legal concept is a relatively new phenomenon that is historically based on laws against infanticide. This chapter examines these historical roots and describes the legal concepts of corporal punishment, criminal procedure relative to child abuse, and modern child protection laws. Against this background, nursing responsibilities to the child and the community within the judicial system are delineated. The nurse's role in testifying in specific cases and the nurse's potential as an expert witness are examined. The latter role is advocated as an important contribution that has not been previously used in the spectrum of nursing practice.

Infanticide and the Law

Until recently in Western societies, the law has considered children as chattels or near-chattels of their fathers. Children's status is also tied to the relatively low legal status of women. Illegitimate children (children literally without the legal protection of a father) and their unmarried mothers (women without the legal protection of a husband) were particularly at risk in a society that morally condemned their status and left them with few economic opportunities for survival. Under the Law of the Twelve Tables of ancient Rome, a father had life and death power over his children.

It is not surprising, then, that as long as there have been laws against murder, assault, and battery, there has been ambivalence whether they apply when a child is the victim. Infanticide was commonly practiced in ancient Thebes, even though it was a capital offense.[1] Figures of myth, history, and

343

literature were "exposed," or abandoned as infants, including Egypt's Horus, the Jews' Moses, Sophocles' Oedipus, and Romulus and Remus.[2] Throughout history and undoubtedly before, children have been killed for various reasons, with or without the sanction of society. Indeed, "anthropologically, infanticide refers to the killing of a newborn with the consent of the parent, family, or community."[3] This consent takes the form of decree by a group leader, as with the orders of Pharoah and Herod for the slaughter of the innocents, or of the group's tacit acceptance of individual acts. Infanticidal behavior is also found among primates.[4]

Infanticide was also practiced and condoned as a form of population control, particularly in times of famine, war, and social stress. Sometimes unusual births or those resulting in deformed babies were followed by infanticide.[5] The law of ancient Sparta required new parents to bring their infants for inspection by the elders; if an infant was deemed weak or defective, it was cast off a mountain.[6] Infanticide was the legally decreed fate of deformed children under the Roman Law of the Twelve Tables. Martin Luther recommended that mentally defective children, believed to be instruments of the devil, should be drowned.[7] The practice of allowing mentally defective or severely malformed infants to die by withholding food and water or corrective surgery continues. The highly publicized "Baby Doe" cases of the mid-1980s exposed the medical practices of denying food and hydration to seriously malformed neonates, and of withholding simple or sophisticated lifesaving medical and surgical treatments to mentally defective or deformed infants.[8] Advances in medical technology force physicians and parents to make difficult ethical decisions.

Illegitimate children were, and still are, more frequent targets of infanticide. Considering the social ostracism to which their mothers were often subjected and the economic hardships of a single woman, these infants often paid the price of women's low status in society. Traditional recourse for mothers of illegitimate children included concealing the pregnancy and "overlaying" or exposing the infant; paying an unscrupulous midwife to arrange

for the death of the child at birth; hiring herself out as a wet nurse, at the expense of her own child's food supply; and abandoning the infant on a doorstep, at a foundling home, or in the nearest sewer.

Concealing a pregnancy was unlawful in eighteenth century Europe. Unmarried women were required to register their pregnancies, and if they did not have an infant to show at the end of the term, they could be tried for infanticide. The penalties varied from high fines to cruel execution. Although many married women disposed of children they could not handle, only married women were ever acquitted of "overlaying."[9] There were different rules for prosecution of mothers committing infanticide; the law treated mothers under the protection of a husband much more leniently.

Midwives were always available to do indirectly what an unwilling mother risked everything to do directly. Before the professionalization of medicine, midwives were responsible for establishing and reporting the cause of death of infants and children. Thus it was possible for a midwife to kill an unwanted infant, for a fee for her deed and silence.

The notion of foster care is ancient and indeed is mentioned in the Code of Hammurabi and in the Bible.[10] Throughout history fostering served a variety of political and social functions, including strengthening family alliances by an exchange of children for rearing. Some of these arrangements amounted to an accepted form of hostage-holding, deterring different factions from aggression against each other with the threat that such action would result in the aggressor's heir being put to death in retaliation.

The taking in of abandoned children by private individuals and by institutions involved a variety of practices.[11] Our contemporary notion of state-regulated foster care, with theoretically strict standards of medical and legal surveillance, is relatively recent. It would be easy to cite historical and literary examples of greedy guardians, foster parents, and masters killing their wards or apprentices by starvation and ill-usage, while pocketing the fees they received for their care, but even our contemporary systems of supervised foster care fail to protect all children from abuse and neglect.[12]

The wet nurse system operated as another example of a legally condoned method of infanticide. During the nineteenth century in London, 80% of the illegitimate children put out to nurse died.[13] But in societies where putting children out to nurse was the norm for the well-to-do, as it was in the Italian Renaissance, the one who paid for the practice was the nurse's own infant, who generally starved or was in turn put out to nurse while his or her mother cared for the wealthy client's child.[14] The fate of the nurse's child was never discussed and was in fact repressed from the consciousness of a society that needed the nurse's services. Becoming a wet nurse, like becoming a prostitute, was one of the few sources of economic survival open to poor young women who found themselves with an illegitimate child. The interdependence of society on the wet nurse and of the wet nurse on her clients led to a striking situation: while infanticide was punishable by death everywhere in Europe, "it seems that infanticidal mothers were punished by death. Wet nurses were not.[15] Thus the wet nurse was both a "professional feeder and a professional killer,"[16] and in accepting her services society condoned the unfortunate consequences of the system.

The foundling hospitals established in the eighteenth century appeared to present a humane method of dealing with unwanted children. Although the hospitals at first seemed a good idea and gave women somewhere to place the children that they did not want or could not care for, the death rate of these institutionalized infants was alarming. Even at the best hospitals, only about one third of the infants survived to become school age.[17] In addition to the problems of finding adequate wet nurses for all the young patients, undoubtedly many, if not most, of these infants suffered from what later became known as "hospitalism," a type of emotionally induced failure to thrive among the institutionalized.[18] When the hospitals were full, the surplus infants were put out to nurse, with its attendant hazards. Only after World War II were the foundling hospitals abandoned as a type of foster care.[19]

The use of child labor in industry from the eighteenth through the early twentieth centuries also led to deaths of children from starvation, overwork, injury, disease, and suicide. But the industrial revolution provided a market for unwanted children. For years their hardships were disregarded by industrializing societies that must have been aware of the exploitation of these children. Because society needed this cheap pool of labor at the time, it legally condoned this treatment of children.

Corporal Punishment of Children

Corporal punishment of children has long been accepted in most Western societies as necessary to make the child obey and learn. This belief is echoed in the biblical intonation that "he that spareth the rod hateth his son: but he that loveth him chasteneth him betimes."[20] Under the *Patria Potestas* of ancient Rome, the father had the power of life and death over his children, including the right to sell, discipline, abandon, or do whatever he pleased with them. Massachusetts in 1646 and Connecticut in 1651 imposed the death penalty on unruly children, although more often the punishment actually meted out was public whipping.[21] Harsh physical punishment was the usual form of discipline.

Beatings were also administered to "drive out evil spirits" thought to be residing within children because of their "impish" playfulness or affliction with madness or epilepsy. Today nurses in emergency rooms still see badly beaten children of parents who firmly believe religious injunctions to beat their child for disobedience. Sometimes such parents do not or cannot stop until the child is dead. When tried for second-degree murder or for manslaughter, such parents steadfastly maintain that they had to beat the devil out of the child, and they seem somewhat incredulous that society does not agree. Some parents jokingly threaten their children by saying "if you don't stop that, I'm going to beat the devil out of you."

Corporal punishment has been used by parents, guardians, teachers, and masters to whom a child was apprenticed. In the United States parents and teachers in the public schools may legally administer corporal punishment to children. In 1977 the Supreme Court of the United States held that corporal punishment in the public schools was not cruel and unusual punishment under the Eighth Amendment to the United States Constitution, nor was it a violation of a schoolchild's Fourteenth Amendment right to due process of law.[22] Thus a common-law right still exists for teachers (and parents) to punish children with physical force. Until recently children have been completely barred from suing their parents for injuries the parents inflicted on them intentionally or negligently by the doctrine of family immunity from suit. The legal rationale for this common-law rule is that it preserves family harmony; in effect it preserves parental power over children without regard to the consequences. In some jurisdictions parental immunity has been moderated to allow some suits to be brought by children for personal injuries suffered at the hands of parents.

In divorce practice today many child custody orders still award "possession" of the minor children to the father or the mother. Although the term "possession" here is synonymous with "physical custody," it nevertheless reverberates with connotations of the child as chattel.

In addition to corporal punishment and the sometimes sanctioned practice of infanticide, children have been and continue to be mutilated by their caretakers. Footbinding, castration, headshaping, and other practices were considered acceptable in the societies in which they were practiced. In some places, children continue to be mutilated to make them look more pathetic as street beggars. Countless child laborers were maimed and crippled in the machinery of the industrial revolution. Industrialists of the nineteenth century discovered "that children, especially poor ones, constituted the world's most inexpensive and unprotected labor force, that they could be made to substitute for the machine."[23] As a measure of how acceptable child mutilation is today in the United States, note the number of earpiercings practiced on infants, and the fact that circumcisions are now routinely performed on unanesthetized infants by parents who have no religious, ethnic, or medical mandate for doing so.[24]

Medical Model of Child Abuse

The law's historical ambiguity toward children continues today in some of the forms mentioned. The criminal law provides that murder, manslaughter, assault and battery, mayhem, and other crimes apply regardless of the victim, but the idea persists that somehow killing one's own child is different from other homicides. The common-law privilege to use corporal punishment makes it difficult, legally, to decide whether to treat the striking of a child as allowable discipline or forbidden assault and battery. One commentator opens an article on criminal child abuse prosecutions with the statement, "Child abuse differs from other criminal assaults or homicides."[25] Some judges still occasionally dismiss criminal charges in cases resulting in death or serious injury on the basis of parental right to discipline, believing the injuries to be the result of an accident or of "things getting out of hand." At the other extreme, some parents are vigorously prosecuted for far less serious neglect or abuse, usually following intense media exposure of the case. These parents may be society's scapegoats, punished publicly for what the community is evidently powerless to prevent—child abuse.

In the nineteenth century the law began to limit the power of parents over children. Under the doctrine of *parens patriae*, which stated a general guardian of the community could intercede in family matters to protect children, courts began to remove cruelly treated children from their parents. By the end of the nineteenth century, England and France had enacted legislation for the protection of maltreated and abandoned children. At the same time, some cities in the United States were establishing homes for wayward (delinquent) children; such homes also took in abandoned and ill-treated children. The celebrated case of Mary Ellen in New York City in 1874 spurred the development of child protection legislation (see Chapter 5). Today all states have such legislation that provides that the state can become the child's guardian or even remove the child from the parent's care if the child is subjected to cruelty, neglect, an unfit home, or abandonment.

By the late 1960s there was an explosion in medical attention to and knowledge about child abuse.[26] Caffey,[27] Silverman,[28] Wooley and Evans,[29] and Kempe et al.[30] reported their findings to the medical profession, and the "battered child syndrome" became a medical diagnosis. Despite the increased awareness of child abuse, many cases nevertheless went unreported. In 1962 California enacted the first statute requiring physicians to report child abuse, and by 1966 49 states had passed reporting statutes.[31] In response to the states' need for funding to carry out their reporting and treatment programs, the Congress enacted the Child Abuse Prevention and Treatment Act, effective January 31, 1974, which established criteria for state child abuse reporting statutes in order for the state to qualify for federal funds.[32] The states quickly amended their reporting laws in accord with the mandates of the federal legislation, and today all 50 states, Puerto Rico, Guam, and the Virgin Islands have reporting statutes modeled on the federal act.

The states' reporting laws do vary somewhat in their definitions of what should be reported. The categories of abuse and neglect that must be reported have been expanding, partly because of the impetus of the federal act, and partly because of increased medical and public awareness of the various forms of exploitation and maltreatment that children suffer.

For the nurse to deal effectively with the child abuse issues that she or he might face, it is necessary to detail the various situations in which the nurse can come into contact with the legal system.

THE LAW AND VIOLENT FAMILIES

There are three types of laws that can be used in child abuse situations. Parents, legal guardians, and strangers who physically attack children can be criminally prosecuted under existing criminal statutes against murder, manslaughter, sexual assault, assault and battery, and mayhem. Because of the long history of children as legally near-chattels of their parents, it has always been easier to prosecute nonrelated persons for crimes against children.

Persons accused of crimes have constitutional protections against the power of the state. The Fifth Amendment privilege against self-incrimination forbids the state from compelling a criminally accused to testify against himself. It also gives the state the legal burden of providing an accused's guilt. The burden of proof in criminal proceedings is "proof beyond a reasonable doubt," a high standard for the prosecution to meet. The Fourth Amendment protects an accused against any unreasonable searches and seizures. The Sixth Amendment requires that the accused be confronted with the witnesses against him, so that they can be cross-examined. This constitutionally guaranteed right to confrontation is a problem in a criminal prosecution for child abuse when the witness is the child and the child is afraid to testify against the abuser. The Fifth and Fourteenth Amendment guarantees of due process of law provide a number of procedural protections to the accused in a criminal proceeding.

In contrast to the criminal laws, child protection laws are considered civil in nature. The goal is to protect the children, not punish the abuser. Only parents or guardians can be made parties. The burden of proof is generally "proof by a preponderance of the evidence," a much easier standard to meet. Although parents have a constitutionally protected liberty interest in custody of their children, the procedural requirements in a child protection proceeding are less stringent than in a criminal prosecution.

Many child protection laws also allow the child or the child's estate to sue a person who fails to make a required report of child abuse in cases where the child is later reabused or killed. This civil remedy allows the child to collect damages in cases where a report would have prevented subsequent abuse. The burden of proof is "proof by a preponderance of the evidence." This cause of action exists not only to benefit a reinjured child, but it also serves as a civil law mechanism to enforce the reporting statutes. However, it is not frequently used.

When dealing with legal proceedings involving child abuse, it is important to determine which of the three types of proceedings—criminal prosecution of the parent, child protection proceeding, or civil suit for damages for failure to report—is involved, because they have different purposes and different evidentiary and procedural requirements.

CRIMINAL LAW AND CHILD ABUSE AND INFANTICIDE IN THE UNITED STATES

The existing criminal laws against assault and battery, murder and manslaughter, and criminal sexual assault can be used to charge child abusers. In addition to these, there are special statutes on child torture and criminal child neglect in many jurisdictions. If the police are involved in an investigation of child abuse and neglect, they may attempt to have the responsible parent or guardian charged under the criminal law. The implications for the parent are serious. He or she can be jailed until the trial if unable to post bond. The trial can be a humiliating experience, with the sordid details of the crime made public. If the parent pleads guilty to the charge or to lesser charges, he or she then has a criminal record. This record is public, and the parent is obliged to reveal it to all prospective employers. The parent may be placed on probation and have his or her movements and habits controlled by the conditions of probation. The parent may be sentenced to prison if he or she pleads guilty to or is convicted of one or more serious charges.

However, criminal prosecution of child abuse cases is not common. Most commentators recommend that prosecution be used only in cases where the abuse results in serious injury or death.[33] The approach holds that treatment, not punishment, should be the goal of the law. Punishment does not solve the problem of abuse, and when the parent returns home, he or she is likely to be embittered by the experience. This leaves the child at greater risk from a hostile parent. In addition, a parent who is afraid of the possibility of being jailed may be more reluctant to seek necessary medical treatment for injuries he or she inflicts on the child.

It is more difficult to prove child abuse in a criminal proceeding. The prosecutor must establish which parent or other person in the household was the perpetrator, or no one can be charged. The prosecutor (known in some states as the state's attorney,

district attorney, or public prosecutor) has the high burden of establishing the accused's guilt "beyond a reasonable doubt." A jury may have difficulty believing that a parent would actually abuse his or her child. The only eyewitness may be the child victim. If the child is verbal, he or she may have to testify against the parent to obtain a conviction. This may be more damaging to the child and the family than dropping the prosecution.

When only a few child abuse cases are processed through the criminal justice system, there is a danger that this selective enforcement will fall more harshly on one segment of the population, notably the poor. A parent whose case receives extensive media coverage is more likely to be prosecuted than another parent who caused equally serious injury, but whose case does not come under the scrutiny of the press.

When a nonrelated adult member of the household is responsible for the abuse, the policy considerations are different. There is usually no rationale for reuniting a parent's boyfriend or girlfriend with the child. In fact, criminal prosecution may be the only effective way to remove the abuser from the family when the parent is ambivalent and does not take steps to remove the offender.

The consensus that the criminal law should only be used in extreme cases of child abuse overlooks two factors. The first is that the criminal courts have a wide latitude in sentencing offenders. Although a prison term is unlikely to rehabilitate a child abuser, a creative probation order can mandate a treatment plan. If substance abuse is a problem, the court can order attendance at inpatient or outpatient treatment centers. The court usually orders the probationer to undergo counseling or psychotherapy. It can order completion of parenting skills classes. It can also control the contact of the probationer with the child victim, either forbidding it completely or providing that it be under appropriate supervision. The probation officer can refer the probationer for job training skills, budget counseling, and other services designed to help reduce the pressures that may have contributed to the child abuse. Although criminal prosecution may not be a good tool in dealing with some cases, "the *threat* of criminal prosecution may be necessary to induce some parents to have treatment."[34]

The second factor overlooked is that the policy of limiting criminal prosecution to cases of severe injury or death endorses the notion that child abuse *is* different from other forms of violence, a legacy of the centuries-old common-law privilege of parents and teachers to use corporal punishment. The only other circumstances in which an individual is privileged to use force against another are in the case of self-defense, defense of others, and in limited circumstances, defense of property. Someday our society may decide that children do not have to be physically punished to make them obey and learn. Courts may tire of deciding how to differentiate between permitted discipline and assault and battery.

Some special problems have arisen in criminal prosecution of parents for child abuse. Medicine has documented both the effects of painful withdrawal symptoms in drug-addicted neonates and the devastating effects of fetal alcohol syndrome on children since the 1970s. Most states have child protection laws that allow the removal of drug-addicted infants from their parents at birth. However, it was not until the late 1980s and the frustrations encountered in treating babies born addicted to crack cocaine that states considered criminal prosecution of pregnant women for delivering drugs to their fetuses. In 1989 Florida was the first state to obtain a criminal conviction of a pregnant woman for delivery of a controlled substance to her fetus.[35] In Michigan a mother was convicted of delivering crack cocaine to her infant through the umbilical cord in the few moments after birth. In 1991 her conviction was reversed on appeal. Critics of prosecution of drug-addicted pregnant women point out that criminal liability deters pregnant addicts from obtaining prenatal care and drug treatment. In the Florida prosecution, the trial court would not allow the defendant mother to give evidence that she tried to obtain treatment for her crack cocaine addiction but was turned away from treatment centers because she was pregnant.[36] At the time of the Florida and Michigan convictions, there were few or no drug treatment centers that accepted pregnant women.

These cases raise many troublesome policy issues. Criminal penalties are usually intended to prevent certain behaviors, but the practical effect of criminalizing drug abuse by pregnant women does not stop them from using but stops them from seeking prenatal care.[37] Significant damage may have occurred in the developing fetus before the woman is aware that she is pregnant. If the lack of drug treatment programs for pregnant addicts continues, then the criminal statute is merely a punitive measure. In late 1991 genetic researchers published evidence that cocaine abuse by prospective *fathers* can cause birth defects in their offspring. In view of these developments, further discussion is necessary to develop policies, such as effective drug abuse prevention programs, that actually protect children and do not violate constitutional principles of due process.[38]

Modern Child Protection Laws and Procedure in Juvenile Court

State child welfare laws provide for judicial intervention by the juvenile or family court. Because the statutory scheme varies from state to state, it is important for the nurse to obtain a copy of the current law in her or his state. The statutes are usually available in pamphlet form from the local department of social services or child welfare department. State legislatures change and update child welfare laws from time to time, and the changes may have a direct impact on the nurse's function in the system.

Generally, state welfare laws provide a mechanism for bringing cases to the attention of the court. Not all cases uncovered by means of the reporting laws will be brought to court. If parents agree to accept the services of a child protection worker and the risk to the child can be reduced so that the child may remain with the parents while they undergo treatment, there is no need for the court's intervention. If the case does warrant the attention of the court, then the protective services worker or some other authorized person files a petition with the court. Nurses should check to see if they are authorized to bring petitions in their states.

The child welfare laws also provide for a procedure for removal of a child from the home. In emergency situations, children in imminent danger of harm can be removed without a prior court hearing. In such instances there is a provision for a hearing on the removal within a very short period of time. In less threatening circumstances, the children may remain in the home pending the hearing on the petition.

The court procedure is usually divided into two stages: the adjudication (hearing or trial on the petition) and the disposition (hearing on where the child should be placed). There may be a pretrial conference before the adjudication, where all the parties are gathered to determine whether some agreement can be reached between the parties without having to take the petition to trial. One or both of the parents may admit some or all of the allegations in the petition. If so, a hearing is usually unnecessary if the admissions are sufficient to constitute a determination of abuse or neglect under the statutory definitions.[39] If the problems in the home appear to be resolved and court intervention is no longer necessary or appropriate for the protection of the child, the parties may agree to dismiss the petition before adjudication. Then the court would no longer be involved, although the child's protective services worker may continue to work with the family on a voluntary basis.

If agreement cannot be reached at a pretrial conference, the hearing officer (called a referee or master in some states) or judge who is handling the trial sets a date for the hearing on the petition. The parties subpoena witnesses. On the date of the hearing, the witnesses, usually including the petitioner, testify and other matters may be admitted into evidence. In the early days of juvenile court, proceedings were informal and the rules of evidence were not strictly followed. Frequently there were no attorneys representing the various parties. In recent years more careful attention has been paid to parent's and children's rights to counsel and due process of law in general. Proceedings are now more formal, and the rules of evidence are more strictly followed.

At the conclusion of the adjudication hearing, the hearing officer (or jury in states where the child protection statute grants the right of jury trial in child protection cases) must give a decision on whether the allegations in the petition have been proved, usually "by a preponderance of the evidence." If not, the petition is dismissed for lack of sufficient evidence, and the court is no longer involved. However, if the petitioner has met this burden of proof, the court will find that the neglect or abuse has been proved. The children then come under the wardship of the court, and some parental rights are thereby temporarily suspended.

The second stage of the proceedings is the dispositional hearing, which determines where the child should be placed and what treatment plan should be ordered for the family. If the hearing officer has enough information to make a disposition on the date of the trial, an order of disposition can be entered at that time. If further information is needed, then a separate dispositional hearing is scheduled. After testimony at the dispositional hearing, the hearing officer can make various orders. The child may be placed in the parental home under the court's supervision. The court can also place the child with a qualified relative, with a legal guardian, in a licensed foster home, or in a group home, depending on the particular circumstances of the case, the degree of risk to the child, and the available community resources.

When the child remains under the supervision of the court, the court is usually directed by statute to review the parents' progress at prescribed intervals. If the problems leading to the abuse or neglect are resolved, the court can dismiss the case and return the child to the parents. If some progress has been made and it is now safe to return the child to the parents, the court can do so and still keep the child under its supervision.

There are a significant number of cases where the parents make little or no progress during the entire time that the child is not in their custody. Some parents disappear for long periods of time and cannot be located by the court or by the agency supervising the children for the court. In appropriate circumstances, after adequate legal notice and on proof by "clear and convincing evidence,"[40] the court can terminate the parents' rights to the child permanently. "Clear and convincing evidence" is a stricter burden of proof than a "preponderance of evidence," but not as strict a burden of proof as the "evidence beyond a reasonable doubt" required for conviction of a criminal offense.

The various states have left their own criteria for termination of parental rights, but termination is usually done only in cases where the abuse or neglect is severe, repeated, and long-standing, and where there is little likelihood that the parents will become rehabilitated to the extent that the child can safely be returned to their custody. Termination of parental rights is also done in cases of long-term abandonment. Other criteria vary by state. Once the court terminates the parental rights and the applicable appeal period has passed, the child is legally free for adoption.

Although the foregoing description of the procedures in juvenile court is general and somewhat oversimplified, it describes the basic flow of a case through the system. There is some variation among states and even within a state regarding how some aspects of the process are handled. For Native American children, federal law (Indian Child Welfare Act [25 U.S.C.A. Section 1901 et seq.]) applies in child protection proceedings. One of the major ways in which it differs from state law is its requirement of higher burdens of proof to establish court jurisdiction (clear and convincing evidence) and termination of parental rights (proof beyond a reasonable doubt). In many instances the federal legislation preempts state court jurisdiction over qualified children, referring the case to the legal jurisdiction of the child's tribe or band.

The juvenile courts also have jurisdiction over delinquency cases. Many of the delinquent children also came before the court years earlier as abused or neglected children. This relationship needs to be investigated fully, for adequate prevention of and treatment for child abuse and neglect may be the best prevention of juvenile delinquency.

INTERACTION BETWEEN NURSING AND THE LEGAL SYSTEM
The Nurse's Responsibility: Reporting Child Abuse and Neglect

The early reporting laws only required physicians to report suspected child abuse and neglect. By 1974 the list of mandated reporters was extended to include nurses in 21 states.[41] Today all states require nurses to report, either under provisions specifically listing nurses or any person to report.[42]

What must be reported varies to some extent by state. It can also change as reporting laws are amended following a trend to expand the list of situations requiring a report. Generally, a report is required in cases of physical abuse, emotional abuse,[43] some forms of neglect,[44] and sexual abuse.[45] Neglect can include such situations as abandonment; failure to provide food, clothing, shelter; and failure to provide adequate supervision and care (including failure to protect from obvious hazards, failure to seek necessary medical care, or failure to send the child to school).

How certain must the reporter be before a report should be made? State laws vary, using terms such as "has cause to suspect," "has reasonable cause to believe," "probable cause to suspect," "reasonably suspects," and "has reason to believe or suspect." Words such as "probable cause," "reasonable," and "belief" are legal terms of art. Practically speaking, they mean that the reporter does not have to be positive or certain that the child has suffered abuse or neglect; well-founded suspicion is enough. The reporter need not prove the abuse to make a report. Sometimes, however, abuse and neglect will be obvious.

Requiring the report of *suspected* abuse and neglect is important because the reporter may not have access to all the pertinent data on the child. If, for example, a clinical nurse suspects abuse and makes a report to the appropriate child protection authority, that agency must conduct an official investigation. That investigation can gather information unavailable to the reporting nurse. The official investigation can help to confirm or rule out abuse or neglect. At this point, the parent may agree to accept services designed to reduce the risk to the child. If the parent fails to cooperate, court intervention may be necessary to save or protect the child's life or health. If reporters waited until they were *positive* the child was being abused or neglected, many children would slip through the protective net, sometimes with crippling or fatal results.

A report sometimes reveals that the case is already active with a protective services agency or the juvenile court. A report can also uncover patterns of "hospital shopping," as the investigator checks the child's name against the central registry. Furthermore, a reporter is usually not an eyewitness to abuse or neglect. Unless the parents admit abuse to the nurse, or the child is able to talk about the injury, or the pattern of injury is obvious, the reporter generally is less certain that the child's problems are caused by abuse or neglect.

The existence of specific statutory civil penalties for failure to report can make it easier to explain to parents why a report must be made.[46] This can be invaluable to nurses. "For example, nurses frequently relate how the mention of the potential liability for failure to report is the only argument that convinces reluctant hospital administrators to commence protective action."[47] Nurses sometimes face conflict with supervising physicians. A nurse's opinion may be devalued and her or his experience ignored because the nurse is not a medical doctor. However, the particular nurse may actually have more skill than the physician in recognizing some cases of suspected abuse. If the physician refuses to report, or disagrees with the nurse's assessment, the nurse is in a delicate situation. Many hospitals and clinics have established in-house protocols under which only a physician or administrator can make the required report. If the nurse is unable to persuade the designated persons to file the report, what can the nurse do?

One commentator, a nurse, suggests that a nurse in this situation can sometimes remind the physician that the case may be referred to a child protection team physician, or the nurse can, as a last resort, submit an anonymous report.[48] The best solution is to determine a procedure in advance that recognizes the nurse's professional status and skills and the fact that the nurse, too, is subject to penalties for failure to report.

There are some special problems for the nurse in dealing with the reporting laws, in addition to disagreements with physicians and administrators on whether to file a report. For instance, private physicians seem more reluctant to report the people who pay them, or they are reluctant to believe that well-educated, employed parents would actually abuse their children. They may not understand the legal protections given to reporters. Thus a nurse who works for a physician in private practice may have to do some subtle education, remembering that she or he, too, is liable for failure to report.

The visiting or public health nurse is probably in a position to make more reports than nurses with other assignments. In some communities a visiting nurse is assigned to do a follow-up home visit for all new births. At the home visit the nurse can assess the level of care given the new infant. If there are problems, the nurse can provide education to the parents. If education fails to help, or if there are definite signs that the infant is at risk but the parents will not accept voluntary intervention, then the nurse can make a report. If the parents never bring the child for any routine clinic checkups, the visiting nurse may be the only mandated reporter who ever sees the child.

Another problem the nurse may encounter is lack of response from the agency with responsibility to investigate the report. Some protective services departments in large cities are monolithic bureaucracies. They may be inefficient in some investigations, or the investigator may not appreciate the urgency of a situation in the same way the nurse does. In smaller towns and rural areas, there may be a tendency not to report a neighbor, for fear of being branded an informer. The nurse, or the nursing supervisor if necessary, can always contact the investigating worker's supervisor if there is a problem with the worker.

THE ROLE OF THE NURSE IN THE LEGAL SYSTEM
Evidence

The nurse deals with evidence in two ways. First, she or he collects evidence for use in medical diagnosis of child abuse. Second, the nurse's testimony in a child abuse hearing is evidence that can be used to prove child abuse or neglect. How well the nurse collects and records data and observations affects how useful the nurse's testimony will be in court.

Some understanding of the rules of evidence can enable the nurse to record important data for proving child abuse and neglect.

There are two main forms of evidence. *Demonstrative evidence* consists both of things and of the testimony of witnesses about things. In child abuse cases, demonstrative evidence includes photographs of the child's injuries; x-ray films; plotted growth charts; and skin injury maps that chart a pattern of bruises, burns, or other injuries. *Testimonial evidence* includes the statements of witnesses about what they saw, heard, palpated, measured, were told, and in the case of expert witnesses, their opinions.

Evidence can also be characterized as *direct* or *circumstantial*. Direct evidence in child abuse cases includes the testimony of a witness who saw a parent strike a child, the child's testimony that the parent struck him or her, the parent's admission to the witness that he or she struck the child, and the parent's admission in court that he or she struck the child. This kind of testimony is sometimes available in child abuse cases, but not often. It is usually necessary to resort to circumstantial evidence to prove abuse or neglect. The court can infer that the child has been abused from testimony of witnesses who observed the injuries, from testimony of witnesses who observed the behavior of the child, and from various items of demonstrative evidence, such as photographs, x-ray films, and growth charts.

Juvenile courts have also adopted the common-law tort theory of *res ipsa loquitur*, which essentially says that the child's condition speaks for itself, that any unexplained, nonaccidental injury to the child while in the parent's exclusive care can lead the court to conclude that the parent inflicted the injury or allowed it to be inflicted on the child.[49] It should be noted that the doctrine of *res ipsa loquitur* is merely presumptive. It does, however, shift the burden of proof to the parent to disprove the presumption that the injury took place under the control of the parent.

A note about hearsay, which simply means "any statement made out of court," is necessary. When a party calls a witness to testify at a hearing, the other party has an opportunity to cross-examine that person. The purpose of cross-examination is to ask questions to test the witness's credibility. When a witness testifies in court about what another person (called the "declarant") said, there is no opportunity to cross-examine the declarant to determine or assess his credibility. The declarant usually was not under oath when he made the statement. Because such secondhand testimony is deemed inherently unreliable, courts developed the hearsay rule. "Hearsay is a statement, other than one made by the declarant while testifying at the trial or hearing, offered in evidence to prove the truth of the matter asserted."[50] Because some hearsay statements are considered more inherently reliable than others, a list of exceptions to the rule has been developed. If the declarant's statement meets the exceptions, it can be admitted into evidence to prove the truth of what the declarant said.

The nurse encounters admissible hearsay in a number of circumstances. Hospital, clinic, and agency records are admissible under the business records exception. The qualifications for the business records exception include:

1. The business record must be kept in the usual course of business.
2. The person who made the record or the person informing him or her must have firsthand knowledge of the matter, and both must have been acting in their usual business capacity.
3. The entries must be made at or near the time of the event being recorded.
4. The entries must be original entries.

If these criteria are met, the business record is deemed reliable, since persons at the business, institution, or agency rely on the accuracy of the entries made in their records.

Not all parts of a business record are admissible into evidence, and individual information can be challenged regarding its accuracy. Statements that are diagnoses, either by a nurse or a physician, are usually not admitted to prove their truth, since the statement is the maker's opinion and the opposing party has the right to cross-examine the maker regarding how he or she formulated that opinion. If the portions of the medical record fall within another exception to the hearsay rule, then those portions can be admitted to prove the truth of the matter asserted.

A nurse's notes of her or his own observations can be read at the trial if the nurse at the time of her or his testimony cannot remember the contents of the notes fully enough to give accurate and complete testimony.

A child's excited utterances, "statements relating to a startling event or condition made when the declarant was under the stress of excitement caused by the event or condition,"[51] can be testified to by the nurse who hears them. For instance, if an injured and distraught child in the emergency room says to a nurse, "Daddy hurt me," the nurse can testify to what the child said, and the child's statement to the nurse can be admitted as evidence that the father abused the child. The nurse (or other person) who hears the child's statement should enter it verbatim in the child's chart, with quotation marks around the exact words the child uttered, and identify in the chart all staff or others present who heard the child make the utterance. Thus if the nurse who heard the statement leaves the job and cannot be summoned to a hearing to testify, another person who heard the utterances can be called to testify, and the evidence will not be lost.

Statements made for purposes of medical treatment or a medical diagnosis in connection with treatment are also admissible under another exception to the hearsay rule. For example, a child may say to a nurse or physician who examines him or her at a clinic or emergency room, "It hurts where Mommy hit me," or "I got burned when Daddy held my hand on the stove." The person to whom these statements were made can relate them in his or her testimony in court. Some courts allow descriptions of past pain to be admitted, as well as descriptions of present pain. It is important to record the statement accurately, as well as the names of the persons to whom the statement was made.

A statement of a declarant's then-existing state of mind, emotion, sensation, or physical condition (including mental feeling, pain, and bodily health) is also admissible. If a child says, "I don't want to go home; I'm afraid of Daddy," the person who hears the statement can testify as to it, and the statement can be admitted as proof that the child is afraid of the father.

Also admissible are statements made under belief of impending death, or so-called dying declarations. If the child makes such a verbalization, the nurse hearing it can testify regarding the statement. Or if a parent's boyfriend, for example, says to a nurse from his deathbed, "I beat my girlfriend's kid many times, and I'm sorry; I just couldn't seem to stop doing it," that is also admissible in a neglect case to show that the mother failed or was unable to protect the child from a known abuser.

A statement made against interest, where the statement tends to subject the declarant to civil or criminal liability, is also admissible. If the above boyfriend (in good health) says to the emergency room nurse, "I just couldn't seem to help myself; it got on my nerves when the baby cried; all I did was shake the baby and then the baby went limp and stopped crying," this statement is admissible as one made against interest, since the boyfriend can be sued or prosecuted for doing what he said that he had done.

Some out-of-court statements are *not* hearsay. If a party to a child abuse case (as opposed to the boyfriend in the example, who is not a party if he is not legally related to the child) makes an admission that he or she hurt or neglected the child, that statement is admissible and is not considered hearsay. Parties in a child abuse or neglect case (besides the state and usually the child) are parents or legal guardians. If a nurse hears an admission, it is important, as in all the previous instances, to enter the exact words spoken by the parent, and to whom the parent made the statement, into the child's chart. When the parents know that the state can prove that they admitted the abuse, the case generally does not go to trial, saving the court and witnesses time and money, and saving the parents the pain and humiliation of a contested trial they will almost surely lose.

A nurse can testify to a number of her or his observations. The nurse may be needed to describe the child's physical condition, such as skin injuries, height and weight, and general body hygiene. The nurse may also testify as to any parental admissions of abuse or neglect, as well as to any statements the nurse heard that may represent one of the exceptions to the hearsay rule. The nurse may also testify as to the child's behavior (did the child flinch when the blood sample was drawn, or behave stoically during painful procedures?) or as to observations of the interaction between parent and child during visits at the hospital. The floor nurse at a hospital has the time and opportunity to make a number of important observations that the physician is not available to see. Who visits the child? How do the visits go? How does the child react to the visits? How long do the visitors stay?

In some instances nurses may be able to testify as expert witnesses. An expert, as opposed to a mere observer of events, can draw inferences from a set of facts and render an opinion about the facts. To be qualified in court to testify as an expert, the witness must have expertise in the field above and beyond that of a layperson, and the witness must have sufficient skill and expertise in her or his field so that her or his opinion will aid the hearing officer, judge, or jury in its task of determining what happened. Physicians, particularly radiologists, are frequently called to give their opinions whether an injury is the result of nonaccidental means. There is no legal reason why, in appropriate cases, an experienced nurse could not be qualified as an expert witness and render her or his opinion. The only barriers to nurses with appropriate qualifications testifying as experts in certain situations are the reluctance of the courts to hear opinion testimony from other than the traditional medical expert, the physician, and the lack of imagination of tradition-bound attorneys who are overlooking a valuable resource.

The nurse is asked to testify as an objective witness. She or he is to testify to the facts as she or he perceives them, and not as an advocate or adversary. It is important that the nurse appear professional and nonjudgmental in the case, although this is sometimes difficult when the subject is injury to children. As witness, the nurse's role is to give the facts as she or he knows them, but not to judge those facts.

Testifying in Court

Familiarity with the conduct of a child abuse hearing can help reduce some of the witness's anxiety about testifying. There are generally three attorneys involved in a child abuse hearing, each one representing a different party. The nurse may be contacted by an attorney, usually the prosecuting attorney or the attorney for the child, to discuss what evidence may be offered. If no attorney contacts the nurse, and the nurse knows something important that is being overlooked, the nurse can bring it to the attention of the hospital's or clinic's medical social worker assigned to the case or to the nursing supervisor, or even contact the court for the names and telephone numbers of the prosecuting attorney or the child's attorney. Prosecutors often have heavy caseloads, and not all cases are thoroughly prepared. Like all professionals, attorneys vary in their levels of expertise and competence. In our society working with or for children carries low prestige and does not usually pay well, so attorneys who work in child abuse tend to be either very dedicated or very inexperienced.

No one can ignore a subpoena, but many times witnesses are called to testify, only to learn when they arrive at court that the case was settled without a hearing or that the hearing was postponed. If the witness's workplace is relatively close to the court and there is a telephone number where the witness can be reached, the witness can ask to be placed on call. The witness can thus avoid unnecessary trips to court and some of the waiting involved for a case to be called into court.

At the hearing or trial, the attorney who subpoenaed the witness calls him or her to the witness stand. The witness is asked to swear or affirm that she or he will tell the truth. The attorney conducts the direct examination, a series of questions designed to gather testimony on the court record in a coherent and logical manner. The other attorneys cross-examine the witness. Their questions may try to confuse or upset the witness or provoke an argument. They try to note inconsistencies in the testimony already given. In short, their job is to discredit testimony so that the court will not believe the witness.

Most people asked to testify are somewhat nervous. The nurse should take the time needed to answer a question. If the witness does not understand a question, she or he should say so. Attorneys are not always articulate. The witness can ask to have a question rephrased or repeated. If the witness answers "yes" or "no" to a question that she or he does not understand, she or he may have inadvertently placed an opposite meaning to her or his testimony. If the witness does not know the answer, she or he should say so.

In a well-prepared case the nurse will have discussed the proposed testimony with one or more attorneys. The nurse should not be afraid to say so if asked in court whether she or he discussed the proposed testimony with anyone before coming to court. The attorneys to whom she talked acted appropriately in preparing their cases by contacting the witnesses before trial.

If the nurse is asked a question, she or he should answer it even if she or he believes the answer will involve hearsay or other inadmissible evidence. As discussed, hearsay is admissible under a number of circumstances. Even technically inadmissible hearsay or other testimony is admitted into evidence if no attorney objects to its admission. The parents' attorney may have a strategic reason to allow such evidence. Therefore the nurse should follow the direction of the hearing officer or judge on whether to answer a question to which an attorney has made an objection.

The nurse should make notes from her or his records. A witness who can quickly recite the dates she or he made home visits is more effective and believable than one who shuffles noisily through the chart for information she or he does not remember. The nurse's credibility as a witness rests on how she or he answers questions, as well as on the content of the answers. If the witness appears hesitant, unsure, easily confused, or self-contradictory in answers given, the testimony does not carry as much weight. Preparation can prevent this. If the nurse knows what to expect, she or he can take the time to be prepared. The nurse's self-confidence and professionalism will be evident.

Follow-up

The nurse may be subpoenaed to testify at another stage in the proceedings. The court may order that a visiting nurse be allowed to check on the child regularly as a condition of the child returning home. The nurse may be subpoenaed to testify regarding the child's progress in foster care. She or he may also be assigned to monitor the child's siblings in the parents' home or to file a report of suspected abuse or neglect when a new sibling is born to extremely dysfunctional parents in serious abuse cases.

Nurses may also be used more extensively by the court in treatment functions. Nurses can teach parents informally in the home. They can offer support and counseling to parents who themselves were abused and neglected as children. Nurses can refer parents to various agencies for services and treatment. Pediatric nurse practitioners can fulfill a number of specialized needs in the treatment of abusive families. The juvenile court should be made more aware of all the resources available to it from the nursing profession.

SUMMARY

The nurse is in an excellent position to assist the legal system in detecting, proving, and treating child abuse and neglect. In most states the nurse is required to report cases of suspected child abuse and neglect to the appropriate authorities for investigation. In the record keeping role, the nurse can fully document and preserve valuable evidence of abuse and neglect for trial and treatment purposes. Although courts have traditionally ignored the nurse's expertise as a witness, this will change as courts are made more aware of the education, experience, and specialization of nurses and nurse practitioners. Finally, nurses can fill a number of educational and treatment functions to improve parenting skills to prevent child abuse and neglect or to reunite troubled families. A closer collaboration between the nursing profession and the legal system can aid both in their handling of child abuse and neglect.

REFERENCES AND NOTES

1. Radbill, S. X. (1974). A history of child abuse and infanticide. In R. E. Helfer & C. H. Kempe (Eds.), *The battered child* (p. 14). Chicago: University of Chicago Press.
2. For a historical treatment of child abandonment, see: [Boswell, J. (1988). *The kindness of strangers: The abandonment of children in Western Europe from late antiquity to the Renaissance.* New York: Vintage-Random House.
3. Radbill, p. 8.
4. Piers, M. W. (1978). *Infanticide: Past and present* (p. 34). New York: W. W. Norton.
5. For a review of treatment of unusual births and failure to thrive in folklore, see: Eberly, S. S. Fairies and the folklore of disability: Changelings, hybrids and the solitary fairy; and Munro, J. U. The fairy changeling as a folk articulation of failure to thrive in children: The invisible made visible. Both essays are included in Narvaez, P. (Ed.). (1991). *The good people: New fairy lore essays.* New York: Garland Press.
6. Radbill, p. 8.
7. Radbill, p. 8.
8. In 1984 Congress passed a bill, effective October 1985, to curtail the practice of withholding food, medication, and treatment from selected infants who suffer from one or more serious, although treatable, medical problems. 42 U.S.C. §§ 5101-05 (1984).
   See also: Note (1985). The Child Abuse Amendments of 1984: The infant Doe amendment. *Akron Law Review, 18,* 515-536; and Lund, N. (1985). Infanticide, physicians and the law: the 'Baby Doe' amendment to the Child Abuse and Prevention and Treatment Act. *American Journal of Law and Medicine, 11,* 1-29.
9. Piers, p. 68.
10. Radbill, p. 7.
11. See Boswell for an extended discussion.
12. In *DeShaney v. Winnebago County Department of Social Services,* 489 U.S. 189, 109 S.Ct. 998 (1989), the U.S. Supreme Court ruled that the state, in this case a county child welfare agency, has no affirmative duty to protect a child from an abusive parent under the civil rights legislation of 42 U.S.C. § 1983. The child was inadequately supervised by the agency after being returned to the parents who had been abusive in the past. The child was reabused, and a civil suit for money damages was filed against the agency for negligence in failing to protect the child. The civil suit was dismissed on the basis of the county agency's governmental immunity from lawsuit.
    See: Note (1990). Constitutional law—governmental child abuse—Who watches the watchers, *DeShaney,* etc. *Land and Water Law Review, 25,* 251-265; and Note (1991). Abused children: The Supreme Court considers due process right to protection. (*DeShaney v. Winnebago Co. Department of Soc. Serv.* 489 U.S. 189). *Journal of Family Law, 29,* 679-702.
13. Radbill, p. 7.

14. See: Piers, pp. 45-55, "About wet nurses."
15. Piers, p. 51.
16. Piers, p. 52.
17. Piers, p. 67.
18. See: Chapin, H. D. (1915). Are institutions for infants necessary? *Journal of the American Medical Association, 64,* 1-3; and Bakwin, H. (1942). Loneliness in infants. *American Journal of the Disabled Child, 63,* 30-40.
19. Bakwin, H. (1949). Emotional deprivation in infants. *Journal of Pediatrics, 35,* 512-521.
20. Proverbs 13:23.
21. Radbill, p. 4.
22. See: *Ingraham v. Wright,* 430 U.S. 651, 51 L.Ed.2d 711, 97 S.Ct. 1401 (1977), where the U.S. Supreme Court upheld corporal punishment in the schools, saying "the State itself may impose such corporal punishment as is reasonably necessary for the proper education of the child and for the maintenance of group discipline," 430 U.S. 651, 662. See also: Stoneman, J. P., II. (1980). Corporal punishment in the schools: A time for change. *Journal of Juvenile Law, 4,* 155-169.
    Some states have since passed legislation limiting or forbidding corporal punishment in the public schools.
23. Piers, p. 80.
24. Bridgman, W. E. (1984). Circumcision as child abuse: The legal and constitutional issues. *Journal of Family Law, 23,* 337-358.
25. Plaine, L. L. (1974). Evidentiary problems in criminal child abuse prosecutions. *Georgetown Law Journal, 63,* 257; Note (1988). Sixth Amendment violated by screening children within from accused in courtroom. *Coy v. Iowa,* 108 S.Ct. 2798, *Drake Law Review, 38,* 147-155; Spencer, J. R., & Flin, R. (1978). Child witnesses—are they liars? *New Law Journal, 139,* 1601-1602; Note (1987). Videotaping children's testimony: An empirical view. *Michigan Law Review, 85,* 809-833; Christiansen, J. R. (1987). The testimony of child witnesses: Fact, fantasy and the influence of pre-trial interviews. *Washington Law Review, 62,* 705-721; Warner, K. (1988). Child witnesses in sexual assault cases. *Criminal Law Journal, 12,* 286-302; Ringland, R. P. (1988). Child sex abuse evidence problems update 1988. *University of Dayton Law Review, 14,* 147-164; Graham, M. H. (1988). The confrontation clause, the hearsay rule, and child sexual abuse: The state of the relationship. *Minnesota Law Review, 72,* 523-601; and Note (1989). *Coy v. Iowa,* [108 S.Ct. 2798] Should children be heard and not seen? *University of Pittsburgh Law Review, 50,* 1187-1208.
26. See: Foucault, M. (1975). *The birth of the clinic: An archaeology of medical perception* (A. M. Smith, Trans.). New York: Vintage-Random House; for an analysis of how much of the state's authority and responsibility in controlling citizens was gradually transferred to the domain of medicine as medicine became professionalized.

27. Caffey, J. (1946). Multiple fractures. *American Journal of Roentgenology, Radium Therapy, and Nuclear Medicine, 56,* 163-173.

28. Silverman, F. N. (1953). The roentgen manifestations of unrecognized skeletal trauma in infants. *American Journal of Roentgenology, Radium Therapy, and Nuclear Medicine, 69,* 413-427.

29. Wooley, P. V., Jr., & Evans, W. A., Jr. (1955). Significance of skeletal lesions in infants resembling those of traumatic origin. *Journal of the American Medical Association, 158,* 539.

30. Kempe, C., Silverman, T., Steele, B., Droegemueller, W., & Silver, H. (1962). Battered-child syndrome. *Journal of the American Medical Association, 181,* 17.

31. Freiman, M. R. (1982). Unequal protection and inadequate protection under the law: State child abuse statutes. *George Washington Law Review, 50,* 242-250.

32. Child Abuse Prevention and Treatment Act, 42 U.S.C. §§ 5101-5106 (1976 & Supp. LV 1980), Pub. L. No. 93-247, 88 Stat. 4 (1974).

33. Katz, S. N., Ambrosino, L., McGrath, M., & Sawitsky, K. (1977). Legal research on child abuse and neglect: Past and future. *Family Law Quarterly, 11,* 151-184; Plaine, L.L. (1974). Evidentiary problems in criminal child abuse prosecutions. *Georgetown Law Journal, 63,* 257-273; and Paulsen, M. K. (1980). The law and abused children. In R. E. Helfer & C. H. Kempe (Eds.), *The battered child* (p. 154). New York: Vintage-Random House.

34. Katz et al., p. 156.

35. Roberts, D. E. (1990). Drug-addicted women who have babies. *Trial, 26,* 56-58.

36. Roberts, p. 61.

37. Toufexis, A. (1991). Innocent victims. *Time, 137* (19), 56-60; Wilwerth, J. (1991). Should we take away their kids? *Time, 137* (19), 62-64.

38. Mainor, P. (1990). Fetal protection: Drugs and Pregnancy, the legal impact. *Maryland Bar Journal, 23,* 22-23; Comment (1990), Gestational substance abuse: A call for a thoughtful legislative response. *Washington Law Review, 65,* 377-396; Note (1988). Maternal rights and fetal wrongs: The case against criminalization of 'fetal abuse.' *Harvard Law Review, 101,* 994-1012; Bainham, A. (1987). Protecting the unborn: New rights in gestation? *Modern Law Review, 50,* 361-368; Curriden, M. (1990). Holding mom accountable. *American Bar Journal, 76,* 50-53; Note (1988). Pregnancy police: The health policy and legal implications of punishing pregnant women for harm to their fetuses. *New York University Review of Law and Social Change, 16,* 277-319; Note (1987). Maternal substance abuse: The need to provide legal protection for the fetus. *Southern California Law Review, 60,* 1209-1235; Roberts, D. E. (1990). Drug-addicted women who have babies. *Trial, 26,* 56-58.

39. Or to designate the child a "minor in need of care" or "person in need of supervision," two of the newer terms being used in some states. It is important to repeat that child protection legislation continues to undergo study and revision in the states.

40. *Santosky v. Kramer,* 455 U.S. 745, 71 L.Ed.2d 599, 102 S.Ct. 1388 (1982).

41. Paulsen, p. 161.

42. Freiman, p. 257.

43. Freiman, p. 254.

44. Freiman, p. 254.

45. Freiman, p. 254.

46. Besharov, D. (1978). Legal aspects of reporting known and suspected child abuse and neglect. *Villanova Law Review, 23,* 458, 482.

47. Besharov, p. 482.

48. Bridges, C. L. (1978). The nurse's evaluation. In B. D. Schmitt (Ed.), *The child protection team handbook—a multidisciplinary approach to managing child abuse and neglect* (p. 71). New York: Garland STPM Press.

49. See the opinion of the Hon. Harold A. Felix of the New York Family Court for a good discussion of the application of the doctrine of *res ipsa loquitur* in child abuse cases, *In the Matter of S.* 46 Misc. 2d 161, 162.

50. *Federal Rules of Evidence,* Rule 801 (c).

51. *Michigan Rules of Evidence,* Rule 803 (2).

CHAPTER

14

The Nurse and the Legal System
Dealing with Abused Women

William O. Humphreys *and* Janet E. Findlater

N urses who are informed about the legal system
and the law relating to domestic violence can
be a valuable resource. They can supply general information and support to the battered women they
treat. Nurses who know about the rules of evidence
and confidentiality can be of great assistance to lawyers who work on behalf of battered women.

TRADITIONAL RESPONSE OF THE LAW TO WIFE ABUSE

For the last 15 years, survivors of domestic violence
and their advocates have been working to improve
the response of the legal system to the needs of battered wives.[1] To appreciate how much has been accomplished, and to understand how much remains
to be done, some historical perspective on the law relating to married women is required.

Civil Law

Law both reflects and reinforces the norms of the society in which it is made. Until the mid-nineteenth century, women were regarded by philosophers, theologians, and political theorists alike as inherently
unequal and subordinate to men.[2] This assumption of
sex inequality was embedded in the common law.
Married women had no legal identity separate from
that of the men they married; their legal existence was
regarded as merged into that of their husbands. It is
said that upon marriage, husband and wife became
one, and that "one" was the husband.[3] Married women
could not own or convey property, enter into contracts,
or initiate legal proceedings.[4] Because of the merging
of their legal identities, married women could neither
sue their husbands nor be sued by them.

In the 1840s, state legislatures began passing

statutes, known as Married Women's Property Acts, that were intended to secure for a married woman a separate legal identity and a separate legal estate in her own property. Because these statutes pertained to property, however, courts concluded that they did not alter the common law rule that neither wife nor husband could maintain a cause of action against each other for personal injury.[5]

This vestige of the mystical notion of merged identities became known as the doctrine of interspousal tort immunity. Although the doctrine appears neutral on its face, it is significantly uneven in its application, especially in cases of physical abuse, when wives are more likely to be the victims.

In defending the doctrine of interspousal tort immunity, courts had to devise reasons for it other than the concept of merged legal identities that the Married Women's Property Acts had presumably abolished. Three arguments, none of them persuasive, were routinely made. First, to allow one spouse to sue another would disrupt family harmony. Second, absent a complete bar to these actions, spouses would collude and fabricate false claims in an effort to defraud insurance companies.[6] Third, a tort cause of action between spouses would be superfluous: remedies are available in divorce, in criminal prosecution, or both.

These arguments are specious. First, the physical assault disrupts family harmony, not the court remedy. Second, there are safeguards in the legal system to protect against fraudulent claims; there is simply no evidence that the risk with regard to these claims is higher than it is with regard to other claims.[7] Finally, a criminal prosecution is brought to vindicate society's interest in punishing the wrongdoer, not to remedy harm caused an individual victim. The purpose of divorce is to dissolve the marriage and divide the assets; divorce does not compensate for injuries caused during the marriage[8] and often does not end the violence.[9]

Today interspousal tort immunity has been abolished in most states.[10] Abused wives can bring a cause of action against their husbands[11] for, among others, assault and battery, intentional infliction of emotional distress, or false imprisonment. The impediments to these lawsuits are now practical, not legal. Abused wives can collect monetary compensation only from husbands who have assets. And juries might be reluctant to find in favor of abused wives who are still living with their husbands. Nonetheless, abused wives are with increasing frequency and success using tort law to collect money damages for personal injury from husbands and ex-husbands.[12]

Criminal Law

It is, and has been, a crime to intentionally inflict injury on another person. However, as late as the mid-nineteenth century, a husband was permitted to chastise his wife "without subjecting himself to vexatious prosecutions for assault and battery, resulting in the discredit and shame of all parties concerned."[13] Because of the assumption of sex inequality, a married woman was placed under the authority of her husband, who was permitted to discipline her, using physical force if necessary. The legal system refused to treat wifebeating as a crime.

By 1870 most states recognized that wifebeating was illegal.[14] However, for the next 100 years, few assailants were arrested or prosecuted. It was not until the mid-1970s that battered women and their advocates made an organized effort to have the criminal law enforced against abusive husbands.

Perhaps the most insidious and dangerous consequence of the wife's merged legal identity was that a husband could not be convicted of raping his wife, regardless of how much force he used to accomplish sexual intercourse.[15] A number of rationalizations for this "marital exemption" to the rape law have been offered. First, husband and wife are one, and a husband cannot rape himself.[16] Alternatively (and inconsistently), sex is part of the marital relationship, and, under her marriage contract, a wife gives irrevocable and continuing consent to have sexual relations with her husband.[17] Finally, to prosecute a husband for rape would disrupt family harmony, intrude on family privacy, and deprive the family unit of its breadwinner.

These arguments are easily rebutted. The sexual relations that are part of the marital contract are those of mutual consent, not those that are forced by one spouse on the other. Rape disrupts marital harmony. Safety and physical integrity for abused wives are more important than preserving a concept of family privacy that is nothing more than a screen behind which physical and sexual violence occurs. Although society generally devalues work done by wives, thus rendering them economically dependent on their husbands,[18] the criminal justice system should provide safety for sexually abused wives who seek protection without undue regard to the immediate economic risks posed to the family.[19]

The marital exemption is on the wane. Most states now recognize that it is a crime for a husband to rape his wife.[20] Despite initial cries from critics that recognizing marital rape as a crime would flood the courthouse, relatively few marital rape prosecutions have been brought.[21] In part, this is because it is not generally known that rape in marriage is now a crime. Nonetheless, the importance of this change in the law should not be minimized: wives are no longer regarded by the law as sexual objects who must provide unlimited sexual access to their husbands.

Many of the historical reasons for nonintervention in domestic violence cases continue to influence criminal justice response. Domestic violence is considered a "family matter," to be worked out between the parties. Criminal justice intervention is inconsistent with respect for family "privacy," especially the privacy of the home.[22] Sending an abusive husband to jail is deemed unacceptable; it would destroy the family unit by depriving it of its breadwinner.

If an abused wife seeks to initiate a criminal proceeding on her own, or if her husband has been arrested for assaulting her, many obstacles to prosecution may be encountered. Prosecutors, like police officers, have tended to view domestic violence cases as "family matters," not crimes.[23] When they do decide to proceed, prosecutors are often frustrated. Domestic violence cases can be difficult. There frequently are no witnesses to the abuse, and police reports are not carefully written, if they exist at all. Abused wives do not always seek medical attention; consequently, they lack documentation of their injuries. Bruises, cuts, scratches, and the like have usually healed by the time of trial.[24] Abused wives sometimes ask that charges be dropped, refuse to testify, and fail to appear in court.

To protect against what they perceive as wasting their time on abused wives who ultimately decided not to proceed, prosecutors developed policies and procedures they thought would identify those abused wives who were serious about going forward. Unfortunately, the procedures often exacerbate, rather than remedy, the problem of noncooperation. A mandatory "cooling-off" period, a delay of days or weeks before any official action would be taken, just to be sure the abused wife did not change her mind, only provides the assailant (and his family) more time to pressure the abused wife to drop the charges. The policy that charges would automatically be dropped if the abused wife so requested plays directly into the assailant's hand.

A NUMBER OF INITIATIVES

Wife abuse is a crime, not merely a "family matter." It is a crime with devastating consequences, not only for the family involved, but also for the entire community. Domestic violence is the primary cause of injury to women, producing more injuries to women than rapes, muggings, and automobile accidents combined.[25] In addition to enormous medical costs, domestic violence is responsible for lost productivity at work and considerable public safety expenses.[26] Domestic violence also is a context in which child abuse often occurs.[27]

Over the past 15 years, as public awareness of domestic violence has grown, there have been several significant developments in the law and the legal system designed to provide a more appropriate and effective response to domestic violence. By themselves, new laws cannot end domestic violence, but they can change the legal system's response to the problem and promote safety for abused wives and their children. This section studies a number of these initiatives.

Coordinated Community Response: Abuse of Women Is a Crime

Domestic violence is a pattern of learned behavior. The failure to treat wife abuse as a crime condones and reinforces the assailant's use of violence to dominate and control his partner. Just as it is learned, domestic violence can be unlearned, provided the assailant has sufficient motivation for change. Criminal justice intervention that treats domestic violence as a crime provides that motivation.

The Domestic Abuse Intervention Project (DAIP) in Duluth, Minnesota, developed a model for criminal justice intervention that has been replicated throughout the country.[28] In the DAIP program, all components of the criminal justice system—police, prosecutor, and court—treat domestic violence as a crime. The criminal justice response to the crime of domestic violence is then coordinated with battered women's shelter programs and local human service agencies to provide a comprehensive community intervention in these cases. The responsibility for holding the batterer accountable for his behavior is placed where it should be—on the community, not the victim.[29]

Another example of concerted action is taking place in Michigan. The coordinated community response program in Ypsilanti Township began in 1988. After 3 years, there has been a substantial increase in the number of arrests and convictions of assailants, and a substantial decrease in the number of repeat calls to the same address.[30]

Law Enforcement

A police officer cannot make an arrest without a warrant unless the crime is either a felony, or a misdemeanor that was committed in the officer's presence. Because many wife abuse cases are viewed as misdemeanors, and husbands rarely beat their wives in front of police officers, this rule of criminal procedure presents a serious impediment to effective law enforcement intervention.

States have dealt with this problem in a variety of ways. Some have changed the law to allow arrest in domestic assault misdemeanor cases even though the crime was not committed in the officer's presence.[31] Others have made domestic assault a felony.[32] The California Supreme Court has stated:

> (most interspousal attacks) are usually accomplished with fists and kicking. . . . The severity of the injuries are therefore not always capable of instant diagnosis. . . . An officer responding to a wifebeating case

would ordinarily, in the exercise of caution and to avoid a charge of false arrest, only arrest the husband under the provisions of . . . (the assault law) in extreme cases. Even the infliction upon a wife of considerable traumatic injury would tend to be treated by the arresting officer as a misdemeanor which would produce the consequences of the wife's being left in the home to face possible further aggression. But an officer given the alternative of arresting for a felony under the . . . (spouse abuse law) may do so. . . .[33]

For a full description of law enforcement response to domestic violence, see Chapter 12.

Prosecutor

Increased public awareness about the seriousness of wife abuse has caused many prosecutors to reassess their priorities and more vigorously prosecute these cases. A number of steps have been taken to provide the victim the information and support she needs to get through the criminal process.

It is a basic tenet of the criminal law that a crime is an offense against society, not the individual victim. It is the prosecutor who decides whether to charge someone with a crime, and it is the prosecutor, not the victim, who should decide whether charges will be dropped. "By setting a policy that charges will not be dropped at the request of the victim, these prosecutors prevent battered women from repeatedly testing their resolve to go to court."[34] In addition, a "no-drop" policy reduces the incentive for the batterer to threaten and intimidate the victim; the decision to proceed is not hers.

To protect the victim against harassment, the prosecutor can request that the court only release the batterer from custody after arrest on the condition that he have no contact with the victim.[35] Any violation of the condition of release would result in a return to jail.

The criminal justice system is complex and can be intimidating for someone not familiar with it. Victims unprepared for the possibility of delays and numerous court appearances can become frustrated and discouraged. Uninformed victims can have unrealistic expectations and concerns about the outcome of the proceedings. For example, abused wives often worry that their husbands will spend years in prison if they are convicted. In fact, a batterer convicted the first time of a misdemeanor is rarely sentenced to jail. Instead, he is more likely to be put on probation, and ordered to attend a counseling program for assailants.

An important change in policy is the effort to inform the abused woman about the criminal process. Some prosecutors have programs in their offices that provide information and support to battered women.[36] Others allow advocates from battered women's shelter programs to work with the women throughout the criminal proceedings.[37]

Improvements in the prosecutor's response to domestic violence support similar efforts by police officers. An enhanced priority for domestic violence cases encourages more assertive police action and provides greater protection for battered women.[38]

Restraining Orders

An abused wife can petition a court to issue an order directing her abuser to do any number of specific things, such as stop assaulting her, move out of the house, have no contact with her, and pay support. The terminology used to describe these orders and the requirements for obtaining them vary from state to state. In addition to "restraining orders," they are commonly referred to as "orders of protection" and "injunctions."

The consequences for an assailant who violates a restraining order depend on the type of order. Usually, the assailant will be served with another order (obtained by the wife's lawyer) to appear in court for a hearing to determine whether the assailant should be found in contempt of court. If so found, he can be fined, sent to jail, or both.

However, courts in many states now have the authority to issue restraining orders that allow the police to arrest an assailant for violating the order.[39] These orders are often narrow in scope, limited to, for example, not assaulting the wife, and staying away from the home.[40] But they have the advantage of immediate law enforcement intervention and removal of the abuser, which is important for the woman's safety. As with other restraining orders, a court hearing is held to determine whether the assailant should be held in contempt.

Abused wives can obtain temporary restraining orders, including those that provide for arrest for violation, ex parte. This means that the temporary restraining order can be issued without a hearing. Thus protection is available almost immediately upon application to the court. A hearing is held before the restraining order becomes permanent.

Defending Battered Women Who Kill Their Assailants

When abused women kill to protect themselves, they are often charged with murder. There have been a number of significant changes in the criminal law used to defend them.

Self-defense is a "state of mind" defense. The law provides that a person who is not the aggressor is justified in using deadly force if he reasonably believes that he is in imminent danger of death or great bodily harm.[41] Cases often are determined on the basis of whether the jury finds that the defendant believed he or she was in imminent danger, and whether that belief was reasonable.

The problems presented to the abused woman who has killed her assailant are many, especially when she has killed him while he is not, at the moment, assaulting her. Generally, the decision about imminent danger is made by viewing the incident in isolation, as if it were a photograph. So limited, juries have difficulty understanding why an abused woman would think that her life was in imminent danger at the time she killed.

Most states now permit the defendant in these cases to present all the circumstances of the abusive relationship, and introduce expert testimony about the "battered woman's syndrome".[42] Expert testimony informs the jury about the dynamics of domestic violence, and assists the jury in understanding the defendant's state of mind and the reasonableness of her belief that this time she had to kill to save her life.[43] It is especially helpful in overcoming attitudes that the jury may have about battered women, such as the myth that any woman in fear of her husband would call the police or leave.

Finally, a number of courts have recognized that to determine "reasonable" by a "reasonable man" or even a "reasonable person" standard precludes consideration of a woman's perception of danger.[44] The implications of this insight are significant for defending battered women who have killed.

Task Forces on Gender Bias in the Courts

More than half the states have established task forces to determine the nature and extent of gender bias in their courts and to make recommendations for eliminating it.[45] Issues concerning battered women are an important focus of this work. Task force recommendations have included a number of the issues previously discussed: treat domestic violence as a crime; adopt policies and procedures that make domestic violence cases a priority for prosecutors; permit experts to testify about the battered woman's syndrome; make orders of protection available to battered women; and eliminate the marital rape exemption.[46] The next step is implementation of these and other changes throughout the country as part of the effort to provide safety for battered women by ending the violence.

THE NURSE IN THE LEGAL SYSTEM

An attorney usually proceeds with a case only if she or he thinks it can be won. The decision to go forward depends on the availability of credible witnesses and other evidence.

A battered woman who seeks medical attention has contact with the nursing profession almost immediately after the violent episode. Because of this, the nurse is in a unique position to aid the attorney by carefully documenting a woman's injuries and writing down any statements she might make in a case that appears to be the result of battering.

Rules of Evidence

"Evidence" means testimony, writings, material objects, or other things presented to the senses that are offered to prove the existence or nonexistence of facts.[47] There are two fundamental types of evidence. The first, *direct evidence*, sometimes termed "eyewitness" evidence, proves a proposition directly rather than by inference. The second, *circumstantial evidence*, depends on inferences for its relationship to the material issue to be proven.

To safeguard against false accusations and to expose inaccuracies, the American legal system requires a witness to testify under oath in court and be subjected to cross-examination.[48] Testimony based on a witness' personal (direct) knowledge of the facts is generally admissible because the witness can be cross-examined about what he or she knows.

A witness can testify to the truth of only firsthand knowledge. Thus testimony that the witness was told something by someone else is admissible to prove that the statement was made (the witness can be cross-examined about this), but not to prove the truth of that statement (the witness has no direct knowledge of this and therefore cannot be cross-examined about it.) This, essentially, is the hearsay rule. Statements made outside the courtroom cannot be offered at trial to prove the truth of the matter they assert.[49] The inability to cross-examine the person who made the out-of-court statement renders the statement unreliable and therefore inadmissible.

It is important for nurses to understand the hearsay rule. Nurses rarely see the injury take place, and therefore have no direct knowledge of how the injury occurred or who inflicted it. Any information they obtain about how the injury happened is usually supplied by the battered woman. Under the hearsay rule, a nurse is not able to testify about what the woman told her as a way to establish what happened.

There are, however, a number of exceptions to the hearsay rule that are important for nurses who treat battered women. Since credibility is the main issue in most hearsay problems, the court has made exceptions in instances when something in the statement's content or in the circumstances of its utterance guarantees its trustworthiness.

One such exception is for a statement made while under the influence of a startling event. This "excited utterance" is important to the nurse because she is usually one of the first persons to encounter the abused wife and therefore is present while the woman is still under the influence of the violent episode. The two requirements for an excited utterance are satisfied: a startling event, and a statement made while still under the stress of the event and before time for reflection.[50]

A second exception is recognized for statements made while in fear of impending death.[51] A "dying declaration" is considered trustworthy because people do not wish to die with a "lie on their lips." Thus if the abused wife, conscious that death is near, says "My husband beat me up," this is admissible. If a husband shot by his wife states "I've hit her for so many years and she never fought back before," his statement might be admissible to aid in her defense.

Another exception to the hearsay rule is for "regularly kept records."[52] The reason for this exception is that business records should be admissible when the sources of information, and the method and time of preparation, indicate their trustworthiness.

The nurse has a duty to record certain facts in the patient's medical records. These records are standardized and routinely used to make decisions on which the health and life of the patient depend. Their trustworthiness seems assured.[53] They must, however, reasonably relate to the diagnosis and treatment of the patient's condition.[54] For example, entries in hospital records as to who hit her may be held unrelated to the woman's treatment. However, in cases involving battered women, the cause of injury is important to diagnosis and treatment.

For these exceptions to the hearsay rule to be allowed, it is critical that the nurse keep accurate and complete records. The nurse should record exactly what was said by the battered woman. The use of quotation marks for direct statements is a good practice in such cases.

The importance of preserving and recalling vital facts should not be underestimated. Accurate record keeping and documentation is important to the lawyer who needs to determine how to present the evidence so that it is admissible in court.

The nurse may be called to testify about facts of which she has direct knowledge. Testimony about the woman's physical condition (that is, scars, cuts, bruises) or how she relates to her husband at the hospital is direct evidence, not hearsay, and therefore admissible.

Confidentiality

A nurse-patient privilege of confidentiality, unlike the doctor-patient privilege, is not universally recognized. However, even in those states that do not have a nurse-patient privilege, statements made by an abused woman to a nurse still might be confidential because they are protected by another privilege.

For example, when the nurse is acting as an assistant to a physician, the doctor-patient privilege protects statements relating to diagnosis and treatment made by the patient to the nurse.[55] Any information provided by the patient that is required to enable the nurse to assist the physician is within the privilege. Therefore it appears that statements made by patients to nurses working in emergency rooms or offices of private physicians are covered by the doctor-patient privilege.

Similarly, the doctor-patient privilege protects statements made by the patient that relate to diagnosis and treatment and are entered into hospital records by the nurse.[56] Although "regularly kept records" are admissible as an exception to the hearsay rule,[57] the patient could use the doctor-patient privilege to prevent the admission of any confidential statements contained in those records.

The doctor-patient privilege of confidentiality protects only communications necessary to enable nurses to act in their professional capacity; it does not cover conversations or observations unrelated to treatment and care. Thus a nurse is able to testify that a patient was mentally alert and his memory was good without violating the patient's privilege.[58]

Expert Testimony

Finally, if the nurse has sufficient skill, knowledge, or experience regarding abused women, she may be called to testify as an expert witness. Most states allow the use of expert testimony about the "battered woman's syndrome" in cases where the woman has killed her abuser and is charged with homicide.[59]

SUMMARY

Changes in the law and the response of the legal system are being made to provide safety for battered women. However, until sex equality exists in our society, women will continue to face obstacles when they seek redress through the legal system and abuse of women will not be eliminated.

REFERENCES AND NOTES

1. Although some of this chapter focuses on married women, most of its information also applies to abused women who are not married to their assailants.
2. Deborah L. Rhode, *The "No-Problem" Problem: Feminist Challenges and Cultural Change*, 100 Yale L.J. 1731, 1737 (1991).
3. W. Page Keeton et al., Prosser and Keeton on the Law of Torts Sec. 122, at 902 (5th ed. 1984).
4. Id. at 901.
5. Id. at 902.
6. Id.
7. Id. at 902-03.
8. Barbara H. Young, Note, *Interspousal Torts and Divorce: Problems, Policies, Procedures*, 27 J. Fam. L. 489 (1988-89).
9. Women are more likely to be injured or killed when they are attempting to leave or have left their assailants. See Ann Jones, Women Who Kill 298-99 (1980).
10. Robert G. Spector, *Marital Torts*, 15 Fam. L. Rptr. 3023 (1989).
11. A woman can also sue her ex-husband for injury inflicted during the marriage.
12. Spector, supra note 8.
13. Sue E. Eisenberg and Patricia L. Micklow, *The Assaulted Wife: "Catch-22" Revisited*, 3 Women's Rts. L. Rptr. 138, 138 (1977).
14. Elizabeth Pleck, *Wife Beating in Nineteenth Century America*, 4 Victimology 60, 71 (1979).
15. The common law defined rape as "unlawful sexual intercourse with a woman by force and without her consent." The word "unlawful" contained the marital exemption. Rollin M. Perkins and Ronald N. Boyce, Criminal Law 202 (3rd ed. 1982).
16. This is based on the common law concept of merged legal identities. See text accompanying notes 3-4 supra.
17. State v. Smith, 85 N.J. 193, 426 A.2d 38, 41 (1981).
18. R. Emerson Dobash & Russell Dobash, Violence Against Wives 51 (1979).
19. Domestic violence assailants engage in multiple types of abuse, including economic abuse. The assailant often will not allow his partner to work. He controls the family resources as another way to control her.
20. Diana E. H. Russell, Rape in Marriage 21 (1990).
21. Id. at 24.
22. Maria L. Marcus, *Conjugal Violence: The Law of Force and the Force of Law*, 69 Calif. L. Rev. 1657, 1659 (1981).
23. Dobash and Dobash, supra, at 218.
24. Lisa G. Lerman, Prosecution of Spouse Abuse: Innovations in Criminal Justice Response 22 (1981).
25. Teri Randall, *Domestic Violence Intervention Calls for More Than Treating Injuries*, 264 JAMA 939, 939 (1990).
26. Teri Randall, *Domestic Violence Begets Other Problems of Which Physicians Must Be Aware To Be Effective*, 264 JAMA 940, 943 (1990).
27. Maria Roy, Children in the Crossfire 20 (1988).
28. For example, similar projects exist in Ann Arbor, Troy, and Ypsilanti Township, Michigan, as well as in almost two dozen communities in Minnesota.
29. Ellen Pence, Criminal Justice Response to Domestic Assault Cases: A Guide for Policy Development (1985); Ellen Pence, *The Duluth Domestic Abuse Intervention Project*, 6 Hamline L. Rev. 247 (1983). See also R. Emerson Dobash and Russell P. Dobash, Women, Violence and Social Change 146-212 (1992).
30. Susan McGee, Executive Director, Domestic Violence Project/Safe House, Presentation at the Wayne State University Law School (Sept. 11, 1991).
31. Mich. Comp. Laws Ann. Sec. 764.15a (West 1982).
32. Cal. Penal Code Sec. 273.5 (West 1988).
33. People v. Cameron, 53 Cal. App.3d 786, 793, 126 Cal. Rptr. 44, 48 (1975).
34. Lerman, supra, at 44.
35. Id. at 54.
36. For example, The Family Violence Project, San Francisco District Attorney's Office, San Francisco, California.
37. For example, the Domestic Abuse Intervention Project (DAIP), Duluth, Minnesota.
38. Lerman, supra, at 15.
39. See, for example, Mich. Comp. Laws Ann. Sec. 764.15b (West 1982).
40. Id.
41. Joshua Dressler, Understanding Criminal Law 191 (1987).
42. Martha R. Mahoney, *Legal Images of Battered Women: Redefining the Issue of Separation*, 90 Mich. L. Rev. 1, 37 (1991).
43. See, for example, State v. Kelly, 478 A.2d 364 (N.J. 1984).
44. State v. Wanrow, 88 Wash. 2d 221, 559 P.2d 548 (1977); Radtke v. Everett, 189 Mich. App. 421 (1991).
45. Karen Czapanskiy, *Gender Bias in the Courts: Social Change Strategies*, 4 Geo. J. Legal Ethics 1, 1 (1990).
46. Final Report of the Michigan Supreme Court Task Force on Gender Issues in the Courts (December, 1989); *Report of the New York Task Force on Women in the Courts*, 15 Fordham Ur. L. J. 11 (1986-87).
47. Cal. Evid. Code Sec. 140 (West 1966).

48. Edward W. Cleary et al., McCormick on Evidence Sec. 245, at 726-28 (3rd ed. 1984).
49. Id. Sec. 246, at 729.
50. Id. Sec. at 854-55.
51. Id. Sec. 282, at 829.
52. Id. Sec. 306, at 872.
53. Id. Sec. 313, at 882.
54. Id. at 883.
55. Id. Sec. 101, at 250.
56. Id. Sec. 313, at 884.
57. See text accompanying notes 52-54 supra.
58. In re Avery's Estate, 76 N.Y.S.2d 790 (1948).
59. See text accompanying notes 42-43 supra.

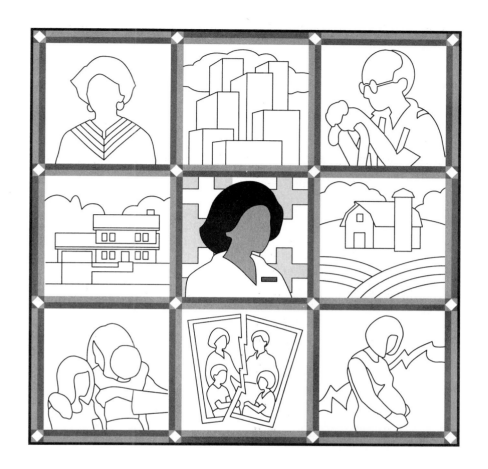

PART

V

Future Directions

Future Directions for Nursing

Janice Humphreys *and* Terry T. Fulmer

"So Many Faces Pass Through This House"
So many faces pass through this house
Younger, older, richer, poorer
Women with bruised marks
surrounding their faces,
Babies with welt scars on
unmentionable places.

Barbee Finer*

The case for violence in families as a health problem of concern to nursing has been made, and the issue now becomes what are the future directions for nursing? Once nursing as a profession acknowledged that family violence can and does happen, what are the requisite policy actions and practice adaptations? What programs of research must be mandated to stem the tide of family violence? This chapter examines the implications of family violence for nursing. The discussion particularly focuses on the application of nursing theory, the generation of new nursing theory, and practice changes as they relate to violence in the family.

*Reprinted from *Every Twelve Seconds*, compiled by Susan Venters (Hillsboro, Oregon: Shelter, 1981) by permission of the author.

NURSING CONCEPTUAL MODEL OF FAMILY VIOLENCE

A nursing theory of family violence currently does not exist. If the definition of a nursing theory given by Fawcett is accepted, that is, "a set of propositions consisting of defined and interrelated units which presents a systematic view of person, the environment, health, and nursing by specifying relations among relevant variables" (Fawcett, 1978, p. 25), it should be clear that much work remains to be done before such theoretical specificity can be achieved. However, it seems possible to make certain statements about the four key concepts—environment, person, health, and nursing.

Newman (1979) defines a conceptual model as "a matrix of concepts which together describe the focus of inquiry" (p. 6). She further states that although a conceptual framework or model is not testable, it does provide direction to the development of research questions and subsequent theories. It is suggested that this book conceptualizes a nursing framework that addresses each of the four key concepts. A delineation of these concepts as they appear throughout the text follows. It is further proposed that these concepts require attention toward describing the nature of the relationships between each.

Environment

The environment in which family violence occurs must of necessity condone, either implicitly or explicitly, aggression against the family system members. Violence cannot exist in a culture that does not allow it. The factors within a society that provide this approval of violence are not altogether clear. The mode of transmission of violence and its cultural tolerance, although tied to the family by some investigators, also exists in the larger sphere of culture.

An environment that condones violence in families has also been shown to selectively allow its commission only against certain members. Clearly gender and age biases play a major role in support of violence. Violence is not experienced equally by all members of the family. The nature of the role that gender and age play, however, is not completely clear and as has been discussed, is not accepted by some investigators. In the presence of repeated evidence to the contrary, some theorists consistently fail to acknowledge that family violence is usually physical aggression directed at women, children, and the elderly by men. Is it possible that the certain aspects of the environment that support gender- and age-biased violence also perpetuate the myths of its nonexistence? These factors need clarification. Guns are outlawed in most European countries and glorified in the United States. Our films, television programs, and magazines reflect a pervasive acceptance of violent activity. The National Rifle Association lobbies effectively against laws that would counter firearm accessibility. Teen gangs in large urban areas describe a "kill or be killed" mentality that

must be countered. Nurses in school-based clinics and in emergency departments know firsthand the outcomes of such philosophies.

Person (Family Systems)

Throughout this text the focus has been on the family. Family has been referred to as the basic unit of nursing. Although the nurse may care for an individual, she does so only within the context of the larger unit, the family system. It has been repeatedly documented that many families are violent, committing numerous and varied aggressive acts against members of their own system. Although child abuse, battering of women, and abuse of the elderly are examined separately, they are really only manifestations of family violence. Clinicians, regardless of setting, practice nursing within the context of families. The theorist and researcher, however, may need to more clearly articulate the position and role of family. Whall (1986), who strongly advocates the family as the basic unit of nursing, has described problems that occur when the profession of nursing "borrows" theoretical frameworks from other disciplines that are not holistic or practice based. Her vision for the integration of family into nursing theory is pressing new boundaries.

The concept of family is further complicated by an inability of theorists and researchers to define *family*. Some omit any attempt at definition, further confusing the application of family theory to systems that might shed new light on family violence. Certainly any definition of family must be broad and flexible enough to include all the relevant members. Families experiencing violence are often experiencing some general alteration of function (Milner & Chilamkurti, 1991).

Health

Definitions of *health* are no clearer operationally than those of family. The World Health Organization has defined health as "a state of complete physical, mental, and social well-being and not merely the absence of disease" (1948). Certain victims of family violence are clearly experiencing physical alterations. This varies across age groups, but it is important to better understand the interrelatedness of health and violence in future research. For example, we know that certain children may be labeled as failure-to-thrive cases, when in fact they are suffering from severe neglect. Elders may be labeled in the exact manner for the same reason, but the concurrent presence of chronic disease and sequelae from associated symptoms may subvert attention from the reason for symptoms to the treatment of symptoms only. Physical damage inflicted on abused family members is the most obvious evidence of impairments to health. Quantifiable bruises, fractures, etc. are clear evidence of health disorders. However, the hidden health impairment rendered by fear of further violence in the family has yet to be measured. Undoubtedly, any 5-year-old child can probably put such fear into words that should jolt the health care system out of the complacency in which it now exists. Simply having a victimology program within a health care system will never suffice. Proactive measures, such as required screening protocols for the detection of mistreatment regardless of age, sex, race, creed, or color, might be a start. Nurses must pioneer in attending not only to the present physical damage but also the long-term psychological, emotional, and spiritual harm.

Smith (1981) describes the eudaemonistic model as "views of human nature that extend the idea of health to general well-being and self-realization" (p. 44). In this model, illness would therefore be any condition that impedes self-actualization. By this definition, the nurse is concerned not only with the bleeding wound but also the potential or actual alteration in the self-concept of the victim. For family violence, such a definition is a necessity.

Nursing

Throughout this text attention has focused on preventing family violence and mobilizing, as well as enhancing, the strengths of individuals and families experiencing all forms of family violence. These ideas are essential to any nursing framework and may even seem too obvious to state. However,

much of the literature on family violence focuses on detection and assessment, rather than prevention and empowerment. It is more common to find theories and articles written about family violence and its attendant causes than on descriptions of family strengths. Clinical practice with families experiencing violence has revealed that both individuals and the family system possess great stamina, creativity, and resiliency (Humphreys, 1989). Yet relatively little research has empirically examined these clinical observations. Professional nursing has not made the contributions that it might to the family violence literature.

The four key concepts—environment, person, health, and nursing—can be applied to help find solutions to the problem of family violence. A nursing framework that addresses family violence must consider the sociocultural condoning of gender- and age-biased violence, the person as a member of the larger family system, health as an integration of strength of body and self-realization, and nursing as a discipline that promotes strengths and prevents violence. This nursing framework is suggested as a starting point for the evolution of a model that can predict individuals at risk for family violence.

NURSING THEORY AND FAMILY VIOLENCE

There has been little research on family violence using nursing theory as its basis. The nursing literature that suggests appropriate nursing interventions does so on the basis of theory from other disciplines. The problems with such interventions are twofold: first, the theory has not been tested in a family violence context, and second, the nurse must generate nursing actions from a nonnursing framework. The body of nursing theory–based research on family violence is growing. Examples are cited throughout this text and appear with regularity in professional publications. However, much of the research remains at the descriptive level. Programs of nursing research of family violence have just begun. Additional research is needed to advance knowledge of nursing theory–based research on family violence.

Nursing interventions described in the literature suffer from the same problems previously identified in research on child abuse and neglect. The literature reports on nursing interventions with victims of family violence tend to use case study or discussion format. The interventions are based on generally accepted principles of nursing, and yet the reader has only the experience and the opinion of the author to support the interventions. Professional nursing has much to do to inform public policy regarding empirically tested intervention models for the prevention of family violence across the life span.

Application of Nursing Theory

The following example illustrates how a nursing theory can be applied to the problem of family violence. The nursing conceptual model developed by Orem (1991) is used as a basis for suggested nursing research related to the area of family violence involving adolescents.

The general theory of nursing set forth by Orem is particularly suited to nursing research related to family violence. Orem's model revolves around the concept of self-care. As such, victims of violence who seek assistance can be viewed as demonstrating both the ability to identify the need for action and the ability to take action to promote life, health, and well-being. The strengths of individuals from violent families are easy to identify in light of self-care. (This model does not address those who are not ready or able to seek assistance, such as the demented elderly person or the child who is too young to articulate the problem.)

Orem's model (1991) lends itself to person-nurse problem solving. Orem defines it as the therapeutic self-care demand. She describes self-care as "the practice of activities that individuals initiate and perform on their own behalf in maintaining life, health and well-being" (p. 117).

According to Orem (1991), the requirement for nursing exists when a client is unable to meet his or her own needs for the basic necessities of life. Nursing interventions must accomplish self-care or assist the individual in the development or regulation of self-care. Self-care has been described by Orem pri-

---

> ### Components of Self-Care Capabilities in Adolescents
>
> 1. Ego strength and health decision-making capability
> 2. Relative valuing of health
> 3. Health knowledge and decision-making experience
> 4. Physical energy levels
> 5. Feelings
> 6. Attention to health

marily in terms of the competent adult. Children and dependent adults are viewed as having some self-care abilities; however, these are not seen as developing and are not clearly described. Subsequent to Orem's early conceptualization, other researchers' have expanded on her model by applying theories of development to self-care (Denyes, 1981, 1982).

Denyes (1981) has developed and tested an instrument to measure self-care capabilities in adolescents. Her findings indicate that adolescents possess interest in their health and self-care. From data on self-care capabilities in adolescence, six components have been identified and are listed in the box above.

Adolescence is a time when various patterns of living are explored and accepted or rejected by the individual. Self-care capabilities need particular attention during the adolescent phase of rapid development and identity establishment. The opportunity to promote self-care practices is particularly pertinent to the self-care–conscious adolescent. Despite recent nursing interest in self-care as a basis for nursing interventions, no research has been conducted regarding the self-care capabilities of the abused adolescent.

Clinical experience with violent families has provided me (Humphreys, 1989) with many opportunities to assess abused adolescents. Observations from experience reveal that adolescents have great interest in their bodies and their health, yet professionals frequently express frustration and mistrust of adolescents as clients. Adolescents who run away from home are frequently maltreated, and females are

---

Possible Research Areas for the Adolescent's Self-Care Strengths

1. How do abused adolescents perceive their self-care capabilities?
2. What differences exist in the degree of perceived self-care capability between abused adolescents and nonabused adolescents?
3. What differences exist in the degree of perceived self-care capability between abused male adolescents and abused female adolescents?
4. What differences exist in the degree of perceived self-care capability between sexually abused adolescents and non-sexually abused adolescents?

---

often sexually abused. The act of "running away from home," rather than being a delinquent action, is an excellent example of self-care. While in the home, the abused adolescent cannot get necessary professional assistance and is a likely subject of repeated parent attacks. By running away, the adolescent immediately stops the abuse and becomes eligible for multidisciplinary assistance. Professionals who work with adolescents who flee their abusive homes often fail to see the strength and resourcefulness of the youth's action and instead treat the child as a juvenile delinquent. Nursing research into abused adolescent self-care capabilities will add to the refinement of the phenomenon. The nurse who works with abused adolescents will be better able to identify and encourage client self-care practices. Knowledge of the abused adolescent's self-care strengths may aid decision making on the part of the professionals who must suggest placement or recommend emancipation.

Nursing research into the adolescent's perceived self-care strengths is needed in many areas. The above box lists several of these topic areas.

Other nursing theories may be used as a basis for nursing research on family violence. Orem's model (1991) has been used as an example. Nursing research based on nursing theory is necessary for advancing the knowledge base of nursing in family violence.

Exploring classic models and their application to the family violence field is also valid. Two examples include Maslow's hierarchy of needs (1954) and Erikson's eight stages of man (1968). In the former, it is important to explore the way victims classify avoidance of victimization in relation to other basic needs. For example, an elderly person might rate safety as secondary to the need for belonging or shelter. If so, prevention strategies might focus on the development of support networks or restraining orders instead of outcomes of violent episodes. Erikson's eight stages might be used to frame longitudinal studies of victimization. In this approach, a child abuse victim might be followed over time to discern patterns of mastery in the eight stages. If the "trust versus mistrust" dilemma is never resolved because of victimization, the other stages may be irreparably unmet at the positive end of the continuum. Theoretical frameworks that are viewed as classics might shed new thinking when applied to family violence research.

NURSING RESEARCH AND FAMILY VIOLENCE

The need for nursing research in the area of family violence is tremendous. Nurses are in an ideal position to make a major contribution to the knowledge base of family violence; however, relatively few nursing studies have been reported. Nursing is not alone in its need to conduct systematic inquiries into family violence. Although other disciplines have conducted and published family violence research, the field is small. All areas of investigation (child, adolescent, women, elderly) describe the problem of poorly designed studies, with small, nonrepresentative samples. There is a dearth of longitudinal or trend analyses.

Another problem is that of excessive use of medical and social service records rather than direct subject contact. Most research does not carefully operationalize definitions to target one specific subcategory, such as neglect, sexual assault, or physical assault. The literature emphasizes definitional issues rather than the intervention and follow-up components that may be able to save lives.

The funneling of money into programs built upon a less than secure base, largely as a result of the lack of solid empirical knowledge, is truly wasted and may even border upon damaging due to its false promises (Bolton, Laner, Gai, & Kane, 1981, p. 538).

An example of generally accepted clinical practices and assumptions being refuted with empirical data is a study by Corey, Miller, and Widlak (1975). The study, involving chart reviews of 48 hospitalized battered children under the age of 6 and 50 randomly selected nonbattered children ($N = 50$), attempted to examine the validity of previous demographic findings as characteristics of abused children.

> Demographic characteristics and the medical history items suggested by some investigators as factors that influence child abuse were shown in the study to be of doubtful value in discriminating between hospitalized battered children and their nonbattered counterparts (Corey, Miller, & Widlak, 1975, p. 294).

The characteristics associated with abuse of children may merely be those associated with hospitalization. In addition, Corey et al. report that the siblings of abused children tended to be abused as well. Therefore nurses cannot relent once they are certain of the safety of one abused child in the family; siblings are likely to be abused as well and even if not, require appropriate nursing interventions (see Chapter 8).

In a review of research in the 1970s on family violence, Gelles (1980), identifies several areas of need. Research must progress beyond mere descriptive efforts toward "a systematic program of research to empirically test theories and also to use available data to build new theories of family violence" (1980, p. 882). Research should test theories, unlike much of the current theoretical knowledge, which is based on post hoc explanations of data. Gelles suggests that longitudinal designs be used to provide greater insight concerning time, order, and causal relationships in family violence research. The use of more nonclinical samples would serve "to overcome the confusion which arises out of confounding factors which lead to public identification of family violence with those factors causally related to violent behavior in the home" (p. 883). Finally,

Gelles recommends that data collection and measurement techniques increase in number and diversity. Researchers no longer need to fear that subjects cannot or will not disclose violence in their family.

Recently Pagelow (1992) summarized what she perceived to be some of the changes in the area of wife abuse as a result of research. She supplemented her summary with conclusions about the general nature of research in the area. Although she noted that progress has been made in the development of knowledge about the causes, circumstances, and outcomes of battering of women, she cautions that governmental funding may affect research findings and their implications. Citing several noteworthy research reviews (Kurz, 1989; Schacht & Eitzen, 1990; Stark & Flitcraft, 1983), Pagelow concludes that "the battered women's movement was deflected from its original feminist goals through government funding of shelters and individualistic solutions. The result is that the state co-opted the battered women's movement's original focus to a new focus: to individualize, professionalize, and depoliticize it" (1992, p. 88). Schacnt and Eitzen (1990) note that "if the government tends to fund research guided by individual explanations, then the resulting policies will be aimed at changing problem people" (p. 12). Pagelow advocates that although additional research is needed, it is important, even necessary, to remember the larger social context of patriarchy and domination of women rather than focusing solely on individuals in the application of research findings.

Horsfall (1991), a nurse theorist, presents a framework for viewing both violence and masculinities that considers the broader social context beyond individual biology or psychology. Research that examines the nature of these relationships, as she advocates, offers exciting possibilities for nursing and survivors of family violence.

Nursing research into family violence is needed in many areas (see the box on the next page.)

NURSING PRACTICE

The professional nurse in clinical practice, regardless of setting, has contact with potential or actual

---

Possible Research Areas in Family Violence

1. Intrafamilial sexual abuse
2. Threats to victim body image from violence
3. Long-term effects of violence on children of battered women
4. Incidence and description of elder abuse
5. Wife abuse and pregnancy
6. Empowerment of battered women
7. Coping strategies of survivors of family violence
8. Relationship between suicide and abuse
9. Relationship between substance abuse and violence against family members
10. Resolution of personal and professional feelings about family violence
11. Nursing interventions with individual survivors of family violence
12. Nursing interventions that assist children of battered women to overcome the intergenerational transmission of family violence

---

family violence. Evidence of family violence may not be readily apparent unless the clinician is highly aware that family violence is a possibility and uses protocols for the assessment of risk factors. Much like the sexual history assessment of the 1960s, the family violence assessment must become a matter of standard nursing practice. The first step toward identifying family violence is for the nurse to be aware of and ask about it as a potential problem. It is hoped that such practice changes will prevent mistreatment of all kinds.

Just as the nurse always asks the client's age, marital status, and date of birth, she should also inquire into family and individual stresses, family conflict resolution, and child-rearing patterns. Clients do not question such nursing assessments and are often pleased to know that a health care provider is interested in more than just their physical health. The nurse also sets the framework for future client interactions. Routine assessment of family functioning lets the client know that such topics are appropriate in client-nurse discussion.

As always, effective nursing care begins with the client or family's concerns. Actual or potential vio-

lence in the family may be a problem; however, it may not be the reason for seeking nursing care. Primary attention given to the clients' concerns indicates that the nurse acknowledges their importance, initiates the process of establishing a trusting relationship, and increases the likelihood of the joint development of an effective plan of care. The collaborative role of the nurse indicates respect for the clients and their freedom to make their own decisions regarding the kind of nursing care they need. Such nursing care therefore logically builds on the strengths of individuals and families. Nursing in this manner can effectively be provided in any setting. The successful development of such nursing in a nontraditional setting was conducted by the editors (Campbell and Humphreys) and is described as an example of its appropriateness for other nurses.

The initial contact took place between Jacquelyn Campbell and the director at the battered women's shelter. At first the staff could identify only the need for occasional first aid, development of emergency protocols, blood pressure screening, and health appraisal form completion as appropriate nursing functions. The agency had only minimal contact with nursing or its services.

The role the nurse played within the agency gradually began to evolve. A sign-up list was established so that any shelter resident could request to see the nurse during her weekly visits. Additional clients might appear at the time of the nurse's established hours. Eventually, some clients began to be referred by the agency staff. Initially only those clients with established medical problems were referred by staff to the nurse. A variety of reasons were given by the residents for wanting to see the nurse. One 9-year-old girl with severe atopic dermatitis referred herself because she wanted to go swimming with the other children. The shelter's staff was fearful that she was "contagious." Another shelter resident, a woman hit in the head with a hammer, sought the nurse because she needed her stitches removed. Many other visits to the nurse were for reasons that can be found in any setting: diarrhea, colds, weight reduction, stress control, pregnancy, infant feeding, sore throats, and headaches. The nurse is called on to be a generalist. Nursing visits were next alternated between the two nurse volunteers with a written record of clients seen, assessment, intervention, and needed follow-up established both in the "nurse's log" and in the individual client's agency record. Additional consultation between the two nurse volunteers occurred by phone.

Through the sharing of experiences at the shelter with the faculty at the College of Nursing, Wayne State University, and the offer of graduate student placement, a master's student in nursing was assigned to the shelter for a clinical learning experience. The student became so intrigued with the opportunities for nursing in such a setting that she continued her involvement even after her course work was completed. The outcome of the student's experience was a master's thesis that investigates the role of play therapy with the children of battered women. The following year, another master's student was placed at the shelter. She too became interested in the women and children and is now a volunteer and engaged in conducting an ethnography into the lives of the battered women and their children in the shelter.

Both authors continue to practice at battered women's shelters. The involvement that began as volunteer work in a shelter has expanded considerably. Both were elected to board of director positions with shelters and other domestic violence groups. Participation also routinely includes speaking engagements on behalf of battered women's shelters, generally on the topic of family violence. Education of health care and other professionals has also become a regular activity.

The purpose of this discussion has been to suggest that in addition to nursing practice with violent families in traditional settings, there is tremendous opportunity to shape public policy, especially health policy, by virtue of outcomes determined by excellence in nursing practice. One nurse's offer to volunteer at a battered women's shelter has grown into a relationship between agency (staff and residents) and nursing that strengthens both.

NURSING EDUCATION AND FAMILY VIOLENCE

The nurse who practices in a truly holistic sense must be prepared to deal with family violence regardless of the type or location of practice. Nursing education has generally acknowledged its inability to expose students to every possible health problem or concern. Appropriately, the baccalaureate nursing student is instructed in the basis of all nursing care, the nursing process, and is then familiarized with certain theories or principles. The student is assisted to develop a flexible and inquiring mind so that whatever client alteration is identified, even though previously unencountered, she will be able to systematically assess, plan, implement, and evaluate to the client's greatest benefit. In the case of physical alterations experienced by a client, the nursing student is often admirably prepared to tackle any circumstance. Appropriate nursing interventions when a client's impairment is related to diabetes mellitus, renal failure, or cardiac insufficiency are usually thoroughly familiar to the nursing student. Nursing interventions in family violence situations, however, are probably unmentioned in many nursing programs and likely do not receive nursing educational time equal to their incidence in the general population. The fact that wifebeating occurs more often than diabetes during pregnancy is an excellent example. Many nursing students spend much time both reading and listening to the many problems related to gestational diabetes. The same cannot be said for the study of abuse of women, which occurs even more often prenatally.

The reasons for the lack of nursing education on family violence are as complex as the problem itself. Nursing as a profession exists in the United States within the larger field of health care. Both are in turn subject to the values and culture of the dominant group, white middle-class males. Nursing as a profession, composed in majority by females, exists as an atypical group within the larger patriarchal culture. Nurses (women) outnumber all other health care providers (men) and yet in many ways have been subject to dominance and control by the male minority. This situation is repeated for women in general in the United States.

Nursing continues to strive for its autonomy; however, as predominantly female professionals, nurses must attempt to meet the health needs of their clients while overcoming obstacles other providers have never experienced. For nursing to have neglected family violence as an issue for nursing education is not surprising. Like the battered woman who is continually told she is worthless, stupid, and incapable of having her own ideas or making her own decisions, the nurse has not been regarded as possessing knowledge that is valuable and worthy of respect given to other professionals. Achieving and maintaining feelings of self-worth were and are arduous tasks for both the battered woman and nursing. Until adequate self-confidence in nurses could be achieved, nursing could not acknowledge the health care implications of male domination. Male oppression of women persists as an experience common to both nursing as a profession and to most of its practitioners as individuals. It might be said that the discipline of nursing is disturbingly familiar with the discriminating forces affecting battered women. The reality of prevention of third-party reimbursement for nursing services by physicians, male-controlled insurance companies, and male legislators is much like the reality of the abusive husband who controls every cent received by his battered wife, only on a larger scale. Until nursing recognized its own oppression, it was difficult to acknowledge the oppression of battered women and was therefore easier to neglect the problem.

It should also be noted that many battered women have been so mentally debilitated that they spend large amounts of time determining if something "they did" was wrong and fearing that they are the "only battered women in town." For a long time, nursing may have been too close to the problem to see it clearly. Because of the nature of nursing and its predominantly female constituents, nurses are in an excellent position to be advocates and providers for the dependent female victims of family violence.

Other factors that may have contributed to the general lack of attention given to family violence by nursing concern the characteristics of violence. As discussed in previous chapters, violence in the family is associated with poverty. Poor American populations have typically been underserved in respect to problems associated with their low socio-economic class. In addition, there is often a tendency for society to "blame the poor" for its difficulties. As a member of the larger society, nursing deserves equal responsibility for its neglect of family violence.

The causes of violence in the family are multifaceted and complex. As such, the tendency is sometimes to focus on the physical injury and not on the causes of physical injury. To proceed further is to invite roadblocks in the system as well as bureaucratic structures that do not necessarily enhance the responsiveness of practitioners. One example is the documentation requirements when an individual is suspected to be a victim of elder mistreatment. In most states, lengthy forms are required for processing the complaint of a suspicion of elder mistreatment, and there is little or no feedback from state systems regarding the outcome of the case, which decreases the likelihood that practitioners will see a benefit and therefore continue to report behavior. Nonreporters are at very little risk for penalty except in the most extreme cases, usually those that receive media coverage.

This discussion does not imply that client physical alterations are not important and should not receive so much attention in nursing education. Indeed physical impairments are of great concern to nurses and clients alike. The first step in increasing the nursing assessments of family violence is to raise the profession's awareness of the problem. An ideal method of familiarizing nurses with family violence as a health problem is to include the topic in basic and advanced nursing curricula. Some states now mandate child abuse detection continuing education credits for relicensure, which is an important first step in emphasizing the problem of family violence.

COURSE DESCRIPTION

Because of the concern of the editors of the text (Campbell & Humphreys), a course was developed to prepare senior-level undergraduate students in a midwestern baccalaureate program to provide nursing care to victims of family violence.

Objectives of the Course

The formalized cognitive course objectives were as follows:

1. Analyze theoretical approaches to the problem of violence in the family
2. Analyze the applicability of nursing care measures and community resources designed to assist dysfunctional families for nursing care of violent families
3. Analyze the influence of culture and community on the problems of violence
4. Formulate appropriate nursing interventions for the problem of violence in the family on the primary, secondary, and tertiary prevention levels
5. Utilize the nursing process to provide nursing care to selected families experiencing violence

This course was to provide students with the opportunity to integrate previous learning about families, adaptation, nursing care of children, communication skills, health assessment, and nursing process with new concepts of violence and discrepancies between family resources and demands to provide holistic and comprehensive nursing care to families experiencing violence. The course was a 4-credit-hour elective that combined both formal classroom lecture/discussion (3 hours per week) and individualized student clinical experiences (3 hours per week). The course focused on the causes and extent of violence in the family; the influence of culture and community on violence in the family; and nursing interventions for the problem at the primary, secondary, and tertiary prevention levels. Areas of family violence examined included child abuse, wife abuse, sexual abuse, violence involving adolescent family members, abuse of elderly family members, and homicide.

In addition to providing educational opportunities in the cognitive and psychomotor domains, the course addressed the affective domain of providing nursing care to survivors of family violence. The decision to include learning experiences in the affective domain was based on the theoretical framework presented by Reilly (1978) in her book, *Teaching and evaluating the affective domain in nursing programs.*

Briefly, Reilly describes and supports the notion that nurses as health care providers have a responsibility to deal with all of the needs of clients within the guidelines of the standards of practice and according to the Code for Nurses. Nursing education in turn has an obligation to prepare students to meet this responsibility. Nursing students have been provided with assistance in the areas of cognitive and psychomotor learning. The affective domain, however, remains essentially untouched in nursing education. The general rationale on this subject is that students will learn about this area as they focus on theory and skills. "Events in our society are now convincing educators that the affective domain of learning is not only a crucial component of any program planning which prepares health providers but it demands the same pedagogical considerations as the other domains" (1978, p. 34).

For the learning of values to take place, two criteria must be met in teaching—experience and critical thinking. Teaching strategies suggested by Reilly (1978) that provide both experience and critical thinking include group discussion based on student experiences, multimedia presentations, "exposure to varied value related patterns of behavior and life-styles," and clinical practice with a group and with one family in particular (pp. 43-47). Each of these strategies was incorporated into the senior-level course described. "The primary goal of this educational endeavor (including the affective domain) is in assisting the learners in the development of values that support a self-identity that is compatible with the responsibilities inherent in the role of a health care provider in a complex ever-changing pluralistic society" (p. 35). In view of the factors suggested earlier as possible contributors to the lack of nursing attention to family violence, nursing education is particularly in need of learning opportunities in the affective domain.

In an effort to crudely measure student nurses' attitudes and experience with family violence, both a presurvey and a postsurvey were conducted. Fifteen demographic variables were also included. The small number of students ($N = I 5$) and the short-term nature of the course preclude generalization. Some interesting results, however, were noted.

The majority of the students were aware of their own values and were generally nonjudgmental in their attitudes about victims of family violence. Little to no change was noted in the students' values surveyed from before and after the course. This may have been mainly related to the students' supportive attitude on entering the course.

Of particular note was the finding that almost all the nursing students reported some kind of close personal contact with violence. The majority of students reported that either they had experienced physical abuse as a child or as an adult, or that a close friend had experienced some kind of physical violence. It must be remembered that the course offered was an elective and chosen by the nursing students themselves. However, self-selected or not, experience with personal violence is common and is likely to have been experienced by a large number of nursing students in any class. The need for nursing education focusing on family violence and including learning opportunities in the affective domain becomes even greater.

Additional studies with working nurses and undergraduate students (nursing and nonnursing) provide information about nurses' attitudes toward female victims of violence. In an investigation of staff nurses' reactions to rape victims versus nonsexually beaten victims, Alexander (1980) found no significant difference in the nurses' perception of victim blame for either group. The practicing nurses did not attribute a significant degree of responsibility for the crime to either type of victim. In a different study, Damrosch (1981) found that graduating baccalaureate nursing students were significantly more likely to attach responsibility for rape to the victim if the woman committed a perceived act of carelessness (failed to lock her car door). When the nursing students were told the study results, their reaction was one of surprise, that they, as a group, had discriminated against the careless victim. As Damrosch emphasizes, the key difference between her study sample and that of Alexander's may be the subjects' exposure to victims of violence.

Recently Barnett et al. (1992) reported that in a study of 298 undergraduate students (majors not specified), those students who indicated that they knew a rape victim reported experiencing more empathy with a female rape victim than those students who did not know a rape victim. Interestingly, the students who previously knew a rape victim reported heightened empathic responses not just for other rape victims, but for victims of traumatic events in general. Barnett et al. also reported differences in subjects' responses based on gender. Female subjects were more empathic and rated the female rape victim as more likable than did the male subjects.

Tucker and Werner (1992) surveyed a convenience sample of 156 nurses from metropolitan ($N = 50$) and nonmetropolitan ($N = 106$) hospitals who were currently practicing in emergency room or medical-surgical settings for their perceptions of knowledge and actual knowledge of the responses and care of female sexual assault survivors. The researchers found that although nurses who provide care to sexual assault survivors may be able to reduce the level of revictimization by being knowledgeable about the care of survivors, approximately 80% of their subjects received no special education before providing care for survivors. Furthermore, nurses in their research who provided care to survivors in the emergency room, while perceiving that they had more knowledge about survivors' responses than medical-surgical nurses, actually had greater knowledge only of evidentiary procedures and not of human responses to victimization.

In a study of 277 emergency nurses and physicians, Kramer (1991), a nurse, found that despite previous reports to the contrary, both the nurses and physicians in her study expressed markedly egalitarian attitudes toward women and strong opposition to wife-beating. Female practitioners (nurses and physicians) were more positive toward women, believed more strongly that wifebeating was not justified, held female victims less responsible, and felt more strongly that help should be given than male practitioners. She concluded that the egalitarian attitudes reported by both female and male practitioners were largely related to their education in family violence and previous contact with survivors. Of particular note was the finding that field rotations or workshops seemed to be most predictive of one's attitudes toward women.

All of these research findings support the need for nursing students to have experience with victims of violence as part of their basic education and for practicing nurses to receive specialized education in the needs of survivors. Such education not only acquaints the nurse (student and nonstudent) with the specific health needs of family violence survivors, but also seems to increase their empathy for other clients experiencing traumatic injuries.

NURSING AND PUBLIC POLICY

Professional nurses who conduct research in the area of family violence are in great demand at the local, state, and national levels for participation in advocacy groups, legislative initiatives, national policy forums, and foundation projects that struggle to make inroads into this difficult area. Vehicles such as workshops sponsored by the National Institutes of Health, sponsorship of bills for new laws mandating improvement in the system (such as the mandated child abuse continuing education units for relicensure), and advisory boards all demand a strong nursing presence. It is not sufficient to wait until nurses, as professionals, are invited to such forums. Aggressive lobbying on an individual and collective basis with appropriate political acumen is absolutely essential for inclusion. Professional nursing needs to play a prominent part in the best literature available on family violence. None of us should miss an opportunity to speak, write, or lobby on behalf of victims of family violence. All aspects of the field are open for improvement. As a clinically-based profession, nursing is in a lead position to describe the nature of current practice, define new strategies for intervention, design studies to answer key questions, and publish all aspects of our research. *Healthy People 2000* has understated the role of family violence programs in keeping our society healthy and productive. There is no specialty within the profession of nursing that is unre-

lated to family violence. Where there are people, there is the possibility of victimization.

SUMMARY

This text attempts to combine the three major areas—theory, research, and practice—that give direction to the nursing care of victims of family violence. The book approaches violence from a nursing perspective and examines the problem as it affects individuals and the family as a unit.

The implications of family violence for nursing are great. The nurse in clinical practice is called on to be aware of the problem and the needs of those victims of family violence. The demands on both nursing and families increase as economic cutbacks require that social agency resources decrease. Nursing can meet the demands placed on it in the care of victims of family violence. To better prepare future nurses, educational content on family violence should be included in every nursing program. Nursing research, particularly that based on nursing theory, is still needed to increase the knowledge base of nursing care of victims of family violence. Violence only exists as we as a society and a profession allow it. The existence of violence is never acceptable, especially when it is inflicted within our most basic unit, the family. Nursing as a discipline is challenged to provide leadership in developing theory, research, and effective practice.

REFERENCES

Alexander, C. S. (1980). The responsible victim: Nurses' perceptions of victims of rape. *Journal of Health and Social Behavior, 21,* 22-23.

Barnett, M. A., Feierstein, M. D., Jaet, B. P., Saunders, L. C., Quackenbush, S. W., & Sinisi, C. S. (1992). The effect of knowing a rape victim on reactions to other victims. *Journal of Interpersonal Violence, 7,* 44-56.

Bolton, F. G., Laner, R. H., Gai, D. S., & Kane, S. P. (1981). The "study of child maltreatment: When is research . . . research? *Journal of Family Issues, 2,* 531-540.

Corey, E. J., Miller, C. L., & Widlak F. W. (1975). Factors contributing to child abuse. *Nursing Research, 24,* 293-295.

Damrosch, S. P. (1981). How nursing students' reactions to rape victims are affected by a perceived act of carelessness. *Nursing Research, 30,* 168-170.

Denyes, M. J. (1981). Development of an instrument to measure self-care agency in adolescents. (Doctoral dissertation, University of Michigan, Ann Arbor, 1980). *Dissertation Abstracts International, 41:* 1716-B. (University Microfilms No. 80-25, 672.)

Denyes, M. M. (1982). Measurement of self-care agency in adolescents. *Nursing Research, 31,* 63.

Erikson, E. H. (1968). *Identity, youth and crisis.* New York: W. W. Norton.

Fawcett, J. (1978). The "what" of theory development. In *Theory development: What, why, how?* (pp. 17-34). New York: National League for Nursing.

Gelles, R. J. (1980). Violence in the family: A review of research in seventies. *Journal of Marriage and the Family, 42,* 872-885.

Horsfall, J. (1991). *The presence of the past: Male violence in the family.* North Sydney, Australia: Allen & Unwin.

Humphreys, J. (1989). *Dependent-care directed toward the prevention of hazards to life, health, and well-being in mothers and children who experience family violence.* Unpublished doctoral dissertation, Wayne State University, Detroit, MI.

Kurz, D. (1989). Social science perspectives on wife abuse: Current debates and future directions. *Gender & Society, 3,* 489-505.

Kramer, A. (1991). *Emergency nurses' and physicians' attitudes about women and wife beating: Implication for emergency care.* Unpublished master's thesis. University of Wisconsin, Milwaukee, WI.

Maslow, A. H. (1954). *Motivation and personality.* New York: Harper & Row.

Millor, G. K. (1981). Theoretical framework for nursing research in child abuse and neglect. *Nursing Research, 30,* 78-83.

Milner, J. S., & Chilamkurti, C. (1991). Physical child abuse perpetrator characteristics: A review of the literature. *Journal of Interpersonal Violence, 6,* 345-366.

Newman, M. (1979). *Theory development in nursing.* Philadelphia: F. A. Davis.

Orem, D. E. (1991). *Nursing: Concepts of practice* (4th ed.). St. Louis: Mosby-Year Book.

Pagelow, M. D. (1992). Adult victims of domestic violence: Battered women. *Journal of Interpersonal Violence, 7,* 87-120.

Reilly, D. E. (1978). *Teaching and evaluating the affective domain in nursing programs.* Charles B. Slack.

Schacht, S. P., & Eitzen, D. D. (1990). *Government sponsored research on battered women: Redefining structural outcomes into individual problems.* Paper presented at the annual meeting of the American Sociological Association, Washington, DC.

Smith, J. (1981). The idea of health: A philosophical inquiry. *Advances in Nursing Science, 3,* 43-50.

Stark, E., & Flitcraft, A. (1983). Social knowledge, social policy, and the abuse of women: The case against patriarchal benevolence. In D. Finkelhor, R. J. Gelles, G. T. Hotaling, & M. A. Straus (Eds.), *The dark side of families* (pp. 330-348). Beverly Hills: Sage.

Tucker, S. J., & Werner, J. S. (1992, April). *A survey of emergency room nurses' knowledge of the responses and care of female sexual assault survivors.* Paper presented at the Midwest Nursing Research Society Annual Meeting, Chicago, IL.

U.S. Surgeon General. (1990). *Healthy people 2000: National health promotion and disease prevention objectives.* Washington, DC: U.S. Dept. of Health and Human Services (DHHS), Public Health Service (PHS) No. 91-50213.

Whall, A. (1986). The family as the unit of care: A historical review. *Public Health Nursing, 3,* 240-249.

World Health Organization. (1948).

Index